Healthy Sexuality

Richard Blonna

William Paterson University

Jean Levitan

William Paterson University

WADSWORTH
CENGAGE Learning™

Australia • Brazil • Japan • Korea • Mexico • Singapore • Spain • United Kingdom • United States

WADSWORTH
CENGAGE Learning™

Healthy Sexuality
Richard Blonna, Jean Levitan

Publisher: Peter Marshall

Executive Editor, Health and Human Performance: Nedah Rose

Senior Development Editor: Peggy Williams

Assistant Editor: Andrea Kesterke

Editorial Assistant: Sarah Lowe

Editor-in-Chief: Michelle Julet

Technology Project Manager: Travis Metz

Marketing Manager: Jennifer Somerville

Marketing Assistant: Melanie Banfield

Advertising Project Manager: Shemika Britt

Project Manager, Editorial Production: Teri Hyde

Print/Media Buyer: Rebecca Cross

Permissions Editor: Sommy Ko

Production Service: Martha Emry

Text Designer: Ellen Pettengell

Photo Researcher: Pat Quest, Quest Creative

Copy Editor: Laura Larson

Illustrator: Precision Graphics, Cyndie Wooley

Cover Designer: Lee Friedman

Cover Image: Sarah Leen/Getty Images

Compositor: GGS Book Services, Atlantic Highlands

For product information and technology assista nce, contact us at
Cengage Learning Customer & Sales Support, 1-800-354-9706
For permission to use material from this text or product, submit all requests online at **www.cengage.com/permissions**
Further permissions questions can be emailed to **permissionrequest@cengage.com**

ExamView® and *ExamView Pro®* are registered trademarks of FSCreations, Inc. Windows is a registered trademark of the Microsoft Corporation used herein under license. Macintosh and Power Macintosh are registered trademarks of Apple Computer, Inc. Used herein under license.

Library of Congress Control Number: 20041000840

Student Edition

ISBN-13: 978-0-495-10659-3

ISBN-10: 0-495-10659-3

Instructor's Edition:

ISBN-13: 978-0-534-62263-3

ISBN-10: 0-534-62263-1

Wadsworth
10 Davis Drive
Belmont, CA 94002-3098
USA

Cengage Learning is a leading provider of customized learning solutions with office locations around the globe, including Singapore, the United Kingdom, Australia, Mexico, Brazil, and Japan. Locate your local office at **www.cengage.com/global**

Cengage Learning products are represented in Canada by Nelson Education, Ltd.

To learn more about Wadsworth, visit **www.cengage.com/wadsworth**

Purchase any of our products at your local college store or at our preferred online store **www.ichapters.com**

Printed in the United States of America
4 5 6 7 8 9 10 11 10 09

*To our loving families: Heidi, Will, Mike, Matt, Mike, and Steve,
who put up with the stress of our deadlines and the time spent locked
in our offices working on the manuscript.*

brief contents

contents

v

Chapter 3

Male Sexual Anatomy and Physiology 69

Chapter 4

Sexual Identity 95

Chapter 5

Child and Adolescent Sexuality 127

viii   Contents

Chapter 6

Adult Sexuality 167

Chapter 7

Human Sexual Response 205

Chapter 8

Sensuality and Sexual Behavior 235

Chapter 9

Atypical Sexual Behavior 271

Chapter 10

Intimate Relationships 293

Chapter 11

Sexual Communication 321

Chapter 12

Sexual Dysfunction, Sex Therapy, and Sexual Enhancement 351

Chapter 13

Human Reproduction 389

Chapter 14

Fertility Control 425

Chapter 15

Sexually Transmitted Diseases (STDs) 467

Chapter 16

Sexual Coercion 513

Chapter 17

The Business of Sex 553

preface

As an introductory text in human sexuality, *Healthy Sexuality* is based on the fundamental information and concepts that have evolved from the body of research in this field. We firmly believe in a biopsychosocial model of human sexuality. In this view, humans become sexual beings and evolve as a result of a continual interaction between biological and psychosocial forces.

We also believe that human sexuality is intimately tied to overall health and wellness. Our overall level of health and wellness plays a big part in our sexuality. *Healthy Sexuality* examines how the components of wellness—physical, intellectual, emotional, social, spiritual, and environmental/occupational—influence our sexual health. Additionally, our sexuality is a key component of our health. The book points out how the healthy expression of our sexuality can improve our overall level of health and wellness.

Essential to being healthy, people have to come to grips with themselves as human beings, to make sound sexual decisions and self-actualize their sexual selves. Although we do cover sexual health concerns and risks (unintended pregnancy, sexually transmitted diseases, date rape, and so on), *Healthy Sexuality* takes a pro-sex rather than a problem-oriented approach to sexual issues. We make no apologies for focusing on the positive, life-enhancing aspects of healthy sexuality instead of presenting sexual topics as a series of problems to overcome.

In the spirit of diversity, we have included information relative to differences between races and ethnic groups, as cited in the most current data generated by the Centers for Disease Control. We use the federally sanctioned language in referring to these groups. We have carefully integrated issues of sexual orientation throughout the book wherever appropriate rather than presenting this as a stand-alone topic in a single chapter. We have incorporated sexual orientation issues into the body of the text, through case studies and in illustrations and photographs. In this way, we hope to project the view of sexual orientation as a healthy part of human sexuality not a "problem" to be discussed in a separate chapter.

Features of the Text

- The opening page of each chapter begins with a set of **Student Learning Objectives** designed to put the chapter's content into a meaningful framework, to introduce readers to the content of each chapter and personally connect them to the material.
- **Case Studies** throughout each chapter are drawn from the authors' work with students and clients over the years in a number of settings. The case studies cover

a diverse cross section of people and are designed to illustrate how the material in the chapter connects to real individuals in everyday situations. You'll meet people like Jorge, a college student who learned the meaning of no the hard way. Although the names have been changed, the cases are authentic.

- **Critical Thinking** questions are inserted next to each case study and bring up questions for readers to answer for themselves. In Chapter 15, for instance, you'll be asked to ponder the issue of discussing one's sexual/medical history with a potential sex partner. You'll be asked to assess the pros and cons of this approach and how a person actually goes about such a task. These questions have no right or wrong answers; they are exercises in critical thinking and represent possible topics for the instructor to consider for group discussion.

- **Personal Exploration Activities** in each chapter allow students to participate in a fun and revealing activity, in which they can explore their feelings and opinions on issues of sexuality. In Chapter 4, for example, students can discover all the things they would never do if of the opposite sex.

- **Healthy Sex Hints** within each chapter are practical, step-by-step suggestions for achieving optimal sexual health and well-being related to the accompanying discussion. Healthy Sex Hints cover a broad range of topics from aphrodisiacs in Chapter 7 to how to perform breast or testicular self-exams in Chapters 2 and 3 respectively.

- **Sex in Society** boxes throughout the text present unusual, interesting, and sometimes controversial material related to the discussion. They add interest and expand upon the basic topic. Sex in Society boxes explore a range of topics such as "Body Image as a Lifelong Concern" in Chapter 4 to the "The HIV Highway" in Chapter 17.

- The text includes an integrated discussion of **Sex and Disability** issues as they relate to healthy sexuality. Our emphasis throughout the text has been that wellness is a continuum and throughout our lives our position on it changes. At any given time in our lives we might have high-level wellness across one or more of the six dimensions of health as we struggle with other dimensions. Disabilities, although they challenge us and sometimes limit some of our options and choices, are presented as just one of many factors that affect our place on our continuum. In Chapter 11, for instance, we examine how living with an ostomy impacts one's sexual response and behavior. In other chapters we introduce people with a host of conditions ranging from being in wheelchairs to having Parkinson's Disease and explore how these challenges affect their sexuality.

- Each chapter integrates **Wellness Syntheses** into key content areas throughout the chapter. These are designed to tie the chapter content to the six dimensions of health and wellness—physical, intellectual, emotional, social, spiritual, and environmental/occupational in a meaningful way. A key facet of our text, this feature demonstrates the linkages between sexuality to health and wellness throughout the text.

- Throughout the text, **Marginal Definitions** identify and highlight key terms that are defined in the margins. These marginal definitions are used to clarify the chapter's content and give the student easy access to the meanings of vocabulary essential to their understanding.

- To further personalize learning, we have added **Personal Assessment** activities at the end of each chapter. These assessment activities are tools for readers to use to apply what they have learned to their own lives—and thereby improve their health and well-being. These assessments range from "Things that Turn Me On" in Chapter 7 to a "Sexual Communication Satisfaction Questionnaire" in Chapter 11.

- The **Thought Questions** and **Test Yourself!** quiz at the end of the chapter offer readers an opportunity to assess their mastery of the course material.
- Also at the end of each chapter, a **Media Menu** provides information on all the media assets to be found on the book's companion Web site that are specific to that chapter. Listed here are animations and short films, as well as a list of Internet resources, with annotations. These carefully chosen Web sites direct the reader to further, specific information related to chapter topics. These entries are current and have been verified for authenticity and rigor.
- In the Media Menu you'll also find the **InfoTrac Activity** that links readers via the book's companion Web site to up-to-date articles drawn from the vast InfoTrac collection. These are tied to readings that are mostly drawn from popular magazines and provide a lighter look at some of the subject matter contained in the chapter. These activities provide a rich source of discussion for instructors. Chapter 8's InfoTrac activity, for instance, provides a lighter look at the "gymnastics of lovemaking" (that is, sexual positions).
- Each chapter contains a list of **References** that includes all of the works cited in the chapter. We have tried to blend the classic works in the field with new material from reputable sources.

Besides these features we incorporate data to support the textual presentation through **illustrative tables** and **figures** from the most current sources available, complemented by the classic studies by Kinsey, Masters and Johnson, Laumann and colleagues, and other respected researchers in this field. Finally, the judicious use of **diverse photographs** and **drawings** illustrates important information under the principle that a picture is worth a thousand words.

Ancillaries

To assist the instructor in presenting the course in an interesting and comprehensive way and for the student to get the most out of the class, the following ancillaries are provided without charge to qualified adopters.

An *Instructor Manual* contains the following information for each chapter:
- Detailed outline of the text
- Resource Integration Guide
- Suggested activities
- World Wide Web sites

ExamView, a computerized testbank with the following features:
- More than 800 multiple-choice, matching, and essay questions
- Capability to add or edit test questions in up to 12 formats
- Ability to save and recall previously generated test to create a new version of the test
- An easy-to-use test assessment and tutorial system
- Ability to create multiple versions of the same test

Overhead *Transparency Acetates* of the book's most important graphics to facilitate class instruction and assist in explaining key concepts.

Multimedia Manager, A Microsoft® PowerPoint® Link Tool:
- Includes PowerPoint viewer on CD-ROM, which allows instructors to use without PowerPoint program
- Enables instructors who have PowerPoint to edit presentation to fit their lecture
- Allows the instructor to go back to past chapters and to start at any chapter
- A lecture-oriented presentation containing at least 25 slides per chapter

Student Supplement

Student Study Guide, to help the student study for tests and retain information learned in the course.
- Key terms
- Review of chapter objectives
- Quizzes to help students learn the key learning objectives for each chapter

Healthy Sexuality Book Companion Web Site:
- Electronic access to all teaching ancillaries (instructors only)
- Additional interactive quizzing content for test preparation
- Digital videos highlighting text topics
- Links to additional Web sites

The features and ancillaries outlined here have resulted in a comprehensive course presentation that covers the content in a most expansive way. We developed this book with the student at the forefront. We hope readers will apply the information to their own lives in a positive way, leading to their optimal sexual health and overall wellness.

Acknowledgments

First, I acknowledge two people who were early influences in my development as a human sexuality professional. Drs. Richard Cross and Sandra Leiblum of the University of Medicine and Dentistry of New Jersey first opened my eyes to the field and my own sexuality many years ago in one of their intensive sexuality seminars for medical students and invited professionals. Their ease and professionalism in dealing with sexual matters left a lasting impression on me. They provided my first exposure to the scientific, professional study of sexuality and validated sexuality as a scientific discipline worthy of serious study.

I'd also like to thank my mentor and role model, Dr. Marvin Levy of Temple University, for standing out as the epitome of what I consider a "healthy sexuality professional." With his rugged, athletic masculinity, scholarly wisdom, and health background, Marv created an image in my mind of someone able to place sexuality squarely in the framework of health rather than a series of problems to be addressed and feared. I was lucky to come under his influence at a crucial time in my life as a young husband and developing professional. I'm thankful for his guidance in both areas of my life.

Finally, I thank Clifford G. Freund, my mentor with the New Jersey State Department of Health (NJSDH). Cliff nurtured my early career as an STD professional and supported my initial interests in sexuality and education. He had the faith in my work and the wisdom to give me the freedom to explore issues and develop as a sexuality professional.

—R.B.

Though my graduate school experience was years ago, the training and learning that took place under the mentorship of Deryck Calderwood and the faculty of New York University, along with the incredible work accomplished with classmates, set the foundation for this text. Since then, the professional friendships and constant learning that comes from the Society for the Scientific Study of Sexuality (SSSS) and my network of sexuality educators (ASET) have bolstered my grounding in healthy sexuality.

My gratitude and appreciation extend to Eva Goldfarb, Ernie Green, Konnie McCaffree, Janet Pollack, Donna Ezrol, Arlene Scala, Anthony Nesto, Nancy

Begin, Elizabeth Schroeder, Elizabeth Casparian, Emily Joslin-Roher, and my many students whose openness and sharing not only keep me up-to-date but enrich this book. Sue Scott, Dan and Judy Lyons, and Linda Truesdale helped me with the draft manuscript, enabling me to keep to my deadlines. Finally, the incredible understanding, patience, and support of my family throughout the writing process are beyond measure.

—J.L.

We'd like to thank the following people at Wadsworth Publishing:

We thank Peter Marshall for the opportunity to write this book. Without Peter's vision and belief in us there would be no *Healthy Sexuality*. April Lemons got us started on the right track, and Nedah Rose has carried on the excellent work that April started, and has been a constant champion for our book.

Peggy Williams, or P, as we affectionately refer to her, kept us on task and in line throughout the course of this project. She kept things light with her dry sense of humor, one-word encouragers, patience, and grace under pressure. She also was our greatest advocate and gave us the courage and support to tackle some of the tough material in refreshing ways. Her vision of this project shines through every page.

Martha Emry, our Production Manager, and Teri Hyde, our Senior Project Manager, made sure that Peggy's good work and initial momentum kept moving forward. Their attention to detail and friendly nudges kept us moving in the right direction as we put the finishing touches on the project.

We'd like to thank Jennifer Somerville, Senior Marketing Manager, and Andrea Kesterke, Assistant Editor, for all their help in the initial stages of this project with everything from contracts to setting up the meetings in Philadelphia.

Many thanks to Lillian Cook Carter for her contribution of the *Personal Exploration* activities in the text and in the Instructor's Guide.

To our reviewers and class testers—Scott Acrement, Canyon College; Consuelo Bonilla, Kean University; Carol Chenault, Calhoun State; F. Scott Christopher, Arizona State University; Paul Finnicum, Arkansas State; Kay Foland, South Dakota State; Lois Goldblatt, Arizona State University; Elyse Gruttadauria, State University of New York College at Brockport; Lynne Hamelton, West Chester Community College; Edward Hart, Bridgewater State College; Dianna Hurlbut, Irvine Valley College; Eileen Johnston, Glendale Community College; Andrew Kanu, Virginia State University; Richard Larkin, Harper College; Katrina Lubbers, University of Nebraska; Don Matlosz, California State University–Fresno; Susan Molstad, Northwestern State University of Louisianna; Lin Myers, California State University–Stanislaus; Marilyn Myerson, University of South Florida; Bobby Ogletree, Southern University of Illinois at Carbondale; Christine Osgood, Mesa Community College; Dianna Peck, Western Illinois University; Miguel Perez, California State University–Fresno; Valerie Pinhas, Nassau Community College; Catherine Sherwood-Puzzello, Indiana University; Stanley Snegroff, Adelphi University; Sherm Sowby, California State University–Fresno; Richard Stacy, University of Nebraska; Sonja Swanson, Palm Beach Community College; Tom Tatchell, University of Toledo; Maria Theresa Wessel, James Madison University; William Yurkiewicz, Millersville University—we extend thanks for their time, dedication to thoroughly reviewing the text, and their thoughtful comments that enabled us to improve the manuscript.

Finally, we thank our colleagues in the Department of Community Health for their support on this project and for providing a wonderful work environment.

Richard Blonna
Jean Levitan

about the authors

RICHARD BLONNA, ED.D, CHES, has been teaching human sexuality for more than 20 years. His initial work in the field was in education and control of sexually transmitted diseases. He served as an STD investigator, counselor, supervisor, and trainer for the New Jersey State Department of Health (NJSDH) STD Control Program. He also worked for the NJSDH as a health education consultant for the AIDS and family planning programs. He has taught human sexuality at Temple University and, most recently, William Paterson University, where he also teaches health counseling, epidemiology, and stress management.

JEAN LEVITAN, PH.D., has been teaching human sexuality at the university level for more than 30 years. At William Paterson University she has taught in both the Community Health and the Women's Studies departments. Past activities include teacher training for human sexuality and evaluation of the Family Life Education Program for the City of New York. In addition to teaching human sexuality, she teaches women's health, supervises community health interns, and teaches courses on reproductive rights and on racism and sexism in the United States.

chapter *one*

Exploring Healthy Sexuality

Student Learning Objectives

After reading this chapter, students will be able to

- Define *human sexuality.*
- Define *health* and *wellness.*
- Describe the key components of healthy sexuality.
- Explain how the six dimensions of health and wellness impact one's sexuality.
- Compare and contrast behaviors that enhance or inhibit healthy sexuality.
- Describe the key sources of sexual information.
- Evaluate sources of sexuality information.
- Describe the major findings of the key researchers of sexuality over the past 100 years.
- Describe the components of informed decision making.
- Understand some of the health challenges to sexuality.

Test your understanding of these objectives by taking the end-of-chapter quiz, available online at **http://health.wadsworth.com/blonna1.**

activity teaser: *How "real" are the relationships we see on TV? Find the answer in the Personal Exploration Activity on page 10.*

case study 1.1

Maria

Maria, age 25, identifies as Puerto Rican American.

Maria is a full-time, commuter student in her senior year. She is engaged to Nick, a 22-year-old Italian American, also completing his senior year. Maria was finishing up her final project in Dr. Blonna's Human Sexuality class and came in to discuss her paper.

"I'll never forget this conversation," Dr. Blonna recalled, "because it came from such an unlikely source that it was striking. Maria was the quintessential urban woman; tough, street-smart, wise beyond her years, with a cynicism born from years of living in northeastern New Jersey."

I just finished writing my paper and took some time to think through some of the assessments that I took and the work that we did in class this semester. I can't believe how much I've changed in just 16 weeks. I took this class because I was curious about my sexuality and my relationship with Nick. I was mostly interested in the, you know, the sexual behavior part. I thought that maybe I could learn a few ways to spice up our sex life.

I can't believe how much more I learned about my sexuality and how I never realized how much a part my health played in it. I never even realized what health really was and how things like my spirituality, fitness, and environment influenced it. I took a couple of fitness and body image assessments, and it made me realize that I have never really been comfortable with my body. I guess that is why I have had such a hard time really relaxing with Nick when I am naked and enjoying sex even though he's told me a thousand times he loves my body and likes me just the way I am.

Dr. Blonna asked Maria to tell him about the other parts of her assessment, her spirituality and environmental health.

I rediscovered my spirituality this semester. I guess I had lost touch with it because I'd spent a lot of time over the past few years questioning my faith and the church I grew up in. You helped me realize that it is normal to question our faith and that faith transcends any specific religion. You also made me realize that it was important to not give up my faith as I sorted through my spiritual beliefs and tried to find a connection to something that worked for me. I've kind of started that by doing more things that connect me with nature. I haven't given up on my religion, but I find I am able to think about it differently outdoors than by sitting in church. Nick and I have started getting away from the hustle and bustle of the city on weekends. We've started to drive to the mountains and take long hikes in the woods. We've found some really amazing places within 2 hours from home that are quiet, peaceful, and beautiful. We really felt that "connection" you talked about in class. We've even gone to the beach in the winter and had the whole place to ourselves. Sometimes we just walk hand-in-hand for miles without even saying a word to each other. It's like some bond has developed that transcends us. I don't know, it sounds crazy but it's made me appreciate everything a little more.

I guess that I can see the holistic thing you've been talking about in class and in the textbook. I mean, like I am getting in shape by doing all of this walking and nature stuff. My relationship with Nick has never been better. We have this new connection, and I've got to admit we've found that some of these places are great for spontaneous sex. I also think I am beginning to find some kind of rekindling of my spiritual self. Being outside, quietly taking it all in, feeling in touch with my body, feeling sexy toward my man, all of this stuff just seems to make me feel some connection with something bigger than myself.

Critical Thinking

Maria and Nick are able to escape from the hustle and bustle of their everyday environment and spend time walking in the woods or along the beach. What other strategies could be used to make sure that health needs are met when such escapes are not possible?

Use your Virtual Workbook to explore your answer to this question at **http://health.wadsworth.com/blonna1.**

Maria's case illustrates how one's health plays a crucial role in healthy sexuality. The interplay of the different dimensions of health manifests itself in many ways in our sexuality. As you can see with Maria, often the dimensions of health overlap. Where does our environmental well-being end and our spirituality begin? Where does our physical health stop and our emotional health start? Maria so eloquently describes the interconnections between our health and our sexuality.

As we continue living in the 21st century, students may be struggling to sort out the conflicting messages about "healthy sexuality." Compared to students growing up in the previous century, so much more information is open and accessible. There are choices that are better understood, with the power of the Internet to answer questions that in previous generations may not even have been asked. More and more, individuals are demanding their rights to be who they are in terms of their sexuality.

Sexuality remains a critical force shaping our lives. It is part of how we see ourselves and impacts our **self-esteem.** It is ever-present as we relate to others on both romantic and platonic levels. Students, as well as the population at large, are constantly confronted with media messages on enhancing sexuality through the use of various products. Sexual themes remain prominent in all forms of entertainment, including books, film, television, and music.

Self-esteem A way of looking at oneself; may be high or low

As health educators, we hold to the position that good decision making is grounded in having accurate information, an opportunity to develop a personal value system, and discussion of possible and probable outcomes of behavior. We advocate the accompanying opportunity to become aware of the variety of sexual lifestyles and concerns of those who are unlike ourselves.

Our Sexual Climate

To try to figure out how best to make healthy personal decisions in a climate of contrasts is confusing and problematic. Americans talk about sex and sexuality all the time. It is a favorite subject of the media. Some conservative media pundits criticize our culture for its overemphasis on sex. They claim that sexual themes dominate our culture and the media and that the government has gone too far in allowing the free expression of sexuality. Some liberal commentators say exactly the opposite. They claim that our culture is sexually restrictive and downright puritanical. As examples of a restrictive culture, they cite the continued demand for abstinence-until-married sexuality education in the schools, restrictions on reproductive rights, and resistance to the legalization of domestic partnerships/gay marriage. Still others claim that our culture sends mixed messages about sexuality. It is used to market and sell almost everything, yet most schools are not allowed to teach about sexuality in a comprehensive, forthright way.

The reality is that government and society influence our sexuality in many ways, some positive, some negative, and some ambiguous. We are sexual beings from conception to death, and our sexuality evolves and grows regardless of official sanctions or restrictions. We learn about sex whether we do or do not have sexuality education in our schools. It is not a question of *whether* we learn. It's more a matter of the *quality* of what we learn. A key to understanding sexual learning is to realize that we learn about sexuality and what it means to be a man or woman even if no one ever sits us down and has a heart-to-heart talk about the "birds and the bees." And that classic explanation of where we came from is only a small part of understanding ourselves.

Quality sexuality programs result from well-thought-out curricula, with goals and objectives for student learning. Curricula are based on accurate information, in which the pursuit of knowledge is encouraged rather than restricted. Students have a chance to examine their values and the factors that contribute to healthy and appropriate personal decisions. Eighteen states plus the District of Columbia require schools to provide sexuality education: Delaware, Georgia, Illinois, Iowa, Kansas, Kentucky, Maryland, Minnesota, Nevada, New Jersey, North Carolina, Rhode Island, South Carolina, Tennessee, Utah, Vermont, West Virginia, and Wyoming (Sexuality Information and Education Council of the U.S. [SIECUS], 2001). Other states have varying requirements, from sexuality "units" within health education programs, to focusing on HIV/AIDS but avoiding much discussion about the broad aspects of sexuality. Some topics may even be prohibited from discussion. For example, 15 states do not require schools to provide STD, HIV, and/or AIDS education: Alaska, Arizona, Arkansas, Colorado, Hawaii, Idaho, Louisiana, Maine, Massachusetts, Missouri, Montana, Nebraska, South Dakota, Texas, Virginia—and of those, Arizona, Louisiana, Mississippi, and Texas require that such education teach abstinence but not prevention methods (National Abortion and Reproductive Rights Action League [NARAL], 2001). In our information-rich culture, such censorship further highlights the conflicts students face when attempting to move toward sexual health.

In many ways the sexual learning that takes place outside any classroom is far more influential, as it is constant, both verbal and nonverbal, and often insidious. Students can easily relate the types of misinformation they acquired from friends throughout their childhood and simultaneously often report that their parents didn't talk with them about sexuality issues. In reality, though, parents convey information, impart values, and serve as **role models** whether a formal, face-to-face, serious conversation ever takes place between parent and child. A frown or a raised eyebrow can convey disapproval just as a nod, smile, or laugh indicates support. To be silent on an issue, to omit sexuality from the daily discourse in our lives, to never bring up sexuality as part of the conversation around the dinner table sends a strong message about its being a taboo subject.

Some of what we see and learn, unfortunately, does not present the healthiest picture of sexuality. Sometimes our parents, caregivers, friends, teachers, and media figures do not provide us with the best role models or information for healthy sexuality. The sexual scripts we receive may not promote healthy relationships and in some cases may actually jeopardize our lives. For example, if women are taught that they must be thin to be sexually attractive, what connection might that "lesson" have to eating disorders such as anorexia and bulimia? If men are taught that they are entitled to sex and that women want to be dominated, what connection does that "lesson" have to dating violence and rape? Sometimes the very people and institutions charged with teaching us and nurturing us fail or, worse yet, sexually abuse us.

So what is human sexuality? **Sexuality** is a broad term that refers to all aspects of being sexual. Many people think human sexuality refers to sexual behavior—what people do, how often they do it, and so on. Although sexual behavior is an important part of being sexual, human sexuality encompasses much more than that. Sexuality involves our genetic inheritance, our anatomy and physiology, and the reality of being a sexual creature in a biological sense. It also encompasses our thoughts and feelings about our body and what it means to be a man or a woman. It involves our ethics, values, and the cultural mores we've assimilated through our family, ethnic group, and religious affiliation.

Our sexuality extends beyond the self to encompass our friendships, intimate relationships, and sexual relationships. Lastly, our sexuality does not exist in a vacuum. It is influenced by and influences our environment. Our institutions (schools, governments, and so on), neighborhoods, communities, campuses, states, and countries, and their policies, help shape the person we are and our options as a sexual being.

Factors That Contribute to Our Sexuality

Our sexuality is influenced by many factors throughout our lives, each impacting our development in similar or unique ways. No researcher or theorist has the widely accepted, definitive explanation for how each of us becomes who we are. Some rely heavily on biology, looking to our genetic inheritance as a prescription for how we will develop. Others hold the culture and the socialization process to

Role model A person whose behaviors are imitated by others

Sexuality A broad term referring to all aspects of being sexual be the critical forces that shape our lives. Some believe the psyche processes information as a result of experiences perceived as positive or negative, which in the end cause the individual to become the person he or she is. Finally, some maintain that the person we are is a result of the interaction of heredity/genetics, family socialization, culture, and personal experience.

Without being able to clearly determine which factor is most influential, we do know that we all receive strong and perhaps conflicting messages about sexuality from family, friends, school, media, religion, and the culture. **Sexologists,** those who study sexuality through various rigorous research methodologies, provide input into our knowledge base. Developing a healthy sexuality involves processing that information and, as individuals, internalizing that which is useful.

Family

The family has historically been viewed as a critical force in our development. The examination of family influence can focus on both genetic predispositions as well as scripted ways of behaving. Are our ways of being due, therefore, to "nature," "nurture," or combinations of both? From a biological perspective, family represents those to whom one is related "by blood," and, consequently, we may be like our parents and siblings. Complicating that perspective, however, are the various reproductive technologies available today, redefining aspects of the biological connection to parents.

Are we the persons we are because of how we were reared? In a social sense, the term *family* has taken on broader connotations as people's living arrangements take on a variety of forms. Divorce, remarriage, stepfamilies, blended families, and single families introduce new models. The traditional **nuclear family,** consisting of a married man and woman and their biological children, represents less than half of all households in the United States today. The primary caregiver thus may assume a greater role in a child's development than previously. The challenge comes in trying to evaluate the impact of various family arrangements on a family's members.

The impact of parental influence on sexuality is still open to debate. For example, the societal concern with homosexuality has led courts—almost exclusively, until more recent times—to award children to the heterosexual parent in custody cases resulting from divorce. The concern is that gay or lesbian parents will influence their children to be gay or lesbian. That the heterosexual parents of the gay and lesbian adults were unable to influence their children's orientation is not given the same credibility. As we will discuss later, good parenting skills, rather than the parents' sexual orientation, are key to raising healthy children. The family influences the development of healthy sexuality in numerous ways. Through family, we learn gender roles and expectations, are taught about love and affection, learn patterns of touch, develop a sense of our physical selves, and assume patterns of social interaction. In each of these areas, our experiences can lead to healthy or unhealthy development. In some areas of parenting, a number of approaches can lead to healthy sexual development.

It is generally accepted that parents should be loving and supportive toward their children. Children who receive physical affection will, in turn, be more likely to be able to give affection to others. Embedded in such general advice, however, are individual patterns that may be criticized. For example, research has shown that boy children stop receiving physical

Sexologists Specialized researchers of sexual subjects from a variety of disciplines including psychology, biology, medicine, nursing, and health

Nuclear family A family made up of the mother, father, and their children

Courtesy of the authors

Children learn about sex from their families without it ever being mentioned.

affection earlier than girls, who may continue to be hugged and kissed through-out their lives. Does the change in the type of touch boys receive impact their adult patterns?

In terms of **gender role** expectations, most parents reinforce gender-stereo-typed behaviors very early on. Boys are expected to play aggressively and to enjoy trucks, Legos, action figures, and the like. Girls get socialized to plan for motherhood, beauty, and domestic tasks. The women's movement of the late 1960s and early 1970s questioned the impact of gender stereotyping on the healthy development of boys and girls. Over 30 years later, television commer-cials for children's toys reveal little departure from the traditional gender role ex-pectations. Toy manufacturers, in their defense, claim they are marketing to the children who will buy their products. When they have attempted to market toys in a more gender-neutral manner, their efforts have not been successful. Families have different views on what is socially acceptable and what toys they want to purchase, yet children seem to develop their own preferences regardless.

Gender role The different behaviors and attitudes that society expects of females and males

Friends

One's peer group has always maintained a powerful role in shaping our attitudes and values about sexuality. Depending on the friends with whom we socialize, we have various experiences at different ages. Teens may refer to others as "being in the fast crowd"—which may mean that more sexual activity and drinking take place. Kids may refer to others as "geeks" or "nerds"—meaning that, though smart, they seem to lack social skills and have interests that are "not cool." Re-gardless, peer pressure, social judgments, and opportunities all interact to in-fluence healthy development. At the same time, those very influences can leave a negative mark dominated by low self-esteem, depression, and feelings of inadequacy.

Most students report that the bulk of their sexuality education comes from talks with friends. They say that some friends passed along accurate information, and others spoke with authority while dispensing inaccurate information. Stu-dents have reported that, as children and teens, they saw sexually explicit pic-tures, magazines, and videos at a friend's home—all supposedly belonging to "my friend's dad." The sneaking around and the searching through hidden mate-rial convey a message about sexuality.

As sexuality educators, we have volumes of accurate information available to our own children. Nonetheless, we have been confronted at times with "What do you know?!" and "Why do you have to have all this stuff around?" In some cases, one's friends are perceived as more knowledgeable than parents.

Culture

Culture The sum of the learned set of rules governing the behavior of people, often focused on the influences of race, class, religion, and ethnicity

Anthropologists have defined **culture** as anything and everything that humans learn. Implied within that is a learned set of rules for appropriate behavior. In practice, when addressing issues of culture, what actually may be under study are influences of race, class, religion, and ethnicity.

All cultures have established rules to regulate sexual activity (Mindlin, Wal-lace, & Kapell, 2002). Some are viewed as restrictive, and others are seen as per-missive. Even though Western cultures share certain traditions and values—such as patriarchy, monogamy, having children within marriage—actual behavior varies from one group to another.

As the United States becomes an increasingly pluralistic society, it is forced to confront what may seem to be "foreign" practices. For example, female genital mutilation or female genital cutting (discussed more fully with female anatomy and physiology in Chapter 2) is a custom practiced primarily in parts of Africa.

case study 1.2

Karen, with Eyes Wide Open

Karen, age 24, is white.

I remember, as a kid, traveling with the "in crowd" in middle school. There was a group of about 25 of us, and we started having boy-girl parties around the sixth grade. A couple of girls were considered the "pretty ones," and they had the boyfriends. I always got invited to the parties but ended up "watching" rather than participating. There were kissing games, close dancing, and the girls with developed chests invariably let some of the boys "cop a feel." I remember my mother, in particular, being very concerned that certain kids were "bad influences." Despite her reservations about some of my peers, I wasn't being approached, so there were no decisions for me to make. I was watching and learning . . . just not being asked to participate.

I had one friend who my mother worried was a "bad influence." Her parents were divorced, her father was out of the picture, and she was living with her elderly grandparents. One weekend she invited me to join her on a visit to her mother's apartment in the city. My friend confided that her mother had two different boyfriends; in retrospect, I realize that she slept with both of them. I remember feeling uncomfortable watching my friend's mother walk around the apartment in her underwear, sit on her boyfriend's lap, and kiss him. Somehow I knew that my own mother would have been very upset if she knew what type of education I was getting!

Critical Thinking

Karen was aware that her mother disapproved of her friend. How might a parent encourage better communication so that a child's observations and concerns could be discussed?

Use your Virtual Workbook to explore your answer to this question at **http://health.wadsworth.com/blonna1.**

Today, U.S. health care providers find themselves caring for girls and women who have undergone this mutilating experience.

Newspapers and magazines will report on international cases where punishments are meted out for those individuals whose sexual behavior violates the established culture. One case involved a couple living on the run in England. The woman was afraid that her father or brother was going to kill her because she had defied her culture by choosing her partner. Western ideas of falling in love, being able to decide whom to marry, and the like, were in direct conflict with her Muslim upbringing, which dictated that the bride's father arrange the marriage, with her input having little or no value. In 2003, pressure from outside nations resulted in a Nigerian court saving a woman from being stoned to death. She had given birth to a child as a result of being raped, yet her village court had labeled the crime adultery, requiring her to be punished.

Both cases confront students with cultural practices different from what is common in the United States. Our cultural beliefs have also been cited as justification for involvement in war and have made us the target for terrorism abroad and at home. The wars in Iraq and Afghanistan, the terrorist attacks of 9/11, and the subsequent vulnerability we have felt on our home soil have changed us all forever.

Although the first World Trade Center attack of 1993 and the subsequent bombing of the Alfred P. Murrah Federal Building in Oklahoma City in 1995 put us on notice to the possibility of major terrorist activity on American soil, the events of 9/11 were so horrific, they could not be ignored and will never be forgotten. Repeated television coverage of the terrorists flying American commercial airplanes into the World Trade Center, the Pentagon, and a lonely field in the middle of Pennsylvania brought the horror into everyone's lives. For those with family members and friends working at the various sites, the intensity of their grief was magnified.

The authors work at a university where the World Trade Center and skyline of Manhattan were visible from the highest point on campus. Our students were directly involved with 9/11, some by working and volunteering at the site, and oth-

7

ers connected to those who died. We will never forget that day, how students, faculty, and staff wandered around campus screaming and sobbing, frantically trying to place cell phone calls to loved ones. Dr. Blonna's son, a freshman at the time, recalls sitting on top of the roof of his dormitory building watching in disbelief as the World Trade Center ruins over 25 miles away smoldered long into the night. Students were crying and trying to console each other as they tried to make sense of what had happened earlier in the day.

The impact of that day lingered over the campus for the entire semester like a thick fog. Many students, faculty, and staff barely survived the semester, sometimes just going through the motions. Many class sessions started out with a moment of silence to honor the dead, the missing, and the heroic rescuers. Many professors, like Dr. Blonna, started each class by getting students to form a circle, hold hands, and share their strength with those who were less hardy. Some of our students remain in therapy, a few years after the events of 9/11. Researchers estimate that tens of thousands of New Yorkers suffered from posttraumatic stress disorder (PTSD) in the months following the attack on the World Trade Center (Seong-Ngoo, 2002). Additionally, about 17 percent of the United States population *outside* New York City reported symptoms of PTSD 2 months after the terrorist attacks (Manisses Communication Group, 2002).

Events such as the terrorist attacks of 9/11, war, and chronic and traumatic stress changed the campus and outside culture (Lane, 2002). On campuses around the country, grief counselors were brought in to help students cope with their losses. Campus counseling centers were inundated with students, faculty, and staff seeking help. Students from around the country made a pilgrimage to New York City to help out any way they could (Kirgiss, 2002).

Loss, grief, and fear brought on by the aforementioned events have changed our collective culture and have many implications for personal wellness and sexuality. They affect our trust, our ability to form intimate loving relationships, and our sexual desire (Davey, 2002; Dettmer, 2001). Studies have shown that blood levels of testosterone, the hormone of sexual desire, diminish in response to such events (Tsigos & Chrousos, 1996). Debra Straw (2001), a professor from Burlington, Vermont, writing in *Community College Week*, describes this so eloquently in the following passage: "One young woman, normally an A student, told me last week that she has been getting B's and that she has been taking depression medication and getting therapy as a direct result of what has been happening in the larger world. These young people now live in fear and uncertainty. Their American Dream seems to have been blown away" (p. 3).

The terrorist attacks of 9/11 threatened the diversity that is so vital to a well-rounded college experience (Garmon, 2001). Terror, fear, anger, and suffering impacted the previous level of acceptance and understanding of students from different cultures, particularly those of the Middle East. Some campuses across the nation reported backlash against Middle Eastern students, professors, and staff, and Islamic studies and culture (Boulard, 2001). This creates a campus climate that is not healthy and safe. We firmly believe that for healthy sexuality to occur, one's environment must be safe and conducive to a free expression of ideas and lifestyles. When tolerance and acceptance are replaced by intolerance and rejection, everyone suffers.

Popular Culture

Terrorism and threats of war, however, do not seem to interrupt popular culture's fascination with sexuality. Television programs in the early 2000s increasingly have brought the viewer into the lives and bedrooms of dating couples. People meet on television, date in front of a camera, get sexually involved in front of a camera, and even marry, sometimes to someone either picked by their parents or voted on by viewers. Even the mainstream program *The Today Show* has succumbed to having couples compete for being married on the show, with Internet voting on the clothes to be worn, ring to be purchased, hairstyle and dress for the bride, among other wedding-related activities.

While television has become more direct about sexual humor and sexual content, it has also taken greater responsibility in discussing sexual issues in a more forthright manner. Cable television can be credited for leading the way for greater openness; competition for viewers has brought the traditional networks along. For example, the History Channel developed a few multipart series on sexuality, looking at sexuality in the 20th century and another beginning in ancient times. Viewers

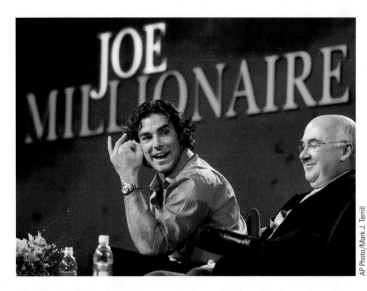

"Reality TV" programs are very popular and bring the viewer into the lives and bedrooms of dating couples.

can also find segments on sexual issues on such news programs as *20/20, Dateline,* and *Primetime,* along with a variety of topics covered by public television stations.

The sexuality of the rich and famous continues to be scrutinized. The years 2002–2003 were witness to Michael Jackson, the pop singer, coming under intense scrutiny for his interest in children, with possible charges of sexual abuse. Catholic priests across the United States were brought to task for the years of sexual abuse covered up by the church hierarchy. Rabbis were arrested for soliciting sex online. As always, the romantic lives of politicians were fair game for media scrutiny. When JonBenet Ramsey was murdered in the late 1990s, not only were people upset at the horror of the death, but they also frequently reacted to the mature look given to this young model and beauty pageant contestant.

A cursory examination of popular magazines today will reveal more and more skin, especially that of women's bodies. The *Sports Illustrated* Swimsuit Issue (winter 2003) is not that different in appearance from a *Playboy* magazine printed decades earlier. Both have well-written articles of interest, yet the sensual photography of the female models makes the magazines big sellers. The lingerie company Victoria's Secret distributes catalogues and designs store windows displaying female underwear in a seductive manner. Abercrombie and Fitch in fall 2003 distributed the *A&F Quarterly—The SEX ED Issue* in which the clothing was the centerfold, with naked male and female models in seductive poses filling the catalogue. The content and images were provocative enough that a paper sleeve surrounded the catalogue, and its purchase was limited to those 18 and older.

Popular music, particularly that focused on youth, has lyrics about sexuality that are explicit, direct, and often angry. Whereas country singers have long shared the details of dysfunctional relationships, the Dixie Chicks raised some eyebrows when they sang about the murder of a man with a history of beating his wife. Rappers sing and shout about reactions to body parts and sexual activity. Women get referred to as "bitches," and young kids will sing along to songs focused on oral sex and sexual intercourse.

U.S. culture is saturated with sexual messages, yet at the same time political leaders debate whether or not honest, factual, information dare be presented to youth.

All That Glitters Is Not Gold

The goal of this activity is to stimulate you to take a critical view of ideas and actions related to sexuality that are presented in the media as normal and healthy. Your task is to determine whether they are healthy or unhealthy for relationships and whether they fit your values.

Gather a few of your friends together to watch one of your favorite television shows that deals with romantic relationships. *Friends* and *Sex and the City* are the kinds of shows that fit well with this activity. Your task while watching the show is to individually list the relationship behaviors as either healthy/realistic or unhealthy/unrealistic. Examples to watch for are couples talking at the same time and never listening to what the other says, one partner treating the other with respect, and similar behaviors. When the show ends, compare your list to the lists of your friends. Do you all see the behaviors in the same way, or do your friends see something as healthy when you think it is unhealthy? If you find differences, explore the reasons for your views with your friends. Ask your friends what healthy/realistic behaviors they would like to have in a loving relationship. Do they think the behaviors we watch in the media hurt the way we relate to one another?

K–12 Schools

Schools are charged as the institutions primarily responsible for transmitting knowledge and helping children learn about the world. As a logical extension, schools are to play a key role in sexuality education. Even so, the debate has raged for decades regarding the role schools should play, the depth of information they should convey, at what ages children should learn information about sexuality, and how, if at all, schools can teach in a "value-free" way. Programs that have been successful have been conducted by working closely with parents, clergy, and community leaders to develop curricula that are acceptable. The efforts in this regard far exceed those in other subject areas such as English or history. Research shows that most parents support sexuality education in the public schools.

The National Guidelines Task Force, under the auspices of SIECUS (1997), identified six key concepts that should be part of comprehensive sexuality education programs: human development, relationships, personal skills, sexual behavior, sexual health, and society and culture. A broad spectrum of professionals, including the American Medical Association, National Education Association, U.S. Centers for Disease Control, and Planned Parenthood Federation of America, to name a few, published *Guidelines for Comprehensive Sexuality Education*, which expands on the teaching of 36 sexuality-related topics presented from an age-appropriate perspective (SIECUS, 1996).

Since the *Guidelines'* publication in the early 1990s, however, opponents to comprehensive sexuality education have seen their position supported with federal funding for programs that teach abstinence until marriage. There is little doubt that concerns about sexually transmitted disease (STD) and HIV infections among young people have fueled the abstinence education movement. In 1997, the federal government earmarked multimillion-dollar grants to the states for the development of **abstinence-based curricula** (see Table 1.1). Such funding was both continued and increased in 2002, with presidential and legislative support.

Nonetheless, the Kaiser Family Foundation (2000) conducted a national study finding that the overwhelming majority of parents, teachers, principals, and students want some form of sexuality education taught in secondary school. The ma-

Abstinence-based curricula School programs that advocate not having sex before marriage

Table 1.1 Federal Guidelines for Abstinence Education

"Abstinence education" means an educational or motivational program which:
A. Has, as its exclusive purpose, teaching the social, psychological, and health gains to be realized by abstaining from sexual activity.
B. Teaches abstinence from sexual activity outside marriage as the expected standard for school-age children.
C. Teaches that abstinence from sexual activity is the only certain way to avoid out-of-wedlock pregnancy, sexually transmitted diseases, and other associated health problems.
D. Teaches that a mutually faithful monogamous relationship in context of marriage is the expected standard of human sexual activity.
E. Teaches that sexual activity outside of the context of marriage is likely to have harmful consequences for the child, the child's parents, and society.
F. Teaches young people how to reject sexual advances and how alcohol and drug use increases vulnerability to sexual advances, and
G. Teaches the importance of attaining self-sufficiency before engaging in sexual activity.

Source: Cited in the *Federal Register, 62* (March 13, 1997), 49.

jority of parents wanted students to learn about HIV/AIDS and other STDs, the basics of pregnancy and birth control, how to deal with the pressure to have sex, the emotional issues and consequences of being sexually active, how to use and get birth control methods and abortion, and issues related to sexual orientation.

The Office of the Surgeon General (2001), under the guidance of then-surgeon general David Satcher, issued a report *The Surgeon General's Call to Action to Promote Sexual Health and Responsible Behavior.* The report summarizes scientific findings about various educational efforts and asks that a mature national dialogue on issues of sexuality, sexual health, and responsible sexual behavior begin. Satcher, along with the professionals from various disciplines who collaborated on the report, recognize that the rates of STDs, HIV/AIDS, unintended pregnancies, sexual violence, and so on, make sexual health an obvious part of public health priorities. The report wisely calls for a variety of educational venues representing the diversity of our culture to positively address sexuality education.

College

Young or old, resident or commuter, full-time or part-time, college students realize that college impacts sexuality in many ways. A college campus is a unique environment. Unlike high school, college is a place of limitless intellectual and personal freedom, where ideas and the pursuit of knowledge reign supreme. It is a place where knowledge, attitudes, and behavior are supposed to be examined and challenged. It is also a place of great personal and intellectual diversity, where people of all walks of life come together to learn and grow. For many of us it is the first time we have ever experienced such freedom and diversity.

The freedom and diversity of college extend into our sexuality. Away from home and in a new environment, we are exposed to people, ideas, experiences, and situations that challenge us and help shape us as sexual beings. The combination of personal freedom and the opportunity to try out new ideas, behaviors, and lifestyles is exciting. Our college years are a time of great personal growth. Many of us develop intimate, loving, sexual relationships in our college years that remain with us for a lifetime.

College life also is a time for making choices. The decisions we make also can remain with us for a lifetime. Our decision-making ability is put to the test on a regular basis. Sexual choices are among the most important decisions we have to make. Decisions about who we are and what it means to be men and women, who we are attracted to, how we want to live and express our sexuality, what our sexual needs and wants are, and how we will fulfill them are but a few of the decisions we will make during our college years.

Evaluating Sexuality Research

Research Methods and Sources of Information

Sexology The discipline that scientifically studies sexuality

As we strive toward a personally healthy sexuality, a critical task for all of us is to evaluate the information we receive. **Sexology,** the discipline that scientifically studies sexuality, is often conducted by researchers, some of whom refer to themselves as *sexologists.* Because the field of sexuality is truly interdisciplinary, researchers may primarily identify as biologists, psychologists, sociologists, anthropologists, health educators, nurses, historians, physicians, and more. Wiederman (2001) identifies 19 professional journals whose primary focus is publishing research on human sexuality. In addition, professional organizations in the field also publish newsletters and reports, which add to the knowledge base.

It has often been difficult for researchers to secure adequate funding for sexuality research. Government funding has been most available if the research agenda can be closely demonstrated to impact public health. To some, however, the very study of human sexuality is suspect; others can appreciate the need to know and how much there is to learn. Table 1.2 profiles some of the more prominent research and researchers. The studies were conducted in different ways—some through questionnaires, some through interviews, some by observation, and so forth—although it would be fair to argue that better funding may have yielded broader samples and more comprehensive information.

As mentioned, a growing number of professional journals are focused on sexuality research. At the same time, there are limitations on the types of research conducted. Although a wide variety of questionnaires have been designed and administered, most sexuality research involves surveying selected populations. Often university academics rely on the input of students, groups who are at the very least better educated and literate. In contrast, it would be far more difficult to assess information from populations who may not speak English, trust researchers, or even communicate about sexuality issues.

Ethical and practical considerations also impact what kinds of research are conducted. Observing and surveying children may be problematic, as parental permission must be secured; determining when an issue may be most related to the developmental stage of the child can become political and contentious. Some research is best conducted as a longitudinal study, where a population can be examined over time; the costs associated with such a design, however, can be prohibitive. In other cases, topics such as understanding sexual functioning related to a particular disease may pose challenges in securing an adequate sample size.

Because disciplines have their own established perspectives, the research presented may have other limitations or biases. Key criteria separate good research from poor research. Issues such as bias, sampling issues, honesty, and access all contribute to the quality of sexuality research findings.

Table 1.2 Contributions of Experts on Sexuality

Researcher(s)	Research	Years	Comments
Richard von Krafft-Ebing	*Psychopathia Sexualis*	1886	Viennese psychiatrist who introduced Victorian public to fetishism, sadomasochism, transvestism, homosexuality
Havelock Ellis	*Psychology of Sex*	1897–1910	Challenged negative views toward masturbation and narrow definitions of normal behavior
Alfred Kinsey and associates	*Sexual Behavior in the Human Male* *Sexual Behavior in the Human Female*	1948 1953	A pioneer undertaking involving thousands of males and females interviewed about their sexual behavior
William Masters and Virginia Johnson	*Human Sexual Response* *Human Sexual Inadequacy*	1966 1970	The first research efforts to photograph and physiologically record thousands of instances of sexual arousal, orgasm, masturbation, and coitus. Followed by brief effective treatment for sexual problems.
Morton Hunt	*Sexual Behavior in the 1970s*	1974	Showed consistencies and changes in sexual behavior a generation after the Kinsey findings
Philip Blumstein and Pepper Schwartz	*American Couples*	1983	Study of sexual and affectional behavior of couples
Shere Hite	*The Hite Report on Female Sexuality* *The Hite Report on Male Sexuality* *Women and Love* *Good Guys, Bad Guys*	1976 1981 1987 1991	Although statistically unrepresentative, an early attempt at qualitative research yielding valuable insights to behavior
Popular culture	Magazine surveys: *Redbook, Cosmopolitan, Playboy*	1980	Surveyed more than 100,000 readers; findings often apply more to magazine's readers than to all adults
Richard Green	*The "Sissy Boy" Syndrome*	1987	Controversial study on the origins of homosexuality
Edward Brecher	*Love, Sex, and Aging*	1984	One of the first large-scale scientific studies of sexuality in older people
John Money Anke Erhardt	*Man and Woman, Boy and Girl* *Gay, Straight and In-between*	1972 1988	Now-controversial study of gender anatomy, and identity. Attempted definitions of the biological and psychological determinants of sex, sexuality, and gender.
Edward Lauman, John Gagnon, Robert Michael, and Stuart Michaels	*The Social Organization of Sexuality: Sexual Practices in the United States*	1994	Comprehensive examination of practices within social settings and their meanings

(continued)

Table 1.2 Contributions of Experts on Sexuality *(continued)*

Researcher(s)	Research	Years	Comments
Vern and Bonnie Bullough	*Sin, Sickness, and Sanity; Women and Prostitution: A Social History; Cross Dressing, Sex, and Gender*	1957–present	Review of extensive historical data on a variety of subjects
Michel Foucault	*The History of Sexuality*	1980	Argues that sexuality is socially constructed, including orientation
Centers for Disease Control	Youth Risk Behavior Surveillance System (YRBSS)	1999, 2002	Federally sponsored ongoing research conducted in collaboration with federal, state, local, and private sector agencies to examine health risk behaviors of youth to develop better health programs. Specific attention paid to tobacco and drug use, diet and exercise, violence and injury, and sexual behaviors connected to STD/HIV and unintended pregnancies.

When applying research findings to one's personal life, practical questions to consider include the following: Are you like most people? If not, how aren't you? If you are part of a sexual minority—identifying, for example, as bisexual—how does this affect your lifestyle? If some expert claims that a sexual behavior is problematic and you engage in it, will your behavior change? Should it? Who *is* this expert when it comes to helping you make decisions about your sexuality?

Sexuality Researchers

Because of the interdisciplinary nature of the field of sexology, individuals and teams of researchers have conducted research exploring various aspects of sexuality. Some of the prominent names in the field have examined human sexual response and subsequently developed strategies to help people respond more fully and positively. Others have focused their work on patterns of behavior, differentiating for gender, race, culture, and ethnicity, where possible. Theorists have worked on questions of gender, orientation, and identity. Others have looked at relationship patterns. Almost all traditional styles of research have been utilized over the years to help provide a fuller understanding of human sexuality. Descriptive research formats have been widely used to survey a myriad of attitudes, values, and experiences. Experimental designs have yielded better understanding of sexual functioning and dysfunction. Qualitative research, in which individuals have been interviewed in depth, has provided the richness and contexts that statistical reports omit.

Each "expert" or group of experts has brought valuable data, theories, and insights into our understanding of human sexuality. What is critical to understand, however, is that the richness and diversity of human sexuality have also posed obstacles to any one theory explaining "it all." A conference held at the famous Kinsey Institute in 1998 brought researchers from different backgrounds together in an attempt to encourage discourse and bridge the gap between those who postulated from a biomedical perspective and those who represented the social constructionist perspective. The participants focused primarily on sexuality across the life cycle, sexual orientation, sexual risk taking, adolescent sexuality, and pol-

sex in society 1.1

Criteria Associated with Good Research

We are bombarded with sexual information every day. Countless studies and reports are released and presented by the media. "Experts" report new findings that challenge our notions about sexual issues. Here are some guidelines for evaluating sources of sexual information and research:

1. **Evaluate the researchers.** Reputable researchers are well known in their fields, have some kind of university or agency affiliation, and are members in good standing in professional organizations, and their research is not connected to or funded by for-profit businesses.
   - Who did the research?
   - Was the study done by reputable researchers?
2. **Evaluate the researchers' track record.**
   - Have they conducted scientific studies before?
   - Is their previous research respected and accepted in the field?
3. **Evaluate the sample.** Two issues related to the population studied will tell you the most about the quality of the study: sample size and randomness.
   - How large is the sample? (In general, the larger the sample, the better the study.)
   - Were the samples chosen randomly (subjects chosen at random from a larger pool of eligible), or were the subjects taken from a convenience sample

(an intact group; students in a certain class—prison population, army recruits, subscribers to a certain magazine, and so on)?
4. **Evaluate the methods.** In general, first-person observable reports (person-to-person interview or direct observation) are better than other ways of gathering data (such as mailed questionnaires and telephone interviews). Sexuality research is unique, though. Anonymity protections in many situations will help guarantee better results. Unfortunately, when facing a questioner, respondents may be sensitive to reactions to their answers and consequently give desired answers rather than honest ones.
   - How was information about the subjects obtained?
5. **Evaluate replication.** Studies that are replicated with different samples and come up with similar findings are more likely to stand the test of time. Research linking smoking to lung cancer, for instance, has been replicated with samples from different countries over the past decade and yielded similar results.
   - Has the study been replicated with a different population resulting in the same findings?
6. **Examine the impact.** Read reviews and reports of the study in reputable journals.
   - Have other researchers in the field received the study well?

icy and culture. Although the work of the researchers added greatly to our understanding of human sexuality, there evolved no shared definition of sexual theory or consensus of perspective (Weis, 2002).

A Wellness Approach to Understanding Sexuality

One way to explain and understand our sexuality is to look at it from a more holistic approach. Think of how Maria from Case Study 1.1 described how the dimensions of health affected her sexuality. A person cannot study something such as body image, for example, without looking at issues related to individual personality, family and peer influences, and societal expectations. The focus of this textbook is on healthy sexuality and strategies for maximizing our sexual potential.

Healthy sexuality enables a person to develop to the fullest potential. It requires being knowledgeable. It involves personalizing information and using it to make informed decisions about your life and the world around you. Making good decisions about yourself and others is an essential part of healthy sexuality.

Healthy sexuality The safe and open exploration and development of our potential as human beings

sex in society 1.2
Diversity in Sex Research

One of the long-standing criticisms of many human sexuality studies is the lack of diversity in their subjects. Most of the classic studies in the field have focused on white, heterosexual, middle-class subjects. The two best-known sexuality works—Kinsey's studies of male and female sexual behavior and Masters and Johnson's work on sexual response—are both based on such a sample. Both were conducted decades ago, when diversity received much less attention. The lack of diversity seems to affect three distinct minority subgroups: lower socioeconomic status populations, racial minorities (blacks, Asians, and Hispanics/Latinos), and gays, lesbians, and bisexuals. To complicate matters, although these three categories of populations are underrepresented in major studies of sexual response and behavior, they are overrepresented in other types of sex research, such as those focusing on STDs and teen pregnancy.

The problem may represent a lack of aggressive recruitment of nonwhite, non-middle-class, nonheterosexual subjects in major sexuality research (particularly studies that are privately funded) and an overreliance on sampling from public clinic populations (people with STDs, family planning), which tend to have higher minority representation.

Studies of gay, lesbian, and bisexual populations also have been clouded by methodological problems associated with sampling. Studies of gay men draw heavily from men who frequent gay bars, subscribe to gay publications, are incarcerated, or attend gay public events. Less is known about lesbian women. A true cross-sectional sample of gay men and lesbians representing various socioeconomic and racial/ethnic lines is needed.

Methodological issues related to sampling and sample size have been cited as the primary problems related to obtaining more diverse samples. It is harder to target recruitment efforts for lower socioeconomic status, minority, and gay/lesbian populations. Targeting narrow segments of these populations (for example, gay men attending gay bars) is easier and has a higher-yield recruitment than mainstream sources such as newspapers, random-digit telephoning, and the like. Narrowing the scope of recruitment, however, means that sampling may miss a true cross section of the population targeted for study.

Can these studies accurately reflect human sexual behavior and response if they omit large segments of the population? Are there differences between and among various racial and ethnic groups, socioeconomic segments, and different sexual orientations that might lend greater insight into the true nature of human sexuality?

Finally, newer research has attempted to draw conclusions and examine differences in attitudes, values, and behaviors of groups drawn from a broader range of backgrounds. Students must remember, however, that the United States has increasingly drawn immigrants into our midst who do not answer surveys, may not speak English, or even feel that sexuality is a topic to be discussed with anyone outside the immediate family circle.

It involves our personal level of well-being, the health of our relationships with others, and the nature of the environment in which everything occurs. The best way to conceptualize this approach to understanding human sexuality is to use a health and wellness model to describe it.

Health Total mental, physical, and social well-being, not merely the absence of disease

Holistic health The process of moving toward optimal functioning across the physical, social, spiritual, emotional, and intellectual dimensions

Health and Wellness Defined

In 1947 the World Health Organization (WHO) defined **health** as "the state of complete mental, physical, and social well-being, not merely the absence of disease" (p. 35). WHO's definition was the first globally accepted conceptualization of health and stood the test of time for more than a decade.

Although multifaceted, this definition of health was flawed, according to members of a new movement called **holistic health.** The holistic health movement came into being in the 1960s as an attempt to expand the view of health that WHO had promulgated.

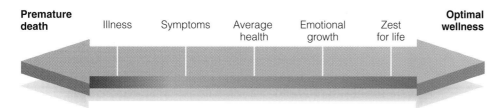

Figure 1.1 *Health and Wellness Continuum* Health can be viewed as a continuum. Where we are on the continuum at any given time is strongly influenced by our lifestyle.

One of the early pioneers in the field, Halbert Dunn (1962), believed that the WHO vision of health characterized it as a static state. Rather than call health a state of well-being, Dunn preferred to view it as a continuum. Developing and maintaining a high level of health means moving toward optimal functioning. Health is a conscious and deliberate approach to life and being, rather than something to be abdicated to doctors and the health care system. Like your health in general, your sexual health is viewed as moving along a continuum, reaching optimal states as a result of your decisions and behavior (see Figure 1.1).

In addition, Dunn recast the notion of well-being to revolve around functioning. How well does the organism function? Dunn viewed functioning as evidence of well-being. Although people will have setbacks in their quest for optimal functioning, the direction in which their lives are moving becomes an important criterion for evaluating their well-being. In this movement, daily habits and behaviors, and overall lifestyle, assumed primary importance.

Originally, the scope of well-being was limited to three dimensions: physical, social, and mental. Adherents of holistic health argued that the mental dimension has two components: the intellectual (rational thought processes) and the emotional (feelings and emotions). Each of these domains deals with a different aspect of psychological well-being. A final dimension, the spiritual, was added because it was thought that humans could not function optimally in a spiritual vacuum. Therefore, the holistic definition of health has five dimensions: physical, social, emotional, intellectual, and spiritual.

In the 1970s and 1980s, the definition of health was expanded once again by the wellness movement (Ardell, 1985). Adherents defined **wellness** as "an active process of becoming aware of and making choices toward a more successful existence" (National Wellness Institute, 2002). Added to the previous dimensions was that of environmental health. Currently, some authors are adding vocational/occupational health to the definition, arguing that one's environment includes the work site and accompanying health issues related to job and career.

What is critical to wellness is to understand that it is a process of becoming healthier. The journey (becoming the best one can be) is more important than the ending. The process of wellness involves becoming increasingly more aware of health and making healthy choices. Success is individually determined and is based on the ability to live life to its fullest.

A key element of the wellness model is striving for balance. When all of the six dimensions are at high levels and in balance, we have optimal health and well-being. When the dimensions are out of balance or one is severely lacking, we have lower levels of health and well-being. Figure 1.2 illustrates this concept.

Wellness The state of optimal health and well-being

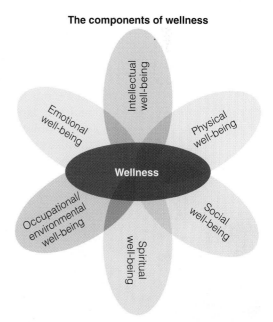

Figure 1.2 *Six-Dimensional Wellness Model* Wellness is a multifaceted phenomenon.

Source: Adapted with permission from Bill Hettler, M.D., 1979; http://hettler.com, 2003.

The average college campus offers many opportunities for engaging in regular physical activity.

Physical well-being A component of wellness reflected in how well the body performs its intended functions

Body composition The fat and nonfat components of the human body; important in assessing recommended body weight

Intellectual well-being A component of wellness referring to the ability to process information effectively and rationally

The Six Dimensions of Wellness

The first dimension, **physical well-being,** is reflected in how well the body performs its intended functions. Absence of disease—although an important influence—is not the sole criterion for health. The physical domain is influenced by one's genetic inheritance, nutritional status, fitness level, **body composition,** and immune status, to name just a few.

Intellectual well-being is the ability to process information effectively. It involves the capability to use information in a rational way to solve problems and grow. It includes issues such as creativity, spontaneity, and openness to new ways of viewing situations. To maintain a high level of intellectual well-being, one must seek knowledge and learn from one's experiences.

Emotional well-being means being in touch with one's feelings, having the ability to express them, and being able to control them when necessary. Optimal functioning involves the understanding that emotions are the mirror to the soul. Emotions help us get in touch with what is important in our lives. Our emotions make us feel alive and provide us with a richness of experience that is uniquely human.

Social well-being involves being connected to others through various types of relationships. Individuals who function optimally in this domain are able to form friendships, have intimate relationships, give and receive love and affection, and accept others unconditionally. They are able to give of themselves and share in the joys and sorrows of being part of a community. This community includes both formal and informal networks. Formal networks include organizations such as churches, professional organizations, fraternities, sororities, and campus groups requiring official membership, dues, and standards. Informal networks such as an intramural sports team do not have rigid rules for membership. In a sense, your social networks are a big part of your environment.

Environmental well-being involves high-level functioning on two levels. The most immediate environment, the **micro-environment,** consists of school, home, neighborhood, and work site. The people with whom we interact in those places link the environment to the social aspects of our health. This environment greatly affects our health and personal safety by influencing whether we are at risk for and fear issues such as theft, crime, and violence. The quality of our air and water, noise pollution, crowding, and other issues that impact our stress levels are also affected. Our social support system is also part of this environment.

The **macro-environment,** the level of well-being at a larger level-state, country, and the world at large—also affects our wellness. The impact of things discussed earlier in the chapter—the wars in Iraq and Afghanistan, the terrorist attacks of 9/11, and other things such as violence, international disputes, racism, sexism, heterosexism, ageism, and so on—all influence us daily to some extent. When we authors were in college, the Vietnam War was going on. College-age men started each day reading the newspaper to see what draft numbers

Friendships are an important part of social well-being.

were being called up (there was a draft, and all draft-eligible men were issued draft numbers) and whether any of their friends were killed or missing in action. Decisions that our political leaders make, such as engaging in wars or determining where we store radioactive wastes, affect the way we think and live our lives. Our ability to stay focused and whole is constantly challenged by the media, which bring the entire world and its problems into our living rooms each night. We need to learn to think globally, act locally, and be happy despite the myriad of problems in the world.

Spiritual well-being involves feeling connected to something beyond oneself. One way to express spirituality is by participating in organized religious activities. This usually means believing in a supreme being or higher supernatural force and subscribing to a formalized code of conduct to live by. In a secular sense, spirituality could manifest itself through connection to something greater than oneself. Whether it is being part of a community, working to save the environment, helping feed the needy, or being committed to world peace, the underlying feeling is a perception of life as having meaning beyond the self.

Finally, **occupational/vocational well-being** involves issues related to job wellness. Occupational/vocational well-being encompasses everything from the safety of our particular work site to the nature of your career. Work site well-being includes physical (air, water, physical plant, machinery, and so on) and social (relationships with coworkers, management, health and wellness facilities and activities) factors. Our personal wellness is affected by the health of our work site. Employers and work sites vary tremendously in relation to health. Some strive for optimal levels, encouraging employees to take advantage of a myriad of health-enhancing programs and services, whereas others meet the minimum acceptable standards for health and safety set by the government.

Besides the specific health of the workplace, different jobs/careers pose varying threats to our well-being as a result of the nature of the work. Some jobs such as police and military service are risky because of possible exposure to hostile combatants. Other occupations such as firefighters, emergency medical service workers, coal miners, and oil rig operators are risky because they place employees in dangerous environments. Other occupations entail high stress due to deadlines, competition, or other factors.

Wellness and Human Sexuality

Our sexuality both contributes to overall health and well-being and is affected by it. High-level sexual health can be a positive force in our lives. It contributes to the full functioning of our body, mind, spirit, and social relationships. When we are engaged in healthy sexual activity and have a healthy outlook concerning our sexuality, we can maximize our potential as men and women. Conversely, our sexuality is affected by our overall level of health and well-being. Sexual response (from desire to arousal and orgasm) is greatly influenced by our overall level of well-being. We simply are less interested in sex and perform poorly when we have low-level health and wellness.

The important thing is to be moving toward optimal health, even if you never achieve it. If your current level of health is lower than you would like, the main thing is to take steps to improve. The experience and process of improving, the journey, is as important as the current level of functioning.

Many of us have limitations that keep us from achieving the high levels of health that others enjoy. A wellness perspective of health and sexuality helps us accept our limitations and maximize the potential within us. You may never have the body of the man or woman of your dreams, but you can enjoy healthy sexuality if you strive to be the best you can be.

Emotional well-being A component of wellness that refers to being in touch with one's feelings, having the ability to express them, and being able to control them when necessary

Social well-being A component of wellness that involves connection to others through various types of relationships

Environmental well-being A component of wellness that reflects our ability to function in our immediate environment, such as home, school, and work, as well as being able to deal with the world at large

Micro-environment The part of one's environment that is immediate and includes living situation, campus, neighborhood, home, and work site and family, friends, and associates who populate these places

Macro-environment The environment that extends beyond the micro and includes one's city, state, country, and the world at large

Spiritual well-being A component of wellness that involves feeling connected to something beyond oneself

Occupational/vocational well-being A component of wellness that reflects our ability to use our unique skills/talents to work that is meaningful and rewarding. Our values are expressed through involvement in paid and nonpaid activities that are personally rewarding for us and make a contribution to the well-being of the community at large.

case study 1.3

Donna's Journey to Sexual Health

Donna, 40, is white.

I'm 40 years old, and I like myself. I accept myself. I can be who I am. But it wasn't always like that. As I look back, I realize that my sexuality has played a very significant role in my life. Sexuality is a significant part of everyone's life, yet if you stray from the center, the average, the expected, then the journey at the very least has more bumps in it than for most.

We can get into a whole list of identities—woman, daughter, lover, student. I see labels as political designations. You try them on to see which ones fit. Can you find "one" that encompasses a total human being? I don't think so. In the last 5 years I've taken "transgendered" as one of my primary identities, yet I am also a mother of two boys. I am committed to a woman as a partner. I am a recent college graduate with a full-time job that isn't what I've always hoped to be doing with my degree, but it pays the bills. And when I clear out some of my debts, I hope to pursue graduate school at some point.

I've always been "inappropriate." My mother was always into dressing me to be the pretty little girl, and in 6 seconds I would destroy her efforts. I wanted to climb trees, play in the dirt, and have fun—all sorts of things you couldn't do in a dress. My hair was always very long to please my mother. My way to manage that was to always keep it in pigtails. Once on my own, I started dressing in drag, with short hair and men's clothing. I came out to my family when I was 16, but to my painful surprise found the reception in the lesbian community most unwelcome. Being butch and dressing like a man back in the 1970s was not "politically correct."

I remedied my sense of not fitting in and trying to sort everything out by marrying a man and trying to live as a heterosexual woman. I was very successful at that game for close to 20 years, being the dutiful wife and mother.

Today it's a 50–50 shot as to whether people think I'm a man or a woman. It used to bother me a lot when people were confused. Now, I find it amusing and really don't care. I have a job where I can be free to be who I am, sharing the ups and downs of my life with people who are friends. I don't fit neatly into the transgendered community, nor do I have "gender dysphoria." My body is my body, and I accept it. I wear men's clothing primarily because they fit better, both body and psyche. I build muscle in "male-patterned" ways, my voice has gotten deeper over time, and my neck is thick. The blood tests I've had in the past all indicate "normal hormone parameters" for a woman.

I feel that I've experimented a lot to find out what is most comfortable and to learn who I am as a sexual person. Not that my journey has ended, but I better understand the road to healthy sexuality. And self-acceptance is a great place to start.

Critical Thinking

How does Donna illustrate some of the problems associated with trying to attach a label to someone's sexuality?

Use your Virtual Workbook to explore your answer to this question at **http://health.wadsworth.com/blonna1.**

High-level *physical well-being* can make us feel better about our bodies and provide the energy and capacity to maximize sexual pleasure and functioning. High-level cardiovascular fitness and muscle tone can enhance sexual functioning and pleasure. When our bodies are healthy and optimally functioning, we feel better about how we look and move and have higher self-esteem—two elements critical to healthy sexuality.

High-level *emotional well-being* can help us understand and cope with the myriad of feelings that being sexual creates. It helps us cope with the emotional roller coaster that most of us face when confronted with issues such as gender identity, sexual orientation, puberty, dating, and preventing unintended pregnancy. A high level of emotional well-being helps us understand and accept our emotions related to these and other sexual issues.

High-level *intellectual well-being* helps us process sexual information, think critically, and make sound decisions regarding our sexual health. The ability to sort through the often-conflicting barrage of sexual information and advice requires an ability to seek out information, evaluate facts, seek clarification of unanswered questions, solve problems, and relate this information to our own needs, wants, and values.

High-level *social well-being* enhances our sexuality and provides a safe forum to explore it and share it with others. Having solid friendships, intimate relationships, and sexual partnerships with people we care about, love, and trust allows us to explore our developing sexuality in a safe way.

Our sexual health is based in our ability to form healthy relationships with others. *Intimacy* is the ability to be open and honest and to feel close with another person. It enhances relationships but is not part of all the relationships we form. For example, you may be open and honest with a college roommate with whom you live day to day. In contrast, you may not find it appropriate or feel comfortable discussing personal concerns with colleagues at work. Relationships that involve an obvious power dynamic—such as boss and employee—often dictate that we are prudent in what we disclose and how intimate we become.

The expression "blood is thicker than water" has been used to explain the support we often expect from family. Friends may come and go, but your family is always your family. In truth, some people have wonderfully intimate relationships with family, whereas others have disengaged from their family or contact them only in times of need. When one's sexual lifestyle is perceived at odds with family expectations, family ties may be strained or severed, with friendships providing the intimacy and support needed.

healthy sex hints 1.1

Making Informed Decisions

The following is a simple decision-making model that may help you make better decisions about your sexuality.

1. *Establish your goal.* Try to put in a broader context the decision you are making about an issue. ("How will this decision affect my goal?")
2. *List the pros and cons.* In two columns on a sheet of paper, list the consequences of saying either yes or no to the question you are trying to make a decision about. Don't scrimp. Put down all of them, no matter how trivial they might seem.
3. *Prioritize the pros and cons.* Rank the pros and cons from most important to least important.
4. *Weigh the pros and cons.* Although one column might be greater than the other (many more pros than cons, for instance), the top one or two items on the shorter list might carry much more weight.
5. *Ponder the results.* Examine the lists, and discuss them with one or two people whose opinions you value.
6. *Listen to your instincts.* Sometimes something may seem to be right for the average person but not feel like the best thing for you. Your rational/intellectual evaluation of your lists and your significant other's advice provides you with two pieces of information; your gut-level intuition provides you with another.
7. *Decide.* Action is important. You must make a decision and move on with your life.
8. *Give it time.* Once you make a decision, give yourself time to experience the effects of that decision. At first it may seem that you made the wrong decision. Only time will tell.
9. *Reevaluate.* Go through this model again to reevaluate your decision once a sufficient amount of time has passed.
10. *Don't beat yourself up!* You are human! Sometimes you will make the wrong decisions. Learn from your mistakes, and try not to make the same ones twice. Persecuting yourself and putting yourself down are not productive and will not help you make better decisions.

Someone once noted that if heterosexual women could relate to their male partners and hold them to the same expectations they have for their female friends, romantic relationships would be in a better state. This observation points to the subtle ways by which we change the script when we look toward developing healthy romantic relationships. Identifying what is unhealthy in someone else's relationship is often easier than seeing the weaknesses in one's own relationships.

High-level *environmental well-being* extends from our personal living space, to our school and work space, to the world beyond. As such, it is often the one area of our health where there is the least personal control. As we age and become independent, our environment extends beyond the family into the immediate community. Community standards for safety and support vary from place to place. Official government, police, and school policies on diverse issues such as treatment of known sexual offenders, sexual harassment in the community, gay rights, sexual abuse, prostitution, prevention and treatment of sexually transmitted diseases, and so on, all influence one's sexual health. Unofficial community standards interact with official policies to create a climate within a community that either supports sexual development and expression or sets up barriers to it.

A primary environment for college students is the campus. Campus policies, especially for residential students, have a great impact on issues related to sexual health. Colleges are becoming increasingly aware of the necessity of formalizing policies on issues such as the prevention and treatment of students with HIV/AIDS, sexual harassment and assault, sexual health services, and so on. The American College Health Association (1996) provides guidance on developing these policy issues. See Table 1.3 for a sample college policy regarding AIDS.

The focus on *occupational/vocational well-being* can be subsumed within a broad definition of *environment*. The jobs and careers we choose reflect who we are as people. They also set the stage for meeting partners and developing relationships that give our lives meaning. As a nation, we are spending increasing amounts of time related to work, both on the job and in commutation. Some individuals find themselves with 2 or more hours needed to "get to work," followed by a full work day, then the advisable 7 hours of sleep, needs for exercise, quality time with family, and so forth; as a result, stress overload becomes "mathematically" apparent. Chemical and radiation exposure at work, along with overall safety of the workspace, affects health in general and aspects of sexual health in particular. Fertility can be affected. Pain and injury can certainly impact sexual functioning.

High-level *spiritual health* connects us with a higher power. It puts our sexuality in a broader context, providing a different perspective from which to view ourselves and our behavior. It also links our lives with a broader purpose and historical continuity that reaches beyond the self and mere personal fulfillment. We feel as though we are part of something that transcends our present place and time.

healthy sex hints 1.2
Creating Healthy Environments

- *Help create a healthy sexual environment within your community.* Be a role model for healthy sexuality. Lead by example, whether through words or actions.
- *Get involved in organizations that actively champion sexual rights.* If you can't or don't want to get publicly involved with them, support organizations financially. Make a contribution to acknowledge and support their work.

- *Be an advocate within any organization in which you are involved,* such as youth sports, church or temple, fraternity/sorority, and the like. If you see or hear things that work against creating or maintaining a healthy sexual environment, speak out.

Table 1.3 Excerpts from a University AIDS Policy

The staggering implications of this country's most life-threatening disease, AIDS, have become part of our nation's consciousness. We must now make the necessary preparations to protect the rights of both those students who have been exposed to or infected by HIV as well as the noninfected members of our University community. Above all, we must train all members of the University community to have a humane, well-informed reaction to those whose lives have been compromised by being exposed to or infected by the virus.

AIDS Advisory Board

WPU [William Paterson University] responded to the AIDS crisis by creating a presidentially appointed 6-member AIDS Advisory Board in 1987. The primary goals of this committee are as follows:

1. To encourage the faculty to include discussions of the social, medical, and economic effects of AIDS in their classes.
2. To offer our students a comprehensive roster of referral sources for their own educational advancement and, if necessary, their own health concerns.
3. To train peer educators to address the social forces that promote behavior that could make them susceptible to HIV infection (alcohol abuse, drug abuse, STDs, etc.).
4. To provide speakers for educational programming.

Guidelines

1. The initial admission decision for applicants will not take into consideration whether the applicant has a positive test to the virus thought to cause AIDS (a + HIV antibody test).
2. Students with the HIV infection will be afforded the same living arrangement as are all other residential students, except in specific cases where the health of the infected student is in jeopardy. Since this virus can be transmitted only by intimate sexual contact and/or by sharing contaminated blood products, the University feels separate housing accommodations are not justified. Individual decisions will be made on a case-by-case basis. It should be noted that the infected student stands a far greater chance of having his/her health compromised by a non-infected roommate through the transmission of the common airborne viruses than would the noninfected student of acquiring HIV through casual contact with his/her infected roommate.
3. Students with HIV infection will be afforded normal classroom attendance, working conditions and participation in cocurricular and extracurricular activities in an unrestricted manner as long as they are physically and psychologically able to do so.
4. Students with HIV infection will have access to all public facilities open to the University community.
5. Programs will not be implemented to require screening of students with HIV infection.

Institutional Responsibility/Confidentiality of Information

The American Council on Education (ACE) recommends that institutions have the responsibility to provide the following:

1. A comprehensive program of education about AIDS.
2. A training program that includes not only information about AIDS but a clear representation of the University's AIDS policy.
3. A system of encouraging people with the HIV infection to inform those who are appropriate of their condition.
4. A means of counseling people with the HIV infection about the facts of the disease and what has to be done to avoid transmission.
5. Regular assessment (every three months) of students with HIV infection to determine health status and psychological needs.

Although this University may be unaware that infected students may be unreasonably engaged in conduct that threatens the health of others, we will attempt to offer protection to the community at large while still protecting the rights of the person with HIV.

Section 504 of the Federal Rehabilitation Act of 1973 prohibits discrimination against individual(s) with disabilities. No qualified student with disabilities at William Paterson University is to be excluded from participation in, be denied benefits of, or be subjected to discrimination under any program or activities of the university community.

The knowledge that a given individual is carrying HIV could have such a profound and possibly irrational effect upon the recipient of this information who then might take steps that could easily compromise the campus life of the individual in question. The likelihood is that such information could not legally be placed in any non-medical files

(continued)

Table 1.3 Excerpts from a University AIDS Policy *(continued)*

without the expressed written permission of the student, according to the Family Education Rights and Privacy Act of 1974. This Act would probably apply to any verbal communication as well, and thus confidentiality must extend to faculty, administrators, other students and even partners.

The diagnosis of HIV or AIDS would occur at a hospital as part of a complete medical work-up and then be reported to the New Jersey State Department of Health, which then should forward the information to the Centers for Disease Control in Atlanta. The hospital or the student may report back the results of such testing, which are confidential, as part of the student health record. Often, a student would continue outside health care and not report to the Student Health Service. Education and counseling are available through the health center and counseling center when requested.

Source: Student Handbook, William Paterson University, 1998–1999. Reprinted with permission.

Health Challenges

As we've pointed out in this chapter, wellness functions along a continuum, with various dimensions impacting our sexual health throughout our lives. Ideally, college students and young adults are not confronted with serious health challenges. In reality, some already have or will find themselves managing chronic, sometimes debilitating illnesses and/or disabilities. Some of those illnesses and disabilities directly affect sexuality, whereas others may do so indirectly. Students have reported problems with substance abuse, eating disorders, and gambling. Others break bones, injure backs, and have accidents that may leave them in a wheelchair. Managing bouts of depression, having panic attacks, or being diagnosed with an obsessive–compulsive disorder all take their toll on socializing and getting close to others. For those who contract an STD such as genital warts, which is viral and long-term, the issue of how and what to tell a future partner adds to the regular issues related to dating.

We take the position that sexual health requires understanding ourselves and others—the people intimately in our lives and those in our communities. Toward that end, when an individual is confronted with health challenges, the specific condition can become a limitation. Although we all have limitations of one kind or another, health challenges become most limiting when they *define* us rather than being viewed as a *part* of who we are. Optimal sexual health requires that we be able to identify available resources and strategies to enable the highest levels of functioning possible.

Table 1.4 provides some of the resources available. Increasingly, the Internet has provided the much-needed link for those who previously may have felt isolated from information and support.

Table 1.4 Resources Available to Support Health Challenges

Professional Journals
Journal of Sexuality and Disability
Sexuality and Disabilities

Selected Web Sites and Phone Numbers
Sexuality and Disability Webliography: www.bccpd.bc.ca
A Web site of suggested readings compiled by the Wellness and Disability Initiative.

Spinal Cord Injury: www.sexualhealth.com
A Web site with information and resources on sex and disability.

Mental Health: http://Ulifeline.org
A Web site designed for college students. Sponsored by the Jed Foundation, named for a college student who committed suicide. The site has linkages to resources related to mental health, suicide prevention, drug abuse, and more.

Depression and Bipolar Support Alliance: www.dbsalliance.org
Web site support for those living with mood disorders.

STDs
American Social Health Association: www.ashastd.org
Provides information and resources about sexually transmitted diseases.

National AIDS hotline: (800) 342-2437

Gay Men's Health Crisis line: (212) 807-6664; www.gmhc.org
These two resources focus primarily on HIV/AIDS.

Chronic Illness/Cancer
Chronic Fatigue: www.chronicfatiguesupport.com
A Web site sponsored by ProHealth, Inc., with an expert medical advisory board.

Testicular Cancer Resource Center: http://tcrc.acor.org
Provides information for patients, caregivers, and physicians.

Susan G. Komen Breast Cancer Foundation: www.komen.org
Provides breast cancer research funds as well as educational and support services.

Drug Use
Bacchus & Gamma Peer Education Network: www.bacchusgamma.org
This is an association of college and university peer education groups focused on alcohol and other safety issues for students.

Alcohol hotline: (800) ALCOHOL

Alcoholics Anonymous: http://alcoholics-anonymous.org
The white pages of phone books list local chapters.

Cocaine hotline: (800) COCAINE

Narcotics Anonymous: www.wsoinc.org
The white pages of phone books list local chapters.

Eating Disorders
National Eating Disorders Association: www.NationalEatingDisorders.org
Provides educational and treatment information on eating disorders.

National Association of Anorexia Nervosa and Associated Disorders (ANAD): www.anad.org
Provides hotline counseling, education, and referrals.

Your responses to the Personal Assessment, Thought Questions, and Test Yourself! quiz questions can be logged online in your Virtual Workbook at **http://health.wadsworth/Blonna1.**

Personal Assessment

1.1 Wellness Lifestyle Questionnaire

Because sexual health cannot be separated from overall health, we would do well to attend to all the dimensions of our well-being. As you answer the items, try to think about how each may have an impact on your sexual health.

Please circle the appropriate answer to each question and total your points as indicated at the end of the questionnaire. Circle 5 if the statement is *always* true, 4 if the statement is *frequently* true, 3 if the statement is *occasionally* true, 2 if the statement is *seldom* true, or 1 if the statement is *never* true.

1. I am able to identify the situations and factors that overstress me.	5	4	3	2	1
2. I eat only when I am hungry.	5	4	3	2	1
3. I don't take tranquilizers or other drugs to relax.	5	4	3	2	1
4. I support efforts in my community to reduce environmental pollution.	5	4	3	2	1
5. I avoid buying foods with artificial colorings.	5	4	3	2	1
6. I rarely have problems concentrating on what I'm doing because of worrying about other things.	5	4	3	2	1
7. My employer (school) takes measures to ensure that my work (study) place is safe.	5	4	3	2	1
8. I try not to use medications when I feel unwell.	5	4	3	2	1
9. I am able to identify certain bodily responses and illnesses as my reactions to stress.	5	4	3	2	1
10. I question the use of diagnostic X rays.	5	4	3	2	1
11. I try to alter personal living habits that are risk factors for heart disease, cancer, and other lifestyle diseases.	5	4	3	2	1
12. I avoid taking sleeping pills to help me sleep.	5	4	3	2	1
13. I try not to eat foods with refined sugar or corn sugar ingredients.	5	4	3	2	1
14. I accomplish goals I set for myself.	5	4	3	2	1
15. I stretch or bend for several minutes each day to keep my body flexible.	5	4	3	2	1
16. I support immunization of all children for common childhood diseases.	5	4	3	2	1
17. I try to prevent friends from driving after they drink alcohol.	5	4	3	2	1
18. I minimize extra salt intake.	5	4	3	2	1
19. I don't mind when other people and situations make me wait or lose time.	5	4	3	2	1
20. I walk four or fewer flights of stairs rather than take the elevator.	5	4	3	2	1
21. I eat fresh fruits and vegetables.	5	4	3	2	1
22. I use dental floss at least once a day.	5	4	3	2	1
23. I read product labels on foods to determine their ingredients.	5	4	3	2	1
24. I try to maintain a normal body weight.	5	4	3	2	1
25. I record my feelings and thoughts in a journal or diary.	5	4	3	2	1
26. I have no difficulty falling asleep.	5	4	3	2	1
27. I engage in some form of vigorous physical activity at least three times a week.	5	4	3	2	1
28. I take time each day to quiet my mind and relax.	5	4	3	2	1

29. I am willing to make and sustain close friendships and intimate relationships.   5   4   3   2   1

30. I obtain an adequate daily supply of vitamins from my food or vitamin supplements.   5   4   3   2   1

31. I rarely have tension or migraine headaches, or pain in the neck or shoulders.   5   4   3   2   1

32. I wear a seat belt when driving.   5   4   3   2   1

33. I am aware of the emotional and situational factors that lead me to overeat.   5   4   3   2   1

34. I avoid driving my car after drinking any alcohol.   5   4   3   2   1

35. I am aware of the side effects of the medicines I take.   5   4   3   2   1

36. I am able to accept feelings of sadness, depression, and anxiety, knowing that they are almost always transient.   5   4   3   2   1

37. I would seek several additional professional opinions if my doctor were to recommend surgery for me.   5   4   3   2   1

38. I agree that nonsmokers should not have to breathe the smoke from cigarettes in public places.   5   4   3   2   1

39. I agree that pregnant women who smoke harm their babies.   5   4   3   2   1

40. I believe I get enough sleep.   5   4   3   2   1

41. I ask my doctor why a certain medication is being prescribed and inquire about alternatives.   5   4   3   2   1

42. I am aware of the calories expended in my activities.   5   4   3   2   1

43. I am willing to give priority to my own needs for time and psychological space by saying no to others' requests of me.   5   4   3   2   1

44. I walk instead of drive whenever feasible.   5   4   3   2   1

45. I eat a breakfast that contains about one-third of my daily need for calories, proteins, and vitamins.   5   4   3   2   1

46. I prohibit smoking in my home.   5   4   3   2   1

47. I remember and think about my dreams.   5   4   3   2   1

48. I seek medical attention only when I have symptoms or think some (potential) condition requires checking, rather than have routine yearly checkups.   5   4   3   2   1

49. I endeavor to make my home accident-free.   5   4   3   2   1

50. I ask my doctor to explain the diagnosis of my problem until I understand all that I care to.   5   4   3   2   1

51. I try to include fiber (whole grains, fresh fruits and vegetables, or bran) in my daily diet.   5   4   3   2   1

52. I can deal with my emotional problems without alcohol or other mood-altering drugs.   5   4   3   2   1

53. I am satisfied with my school/work.   5   4   3   2   1

54. I require children riding in my car to be in infant seats or in shoulder harnesses.   5   4   3   2   1

55. I try to associate with people who have a positive attitude about life.   5   4   3   2   1

56. I try not to eat snacks of candy, pastries, and other "junk" foods.   5   4   3   2   1

57. I avoid people who are "down" all the time and bring down those around them.   5   4   3   2   1

58. I am aware of the calorie content of the foods I eat.   5   4   3   2   1

59. I brush my teeth after meals.   5   4   3   2   1

60. (*for women only*) I routinely examine my breasts.   5   4   3   2   1

    (*for men only*) I am aware of the signs of testicular cancer.   5   4   3   2   1

How to Score

Enter the numbers you've circled next to the question number, and total your score for each category. Then determine your degree of wellness for each category using the wellness status key.

Emotional health	Fitness and body care	Environmental health	Stress	Nutrition	Medical self-responsibility
6 _____	15 _____	4 _____	1 _____	2 _____	8 _____
12 _____	20 _____	7 _____	3 _____	5 _____	10 _____
25 _____	22 _____	17 _____	9 _____	13 _____	11 _____
26 _____	24 _____	32 _____	14 _____	18 _____	16 _____
36 _____	27 _____	34 _____	19 _____	21 _____	35 _____
40 _____	33 _____	38 _____	28 _____	23 _____	37 _____
47 _____	42 _____	39 _____	29 _____	30 _____	41 _____
52 _____	44 _____	46 _____	31 _____	45 _____	48 _____
55 _____	58 _____	49 _____	43 _____	51 _____	59 _____
57 _____	59 _____	54 _____	53 _____	56 _____	60 _____
Total _____	Total _____	Total _____	Total _____	Total _____	Total _____

Wellness Status

To assess your status in each of the six categories, compare your total score in each to the following key:

0–34 Need improvement; 35–44 Good; 45–50 Excellent

Source: Gordon Edlin and Eric Golanty: *Health and Wellness,* 5th edition, © 1998, Sudbury, MA: Jones and Bartlett Publishers. www.jbpub.com. Reprinted with permission.

Thought Questions

1. What is human sexuality? What are its components?
2. What is the definition of *health* according to the World Health Organization?
3. What complaints did the wellness movement have with the WHO conceptualization of health?
4. What is the definition of *wellness*? What are its six components?
5. Define healthy sexuality, incorporating the elements of wellness.

Test Yourself!

1. Which generalization about sexuality in our culture is most accurate?
   a. Our culture is clearly becoming more sexually permissive, as reflected in the content of our television programming.
   b. Our culture is clearly becoming more sexually restrictive, as evidenced by growing financial support for abstinence-until-marriage education.
   c. Our cultural climate has not changed significantly for decades.
   d. Sexual messages in our culture are contradictory and diverse.

2. Guidelines developed for comprehensive sexuality education programs highlight the importance of teaching about all but which of the following?
   a. Abstinence-until-marriage strategies
   b. Human development
   c. Relationship skills
   d. Society and culture

3. In evaluating sexuality research, which among the following is least important?
   a. The size of the sample responding
   b. The gender of the researcher
   c. The professional affiliation of the researcher
   d. How the information was gathered

4. The criticism that there has been a lack of diversity in research subjects is highlighted by the fact that
   a. most subjects are white, heterosexual, and middle class.
   b. most research is conducted on the East and West coasts of the United States.
   c. more research has been conducted on women than men.
   d. few subjects are over 35 years of age.

5. According to Dunn, personal well-being is connected to
   a. regular visits to physicians and other health practitioners.
   b. personal habits and lifestyle.
   c. the health of your parents and other relatives.
   d. age and ethnic background.

6. John feels depressed a lot and is told about a Web site where college students can get information about mental health, along with a referral. By checking the site out, he will be attending to which aspects of his well-being?
   a. Physical and spiritual
   b. Emotional and intellectual
   c. Emotional and physical
   d. Intellectual and environmental

7. Sarah has decided to move into a campus apartment with friends. Her decision should improve which components of her well-being?
   a. Physical and social
   b. Environmental and emotional
   c. Social and environmental
   d. Emotional and physical

8. Students who exercise regularly are more likely to
   a. feel better about their bodies.
   b. get better grades.
   c. have more friends.
   d. gain weight over time.

9. Increasingly, college campuses have policies focused on sexuality-related issues. Policies related to all but which of the following should be expected?
   a. HIV/AIDS
   b. Sexual assault and date rape
   c. Sexual harassment
   d. Premarital sex

10. The model for making informed decisions recommends all but which of the following strategies?
    a. Identify the pros and cons.
    b. Weigh the pros and cons.
    c. Rate what is most important to least important.
    d. Think about what is right, not what your gut instincts tell you to do.

Media Menu

You can link to the following online tools by visiting
http://health.wadsworth.com/blonna1.

Film

Research Methods

 InfoTrac Activity

Kempner, M. E. (2003, February–March). True integration of prevention programs requires broad focus on sexual health. *SIECUS Report, 31*(3), 5.

 Web Resources

American Association of Sex Educators, Counselors, and Therapists

www.aasect.org/

Professional organization devoted to the promotion of sexual health by the development and advancement of the fields of sex therapy, counseling, and education. There is a selection of associated Web links and the "contemporary sexuality" section providing general items of interest on sexuality.

Go Ask Alice

www.goaskalice.columbia.edu/

Columbia University's Health Education Program, offering information and e-mail advice on sexual health, sexuality, communication, and relationships. The primary goal is to make health and wellness a life priority for students, staff, and professors.

Sexuality Information and Education Council of the U.S. (SIECUS)

www.siecus.org

National nonprofit organization that promotes comprehensive education about sexuality and advocates the right of individuals to make responsible sexual choices. This site details information on sexuality, contraception, and sexual abuse and assault.

The Society for the Scientific Study of Sexuality (SSSS)

www.SexScience.org

The Society for the Scientific Study of Sexuality is dedicated to advancing knowledge of sexuality. It believes in the importance of both the production of quality research and the application of sexual knowledge in educational, clinical, and other settings. The site provides links to professional meetings, journals in the field, other SSSS publications, professional contacts, and more.

Discovery Health

http://health.discovery.com/

This the Discovery Channel's health Web page. It has excellent sexual health information (click on sexual health icon on the left side). It also offers an array of online health assessments through the following link: http://health.discovery.com/tools/assessments.html.

National Wellness Institute (NWI)

www.nationalwellness.org/home/definitionofwellness.asp

Founded in 1977, the National Wellness Institute has steadfastly provided health promotion and wellness professionals unparalleled resources and services that promote both professional and personal growth. Besides a membership division, NWI hosts the National Wellness Conference. Held annually in Stevens Point, Wisconsin, at the University of Wisconsin for over 25 years, it is the most highly acclaimed conference for wellness and health promotion professionals.

The Sexual Health Network

www.sexualhealth.com

The Sexual Health Network is dedicated to providing easy access to sexuality information, education, mutual support, counseling, therapy, health care, products and other resources for people with disabilities, illness, or natural changes throughout the life cycle and those who love them or care for them.

Bill Hettler Home Page

http://hettler.com/

Bill Hettler has been providing wellness/health promotion consultations and presentations since 1972. He serves as president of the board of directors and is one of the cofounders of the National Wellness Institute, Inc. He is probably best known as one of the creators of the National Wellness Conference. This week-long conference has influenced the lives of thousands people for more than 20 years.

Online Health Assessments

http://health.discovery.com/tools/assessments.html

Take as many of the additional assessments as you wish. Make sure to explore all of the available assessments under all three menus (general health, personality, nutrition).

References

American College Health Association. (1996). *Policy guidelines for HIV/AIDS on campus.* Washington, DC: Author.

Ardell, D. (1985). *The history and future of wellness.* Dubuque, IA: Kendall/Hunt.

Boulard, G. (2001, December 24). After September 11th students find themselves under a magnifying glass. *Community College Week, 14*(10), 2–4.

Davey, J. (2002, September 30). One day in September. *Community College Week, 15*(4), 4.

Dettmer, J. (2001, October 29). New York shows strength in adversity. *Insight on the News, 17*(40), 13.

Dunn, H. (1962). High-level wellness in the world of today. *Journal of the American Osteopathic Association, 61*, 9.

Garmon, J. (2001, December 24). Making sense, not war. *Community College Week, 14*(10), 4–6.

Henry J. Kaiser Family Foundation. (2000). *Sex education in America: A view from inside the nation's classrooms.* Chart pack. Menlo Park, CA: Author.

Kirgiss, K. (2002, February). Taylor-made service: After the terrorist attacks, 99 students from Indiana's Taylor University drove to New York to help however they could. *Campus Life, 60*(7), 62–64.

Lane, K. (2002, January 21). After the fall: Against the ruined backdrop of Ground Zero, the wounded Borough of Manhattan community college is struggling to rebuild. *Community College Week, 14*(12), 6–11.

Manisses Communication Group. (2002, September 16). Survey finds impact of September 11th stretches across the country. *Mental Health Weekly, 12*(35), 1–3.

Mindlin, A. C., Wallace, E. E., & Kapell, M. (2002). Cultural and religious determinants of sexual behaviors: A crosscultural analysis of the available literature. *Michigan Academician, 34*(1), 6–8.

National Abortion and Reproductive Rights Action League Foundation. (2001). *Who decides? A state-by-state review of abortion and reproductive rights.* Washington, DC: NARAL and the NARAL Foundation.

National Wellness Institute. (2002). Definition of wellness [Online]. Available: www.nationalwellnessinstitute.home.

Office of the Surgeon General. (2001). *The surgeon general's call to action to promote sexual health and responsible sexual behavior.* Washington, DC: U.S. Government Printing Office.

Seong-Ngoo. (2002, May). Psychological burden after September 11th tragedy. *Student British Medical Journal, 138.*

Sexuality Information and Education Council of the U.S. (1996). *Guidelines for comprehensive sexuality education* (2nd ed.). New York: Author.

Sexuality Information and Education Council of the U.S. (1997). Guidelines for comprehensive sexuality education fact sheet [Online]. Available: www.siecus.org/pubs/fact/fact0003.html.

Sexuality Information and Education Council of the U.S. (2001, August–September). Issues and answers: Fact sheet on sexuality education. *SIECUS Report, 29*(6) [Online]. Available: www.siecus.org/pubs/fact/fact0007.html.

Straw, D. (2001, December 24). A separate peace in a wartime classroom. *Community College Week, 14*(10), 4–6.

Tsigos, C., & Chrousos, G. P. (1996). Stress, endocrine manifestations and disease. In C. L. Cooper (Ed.), *Handbook of stress, medicine, and health.* New York: CRC.

Weis, D. (2002, May). Another stab at sexual theory [a review of *The Role of Theory in Sex Research,* edited by J. Bancroft]. *Journal of Sex Research, 39*(2), 158–160.

Wiederman, M. (2001). Why understanding research? In *Understanding sexuality research.* Belmont, CA: Wadsworth.

World Health Organization. (1947). Constitution of the World Health Organization. *Chronicles of the World Health Organization, 1,* 29–43.

chapter *two*

Female Sexual Anatomy *and* Physiology

Student Learning Objectives

After reading this chapter, students will be able to

- Identify and locate the key structures of the female sexual anatomy.

- Describe the main functions of the key female sexual structures.

- Identify and describe the functions of the key female sex hormones.

- Explain the erogenous potential of the female sexual structures.

- Perform a breast self-exam.

- Identify the signs, symptoms, and treatment for common female sexual disorders.

- Describe a variety of screening tests used to diagnose common female sexual disorders.

*Test your understanding of these objectives by taking the end-of-chapter quiz, available online at **http://health.wadsworth.com/blonna1**.*

activity teaser: *How much do you know about female anatomy? Find the answer in the Personal Exploration Activity on page 35.*

"The Vagina Workshop" from *The Vagina Monologues* by Eve Ensler

The subject of this piece is an anonymous woman in her late 30s to 40s.

Ensler prefaces this piece as belonging to one of the women she interviewed from a group in their late 30s and early 40s. The woman had learned about her body and orgasm at one of the body workshops taught by Betty Dodson.

> . . . *I found it quite unsettling at first, my vagina. Like the first time you see a fish cut open and you discover this other complex world inside, right under the skin. It was so raw, so red, so fresh. And the thing that surprised me most was all the layers. Layers inside layers, opening into more layers. My vagina, like some mystical event that keeps unfolding another aspect of itself, which is really an event in itself, but you only know it after the event.*
>
> . . . *It was better than the Grand Canyon, ancient and full of grace. It had the innocence and freshness of a proper English garden. It was funny, very funny. It made me laugh. It could hide and seek, open and close. It was a mouth. It was a morning. And then it momentarily occurred to me that it was me, my vagina: it was who I was. It was not an entity. It was inside of me.*

Critical Thinking

Is it comfortable for you to examine your genitalia? Why is it important for women to look and understand how they are built?

Use your Virtual Workbook to explore your answers to these questions at **http://health.wadsworth.com/blonna1.**

Many of the structures and functions of sexual anatomy are really quite similar when comparing females and males. Indeed, an underlying theme in this book is the emphasis on how women and men are more similar than different. That being said, however, women's unique role in reproduction and the experiences associated with monthly menstruation across much of a woman's life require women to be aware of their bodies in a way different from men. Those experiences also make it challenging to separate the sexual from the reproductive function of the anatomy.

External Female Sexual Structures

Vulva The external female genitalia

The formal term used to describe all of the external female genital structures collectively is the **vulva.** The vulva includes the mons pubis (also known as *mons veneris*), labia majora and minora, clitoris, hymen, introitus, and vestibule. These are shown in Figure 2.1.

Mons Veneris

The mons veneris is named after the Greek goddess of love. In Latin, *mons veneris* means "the mound of Venus." The mons veneris, commonly called the pubic area, is the softly protruding cushion of fat, skin, and pubic hair that covers the pubis symphysis, the juncture of the pubic bones of the pelvis. Although it serves no reproductive function, the mons is sensitive to stimulation during sexual arousal. Its pad of fatty tissue provides a soft cushion to maximize pleasure during sexual activities, particularly those involving grinding circular movements.

Labia Majora

Labia majora The larger, outer vaginal lips

The two **labia majora** form the outermost vaginal lips. The labia are folds of skin covering fatty tissue and are covered with hair on the outside. The inner portion of the labia majora is covered with numerous sweat and oil glands.

What Do You Know?

After drawing and labeling the female sexual anatomy, you will be able to identify what is accurate and inaccurate about your knowledge of the female anatomy.

Before reading this chapter on female anatomy, take a few minutes to see how much you know or don't know about the female sexual anatomy. Take a sheet of paper and draw from memory the internal and external female sexual anatomy. If possible, get one of your friends of the opposite sex to team up with you to do this drawing. This will be more fun and will show which sex has the most knowledge of the female anatomy. Once you have drawn the anatomy, label the following parts: clitoris, ovaries, uterus, vagina, cervix, labia majora, labia minora, mons pubis, urethra, ureter, fimbria, and bladder.

When you have finished, compare your drawing to the one in this chapter. Are you surprised by how little or how much you know? How comfortable were you drawing this sexual anatomy? Ask one of your friends to do this activity. Does your friend's drawing indicate that they have good knowledge of the female anatomy? How comfortable were they drawing the sexual anatomy?

In the unaroused state, the labia majora remain closed, providing protection for the vaginal opening and clitoris. The skin of the labia, like that of the male scrotum, is normally darker in color than the rest of a woman's body. During sexual arousal, underlying erectile tissue engorges with blood, causing the labia to swell, deepen in color, and open like "the petals of a flower" (see "Betty Dodson's Art"), exposing the vaginal opening and clitoris.

The sweat and oil secretions of the labia majora are capable of producing a cheesy substance called *smegma*. Good hygiene involving washing of this area with soap and water can prevent unhealthy buildup of this material and ensure cleanliness.

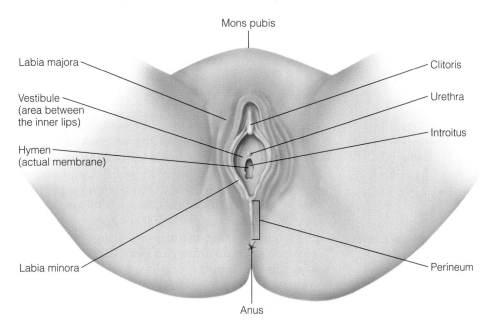

Figure 2.1 *The External Genitalia*

Susan Lerner 1999/Joel Gordon Photography

The appearance of the vulva varies woman to woman.

Labia Minora

Labia minora The smaller, inner vaginal lips

Bartholin's glands Small glands adjacent to the vaginal opening that secrete a mucus-like lubricant during arousal

Clitoris A small, highly sensitive, organ located at the top of the labia minora

The **labia minora** are a second set of vaginal lips located within the larger labia majora. Thinner than the labia majora, the labia minora have spongy tissue containing oil and sweat glands and are richly endowed with blood vessels and nerve endings. The top portion of the labia majora fuse to form the clitoral hood, or *prepuce*. Unlike the labia majora, the minora are hairless. In the unaroused state they, too, remain closed, providing a second line of protection for the vaginal opening and clitoris.

The labia minora are highly sensitive to sexual stimulation and engorge with blood during sexual stimulation, opening up and exposing the vaginal opening and clitoris. Within the labia minora are **Bartholin's glands,** which secrete a mucus-like lubricating fluid during sexual arousal. Once thought to provide the major portion of lubrication during arousal, it is now understood that vaginal lubrication comes from the walls of the vagina, rather than any significant amount of secretion from these glands. Bartholin's glands are homologous in structure and function to the bulbourethral (Cowper's) glands in males.

Clitoris

The **clitoris** is a small structure made up of erectile tissue located at the top of the vestibule where the labia majora join. It is made up of three parts—the glans, the shaft, and the root, or *crura*, and evolves from the same tissue that develops into the penis on the male. The glans of the clitoris is exposed by retracting the prepuce or clitoral hood.

The clitoris is a structure solely designed for sexual pleasure; it has no urinary or reproductive function. It is not involved in the passing of any body fluid, in contrast to the penis, which has a role in sexual response, reproduction, and urination. Because of this, many girls don't discover their clitoris until preadolescence or older. Figure 2.2 depicts the clitoris.

Labia majora

Prepuce or foreskin ("hood")

Urinary metus (opening)

Clitoral shaft (covered by prepuce)

Clitoral glans

Labia minora

Figure 2.2 *The Clitoris*

Betty Dodson's Art

The vulva has long been the subject of artistic expression. The vulva has often been portrayed as a flower, with the labia representing its petals, moist with the dew of sexual arousal, unfolding to reveal the secrets of love and lust contained within.

For more than 30 years, author, artist, and lecturer Betty Dodson has been celebrating female form and function. She has had over 100 exhibitions, and her artwork has adorned countless galleries throughout the world. Her sketches of the vulva capture the variety and uniqueness of female external genitalia. She combines artistic expression with sexual health activism.

Her book *Sex for One: The Joy of Self Loving* is a celebration of female sexuality. In the book, Dodson chronicles her own personal journey from a woman who questioned her own sexual response and ability to enjoy orgasm to a champion of women's sexual health. For decades, Dodson has run workshops devoted to helping women become orgasmic by using masturbation to liberate their sexual energy. Her artwork adorns her book, illustrating the sensual nature of female sexuality.

Source: From *Sex for One: The Joy of Self Loving* by Betty Dodson, copyright © 1974, 1983, 1987 by Betty Dodson. Used by permission of Harmony Books, a division of Random House, Inc., and Betty Dodson.

The clitoris is richly endowed with nerve endings. Although it appears externally as much smaller than the male penis, the clitoral glans has a comparable number of nerve endings. Because of its dense concentration of nerve endings, the clitoris is sensitive to overstimulation, and the prepuce will move forward to cover and protect it from excessive stimulation.

In the unaroused state, the clitoris is hidden by the prepuce. During sexual arousal, the spongy tissue of the clitoris engorges with blood, causing the clitoris to grow, become erect, and protrude from the prepuce, which retracts as the labia minora unfold. The clitoris is highly sensitive to sexual stimulation. Adequate clitoral stimulation plays a key role in female sexual response.

Women often find that certain forms of sexual activity do not always produce the correct form and amount of stimulation necessary for them to reach orgasm. Manual, oral, and mechanical stimulation of the clitoris, as well as female-on-top intercourse positions, seem to be the most effective for clitoral stimulation.

Discussion of the clitoris has often been missing from the education of young women. Undergraduate women have consistently reported that they didn't fully understand how the clitoris worked until college. Although a minority of women learned about the clitoris in high school, few, if any, learned about it in elementary school, when they were first taught about the vagina and uterus. The clitoris is the center of sexual arousal, and U.S. culture has historically been reticent to discuss sexual pleasure with young girls.

Vestibule

Vestibule The area within the labia minora that includes the hymen, introitus, and urethral opening

The **vestibule** is the area between the labia minora that is covered with the hymen and contains the openings to the vagina and urethra. In a sense, the vestibule represents the entrance to the vagina. During sexual arousal, the vestibule is sensitive to stimulation of all kinds. Like the labia and clitoris, it is richly endowed with nerve endings.

Urethral Opening

Urethral opening The opening to the urethra, lying behind the clitoris and in front of the vaginal opening

The **urethral opening** in the female lies behind the clitoris and in front of the vaginal opening. Because it is difficult for a female to see and locate, some people have mistakenly thought that a female urinates out the vagina. The urethra itself is an internal structure.

Hymen and Introitus

Hymen The membrane that lines the introitus

Introitus The vaginal opening

The **hymen** is a thin mucous membrane that covers the vestibule and **introitus** (vaginal opening). The hymen is intact at birth but typically becomes perforated by the time a young woman reaches puberty, allowing the passage of menstrual flow. Various activities ranging from sports and exercise to inserting fingers or other objects into the vagina during masturbation are capable of perforating the hymen.

Although the hymen is durable, its opening is capable of being stretched or enlarged through intercourse, masturbation, or insertion of a tampon. Some mothers discourage their daughters from using tampons for fear of ruining the hymen, yet that fear is unwarranted (Stewart & Spencer, 2002). Many people believe that the presence of a hymen is proof of a woman's virginity. This belief also is not true.

Figure 2.3 illustrates the three main types of hymens. The most common is the *annular,* in which the tissue surrounds the entire opening of the vagina and is open in the middle. The *cribiform* hymen has a web of tissue over the introitus and several small openings. The *septate* has a single band of tissue that divides the introitus into two parts. In rare occurrences, girls are born with the hymen completely covering the opening of the vagina, which is not discovered until she starts menstruating. This causes the fluid to build up in the vagina. When this happens, a physician must make a small opening to allow the menstrual flow.

If the hymen is still present at the time of first intercourse, penetration by the penis can produce some discomfort or even bleeding if the hymen is torn. The

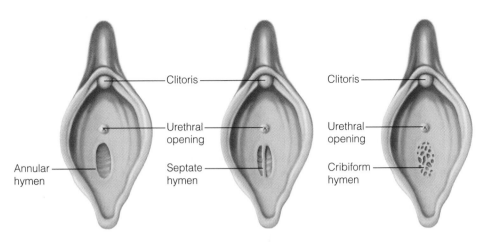

Figure 2.3 *Types of Hymens*

hymen can be gradually widened by inserting fingers into the opening, or a physician may also cut the hymen or stretch it with dilators. Generally, there is little trouble inserting the penis through the hymen if the male is gentle and the female adequately lubricated.

Perineum

The female **perineum** is the area between the thighs bounded in the front by the pelvis joint (the *symphysis pubis*) and in the rear by the coccyx (tailbone). The muscular tissue is covered by a layer of skin. Although it is not normally considered part of the female sexual anatomy, the perineum plays a part in sexual response because the entire area is endowed with nerve endings and is highly responsive to sexual stimulation. As with men, the nature and intensity of stimulation desired in this area varies from woman to woman and encounter to encounter.

The major difference between the perineum in women and men is its role in childbearing. The perineum of pregnant women is subject to tearing of the skin and muscle tissue during childbirth. This is usually the time when they first become aware of this region. During delivery, pressure from the emerging fetus can exert a tremendous force on the perineum, first stretching, then tearing, the muscle and skin. The muscles and skin will heal, although some women report less sensitivity, as nerve endings can be injured and require additional time to recover. Jagged tears are more likely to result in scar tissue, which can reduce the sensitivity of nerves in the area.

Two schools of thought have emerged concerning how to minimize damage to the perineum during childbirth. To avert tearing, obstetricians often perform a surgical procedure called an **episiotomy** to enlarge the opening, which facilitates the birth of the fetus. Midwives try to avoid performing episiotomies whenever possible. They encourage pregnant women to massage the perineum with oil during pregnancy and labor to help deliver their babies without an episiotomy. Sometimes the massage will help minimize the tear.

Anus

The anus in women is exactly the same as in men and, as such, is capable of similar responsiveness during sexual activity. Sexual stimulation can be enjoyed manually, orally (**anilingus**), and through anal intercourse. Some women use anal intercourse as an alternative to vaginal coitus because they think that by doing this, they can "preserve their virginity" and still enjoy sex.

Perineum The area of muscle and skin between vagina and anus

Episiotomy A surgical procedure that facilitates childbirth by enlarging the vaginal opening through cutting the perineum

Anilingus Oral stimulation of the anus

sex in society 2.2

Female Genital Cutting

The practice of female genital cutting (FGC) is a centuries-old tradition in some cultures, primarily in 26 of 43 African cultures, some parts of the Middle East, and areas of western and southern Asia (Chelala, 1998). The practice has been referred to as *female genital mutilation* (FGM) and *female circumcision*. Referring to the array of practices as FGC removes the value judgments associated with what is being done to the female body.

It is estimated that 2 million girls and women undergo the procedure annually (Chelala, 1998), with between 100 million and 180 million having undergone the procedures worldwide (PLANetWIRE, 2002). The procedure ranges from cuts around the clitoris to, more commonly, removal of the clitoris, removal of the clitoris and labia minora, or removal of the clitoris and entire labia with the area stitched closed. Although the procedure is most commonly performed between the ages of 2 and 15, some girls have had it done within the first week of life (Rising Daughters Aware, 1999). This cultural and religious custom has been done to reduce females' ability to experience sexual pleasure and ensure marital fidelity. The cultures that practice FGC do not believe a woman should derive pleasure from sex.

In recent years many organized groups, most prominently the World Health Organization and the United Nations Children's Fund, have condemned this treatment of females and are continuing to pressure the countries and cultures that still practice genital mutilation to end it. U.S.

representatives to the World Bank and other financial institutions oppose loans to countries that widely practice genital cutting and have no anti-FGC educational programs. Recently, efforts in Kenya and Uganda to celebrate the pubescent girl without FGC are slowly gaining acceptance (Chelala, 1998). A study of Nigerian women who have undergone FGC revealed that they were as likely as those who had not been cut to achieve orgasm during sexual intercourse, yet they reported that their breasts rather than clitoris were the most sensitive part of their bodies. Cut women, however, were significantly more likely to experience reproductive tract infections (Coren, 2003).

In the United States, the Federal Prohibition of Female Genital Mutilation Act of 1995 passed in September 1996, provides for prison sentences for anyone who performs this procedure on a female under 18 years of age. That law does permit the surgery if it is "necessary to the health of the person on whom it is performed." Other countries that outlaw the procedure include England, Canada, France, Sweden, and Switzerland.

U.S. health care professionals see the effects of genital mutilation on females emigrating to the United States, as well as those born to women here who follow the cultural practice. According to Carmen Retzlaff (1999), using 1990 census data, an estimated 168,000 girls and women living in the United States either have had or may have been at risk for FGC.

Underlying Structures

Although only the vulva is visible, there are underlying structures that are important to sexual arousal (see Figure 2.4). The area is rich in erectile tissue, with a network of nerves and blood vessels that become engorged, comparable to the spongy tissue of the penis. The vestibular bulbs run along the vagina, with the crura of the clitoris extending up toward the pelvic bone. The structures engorge with blood during sexual arousal, causing the labia, clitoris, and vagina to enlarge, swell, and deepen in color.

The muscles in the area also play a significant role in arousal. As discussed in Healthy Sex Hints 2.1, strengthening the pelvic floor muscles through Kegel exercises has clear health benefits.

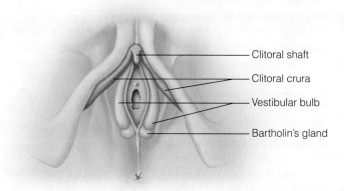

Clitoral shaft

Clitoral crura

Vestibular bulb

Bartholin's gland

Figure 2.4 *Underlying Structures*

Breasts

Although the main function of the female breast is **lactation,** it has taken on erotic and sexual significance in American and other cultures. Breast size and shape have become markers for attractiveness, sexiness, femininity, and motherhood, as well as disease. The breasts are composed of mammary glands, fatty tissue, the nipple and areola, and underlying muscle and ligaments.

Increasingly, women—even teen girls—are choosing to surgically alter their breasts. Large-breasted females may choose reduction surgery, as did Denise in Case Study 2.2. Her concerns focused on her appearance and breast changes after giving birth. For others, breast reduction is chosen not only for appearance issues but also due to back pain from the sheer weight of the breasts.

Lactation The process of producing and secreting milk from the breasts

Mammary Glands

The **mammary glands** are divided into 15 to 20 lobes or compartments separated by fatty tissue. Each lobe is made up of several smaller components called *lobules.* Imbedded in the lobules are milk-secreting cells called *alveoli.* Following childbirth, special hormones trigger the production and secretion of milk from the alveoli. Milk secreted from the alveoli is stored in chambers called *mammary ducts* and are drained through nursing.

Swelling of glandular tissue and storage of milk typically cause the breasts of nursing women to enlarge significantly. Breast size returns to normal after nursing ceases. (We will discuss lactation and nursing more fully in Chapter 13.) Breast swelling, and in some cases painful tenderness, often precedes menstruation, as the breasts (like the uterus) prepare for potential pregnancy.

Mammary glands Glands within the breasts that produce milk for lactation

Fatty Tissue

Breast size and shape in a woman who is not nursing are determined primarily by heredity and the amount of adipose or fatty tissue present in the breast. Heredity and overall percentage of body fat influence the amount of fatty tissue.

The female breast comes in a variety of shapes and sizes.

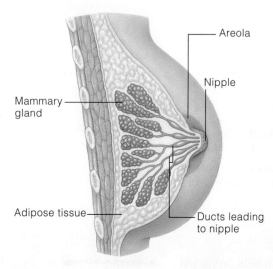

Figure 2.5 *Structures of the Female Breast*

Changing hormonal levels also can influence breast size. A common side effect of using hormonal contraceptives is a larger breast size. Figure 2.5 highlights the different structures of the breast.

Because of the cultural emphasis on breast size, surgical breast augmentation (enlargement) and reduction procedures have become much more common than before. In 2001, approximately 219,880 women had breast implant surgery, compared to 99,428 who had breast reduction surgery (American Society of Plastic Surgeons, 2003). The number of augmentation procedures had been as low as 32,000 in 1992, the year the Food and Drug Administration (FDA) banned silicone implants because of the problems associated with leakage and the subsequent development of cancer and other health problems. Cosmetic surgeons began to substitute medically safe saline-filled forms for silicone. However, because the quality of silicone breasts is seen as superior to other materials, and researchers debate silicone's negative side effects, there have been increased efforts to make silicone breasts available once again.

Breast augmentation and reduction procedures are not without problems. Both procedures carry a risk of scarring and loss of sensation in the nipples. Both procedures also can result in the inability to breastfeed. Major weight gain can influence both procedures and undo the effects of breast reduction.

Physical and Emotional Wellness

Concern for the appearance of one's breasts highlights how the emotional dimension of health interfaces with the physical dimension. Case Study 2.2 focuses on breast reduction, yet many females spend money to increase the size of their breasts with implants. Plastic surgeons are available to make breasts smaller, larger, more even, or higher and/or to replace one or both that may have been removed due to disease. Because breasts in American culture are sexualized and significant to women's sense of being attractive, focusing on breast health from the physical perspective may become secondary to a woman's concern that her breasts are "acceptable."

The physical dimensions of breast health can change with menstruation, pregnancy, breastfeeding, menopause, and aging. Some females are prone to breast cysts related to their menstrual cycles. Some are amazed at the changes in the breast when they breastfeed, whereas for others concerns over breast changes can stand as an impediment to their desire to breastfeed. Breast health requires paying attention to the breasts and their changes and ensuring that emotional concerns do not get in the way of proper care.

Areola and Nipple

Areola The brownish or pink ring of tissue surrounding the nipple of the breast

At the end of the breast is a ring of darker skin called the **areola.** In the center of the areola is the nipple. The areola is slightly rougher in texture than the rest of the breast because it contains oil glands that help lubricate the nipples during breastfeeding. The areola also contains small muscles and many nerve endings. This makes it highly responsive to sexual stimulation. Nursing mothers also report that suckling their babies can cause sensual feelings that can be a source of confusion.

Breast Reduction

Denise, age 35, is white.

Denise has two children and is finishing her degree in psychology part-time at night. She discussed her breast reduction surgery in a small group in a human sexuality class.

I couldn't wait to get my breast reduction surgery. I could never understand why some women want large breasts. I've had them since puberty, and they've been nothing but a pain in the neck. Ever since middle school, it seems that boys, and later men, would gawk at my breasts.

It's not like I ever did anything to invite this. I've always dressed conservatively and never flaunted my breasts (size 38DD), but it's hard to conceal them. Lord knows I've tried, but after a while I just got disgusted trying to hide them and figured there was nothing I could do about them until I got older and could think about surgery.

A lot of guys thought that just because I had big breasts, I was loose and interested in them sexually. That pretty much stopped after a couple of guys I dated in high school got the word out that I wasn't "one of those girls."

Anyway, I met my husband in my junior year of high school, and we've been together ever since. We got married in our sophomore year in college and had kids right away. We decided that after the kids were out of diapers and we decided we didn't want any more, we'd talk about my surgery.

I breastfed each of my kids for more than a year, and that solidified my decision. My breasts were absolutely ponderous when I was nursing. As soon as our second child was 3, we made the arrangements to get the surgery done. Everything went well, but the postoperative healing was a little painful and took longer than I expected. I even lost some sensation in my nipples and breasts for about a year. That's come back now, and I love my smaller, firmer breasts. I can jog and go braless—something I never did before the operation—and my husband still thinks my breasts are great. I'm happy I had it done.

Critical Thinking

What were the benefits Denise experienced as a result of having had breast reduction? Do you think her decision was a wise one?

Use your Virtual Workbook to explore your answers to these questions at **http://health.wadsworth.com/blonna1.**

The nipple is located within the areola and contains smooth muscle fibers, milk ducts, and many nerve endings. The nipples and areola are highly sensitive, and their smooth muscle fibers can contract upon stimulation, causing them to stiffen and become erect. Nipples also can stiffen and become erect in response to cold and nonsexual tactile stimulation.

Digital Vision /GettyImages

Breastfeeding is strongly encouraged as a healthy and economical way to nourish a baby.

43

Internal Female Sexual Structures

The internal structures of the female anatomy include the vagina, uterus, cervix, fallopian tubes, and ovaries (Figure 2.6). The urethra in the female lies outside the reproductive system, yet, along with the bladder, it is affected by pregnancy, menstruation, and sexual behavior.

Urethra

Cystitis Bladder infections

The urethra in the female runs from the bladder to the vestibule, and it is much shorter than that of the male (1 inch compared to 9 inches in the male). It is relatively easy for bacteria from outside the body to enter the urethra and lead to bladder infections known as **cystitis** (Starr & McMillan, 2003). *Escherichia coli* bacteria from the rectum and sexually transmitted infections can move to the urethra, necessitating antibiotic treatment. Drinking plenty of fluids and practicing good hygiene enhance urinary health.

Bladder

The bladder in the female lies next to the anterior wall of the vagina and in close proximity to the uterus. Because of its location, women's sense of needing to void can be affected by menstruation, pregnancy, lovemaking activities, and pelvic exams.

The rituals around the use of public restrooms differ for males and females. Anecdotally, women have complained of waiting on long lines, particularly when rushing during the intermissions at theatrical, film, or musical performances. Women argue that clothing issues and the custom of requiring privacy necessitates making more stalls available. Some theaters and stadiums have redesigned their restrooms in response to women's concerns.

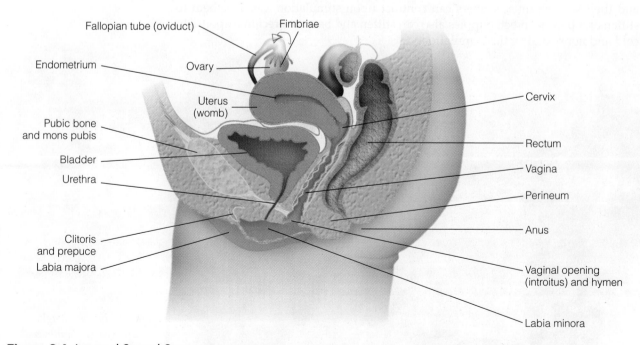

Figure 2.6 *Internal Sexual Structures*

Vagina

The **vagina** is a thin-walled muscular tube, about 3 to 4 inches long, lying between the bladder and the rectum, which connects to the cervix at one end and opens up to the outside of the body at the other. The vagina is tilted upward at a 45-degree angle extending toward the small of the back.

The walls of the vagina contain an outer layer of muscular tissue and an inner layer of mucous membrane. The mucous membrane tissue produces a thin, clear, moderately acidic (pH 3.5–4) discharge that provides an efficient self-cleaning mechanism. During sexual arousal, these same tissues engorge with blood, producing a thin, slippery lubrication that reduces friction and facilitates intercourse.

The outer third of the vagina contains the most muscle tissue and nerve endings. The interior and rear part, which connects with the cervix, is relatively devoid of nerve endings. In the unaroused state, the vagina resembles a collapsed space similar to a balloon without air in it. During sexual arousal the vagina expands, accommodating objects of varying sizes ranging from a tampon, penis, or sex toy to a newborn's head. Myths and stories exist, nonetheless, alluding to male or female partners being incompatible: "He's too big for me," "She's too loose for him," and so on. Women can improve the tone of the vaginal and pelvic muscles used during sex by doing Kegel exercises (Kegel, 1952). As will be discussed relative to sexual dysfunctions, some women require therapy to relax the vaginal muscle to allow for penetration.

On the front wall of the vagina, midway between the introitus and cervix, is an area known as the **G-spot,** or Grafenberg spot, named for the physician who first identified that portion of the vagina as having erotic potential. Research conducted in the 1980s brought discussions of the G-spot into analyses of female sexual response, with debate focused on whether all women had such a spot, found stimulation to the area arousing, and what exactly was the chemical makeup of the fluid propelled from the urethra in some women at the time of orgasm. Deep manual stimulation or penile stimulation can cause the area to swell, leading to

Vagina A tubular organ connecting to the uterus, which serves both reproductive and erotic functions

G-spot An area on the front wall of the vagina

healthy sex hints 2.1

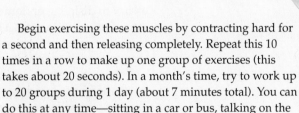

Pelvic Floor (Kegel) Exercises

You can practice contracting your pelvic floor muscles to prevent or reduce sagging of the organs and urinary incontinence (losing urine when you cough, sneeze, or laugh), to strengthen your orgasms, and to prepare for childbirth. If done regularly, these exercises can help prevent prolapse of the uterus (falling uterus into a stretched vagina, which has lost its muscle tone), cystocele (a bulge of the bladder into the vagina), and rectocele (bulge of the rectum into the vagina).

A good way to locate these muscles is to spread your legs apart while urinating to start and stop the flow of urine. Your ability to do this is one indication of how strong your muscles are. Another method is to try tightening against a man's erect penis during intercourse (this can feel pleasant to both partners).

Begin exercising these muscles by contracting hard for a second and then releasing completely. Repeat this 10 times in a row to make up one group of exercises (this takes about 20 seconds). In a month's time, try to work up to 20 groups during 1 day (about 7 minutes total). You can do this at any time—sitting in a car or bus, talking on the telephone, or even as a "wake-up" exercise.

Some of us have noticed improved muscle tone (and occasionally increased pleasure during intercourse) in just several weeks. For more detailed instruction on Kegel exercises, consult your local childbirth group.

Source: A. Kegel, "Sexual Function of the Pubococcus Muscle," *Western Journal of Surgery, Obstetrics, and Gynecology, 60* (1952), 521–524.

an orgasm that has a strong, vaginal component. Overall, research on the G-spot has been related to discussions of female ejaculation, tissue referred to as a female prostate gland, and a redefining of the components of female orgasm (Zaviacic & Whipple, 1993).

The vagina is also known as the *birth canal* because of its function as the exit point for the newborn during childbirth. The vagina has both reproductive and sexual pleasuring functions. Unlike the penis, the vagina is not involved during urination. Urine is excreted through the urethra, whose opening is located above the vaginal opening in the introitus.

The vagina is actually a self-cleansing structure. To ensure vaginal health, the average, healthy woman needs to do nothing more than shower or bathe daily (making sure to wash the vulva). She has no need to douche, wear minipads (if not menstruating), or use feminine hygiene sprays to perfume the vaginal area.

The walls of a normal, healthy vagina produce a thin, clear, slippery discharge that cleanses the vaginal lining. This discharge turns brownish when exposed to air. A small amount of this brownish discharge seeps out of the vagina and can be noticed on underwear. This does not indicate any problem. The discharge and the vagina in general have a characteristic musky odor. Sex partners often consider this odor erotic.

Changes in the amount, consistency, color, and odor can be used to assess whether you have a vaginal infection. If the amount of discharge increases, changes in color (from clear to yellow, green, or white), consistency (from thin and slippery to thick and curdish), or odor (becomes foul smelling), it could indicate a vaginal infection.

Uterus

Uterus Also called the womb, a fist-sized muscular structure that houses the developing fetus during gestation

The **uterus** is an organ that is sized and shaped like a pear. It is connected to the vagina at its narrow end. The end, or cervix, of the uterus is attached to the vagina and protrudes into the end of the vaginal canal. The wider end (the fundus) extends backward and is held in place by a broad uterine ligament. The uterus is tipped slightly forward.

The uterus is composed of three layers of tissue. The innermost layer, called the **endometrium,** undergoes a cycle of transformation each menstrual period as it prepares for implantation of a fertilized egg. The endometrium is where a fertilized egg implants and grows during pregnancy. If fertilization does not occur, the endometrium breaks down and is shed during menstruation.

Endometrium The inner blood lining of the uterus

Myometrium The muscular, middle layer of the uterus

The next layer of tissue, the **myometrium,** makes up the bulk of the uterus. This is thick muscular tissue capable of providing the powerful contractions necessary to dislodge endometrial tissue during menstruation or deliver a developed fetus during childbirth. This layer is capable of expanding the size of the uterus from that of a pear, prepregnancy, to a small watermelon during pregnancy, and then returning to near its original size within 2 months after birth.

Often, the myometrial contractions associated with menstruation can cause dysmenorrhea, which results in severe cramping and pain. At the end of this chapter, we will discuss self-help strategies to reduce these and other symptoms associated with menstrual discomfort. The third and outermost layer of uterine tissue is called the **perimetrium.**

Perimetrium The outer lining of the uterus

Cervix

Cervix The neck of the uterus, which extends into the inner end of the vagina

The **cervix** is described as the neck of the uterus. It resembles a small ring or button, the center portion tightly contracted and blocked with a plug of mucus. Running through the cervix is the cervical canal, a small passageway connecting the vagina to the uterus. It is filled with irregularly shaped spaces called *crypts*. The cervical opening, or *cervical os*, remains closed and blocked with mucus during most of a woman's menstrual cycle. As a woman's fertile time approaches, the mucous plug thins, allowing a passageway through the cervix into the uterus. Figure 2.7 shows the cervix and related structures.

During adolescence, the tissue of the cervix changes or transforms. This transformation zone is referred to as the **T-zone.** Cervical tissue (columnar epithelial tissue) is different from vaginal tissue (squamous mucous membrane tissue). During childhood, a young girl's cervix is covered with more columnar epithelial tissue than squamous tissue. As she matures, the amount of exposed columnar epithelial tissue decreases. The T-zone becomes smaller, encompassing the cervix and cervical canal. The T-zone is the area most commonly infected by gonorrhea, chlamydia, and other STDs during unprotected vaginal sexual intercourse. Because columnar epithelial tissue seems much more susceptible than squamous tissue to STD infection, all women (particularly young women) who are having vaginal intercourse should protect this area with barrier contraceptives.

The cervix is also a common site for the development of cancer in women. STD infection of the T-zone in young women can be a precursor of cervical cancer in later life. This is particularly true of infection with viral organisms (human papilloma virus, herpes simplex virus) introduced into the cervix during adolescence. It literally lays the seeds for the development of cervical cancer that appears a decade or more later.

T-zone Transformation zone of the cervix, where columnar epithelial tissue of the uterus meets with squamous tissue of the vagina

Fallopian Tubes

The two **fallopian tubes,** also known as *oviducts* and *uterine tubes,* approximately 4 inches long, stretch from either side of the fundus of the uterus to the ovaries. Unlike the male vas deferens, which connects to the epididymis, the fallopian tubes do not actually connect with the ovary. Each fallopian tube stops just short of the ovary and is held in place with ligaments that attach it to the peritoneum cavity. The open end of the fallopian tube is funnel shaped, with fingerlike projec-

Fallopian tubes Also called oviducts, extending from the fundus of the uterus to the ovaries; serve as the passageway for the ova

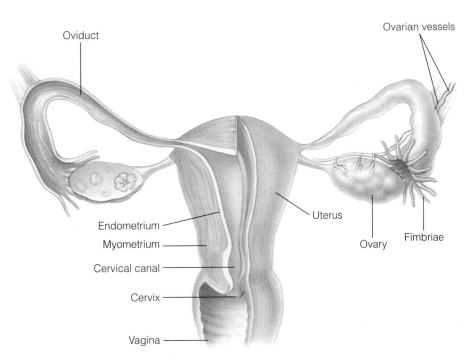

Figure 2.7 *The Cervix and Related Structures*

Follicle development

Ovulation

Figure 2.8 *Movement of the Egg*

tions called *fimbriae,* which shroud but do not connect with the ovaries. The fallopian tubes are made up of smooth muscle tissue and are lined with hairlike projections called *cilia.*

During ovulation, an egg released from the ovary is drawn into the fimbriae of its surrounding fallopian tube. No one knows for sure how this happens, but once inside the tube, the egg is whisked along by a combination of smooth-muscle contractions and the wavelike action of the cilia. For the egg to be fertilized and implanted within the uterus, a ripe ova must reach a viable sperm within 24 hours. Figure 2.8 shows how the female egg develops and moves.

Fallopian tube cilia are highly susceptible to destruction from infection. Destruction of these cilia is a common byproduct of infection with gonorrhea or chlamydia. Once the cilia are destroyed, they do not grow back. This can result in infertility or **ectopic pregnancy.** The term *ectopic* refers to the process in which the fertilized egg implants in a part of the body other than the uterus, most often in the fallopian tubes. Fertilized eggs have been known to implant in the abdominal area or cervical canal. Ectopic pregnancies cannot go to term and, if not treated promptly, can be life-threatening. Symptoms of an ectopic pregnancy include sharp constant abdominal pain and possible slight bleeding (Carlson, Eisenstat, & Ziporyn, 1996).

Ovaries

The **ovaries** are the size and shape of almonds. Each is located adjacent to a fallopian tube and is held in place in the peritoneum by connective tissue that anchors them to the broad uterine ligament. Like the male testes, the ovaries have two primary functions: fertility and hormone production. The ovaries produce ova (eggs) and the two important female sex hormones, estrogen and progesterone.

Reproductive Physiology

Two distinct cycles—the menstrual (also known as *uterine*) and ovarian—work in concert to control reproduction. Each cycle is regulated by hormones secreted by various endocrine glands. These cycles and their respective hormones are introduced here and described in greater detail in Chapter 13, "Human Reproduction."

Menarche is the term to define the onset of the menstrual cycle in girls. The age of menarche has been getting earlier, with an average of 12.2 for African American girls and 12.7 to 12.8 for white girls in the United States (Graber & Brooks-Gunn, 2002).

Menopause has become a term somewhat harder to define, yet the traditional epidemiological definition is 12 consecutive months of amenorrhea, meaning the absence of a period, without a woman having had surgery or any medical treatment that stops menstruation. The median age for menopause is 50 to 52 (Avis, Crawford, & Johannes, (2002). Overall, females menstruate approximately 13 times a calendar year, over a 40-year time frame, minus pregnancy. Consequently, menstruating is a fundamental part of being female, occupying a significant part of a woman's life.

Ovarian Cycle

Unlike male sperm, which are freshly produced in unlimited numbers, women are born with approximately 400,000 immature ova. The health and viability of the ova are affected by age and various environmental factors. Exposure to radiation, toxic chemicals, and other hazards can impair the health of the ova. In general, the viability of ova declines with age.

In a normal cycle, one immature egg matures, is released, and either is fertilized or dies and is discarded with the menstrual flow. This three-phased process

Ectopic pregnancy Implantation of an egg outside the womb

Ovaries Two almond-shaped structures that contain and release ova and secrete the hormones estrogen and progesterone

Menarche The onset of the menstrual cycle in girls

Menopause The absence of a period for 12 consecutive months, without surgery or medical treatment

healthy sex hints 2.2
Taking Care of Your Reproductive Health

For many women, going to the gynecologist or other reproductive health care provider is a visit they don't look forward to. In particular, the pelvic exam tends to arouse the most anxiety and discomfort. Draped from the waist down, lying on their back on the exam table with their feet in stirrups, legs spread wide apart, vulva completely exposed, they wait, feeling vulnerable.

Even when performed by the most sensitive of clinicians, the pelvic examination can be uncomfortable. The examination is designed to allow the clinician to examine visually and manually a woman's internal and external sexual anatomy. To facilitate this examination, a speculum is used to spread the walls of the vagina, and a light is used to illuminate the vaginal walls and cervix.

The examination consists of looking at the vulva and internal structures for any abnormalities—unusual growths, erosions, lumps, rashes, or discharges. After visually examining the area, the clinician manually probes the various structures, feeling for any changes in size or shape. A *bimanual examination* means using two hands to palpate structures such as the cervix, uterus, fallopian tubes, and ovaries. During this procedure, the clinician places one hand on the patient's abdomen and inserts two fingers from the other hand into the vagina. The clinician then feels for any abnormalities. Often these palpations will cause pain if disease is present.

Patient-centered clinicians take extra time and care to prepare patients for what is about to happen. They explain each procedure before it is done, helping the patient adjust to the probes and prods that are part of the examination. They also offer patients the option to see what is happening through the use of floor and handheld mirrors. Little things such as warming a speculum before inserting it and helping patients relax with breathing exercises can go a long way toward making the examination less offensive.

Women are encouraged to understand their bodies, prepare for the exam by thinking through the questions that they have, and make sure their concerns are dealt with in a sensitive manner. Three excellent reference books to have in your home library include these:

The V Book: The Doctor's Guide to Complete Vulvovaginal Health, Elizabeth Stewart and Paula Spencer (New York: Bantam, 2002)

The Harvard Women's Health Guide, Karen J. Carlson, Stephanie A. Eisenstat, and Terra Ziporyn (Boston: Harvard University Press, 1996)

The New Our Bodies, Ourselves, Boston Women's Health Book Collective (New York: Simon & Schuster, 1998)

Ovarian cycle A three-phased period of time covering maturation of a follicle, release of ovum, and secreting role of corpus luteum

Follicle An egg sac in the ovary

Corpus luteum The follicle after it has released its ovum and begins to produce progesterone

is called the **ovarian cycle** (see Figure 2.9). Each cycle has a follicular, ovulatory, and luteal phase. For purposes of illustration, a typical 28-day cycle is used here. Women's cycles can vary significantly; hormonal changes, stress, weight loss, exercise, and other factors can all impact cycle length. A woman who is monitoring her body to determine ovulation needs to understand that ovulation occurs 14 days from the end of the cycle. While the follicular phase can vary in length, the luteal phase tends to be consistently 2 weeks in length.

1. The *follicular phase* consists of the first 10 days. During this time, a **follicle** grows, preparing to release a mature egg.
2. The *ovulatory phase*, days 11 to 14, consists of final preparation for and release of a mature egg.
3. The *luteal phase*, days 14 to 28, revolves around the activity of the **corpus luteum.** The corpus luteum's role of secreting progesterone to sustain the rich endometrial lining necessary for implantation varies depending on whether fertilization occurs.

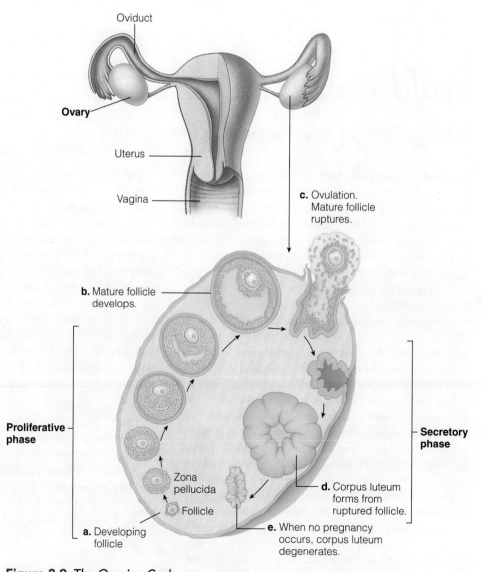

Oviduct

Ovary

Uterus

Vagina

c. Ovulation. Mature follicle ruptures.

b. Mature follicle develops.

Proliferative phase

Secretory phase

Zona pellucida

Follicle

a. Developing follicle

d. Corpus luteum forms from ruptured follicle.

e. When no pregnancy occurs, corpus luteum degenerates.

Figure 2.9 *The Ovarian Cycle*

Menstrual or Uterine Cycle

Although the main function of the uterus is to house the implanted and developing embryo, the cyclic nature of reproduction allows this for only a few short days each month. The menstrual cycle coincides perfectly with the ovarian cycle to ensure the union of sperm and egg at the best possible time to enhance successful implantation in the endometrium. The phases of the menstrual cycle are depicted in Figure 2.10.

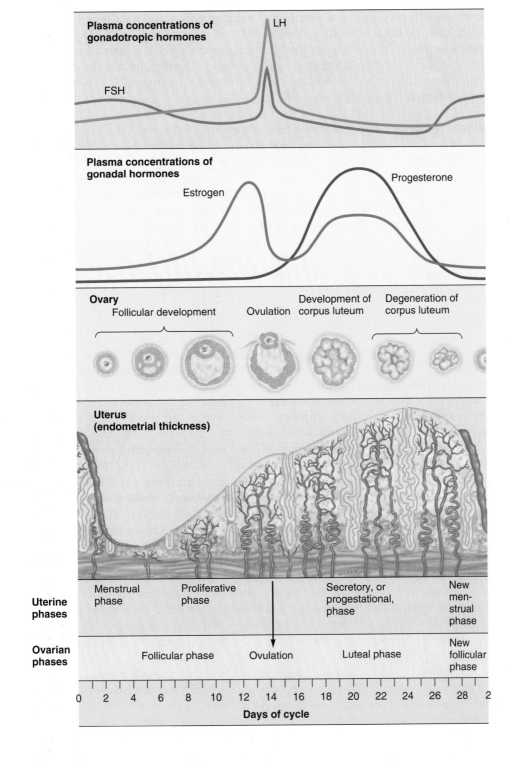

Figure 2.10 *The Menstrual (Uterine) Cycle*

Menstrual Phase   During the menstrual phase, which lasts approximately 3 to 5 days, the uterus sheds its endometrial lining. The strong muscles of the uterus contract and slough off the rich network of tissue and blood vessels built up to support fetal implantation and development. The cervix dilates to allow the bloody menstrual flow to work its way out of the uterus and through the vagina. For menstrual hygiene, females can use internal tampons to absorb the blood, or sanitary pads worn externally.

Proliferative Phase   During this phase of the menstrual cycle, the uterine lining rebuilds. The endometrium literally proliferates with a rich network of tissue and blood vessels, preparing the uterus for pregnancy. To support a pregnancy, the lining must be thick enough and endowed with the complex network of blood vessels necessary to sustain successful implantation and development of an embryo for the 9 months of prenatal development. During the buildup, the endometrium relies on a constant source of the hormone estrogen. This phase takes about 9 days and ends with ovulation.

Secretory Phase   The secretory phase begins with ovulation and lasts about 14 days or until the onset of the menstrual phase. The secretory phase is divided into two parts. During the first half of the phase, the uterus prepares for implantation of a fertilized ovum. Luteinizing hormone (LH), secreted by the pituitary gland, triggers the ruptured ovarian corpus luteum to secrete high levels of progesterone. This extra progesterone mixes with estrogen, causing the endometrium to thicken even more and become engorged with blood vessels.

If fertilization does not occur, the second phase of the secretory cycle begins with a decline in estrogen, LH, and progesterone levels. The corpus luteum degenerates, and the endometrium begins to die, ultimately leading to its sloughing off during the menstrual phase.

Menopause

The cessation of the menstrual period, called *menopause*, generally occurs between ages 45 and 55. Women typically experience 5 to 10 years of what is termed **perimenopause,** a period of gradually declining estrogen levels produced by the ovaries, culminating in no more menstrual periods. As the body works to adjust to changing hormone levels, women can experience a variety of physical symptoms. The most well known is the "hot flash," during which the upper portion of the body becomes flushed and the woman breaks out in a sweat. In 2003, Jeanie Linders wrote *Menopause, the Musical*, subtitled "The hilarious celebration of women and The Change." By parodying popular music and relying on humor and shared experiences, the cast sang about flashing, changing, and the overall need to maintain a positive attitude about it all.

In addition to hot flashes, other troubling symptoms can include changes in vaginal lubrication, sexual interest, and irritability. Postmenopausal women are at greater risk for heart disease, breast cancer, and osteoporosis.

Declining estrogen levels have been related to higher rates of osteoporosis and heart disease in postmenopausal women. With that information, women for years were prescribed either estrogen replacement therapy (ERT) or hormone replacement therapy (HRT), which is a combination of estrogen and progesterone. In addition, some hormone protocols include testosterone replacement therapy, which can help improve sex drive.

The Women's Health Initiative, a government-funded research project, increased the much-needed scientific study of how women's health is impacted during midlife and beyond. In 2002, research was released indicating that not only were many of the touted benefits of HRT questionable, but some were more dangerous than ever suspected (Writing Group for the Women's Health Initiative, 2002). Women had been

Perimenopause A period of gradually declining estrogen levels produced by the ovaries taking HRT for the relief of menopausal symptoms, with the added benefit of lowering their risk of heart disease. It was found that HRT actually increased the risk of heart disease, leading to many women discontinuing their use of the supplements.

The importance of sound scientific research to medical practice is clear, yet in practical terms, some women have been left at a loss as to how to handle menopausal discomforts. Women are increasingly finding healthful strategies such as changes in diet, exercise, yoga, massage, and attitude can increase their sense of comfort with this stage of life. Simultaneously, some physicians and women have chosen to continue using HRT for severe menopausal symptoms. With continued careful monitoring, the immediate benefits for some outweigh the possible risks to health.

Emotional and Social Wellness

Because the menstrual cycle is such a fundamental part of being female, it is important that women learn to manage this part of their health. For some, menstruation means little more than remembering to carry the necessary hygiene products. To others, however, each cycle can be fraught with intense pain, mood swings, irritability, and an overall desire to be left alone.

The cessation of menstruation can bring relief and joy to some women. No more cramps. No more hassles. For others, however, menopause is associated with aging and the myriad possible health changes that occur. Because menopause occurs at midlife, it becomes important for women to find medical and social supports to make the transition easier.

Interacting with Health Care Practitioners

The medical specialty focused on women's reproductive health is called **gynecology.** In practice, many physicians who specialize in gynecology also complete a residency in **obstetrics,** a specialization focused on pregnancy and childbirth. **Family practitioners** offer comprehensive health care, including monitoring pregnancies and delivering babies. Women's reproductive health can also be monitored by nurse midwives and nurse practitioners.

A woman's health requires that she take care of her total body. Unfortunately, some families connect reproductive health to sexual behavior, as in "If you're using that part, take care of it." Young women may be discouraged from seeking gynecological care when they need it, especially if going to the doctor is interpreted as an admission of sexual activity. Older women sometimes neglect their reproductive health once they see themselves as "finished having babies." Lesbian women may avoid reproductive health care, sometimes because of their discomfort in dealing with a health care system that has historically assumed women are heterosexual and want children, or because of the misguided idea that without engaging in sexual intercourse, such care is less necessary.

Women need annual gynecological exams. The guidelines for getting a Pap test (or Pap smear, discussed in more detail later) to check for cervical cancer have been revised from the earlier prevailing wisdom that women needed an annual screening by age 18 or the age of onset of sexual intercourse, based on whichever was first. The American Cancer Society in late 2002 revised its guidelines regarding the timing of the Pap test. Women should have their first Pap test approximately 3 years after the onset of vaginal intercourse but no later than 21 years of age. Subsequent Pap tests should be performed annually until age 30; after that, for women who have had three consecutive negative test results, guidelines are for continued screenings every 2 years (Smith, Cokkinides, & Eyre, 2003).

Gynecology The medical specialty focused on women's reproductive health

Obstetrics A specialization focused on pregnancy and childbirth

Family practitioners Physicians who offer comprehensive health care, including monitoring pregnancies and delivering babies

sex in society 2.3

Disparities in Reproductive Health Care

Both national and international concerns about HIV/AIDS have generated attention to an overall lack in reproductive health care for women of color. Groups at both levels have sought to frame women's health as a women's rights issue. As such, women need to be treated fairly by the health care system, with adequate information, services, and treatments being available.

In the United States, the SisterSong Women of Color Reproductive Health Project was founded in 1998 to address how racial, gender, and economic discrimination impact the reproductive rights of women of color. The four primary ethnic populations represented are black/African American, Latina/Hispanic, American/Indigenous, and Asian/Pacific Islander. Within the project are a number of women-of-color organizations that conduct research, provide direct services, and/or work to develop and implement advocacy strategies.

In the United States, it is estimated that of 36 million women of color, almost one-fourth are uninsured. Native American women have the lowest screening rates for cer-

vical cancer among all ethnic groups. Asian/Pacific Islanders living in the United States often confront language barriers that impede adequate health care delivery. Their cultural values also put them at odds with ideas that they should feel in control of their bodies. Latina women traditionally seek advice from family members before turning to professionals, which has contributed to delayed utilization of health care services. They have higher rates of cervical cancer, cesarian deliveries and sterilization abuse. African American women have high rates of cervical and breast cancer, yet they typically have not been adequately screened by Pap smears and mammograms (Ross, Brownlee, Diallo, Rodriguez, & the Latina Roundtable, 2001). Attempts to provide adequate health care must incorporate the sometimes-unique concerns that race, gender, sexual orientation, and poverty create.

Source: Adapted from L. J. Ross, S. L. Brownlee, D. D. Diallo, L. Rodriguez, and the Latina Roundtable, "The SisterSong Collective: Women of Color, Reproductive Health and Human Rights," *American Journal of Health Studies, 17*(2) (Spring 2001), 79–89.

Health concerns related to menstruation through menopause are in the domain of the gynecologist. Described later in this chapter is a sampling of reproductive health concerns that would most likely be detected by the gynecologist and subsequently treated.

Physical and Intellectual Wellness

Women often learn to associate health and prevention with sexual activity: "If I'm not sexually active or pregnant, I don't need to see my physician or get a Pap smear." To ensure optimal physical well-being, girls should be taught about their body and understand issues such as proper hygiene and care and protection of their genitalia. As girls approach puberty, they need to be aware of the changes that will take place in their body and their sexual anatomy and physiology. They need to understand the changes associated with menstruation and fertility, increasing sexual desire, hygiene, prevention of sexually transmitted disease and unintended pregnancy, and breast self-examination.

As women age, fitness, proper nutrition, and weight management all become increasingly important for optimal sexual health. Throughout adulthood, proper functioning of female sexual anatomy, positive body image, and other sexual health issues are affected by the level of physical well-being. So much information is available through publications targeted at women as well as the tremendous resources of the Internet that becoming an informed consumer is both easy and expected.

Common Disorders of Female Sexual Anatomy

A variety of disorders can affect female sexual anatomy and physiology. Among the most common are endometriosis, uterine fibroid tumors, fibrocystic breast disease, breast cancer, vaginitis, premenstrual syndrome (PMS), and dysmenorrhea. Some women develop cancer of the cervix, endometrium of the uterus, or ovaries, resulting in the removal of those structures.

Endometriosis

Endometriosis is a disorder of the endometrium resulting from migration of the byproducts of menstruation into the fallopian tubes, ovaries, and abdominal cavity. The shed endometrial tissue, called *implants,* adheres to these structures and continues to respond to the effects of hormones during the menstrual cycle. They swell, bleed, and may form **cysts** that can burst, resulting in scar tissue and painful **adhesions.**

The most common symptoms of endometriosis are sharp pain, cramps, and heavy bleeding during menstruation. Some women have chronic pelvic or low-back pain or a feeling of pressure during sexual intercourse. If the endometrial implants spread to the bladder or bowel, this condition can cause painful elimination and blood in the urine or feces. In some cases, endometriosis can cause infertility.

Endometriosis is diagnosed through a combination of history of signs and symptoms and visual examination. An instrument called a **laparoscope,** a flexible tube with a light, is used to locate and examine the implants internally. The abdomen is inflated with carbon dioxide gas, a small incision is made near the navel, and the tube is inserted. The physician can examine the abdomen through the laparoscope, find the exact location of the implants, and determine the extent of the problem.

Several forms of treatment are available for endometriosis. They depend on the extent of the problem, the woman's age, and several other considerations. The least invasive treatments involve hormonal or drug therapies to halt temporarily ovulation and menstruation, resulting in the shrinkage and eventual disappearance of the implants. Surgical removal of the implants and the scar tissue is a more invasive treatment. In extreme circumstances, radical surgery is done to remove the uterus, ovaries, and fallopian tubes.

Uterine Fibroid Tumors

Uterine fibroid tumors are masses of muscle and connective tissue growing in the uterus. These noncancerous tumors are one of the most common disorders of female sexual anatomy in the United States and may be associated with heavy bleeding, difficulty urinating, and pelvic pain. Small tumors usually do not produce noticeable symptoms. As they grow, they begin to take up more space within the uterus and begin to produce symptoms. The most common symptom of fibroid tumors is unusually heavy menstrual bleeding, followed by pressure or pain in the abdomen. If the tumor gets very large (tumors can grow to be as large as a softball), it begins to put pressure on the bladder, causing urinary problems. The tumor can actually push against the stomach, making the woman look pregnant. Large tumors, and the heavy and prolonged bleeding they cause, can cause anemia, resulting in fatigue and other symptoms.

Uterine fibroid tumors are diagnosed in a variety of ways, depending on their location and size. A routine pelvic exam can detect some fibroid tumors. Ultrasound, X ray, laparoscopy, and a variety of other diagnostic procedures are used

Endometriosis A condition in which pieces of the endometrium migrate to the fallopian tubes, ovaries, or abdominal cavity

Cysts An abnormal condition of fluid-filled sacs that can burst and cause pain and scarring

Adhesions Spider-web-like bands of scar tissue that painfully bind internal organs to each other or the abdominal wall

Laparoscope A medical instrument made up of a tube with a light that permits examination of reproductive structures, requiring only a small abdominal incision

Uterine fibroid tumors Noncancerous solid growths on the endometrium or in the walls of the uterus to diagnose the rest of the cases. One in four women is affected, with uterine fibroid tumors being a primary reason why women have hysterectomies. Treatment depends on a variety of factors, including the size of the tumor, its location, the woman's age, the woman's desire to bear children, and others. Drug therapies that block the production of estrogen may be used. These treatments mimic the effects of menopause, which seem to have a beneficial effect on fibroid tumors. Fibroid tumors may grow less rapidly and shrink during menopause because estrogen production ceases. Unfortunately, the tumors begin to grow back once the therapy is discontinued and estrogen production resumes.

Women's health experts continue to debate the role of **hysterectomy,** the surgical removal of the uterus, as the best treatment option when fibroid growths are causing problems. A less radical procedure, **myomectomy,** involves removing the fibroids but preserving the uterus, thereby allowing for subsequent pregnancy. A newer procedure, *uterine artery embolization* (UAE), involves reducing the blood flow to the fibroid, which in turn significantly reduces blood loss and saves the uterus (American College of Obstetricians and Gynecologists, 2003). Heavy menstrual bleeding can

Hysterectomy Surgical removal of uterus. In practice, a hysterectomy often is accompanied by surgical removal of fallopian tubes and sometimes also the ovaries

Myomectomy A surgical procedure that removes fibroid tumors without removing the uterus

healthy sex hints 2.2

Being Familiar with Your Breasts

Despite the controversy surrounding the effectiveness of breast self-exam (BSE), we recommend that women remain familiar with their breasts.

How to Examine Your Breasts

1. Lie down with a pillow under your right shoulder, and place your right arm behind your head.
2. Use the finger pads of the three middle fingers on your left hand to feel for lumps in the right breast.
3. Press firmly enough to know how your breast feels. A firm ridge in the lower curve of each breast is normal. If you're not sure how hard to press, talk with your doctor or nurse.
4. Move around the breast in a circular, up-and-down line or a wedge pattern. Be sure to do it the same way every time, check the entire breast area, and remember how your breast feels from month to month.
5. Repeat the exam on your left breast, using the finger pads of the right hand. (Move the pillow to under your left shoulder.)

6. If you find any changes, see your doctor right away.
7. Repeat the examination of both breasts while standing, with your one arm behind your head. The upright position makes it easier to check the upper and outer part of the breasts (toward your armpit). This is where about half of breast cancers are found. You may want to do the standing part of the BSE while you are in the shower. Some breast changes can be felt more easily when your skin is wet and soapy.

For added safety, you can check your breasts for any dimpling of the skin, changes in the nipple, redness, or swelling while standing in front of a mirror right after your BSE each month.

*Please note that a breast self-examination should not be considered a substitute for a regular mammogram.
Source: American Cancer Society, Atlanta, GA. Reprinted with permission.

also be treated through endometrial ablation. In 2001, the FDA approved NovaSure, which relies on the use of a wand, mesh that fills the uterine cavity, and a brief electrical current to destroy the endometrial lining (Novacept, 2003).

Fibrocystic Breast Disease

Fibrocystic breast disease is a disorder involving the swelling, and resulting "lumpy" configuration, of breast tissue. The breasts, like the uterus, change as ovulation and menstruation approach. The secretory cells surrounding the mammary ducts secrete fluids that seep into the fibrous connective tissue in the lower parts of the breast, and breast tissue swells. This fluid sometimes creates pockets of fluid that appear to be cysts.

Normally, the fluid in these pockets drains from the breast tissue through the lymph system and **lymph nodes** under the breast. Fibrocystic breast condition occurs when the breasts are unable to drain this fluid fully. It results in swollen, firm, or hardened fibrous breast tissue.

Lymph nodes The main drainage and filtration sites in the lymph system

Looking
Stand in front of a mirror with your upper body unclothed. Look for changes in the shape and size of the breast, and for dimpling of the skin or "pulling in" of the nipples. Any changes in the breast may be made more noticeable by a change in position of the body or arms. Look for any of the above signs or for changes in shape from one breast to the other.

1. Stand with your arms down.

2. Raise your arms overhead.

3. Place your hands on your hips and tighten your chest and arm muscles by pressing firmly.

Feeling

1. Lie flat on your back. Place a pillow or towel under one shoulder, and raise that arm over your head. With the opposite hand, you'll feel with the pads, not the fingertips, of the three middle fingers, for lumps or any change in the texture of the breast or skin.

2. The area you'll examine is from your collarbone to your bra line and from your breastbone to the center of your armpit. Imagine the area divided into vertical strips. Using small circular motions (the size of a dime), move your fingers up and down the strips. Apply light, medium, and deep pressure to examine each spot. Repeat this same process for your other breast.

3. Gently squeeze the nipple of each breast between your thumb and index finger. Any discharge, clear or bloody, should be reported to your doctor immediately.

Fibroadenomas Benign, solid tumors associated with fibrocystic breast disorder

Sometimes the inability to drain the breasts fully results in permanent cysts or tumors. Of all cysts and tumors, most are benign (noncancerous). Cysts, also known as **fibroadenomas,** are less common than tumors. These lumps are small, round, and move around freely under the skin. Even though fibroadenomas are noncancerous, they can be a source of distress for women because they are often confused with cancerous lumps. Depending on their size and number, the lumps can cause symptoms ranging from tenderness and mild discomfort to severe discomfort (Carlson et al., 1996).

Fibrocystic breast condition and fibroadenomas are diagnosed through physical examination and laboratory testing. All swelling and lumps should be approached as potentially cancerous until cancer is ruled out when the lumps disappear or biopsy and testing proves negative. This is often difficult for women to do because of the fear associated with breast cancer and the tendency to deny that the lumps exist, despite the fact that more than half of all women have them.

Breast Cancer

Breast cancer develops when cancerous cells proliferate, causing one or more tumors. Because breast cancer cells are of different types, the form of cancer a woman has may have more to do with her survival than how early or late her cancer has been detected. Tumors may metastasize, with malignant cells spreading throughout the body in lymph fluid and the bloodstream.

Breast cancer is the second leading cause of deaths from cancer in women, surpassed only by lung cancer. An estimated 211,300 new cases of breast cancer will be diagnosed in U.S. women in 2003, with 39,800 women dying of the disease. Over time, there has been a noted increase in the incidence of breast cancer, but what is encouraging is that the number of deaths has decreased (American Cancer Society, 2003b).

Robin Nelson/PhotoEdit, Inc.

A mammogram can detect lumps too small to feel during breast self-exam.

The major risk factors for breast cancer in women are family history of breast cancer (mother or sister infected with the disease), family history of other cancers, and previous personal history of cancer. Other risk factors include late childbearing (first child after 30 years old), never having a baby, early onset of menstruation, late menopause, and a history of fibrocystic breast disease. Risk factors that are less strongly associated with breast cancer are a diet high in saturated fat, body composition (excess fatty deposits in waist and hips), excessive alcohol consumption, and hormone replacement therapy.

Genetic researchers have found that a woman who carries mutations of either BRCA1 or the BRCA2 gene may be at great risk for developing either breast or ovarian cancer. It is estimated that only 10 to 15 percent of breast cancers can be traced to mutations of these genes; women with the mutations, however, have a 50 to 85 percent chance of developing breast cancer (American Cancer Society, 2003b). Some women, in response to the discovery of the BRCA1 and BRCA2 mutations, have opted for prophylactic mastectomy and hysterectomy, a radical attempt at maintaining health.

Women need to play an active role in maintaining the health of their breasts. Menstruation, pregnancy, and menopause can all affect how the breast appears and feels. To check for the possibility of breast cancer, women need to learn to conduct a breast self-exam (BSE). The prevailing wisdom has been that women conduct BSE monthly.

The American Cancer Society has recommended that women 20 to 39 years of age have a clinical breast exam performed by a health care professional every 3 years. Mammograms, which are X rays of the breast, are recommended annually for women 40 years of age and older.

Recent research has suggested that both BSE and mammography may not be particularly useful, especially for young women. The concern with BSE is that by the time a lump is palpable, it has been growing for years, in addition to the fact that survival is more correlated with the aggressiveness of the type of cancer rather than the timing of detection. Although the technology has improved for mammography, younger, premenopausal breast tissue tends to be too dense to make detection accurate (American Cancer Society, 2003a).

If breast cancer is diagnosed, women should discuss the various treatment options with their physicians. More and more women are able to have a *lumpectomy,* which is removal of the tumor, rather than a *mastectomy,* which is removal of the breast. Both treatments may require radiation therapy and chemotherapy afterward to help prevent further spread of any errant cells. Two drugs, tamoxifen and letrozole, have been found to greatly reduce breast cancer reoccurrence, although the ideal usage protocols are still under study (Goss et al., 2003). Breast reconstructive surgery is utilized after mastectomies are performed for the treatment of breast cancer. Women have chosen implants or had flap surgery, utilizing their own muscle and fat tissue to create a replacement breast.

Vaginitis

In **vaginitis,** the vagina becomes inflamed, resulting in one or more of the following symptoms: discharge, dryness, burning upon urination (if the inflammation spreads into the urethral opening), and pain during intercourse. The discharge associated with vaginitis is often overlooked or mistaken for a woman's normal vaginal fluid. Three characteristics of vaginal discharge—quantity, color, and odor—can vary in response to vaginitis. The discharge associated with vaginitis is usually profuse (quantity), ranging from frothy white to greenish yellow (color), and changes from a woman's normal scent to a foul, even fishy-smelling

Vaginitis Inflammation and irritation of the vagina

healthy sex hints 2.3
Promoting Optimal Vulvovaginal Health

1. Do not make your private parts private to you. Examine yourself.
2. Get involved in your health care. Go on the Internet. Get information. Ask questions.
3. Wash the vulva daily with warm, soapy water.
4. Avoid douching. The vagina is a self-cleansing organ. Douching does not prevent pregnancy or infection and can destroy healthy bacteria present in the vagina.
5. Avoid scented products such as vaginal hygiene sprays and perfumed soaps. Do not use talcum powder on the vulva.
6. Be careful about what you insert into your vagina (make sure all sex toys and other objects are safe and clean before inserting them).
7. Do not progress from anal intercourse to vaginal intercourse (a common way to transfer germs from the rectum to the vagina) without first washing your partner's penis.
8. Never force vaginal penetration (make sure your vagina is well lubricated before inserting anything into it).
9. Become familiar with the amount, consistency, color, and odor of your normal daily discharge.
10. If the discharge changes, see a health care provider.

Source: Elizabeth G. Stewart and Paula Spencer, *The V Book: A Doctor's Guide to Complete Vulvovaginal Health* (New York: Bantam, 2002).

odor. Sometimes vaginitis causes vaginal dryness instead of discharge. This unusual dryness results in pain.

The urethra can become inflamed as a result of either the discharge or unusual dryness. When the urethra is inflamed, urination is painful. Painful intercourse is another common symptom of vaginitis.

Vaginitis is diagnosed through a combination of clinical examination and laboratory tests. Various forms of vaginitis have different combinations of symptoms. An experienced clinician often can make the diagnosis based on the symptoms. Microscopic examination of vaginal fluids makes the diagnosis more precise and allows the clinician to treat the patient more effectively. In some cases, a specimen is taken from the vagina or cervix and is grown on a biological culture plate, with the results available within 1 week.

Various prescription drugs and over-the-counter medications are available to treat the different forms of vaginitis. Antibiotics are used with vaginitis caused by bacteria (*E. coli*, gonorrhea). Antifungal agents are used to treat vaginitis attributable to yeast overgrowth (monilia, *Candida albicans*). Other agents (*Trichomonas vaginalis*) necessitate the use of other types of drugs. Self-treatment of vaginitis (especially involving douching) is not recommended without an accurate diagnosis of the condition.

Cervical Cancer

Cervical cancer is the end stage of cervical dysplasia. *Cervical dysplasia* refers to the presence of abnormal or precancerous cells at the cervix. Also known as *cervical intraepithelial neoplasia* (CIN), it is more common than both breast and uterine cancers. The good news is that it is almost 100 percent curable if detected early. Early detection of cervical cancer also can prevent its spread into the uterus. Early changes in the cells lining the cervix can be detected through a procedure called the *Pap test*. Pap test results are graded on the following 5-point scale:

Class 1: no abnormalities
Class 2: atypical benign symptoms of early CIN
Class 3: advanced CIN
Class 4: cancer *in situ*
Class 5: invasive cervical cancer

healthy sex hints 2.4
Reducing the Risks for Cervical Cancer

The major risk factors for cervical cancer are

- early onset of intercourse (beginning in early adolescence);
- lifetime number of sexual partners (risks increase as numbers increase);
- history of STD infection (particularly viral STDs such as HPV and HSV);
- not using barrier contraception (condoms, diaphragm).

To lessen your risk:

1. Delay onset of intercourse (women who begin having intercourse after age 20 have a lower risk).
2. Reduce your number of total sexual partners (having one, uninfected sex partner is lowest risk).
3. Use barrier contraceptives (male and female condoms work best) to protect the T-zone.
4. Starting at age 18 or once you've begun having intercourse (whichever comes first), have an annual pelvic examination that includes a Pap test (this will ensure early detection and treatment of cancer).

The Pap smear is the most reliable tool for detecting cervical cancer early. A Pap smear involves taking a specimen of cells from the cervix and usually is included as part of a routine pelvic exam. Cells are obtained by gently scraping the cervix with a small wooden spatula to dislodge the tissue and then smearing it onto a microscope slide. The slide is stained and examined under a microscope for abnormal cellular changes (Boston Women's Book Collective, 1998).

Uterine Cancer

Uterine cancer usually affects the endometrial lining. Early symptoms include abnormal bleeding or spotting. An estimated 39,300 new cases were estimated to be diagnosed during 2002 (American Cancer Society, 2003d). Risk factors for uterine cancer include estrogen replacement therapy (ERT) used during menopause, early menarche, late menopause, never having had children, and history of failure to ovulate. Pregnancy and the use of oral contraceptives provide protection against endometrial cancer.

The Pap test rarely detects endometrial cancer. Consequently, annual pelvic exams and the use of endometrial biopsy around the time of menopause are relied on for diagnosis. If endometrial cancer is found, hysterectomy, radiation, and chemotherapy are the preferred treatments.

Ovarian Cancer

Even though ovarian cancer accounts for only 4 percent of all cancers among women, it results in more deaths than any cancer of the reproductive system because symptoms do not appear until later in its development. Women may experience abdominal enlargement and digestive disturbances such as persistent stomach discomfort and gas that cannot be explained by other causes.

An estimated 25,400 new cases were projected for U.S. women in 2003 (American Cancer Society, 2003c). The early and well-publicized experiences of comedienne Gilda Radner, a popular figure on the television program *Saturday Night Live*, did much to bring public attention to this disease.

As with breast cancer, current research is focusing on mutations in the BRCA1 and BRCA2 genes as risk factors for ovarian cancer. Pregnancy and the use of oral contraceptives are thought to reduce the risk of developing ovarian cancer. Once diagnosed, women undergo a hysterectomy, followed by radiation and various chemotherapy regimens.

Premenstrual Syndrome (PMS)

Premenstrual syndrome (PMS) is characterized by a myriad of physical and psychological symptoms that appear anywhere within 2 weeks of the onset of menstruation. Psychosocial symptoms include negative emotions such as anxiety, irritability, depression, anger, insomnia, confusion, and social withdrawal. Physical symptoms include fluid retention, breast tenderness, weight gain, headaches, dizziness, nausea, increased appetite, and craving for sweets. Because of the range of symptoms associated with PMS and the number of women affected (between 20 and 75 percent), many women's health experts are beginning to question whether the syndrome really exists or whether these are just the normal parameters of the menstrual experience. It is not unusual to hear women claim to be "PMSing" to explain even general stress overload.

Research into the causes, nature, and treatment of PMS lacks consistency. Although most PMS researchers believe that shifting hormonal balances play a key role in the condition, the specific hormones and exact mechanisms of action are unclear. The ratio of estrogen to progesterone has been implicated, along with the

Premenstrual syndrome (PMS) A condition preceding menstruation, characterized by a myriad of physical and psychological symptoms level of mineral corticoids that control fluid retention. Still other theorists postulate that the key hormones involved are those of the brain that influence mood.

An interesting aspect of PMS is the relationship between women's moods, attitudes, and emotions and the physiological symptoms that characterize the syndrome. Researchers are still trying to ascertain whether negative emotions about menstruation and PMS are what trigger the hormonal and other physiological changes associated with the syndrome or whether the physical discomfort is what precipitates the psychological and social distress.

Dysmenorrhea

Dysmenorrhea Painful menstruation

Often, the myometrial contractions associated with menstruation cause **dysmenorrhea,** which results in severe cramping and pain. As you might recall from our discussion earlier in this chapter, the myometrium is a thick layer of muscular tissue capable of providing the powerful contractions necessary to dislodge endometrial tissue during menstruation or expel a developed fetus during childbirth. Myometrial contractions are triggered by the release of powerful hormones called **prostaglandins.** Dysmenorrhea is often caused by excessively high levels of prostaglandins. This can cause more intense contractions that last longer than usual.

Prostaglandins Hormones that can cause muscle contractions and have been associated with menstrual pain

Toxic Shock Syndrome

Toxic shock syndrome (TSS) is caused by infection with the *Staphylococcus aureus bacterium,* an organism that can live in the vagina without threatening a woman's health. Overgrowth of the bacteria, however, can result in TSS, which *is* life-

healthy sex hints 2.5
Self-Help for PMS

Various treatments are available to help women who have PMS. For years, stress management and dietary changes have been advocated as part of a comprehensive PMS treatment program. Recently, prostaglandin inhibitors have been recommended. The following are some strategies that might work for you:

1. Eat a well-balanced diet high in complex carbohydrates, low in fat, and containing moderate protein. Eat at least three meals a day (it may be preferable to eat many smaller meals). This will provide the best fuel and an even release of energy throughout the day.
2. Avoid excess sugar and snacks high in sugar and fat. This step, coupled with tip 1, will help avoid the extreme high and low blood sugar levels associated with mood swings.
3. Avoid excess sodium intake (table salt and salt in food), which will help reduce bloating related to fluid retention.

4. Have an orgasm. This activity can help release pent-up vaginal and uterine muscle tension.
5. Try relaxation activities such as diaphragmatic breathing, imagery, meditation, and systematic muscle relaxation. These activities can help reduce stress and induce relaxation.
6. Have your partner (or a professional) give you a lower-back massage. It will help relieve muscle tension and induce relaxation.
7. Soak in a warm bath, Jacuzzi, or hot tub, or apply heat to the abdominal area with a heating pad or water bottle. The warmth will help you relieve muscle tension and induce relaxation.
8. Try antiprostaglandin medications. Prostaglandin inhibitors reduce the intensity and duration of cramps. Mild prostaglandin inhibitors include ibuprofen (marketed as Motrin). Stronger prescription medications include naproxen (Naprosyn), naproxen sodium (Anaprox), and mefenamic acid (Ponstel).

threatening. Toxins produced from TSS infection produce initial symptoms including a sudden high fever (101 degrees Fahrenheit or higher), headache, sore throat with swelling of the mucous membranes, diarrhea, vomiting, muscle aches, and a sunburnlike rash. If untreated, TSS can cause kidney or liver failure, resulting in death in about 10 percent of all cases. If diagnosed early, TSS is easily treated with broad-spectrum antibiotics.

Initial research found that TSS was associated with tampons, especially the superabsorbent type. This finding led to the removal of Rely brand tampons from the market. Subsequent studies found that cervical caps, diaphragms, and contraceptive sponges also pose a risk for developing TSS if they are used during menstruation. Since first being reported in 1980, the incidence of toxic shock syndrome has continued to decline.

To reduce the risk of TSS, it is recommended that women not use superabsorbent tampons, frequently change the ones they do use (at least three times per day), use a sanitary pad at least once in a 24-hour period, and when menstruating do not use a cervical cap, diaphragm, or the contraceptive sponge.

Health Challenges

As we've said, it is important to understand how the body functions and what will promote optimal health. At the same time, some individuals are born with health challenges, and others "acquire" them through aging, diagnosis and treatment of illness, and accidents.

Researchers have examined the impact of spinal cord injury (SCI) on sexual functioning, finding that women can menstruate, conceive, give birth, get sexually aroused, and achieve orgasm (Whipple, Gerdes, & Komisaruk, 1996). Looking at the impact of multiple sclerosis on female functioning, researchers found that women reported changes in frequency of sexual activity along with a change in activities, yet sexual activity was defined primarily as sexual intercourse (McCabe et al., 1996).

When confronted with health conditions that leave the woman with chronic pain, it is certainly understandable that sexual desire and enjoyment may be affected (Schlesinger, 1996). Some women feel less sexual after surgery that involves loss of a body part, whether visible, as in the breast, or fertility related, as with the uterus.

All told, sexual functioning is possible on many levels. Our definitions of what may be considered "sexual" also need expanding so that variations in health and physical functioning do not lead to negative perspectives.

Your responses to the Personal Assessment, Thought Questions, and Test Yourself! quiz questions can be logged online in your Virtual Workbook at **http://health.wadsworth.com/blonna1.**

Personal Assessment

2.1 Body Image: Female

Body image refers to our evaluation and perception of our body, specific body parts, and their functioning. It includes the messages (positive and negative) that we tell ourselves about our bodies, our self-esteem, and the behaviors and choices we make as a result. The following inventory will help females assess their body image.

Rate each body part listed here using the following scale: extremely satisfied = 5; satisfied = 4; neutral = 3; dissatisfied = 2; extremely dissatisfied = 1.

1. eyes _____
2. ears _____
3. nose _____
4. hair _____
5. teeth _____
6. mouth _____
7. weight _____
8. face _____
9. shoulders _____
10. breasts _____
11. arms _____
12. calves _____
13. hands _____
14. height _____
15. stomach _____
16. buttocks _____
17. hips _____
18. thighs _____
19. feet _____
20. sex organs _____
21. overall body _____

Scoring:

105–80 Very positive body image	20–40 Negative body image
60–80 Positive body image	0–20 Very negative body image
40–60 Ambivalent about your body	

Rate each item below, using the following scale: very comfortable = 5; comfortable = 4; neutral = 3; uncomfortable = 2; very uncomfortable = 1.

_____ 22. Looking at my nude body in the mirror

_____ 23. Performing self-examinations of my nude body

_____ 24. Being nude when I am alone

_____ 25. Being nude when I am with my lover

_____ 26. Being nude when I am around my kids

_____ 27. Sunbathing in the nude

_____ 28. Swimming in the nude

_____ 29. Walking around the house nude

Scoring:

32–40 Very comfortable with nudity	12–16 Uncomfortable with nudity
21–32 Comfortable with nudity	0–12 Very uncomfortable with nudity
16–21 Ambivalent about nudity	

Complete the following sentences:

30. The thing I like best about my body is _____

31. The thing I dislike most about my body is _____

Thought Questions

1. What is the proper term for the external female genitalia?

2. What are the components of the external female genitalia?

3. What is the nature of the hymen?

4. What are the internal structures of the female sexual anatomy?

5. What are the characteristics of the vagina in the normal and aroused states?

6. What is the best way to ensure good vaginal health?

7. (a) What are the cervical crypts and the transformation zone?

   (b) Describe their significance in the transmission of STDs.

8. How are the ovaries and testes alike and different?

9. What are the phases of the menstrual cycle?

10. What is the role of female sex hormones in female sexuality?

Test Yourself!

1. Which part of female anatomy is *not* considered part of the vulva?
   a. Labia majora
   b. Vagina
   c. Mons pubis
   d. Clitoris

2. The structure most critical for female sexual arousal is the
   a. uterus.
   b. vagina.
   c. clitoris.
   d. mons pubis.

3. Female genital mutilation is a practice
   a. widely found among immigrants to the United States.
   b. designed to enhance female fertility.
   c. supported by the United Nations.
   d. rooted in religious and cultural customs.

4. All but which are true regarding the size of a woman's breasts?
   a. Size is correlated with sexual pleasure.
   b. Size is related to heredity and body fat.
   c. Size can be temporarily affected by pregnancy and lactation.
   d. Cosmetic surgery can be used to increase or decrease breast size.

5. A woman's menstrual blood includes tissue from which part of the uterus?
   a. Cervix
   b. Endometrium
   c. Myometrium
   d. Os

6. Females are born with approximately how many immature ovarian follicles?
   a. 40,000
   b. 40 million
   c. 400,000
   d. 400

7. Which term refers to the cessation of menstruation?
   a. Menarche
   b. Dysmenorrhea
   c. Endometriosis
   d. Menopause

8. Young women are advised to have a pelvic exam
   a. only if having vaginal sexual contact.
   b. by age 18 or upon initiating vaginal sexual contact.
   c. only if heterosexual.
   d. once they get married.

9. The Pap test is designed to detect cancer of the
   a. cervix.
   b. vagina.
   c. breast.
   d. colon.

10. Female deaths associated with reproductive cancers are highest when cancer is found in the
   a. cervix.
   b. uterus.
   c. fallopian tubes.
   d. ovaries.

Media Menu

You can link to the following online tools by visiting
http://health.wadsworth.com/blonna1.

Face to Face Video

Dr. Lisa McIntosh speaks on female sexual dysfunction.

Animation

Female Reproductive System
Female Reproductive Function

 InfoTrac Activity

Davis, S. (2002, Spring). Loose lips sink ships. *Feminist Studies, 28*(1), 7(30).

 Web Resources

National Women's Health Information Center

www.4woman.gov

Developed by the U.S. Department of Health and Human Services, this site provides up-to-date research and information related to a wide variety of women's health concerns.

National Women's Health Network

www.womenshealthnetwork.org

A clearinghouse for a variety of women's health topics. It produces a bimonthly newsletter, *The Network News*, and works as a major advocacy group for women's health issues.

Harvard Women's Health Watch

www.health.harvard.edu

This group interprets medical information for the general reader. A monthly newsletter is also available.

OBGYN.net Women and Patients

www.obgyn.net/women/women.asp

Valuable information concerning all areas of women's health with links to many sites. Information covered in this site includes diseases and conditions, interactive tools, health information resources, forums, directories, organizations, publications, and international resources.

Food and Drug Administration

www.fda.gov/cdrh/mammography/certified.html

Federal Drug Administration–certified mammography facilities by region in the United States.

Susan G. Komen Foundation

www.breastcancerinfo.com

An interactive Web site providing breast cancer screening and treatment information. It includes conversations with survivors, searchable A–Z guide, after-treatment care, insurance issues, and more.

References

American Cancer Society. (2003a). Can breast cancer be found early? [Online]. Available: www.cancer.org.

American Cancer Society. (2003b). What are the key statistics for breast cancer? [Online]. Available: www.cancer.org.

American Cancer Society. (2003c). What are the key statistics for ovarian cancer? [Online]. Available: www.cancer.org.

American Cancer Society. (2003d). What are the key statistics for uterine sarcoma? [Online]. Available: www.cancer.org.

American Cancer Society. (2003e). What are the risk factors for breast cancer? [Online]. Available: www.cancer.org.

American College of Obstetricians and Gynecologists. (2003, August). ACOG statement on alternatives to hysterectomy [Online]. Available: www.acog.org.

American Society of Plastic Surgeons. (2003). www.plasticsurgery.org.

Avis, N. E., Crawford, S., & Johannes, C. (2002). Menopause. In G. M. Winwood & R. J. DiClemente (Eds.), *Handbook of women's sexual and reproductive health*. New York: Kluwer Academic/Plenum.

Boston Women's Book Collective. (1998). *The new our bodies, ourselves*. New York: Simon & Schuster.

Carlson, K. J., Eisenstat, S. A., & Ziporyn, T. (1996). *The Harvard guide to women's health*. Cambridge, MA: Harvard University Press.

Chelala, C. (1998, September 16). New rite is alternative to female circumcision. *San Francisco Chronicle* [Online]. Available: www.fgm.org.

Coren, C. (2003, March). Genital cutting may alter, rather than eliminate, women's sexual sensations. *International Family Planning Perspectives, 29*(1).

Dodson, B. (1996). *Sex for One*. New York: Three Rivers Press.

Ensler, E. (1998). The vagina workshop. In *The vagina monologues*. New York: Villard.

Goss, P., Ingle, J., Martino, S., Robert, N., Muss, H., et al. (2003). A randomized trial of letrozole in postmenopausal women after 5 years of tamoxifen therapy for early stage breast cancer. *New England Journal of Medicine, 349*(19), 1793–1802.

Graber, J. A., & Brooks-Gunn, J. (2002). Adolescent girls' sexual development. In G. M. Winwood & R. J. DiClemente (Eds.), *Handbook of women's sexual and reproductive health*. New York: Kluwer Academic/Plenum.

Kegel, A. (1952). Sexual functions of the pubococcus muscle. *Western Journal of Surgery, Obstetrics and Gynecology, 60*, 521–524.

McCabe, M., McDonald, E., Deeks, A., Vowels, L., & Cobain, M. (1996). The impact of multiple sclerosis on sexuality and relationships. *Journal of Sex Research, 33*(3), 241–248.

Novacept. (2003). The NovaSure system [Online]. Available: www.novacept.com.

PLANetWIRE. (2002). Saving women's lives [Online]. Available: www.planetwire.org.

Retzlaff, C. (1999, May). Female genital mutilation: Not just over there. *Journal of the International Association of Physicians in AIDS Care, 5*(5).

Rising Daughters Aware. (1999). The basics: What is FGM? [Online]. Available: www.fgm.org.

Ross, L. J., Brownlee, S. L., Diallo, D. D., Rodriguez, L., & the Latina Roundtable. (2001, Spring). The SisterSong Collective: Women of color, reproductive health and human rights. *American Journal of Health Studies, 17*(2), 79–89.

Schlesinger, L. (1996). Chronic pain, intimacy, and sexuality: A qualitative study of women who live with pain. *Journal of Sex Research, 33*(3), 249–256.

Smith, R. A., Cokkinides, V., & Eyre, H. J. (2003). American Cancer Society Guidelines for the early detection of cancer, 2003. *CA: A Cancer Journal for Clinicians, 53*, 27–43.

Starr, C., & McMillan, B. (2003). *Human biology* (5th ed.). Pacific Grove, CA: Brooks/Cole.

Stewart, E. G., & Spencer, P. (2002). *The V book: A doctor's guide to complete vulvovaginal health*. New York: Bantam.

Whipple, B., Gerdes, C., & Komisaruk, B. (1996). Sexual response to self-stimulation in women with complete spinal cord injury. *Journal of Sex Research, 33*(3), 231–240.

Writing Group for the Women's Health Initiative Investigators. (2002, July 17). Risks and benefits of estrogen plus progestin in healthy postmenopausal women. *Journal of the American Medical Association, 288*(3).

Zaviacic, M., & Whipple, B. (1993). Update on the female prostate and the phenomenon of female ejaculation. *Journal of Sex Research, 30*, 148–151.

chapter *three*

Male Sexual Anatomy *and* Physiology

Student Learning Objectives

After reading this chapter, students will be able to

- Identify and locate key structures of the male sexual anatomy.

- Describe the main functions of the male sexual structures.

- Identify and describe the functions of the key male sex glands.

- Explain the erogenous potential of the key male sexual structures.

- Perform a testicular self-exam.

- Identify the signs and symptoms of, and treatment for, eight common male sexual disorders.

- Describe a variety of screening tests used to diagnose common male sexual disorders.

- Describe a variety of disabilities and their effects on male sexuality.

Test your understanding of these objectives by taking the end-of-chapter quiz, available online at **http://health.wadsworth.com/blonna1.**

activity teaser: *How much do you know about male anatomy? Find out in the Personal Exploration Activity on page 81.*

Penis Size and Self-Esteem

Jordan, 19, gay, identifies as African American.

Jordan, a sophomore, attends a large urban northeastern university.

For the longest time I can remember being hung up on the size of my penis. I remember, as a kid, getting my mom's tape measure and measuring the length and circumference of my penis. I never talked to my friends about size because I was convinced mine was smaller than theirs.

My dad used to kid me about how small mine was when he'd see me in the shower. I'd get intimidated by his because it seemed so big. I probably should have talked to him about it, but I couldn't. He wasn't so approachable, and, like I said, he always seemed to be making fun of mine. Maybe this was his way of trying to break the ice and get a conversation going. I don't know. I doubt it.

Anyway, I guess I just kind of felt that mine was small, and if I tried to bring it up with my friends, they'd laugh at me or, worse yet, I'd find out that theirs were really bigger than mine. I sent away for this stuff from the back of a magazine that was "guaranteed" to make your penis grow. The only thing it did was make my penis burn. It must have been some kind of liniment or something. I decided from that point on that I'd have to be satisfied with what I have. My current lover thinks my penis is big enough to satisfy him and that has really put me at ease.

Critical Thinking

How far would you go to change a feature of your body that you currently are dissatisfied with?

Use your Virtual Workbook to explore your answer to this question at **http://health.wadsworth.com/blonna1.**

One of the more interesting things about healthy sexuality is the great diversity we are capable of bringing to our sexual response. Whether we are straight or gay, male or female, our bodies are capable of responding in a myriad of pleasurable ways if we take the time to understand them and explore their potential. After our discussion of female anatomy in Chapter 2, we will now focus on male anatomy and physiology as an additional step in understanding our bodies.

Much of male sexual anatomy is external. Most men touch their genitals frequently during urination, and because of this, men tend to be familiar with the external parts. Even though men tend to be comfortable with their external sexual anatomy and physiology, sexual health extends to understanding the proper functioning of the internal structures also.

Many of the internal and external sexual structures of both men and women are capable of responding sexually. Proper stimulation can provide intense sexual pleasure. We vary tremendously in how we like to stimulate (and have our partners stimulate) these structures. We will discuss this further at various points in this and other chapters.

External Male Sexual Structures

The external structures of the male sexual anatomy (see Figure 3.1) include the penis and scrotum, as well as the perineum, anus, and breasts. The last three, although not traditionally considered parts of sexual anatomy, are included here because of their potential as **erogenous** structures.

Erogenous Capable of producing sexual excitement

Penis

Like many structures in the human body, the penis has more than one function. Both sperm and urine pass through the penis on their way out of a man's body. The same organ used to pass liquid waste is capable of providing exquisite sexual pleasure. This duality of function is often cited as a reason for feeling squeamish about engaging in **fellatio.**

Fellatio Oral stimulation of the penis

Structure of the Penis The penis (Figure 3.2) consists of two main parts: the shaft and the glans. The shaft of the penis consists of two cylinders of spongy tissue—the larger cavernous body (*corpora cavernosa*) and one smaller spongy body (*corpus spongiosum*)—wrapped in thick membrane sheaths. Similar to a common household sponge, this cylindrical tissue has many pockets of open space or cavities that are richly endowed with blood vessels, allowing them to fill with blood during sexual arousal. This is how a penis becomes erect during sexual arousal.

A key to understanding this is to visualize how a sponge expands as its cavities fill with water. Contrary to popular belief, the penis has no bone or cartilage and very little muscle tissue. Slang terms such as *boner* and *hard-on* derive their origin from the firm, protruding nature of the spongiosum during erection. The spongy cylinders are held together by **connective tissue** attached to a loose wrapping of skin. The penis is capable of great expansion and changes in size because of its spongy tissue and loose covering of skin.

The corpora cavernosa run side by side along the entire length of the penis, attaching to the abdominal cavity by their roots, the *crura*. The cavernous body lies above the corpus spongiosum and wraps around it, appearing to create two cylinder-like structures on either side. The corpus spongiosum also runs the entire length of the shaft, forming the head or **glans penis.** When the penis is erect, the corpus spongiosum is what gets hard and protrudes, forming a pronounced ridge along the underside of the penis. The **urethra** runs through the corpus spongiosum.

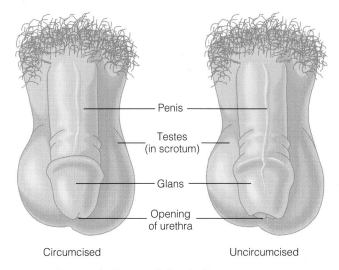

Figure 3.1 *Male External Genitalia* The male external genitalia includes the penis, scrotum, and perineum.

Connective tissue Tissue that supports or binds other tissue

Glans penis The end of corpus spongiosum, which is composed of the head of the penis and the urethral opening

Urethra The tube that transports urine and ejaculate through penis

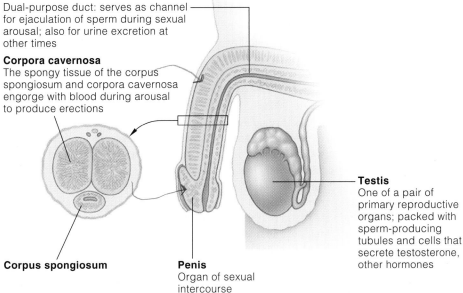

Urethra
Dual-purpose duct: serves as channel for ejaculation of sperm during sexual arousal; also for urine excretion at other times

Corpora cavernosa
The spongy tissue of the corpus spongiosum and corpora cavernosa engorge with blood during arousal to produce erections

Corpus spongiosum

Penis
Organ of sexual intercourse

Testis
One of a pair of primary reproductive organs; packed with sperm-producing tubules and cells that secrete testosterone, other hormones

Figure 3.2 *The Structure of the Penis* The penis consists of three cylinders of spongy tissue wrapped in a muscular sheath.

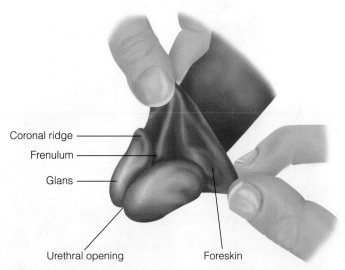

Coronal ridge

Frenulum

Glans

Urethral opening

Foreskin

Figure 3.3 *Glans and Foreskin* The frenulum, located on the underside of the glans, is the most sensitive part of the penis.

The entire penis is responsive to touch. The amount and type of touch that men like vary from man to man and sexual encounter to encounter. Even though the entire penis is responsive to touch, the greatest concentration of nerves is on the glans penis, illustrated in Figure 3.3. Two regions of the glans in particular—the coronal ridge and the frenulum—are the most richly endowed with nerve endings and capable of providing the greatest pleasure.

The *coronal ridge* forms the mushroom-like cap of the penis, separating it from the shaft. The *frenulum* is the triangular patch of tissue on the underside of the penis where the ridge pinches in to give the glans its distinctive shape. Both the corona and the frenulum are involved during arousal but are stimulated more precisely through oral sex and manual stimulation. The latter two forms of stimulation allow more individual control over the type and amount of pressure and stimulation than through intercourse.

The loose layer of skin that covers the shaft of the penis attaches at one end to the base of the penis near the abdomen and at the other end just behind the coronal ridge of the glans. The skin continues forward, extending beyond the glans penis, forming the prepuce or *foreskin*. In the unaroused state, the foreskin extends over the glans, covering and protecting it. During arousal, as the penis grows and expands, the foreskin retracts and stretches backward, exposing the glans for sexual activity.

Social and Spiritual Wellness

The issue of circumcision clearly illustrates how the social and spiritual dimensions of wellness impact men's sexual health. Our parents or caregivers, the core of our social network when we are infants, are our initial resource and primary sex educators. They make the initial decisions regarding our sexual health and provide us with guidance in developing healthy lifestyles that optimize sexual functioning. Parents are charged with the responsibility of making decisions about issues like circumcision. After the decision is made, they are responsible for teaching their sons about the proper hygiene and care of their circumcised penises.

Our parents are influenced by their social milieu. They are products of a culture (and subculture), and their decisions regarding our health are influenced by this. Their social well-being is also affected by their socioeconomic status and religious/spiritual beliefs. Spirituality and religiosity influence sexual health and anatomy and physiology. Circumcision often is part of a religious tradition. Most circumcisions are performed for religious and cultural beliefs and not because of purely intellectual decisions.

As men age, their parents' influence is supplanted by that of friends, peers, teachers, coaches, and intimate partners. These people in their social environment often give advice, share information, and in a direct or indirect way help put sexual health issues into a broader perspective. For instance, an uncircumcised boy may begin to have doubts about his penis if most of his peers are circumcised. This might make him uncomfortable in social settings such as a locker room. Later in his sexual development, the preferences of his intimate sex partner(s) may impact his happiness at being circumcised or uncircumcised.

case study 3.2

A Tough Decision

Jeno, 54, Jaana, 52, married to each other, both identify as Polish American.

Jeno and Jaana emigrated to the United States in 1973 and attended medical school together. They chose not to circumcise their son Jon (age 20) when he was born, but he has since been circumcised.

JAANA: Jon was born in a hospital birthing center within a major metropolitan hospital where Jeno and I had done our residency. After reading the literature on circumcision, doing rotations through labor and delivery, and discussing it with the other residents, we decided against having the procedure done.

JENO: I was raised a Roman Catholic, and Jaana and I are very religious, but our religious beliefs really had nothing to do with our decision. Being born in Poland and living in several Eastern and Western European countries growing up [his father was a diplomat], most of my friends were uncircumcised. I was concerned about my son's experiences in America where circumcision was the norm. Many of the things I had read in the 1970s and 1980s projected that the rate of circumcision would drop dramatically in the coming decades. We figured that by the time our son was in school most of his friends would be uncircumcised.

JAANA: Unfortunately, it didn't work out that way. In fact, it was just the opposite. Jon was usually the only boy in his class who was uncircumcised. None of his friends were uncircumcised, and he felt very self-conscious about it. He started to develop anxiety about going to gym class and participating in sports that required him to shower and change among his peers.

JENO: After much soul searching, Jaana and I decided to have Jon circumcised at age 12. We didn't want him to go through puberty and then have the procedure done. Fortunately, everything went smoothly, and his recovery was uneventful.

I thought that not having him go through the procedure at birth would save him from unnecessary surgery, but as it turned out, he had the procedure done anyway. He is glad he had it done and says he understands why we decided what we did.

Critical Thinking

How would your culture, social relationships, and spirituality influence your sexual health decision making regarding having your son circumcised?

Use your Virtual Workbook to explore your answer to this question at **http:// health.wadsworth.com/ blonna1.**

Circumcision In most cultures and parts of the world, the foreskin is viewed as a normal part of male sexual anatomy, is left intact, and receives little attention. In the United States, the foreskin is usually removed during the first few days following birth through the surgical procedure called **circumcision.** The two most common methods of circumcision are the clamp and the plastibell. Two types of clamps, the Gomco and Mogen, are used with the clamp procedure (Peleg & Steiner, 1998). The carbon dioxide laser circumcision has also been available for use since the 1980s. Because this method results in minimal blood loss, it is the preferred method when the patient has a blood-clotting disorder such as hemophilia (How, Ong, Jacobsen, & Joseph, 2003). Surgical outcomes associated with laser circumcision are comparable to the traditional methods (How et al., 2003). Removal of the foreskin leaves the glans penis exposed.

Most circumcisions done today are for religious, cultural, or aesthetic reasons. Circumcision is an important, required ritual in Judaic and Islamic religious practice. Prior to 1971, the American Academy of Pediatrics (AAP), the nation's foremost pediatric professional organization, had recommended circumcision of

Circumcision Surgical removal of foreskin of penis

newborn males for health concerns associated with smegma and its supposed links to cervical cancer in women and penile cancer in men. *Smegma* is a mixture of oily secretions from sebaceous glands on the skin of the penis, dead epithelial cells, dirt, bacteria, and sweat. Smegma buildup is prevented through simple washing with soap and water and pulling the foreskin back to cleanse this area of the penis. It can be compared to other routine procedures such as washing behind the ears regularly.

Beginning with the 1971 edition of its procedures manual and reiterated in subsequent revisions in 1975 and 1983, the American Academy of Pediatrics Task Force on Neonatal Circumcision found no absolute indication for routine circumcision. In 1999, the task force reexamined the issue in light of new research on circumcision status and urinary tract infections and sexually transmitted diseases. It concluded at the time that newborn male circumcision had potential medical benefits and advantages as well as disadvantages and risks.

The most recent report and recommendations of the American Medical Association (AMA) support those of the AAP Task Force on Neonatal Circumcision released on March 1, 1999. The Council on Scientific Affairs of the AMA reports that although circumcision decreases the incidence of urinary tract infection in the first year of life, the low incidence of this condition minimizes its potential benefits compared to the risks inherent in circumcision (AMA, 2003). This reinforces the Academy of Pediatrics' position, based on 2 years of study of the most recent data available concerning neonatal male circumcision. The AAP (1999) report states that existing scientific evidence demonstrates potential medical benefits of routine newborn male circumcision; however, these data are not sufficient to recommend routine neonatal circumcision. Parents should determine what is in the best interests of their child.

There is an association between circumcision and HIV risk. Studies have shown that uncircumcised men have a two- to eightfold increased risk of HIV infection compared to circumcised men (*AIDS Weekly* Staff, 2002). The increased

healthy sex hints 3.1

Deciding on Circumcision

Parents of newborn males must decide whether to have the infant circumcised. Recommendations about circumcision vary from state to state and medical facility to facility. In 1971, the American Academy of Pediatrics (AAP) removed its recommendation that male babies be routinely circumcised. The AAP now finds circumcision to be unnecessary to safeguard the health of newborn males except under special health circumstances. Although the number and percentage of circumcisions have decreased since the AAP dropped its recommendation, most parents still opt for this procedure. The following facts are intended to help you make an informed choice about circumcision for your child.

1. Circumcision is not required as a routine procedure.
2. The AAP no longer recommends circumcision as a routine procedure.
3. As with any surgical procedure, circumcision involves a small risk for the newborn.
4. Research indicates that uncircumcised boys have a slightly higher rate than circumcised boys of urethral infection.
5. Many fathers prefer that their son's penis look like theirs.
6. No evidence is available that uncircumcised sons of circumcised fathers suffer any psychological distress over this difference.
7. If you opt to have the procedure done, you have the right to indicate who will perform your son's circumcision.

Based on this information, if you had a newborn son, would you have him circumcised?

risk is attributed to the nature of the cells in the mucosal lining of the foreskin. When exposed to HIV in laboratory settings, this tissue was infiltrated at a much greater intensity than other tissue. The increased sensitivity of foreskin tissue to HIV is the suspected link to the increased risk. This link is currently being explored by Dr. Robert Bailey, from the University of Illinois, in a prospective study of 1,400 African American men (*AIDS Weekly* Staff, 2002).

Penis Size   The average penis is approximately 3 to 4 inches when flaccid (soft). In a recent study of penis size, when erect, the average length among subjects was found to be 6.02 inches, with a variation from 3.4 to 9.44 inches. Average penis girth (circumference) at erection was found to be 4.96 inches with a variation from 2.24 to 7.4 inches (Harding & Golombok, 2002). Most of the variation in penis size occurs during erection. **Erection** has been called "the great equalizer" because smaller penises seem to grow more during erection than larger ones, so the extremes tend to equalize when erect.

> **Erection** Filling of the penile spongy tissue with blood during vasocongestion, resulting in a hard, erect, penis

Obsession with penis size has a long history. Most young boys are curious about their penis size and use rulers and tape measures to actually measure their penises. They are concerned that their penises are smaller than their peers'. By late adolescence, most boys grow out of their fears and obsessions about the size of their penises.

Much of the adult male concern about penis size stems from the perception promoted through inaccurate media coverage suggesting that size equates to virility and sexual performance. Penis size is a central theme in both straight and gay erotica and pornography. Male pornographic actors are recruited as much for the size of their penises as their ability to act.

Researchers Masters, Johnson, and Kolodny (1996) found that penis size had little physiological effect on women's sexual response. The vagina, they point out, is capable of adjusting to penises of varying sizes from small to large. The inner depth of the vagina can be reached by a man with an average-size penis by using intercourse positions (such as rear entry) that facilitate deeper penetration. An unusually long penis can extend beyond the depth of the vagina. A slightly shortened vagina also can be the byproduct of a hysterectomy. Partners can accommodate for any discomfort by adjusting intercourse positions and avoiding those that facilitate deeper penetration.

The inner depths of the vagina, the area stimulated by the probing of a larger penis, is relatively devoid of nerve endings. Most of the nerve endings in the vagina are located in the outer third, thereby accessible to all sizes of penises. The most sensitive area for sexual stimulation is actually the clitoris, not the vagina. Female arousal is related to adequate clitoral stimulation; clitoral stimulation is not contingent on penis size (or even the presence of a penis) at all.

The relationship of penis size to anal sexual intercourse is similar to that of vaginal sex. The length of the rectum and bowel is longer than the vagina, allowing for either deeper penetration or a longer penis. Unlike the vagina, the rectum does not produce lubrication. Men and women who engage in anal intercourse should use water-based lubricant to facilitate ease of penetration and thrusting. In Chapter 7 (sexual behavior), we offer a full range of health hints associated with anal sexual activity.

Although penis size has little physiological relationship to sexual response, it can play a big part in one's psychological functioning. Men, whether straight, gay, or bisexual, who are overly concerned with or anxious about the size of their penis seem to be more likely to develop sexual disorders than men who don't share this concern (Masters et al., 1996). Men who are overly concerned about their penis size can become anxious about sexual relations and develop sexual arousal disorders and even inhibited sexual desire.

sex in society 3.1

Penis Size Throughout History

People have been preoccupied with penises and penis size throughout time. Penis artifacts, ranging from pottery to temple decorations to statues with grinning characters possessing huge penises, have been recovered across the globe. Nearly 2,000 years ago, the Romans worshipped Priapus, the god of fertility. Priapus symbolized both passion and fertility. Although small in stature, Priapus had a huge penis. Every bride of the Roman aristocracy was supposed to lose her virginity by sacrificing it on the altar of Priapus.

In Greece, giant penises adorned the classic columns used to support its massive structures. In India, the temple of Kama Sutra is decorated with characters having oversized penises. The erotic pen-and-ink art of Japan has, as its focal point, couples lost in their passion, their elaborate silk robes parted, capturing their genitalia. The men all

Priapus was always portrayed with an unusually large penis.

possess oversized penises that they are thrusting into their enraptured lovers.

No wonder that men are convinced that the size of their penises determines their masculinity.

Scrotum

Scrotum A double-chambered pouch of tissue that hangs loosely from the base of the penis, containing the testicles

The **scrotum** is a sac or pouch with two chambers that house the testes. Each testicle is cradled in its own scrotal pouch, suspended by a *spermatic cord* and *cremaster muscle.* A midline, or *raphe,* divides the scrotum into left and right halves. The scrotum has a sparse covering of hair and is usually darker in pigmentation than skin elsewhere on the body.

The scrotum normally hangs loosely, away from the body. This provides an optimal temperature of about 93 degrees Fahrenheit for the testicles. In a sense, the scrotum acts like a thermostat, regulating temperature by pulling the testicles closer to the abdominal cavity in colder temperatures and letting them hang loosely and away from the body under warmer circumstances.

The scrotum is composed of a thin layer of muscle tissue called the *tunica dartos* covered by skin. The skin attaches to the body at the base of the penis. During sexual arousal, exposure to cold, or threat of physical harm, the tunica dartos contracts and works together with the cremaster muscle to pull the testicles closer to the abdominal cavity for warmth and protection. In doing this, the scrotal sac shrinks and becomes taut.

Like the penis, the scrotum is responsive sexually to various forms of stimulation and pressure. When stimulating the scrotum, care must be taken since each man varies in sensitivity to stimulation.

Perineum

Perineum The erogenous area of skin extending from the base of testicles to the anal opening

The **perineum** is an area between the thighs, bounded in the front by the pelvis joint (symphysis pubis) and in the rear by the coccyx (tail bone). The perineum can be divided into two triangles of muscle tissue, the first containing the base of the penis and the scrotum and the second containing the anal opening. The muscular tissue is covered by a layer of skin. Although not normally considered part of male sexual anatomy, the perineum plays a part in the male sexual response because the entire area is endowed with nerve endings and responsive to stimulation. Again, the nature and intensity of stimulation to this area vary from man to man and encounter to encounter.

Anus

The **anus,** or opening of the bowel, is another body part with multiple functions. Although the primary function of the anus is to eliminate solid waste from the body, it also serves as a part of male sexual anatomy.

The anal canal is about 11.5 inches long and is composed of two sets of sphincter muscles. The internal anal sphincter muscle is made up of smooth muscle tissue, and the external anal sphincter is composed of skeletal muscle. The anal sphincters act like the strings of a purse to open and close the anus. The anus is normally closed, except during defecation and sexual stimulation. Anal tissue is slightly elastic. The bowel or anus produces no natural lubrication.

The anus is richly endowed with nerve endings, can be stimulated manually or orally, and is enjoyed sexually by gay and straight men alike.

As a result of the AIDS epidemic, this behavior is being talked about more openly. Gay and straight couples have discovered that sex toys can be inserted into the anus to provide sexual pleasure that entails less risk than anal intercourse. We will discuss this in greater detail in Chapters 7 and 15.

Anus The opening of the bowel, through which fecal matter is eliminated from the body

Breasts

The breast is not usually discussed as a part of the male sexual anatomy. Although men's breasts are not typically thought of as erogenous, heterosexual women and gay men find the sight and feel of men's breasts to be sexually appealing. In addition, many men enjoy having their breasts stimulated manually or orally during sexual contact.

Structurally, men's breasts have the same components as women's: nipple, areola, fat, and glandular tissue. Men's breasts, however, have much less underlying fatty and glandular tissue than women's do, and men do not lactate. Men's breasts normally do not enlarge during puberty. A small percentage of men develop a condition known as *gynecomastia,* which will be discussed in greater detail later in the chapter.

Breast size and concerns about other external sexual anatomy and body shape in general are a source of stress for many men. A "manly" torso, with well-developed pectoral (chest) muscles, broad shoulders, and a tapered waist, is the ideal that the media and society present to us. Many men become obsessed with trying to achieve the perfect body and, toward that end, try everything from binging and purging to taking steroids. Separating good health from physical perfection is something we have to learn.

The standards for male perfection promoted by media images are often unattainable for the vast majority of men.

Competing with Mr. America

Noredeen, 45, a nontraditional student, identifies as Algerian American.

Noredeen has returned to college to complete his second degree, this one in accounting.

I remember being a kid and reading the ads in the back of comic books for muscle-building equipment. There was always this picture of some well-developed guy kicking sand in the face of a scrawny kid as this really foxy woman watched and laughed at the kid. The ad went on to describe how "you, too, can have a body like this and keep the bullies from kicking sand in your face."

I was that kid. I would die a thousand deaths every time I looked at it, because it rang so true for me. I did get picked on a lot by bullies, and I was small and scrawny. I was always embarrassed to take off my shirt and run around in a swimming suit. Needless to say, I didn't date much, and none of the sexy girls wanted to be around me.

I remember cutting out that picture and dreaming about saving enough money to send away for the muscle-building program that would transform me into the kind of man sexy women want. I really felt that if I could just have a body like that, I'd get respect and the girls would go crazy after me.

It was years before I realized that the muscles were nice, but it was the person inside of the muscles that really mattered. I eventually developed enough self-confidence to start asking girls out more often, and I found that there actually were girls in high school who liked me for who I was, not who I wasn't. Eventually I became more interested in sport and fitness and filled out a little. It didn't seem to matter as much as it did when I was 13. I guess I never had the desire to invest the time it takes to build a body like the guy in the comic book.

Critical Thinking

Does the end justify the means regarding Noredeen's quest for a more muscular physique? In other words, even though his motivation for engaging in exercise is not better health, are his actions acceptable to you?

Use your Virtual Workbook to explore your answers to these questions at **http://health.wadsworth.com/blonna1.**

Physical Wellness

Physical wellness affects men's sexual health from conception until death. A mother's physical health and lifestyle affect the normal development of her baby. Factors such as prenatal nutrition, drug and alcohol use, and weight management can influence fetal structural development. To ensure optimal physical well-being, boys must be taught about their bodies and understand issues such as proper hygiene and protection of their genitals during sports and other activities. To protect the genitals against injury from trauma, all male athletes participating in contact sports should use a plastic protective cup within their athletic supporters.

As boys approach puberty, they need to be aware of the changes that will take place in their bodies and their sexual anatomy and physiology. They need to understand issues such as nocturnal emissions and ejaculation, increasing sexual desire, hygiene, prevention of sexually transmitted disease and unintended pregnancy, and testicular self-exam. Fitness, proper nutrition, weight management, not smoking or abusing drugs and alcohol—all become increasingly important in sexual health as males age.

Often, physical and other disabilities impact on physical well-being. Rather than respond to all disabilities in a stereotypical way, we need to understand the extent of any limitations the disability imposes and strive to maximize all remaining functions.

Internal Male Sexual Structures

The internal male sexual structures are illustrated in Figure 3.4.

Testes

The **testes** are oval-shaped male **gonads** housed in the scrotum. During the third trimester of fetal development, the testes form inside the abdominal cavity and descend into the scrotum. The testes are held in place within the scrotal sac by the spermatic cord, which passes through the inguinal canal attaching to the wall of the abdomen and the cremaster muscle, which connects with the lower part of the internal oblique abdominal muscle (see Figure 3.5).

When one or both testicles have not descended by birth, the infant is diagnosed with **cryptorchidism.** In most cases the testicles will descend by the end of 5 years. If they do not descend by this time, surgical or hormonal treatment may be necessary to get them to fall into place. Undescended testicles are a risk factor for infertility, inguinal hernia, and testicular cancer.

The testes have two primary functions: sperm production and hormone production. Each oval-shaped (1.5 inches long by 1 inch in diameter) testis is divided into 300 to 400 cone-shaped lobules. Each lobule contains two to three tightly coiled *seminiferous tubules* and endocrine cells called *interstitial* or *Leydig cells*. **Spermatogenesis** occurs within the seminiferous tubules. The Leydig cells produce the male sex hormone testosterone. If laid end to end, the seminiferous tubules (each between 1 and 3 feet long) from both testicles combined would stretch almost 0.5 mile.

Testes Two almond-shaped male gonads responsible for sperm and hormone production

Gonads The primary endocrine glands in men (testes) and women (ovaries) that influence sexuality

Cryptorchidism Undescended testicle(s)

Spermatogenesis Sperm production

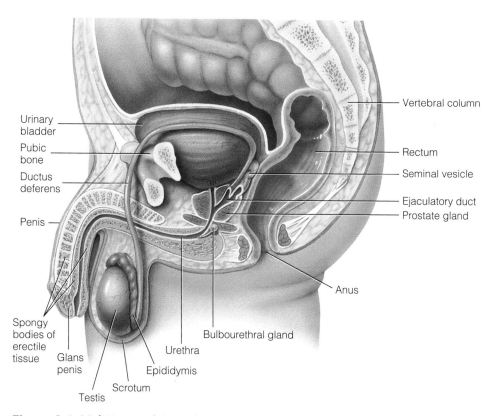

Figure 3.4 *Male Internal Sexual Structures* The male internal sexual structures have reproductive and sexual arousal functions that are similar to female internal structures.

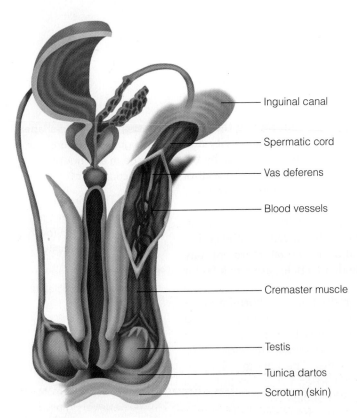

Sperm production begins at puberty and can continue until death, although the rate of production does diminish with aging. Some men fear "running out" of sperm. In fact, sperm are produced on an ongoing basis. Many things can interfere with sperm production, resulting in a low sperm count. Examples of the range of conditions that can lower sperm production as a result of damage to the testicles are injuries incurred during participation in sports and other circumstances, tight clothing, and exposure to toxic chemicals.

Testosterone, the main hormone associated with sexual desire, also is produced first during puberty, and its production ends with death. No evidence shows that sperm have anything to do with energy production and loss. Many men (including athletic coaches, trainers, and associated personnel) erroneously believe that depletion of sperm (through sexual activity) will weaken athletes and hamper their performance. Because of this, coaches sometimes sequester their teams before games or matches to prevent these athletes from having sex. We will discuss the influence of testosterone and other hormones on sexual response in greater detail in Chapter 7.

Figure 3.5 *Testes and Spermatic Cord* The testes are anchored to the abdominal wall by muscles in the spermatic cord.

- Inguinal canal
- Spermatic cord
- Vas deferens
- Blood vessels
- Cremaster muscle
- Testis
- Tunica dartos
- Scrotum (skin)

Testosterone The main male hormone associated with sexual desire

Epididymis A comma-shaped structure that sits along top of each testicle and serves as storage chamber for immature sperm

Vas deferens A tube extending from testicles to prostate gland, where it converts into urethra; responsible for transporting sperm and other ejaculatory fluid

Vasectomy A male contraceptive method resulting in sterilization by cutting the vas deferens

Epididymis

The **epididymis** is a *C*- or comma-shaped, coiled duct that sits on top of and extends along the back of each testis. Each of its heads merges the sperm-producing seminiferous tubules, and each tail connects with the vas deferens (*ductus deferens*). Within the coiled, 20-foot-long epididymis, immature sperm produced in the seminiferous tubules become motile and fertile. The journey of the sperm from head to tail takes about 20 days. During this time, the sperm receive nutrients and mature fully, and the inactive sperm undergo a quality control procedure. Defective and immature sperm are "weeded out" before they are able to be ejaculated. This process helps ensure that only healthy, viable sperm are available for potential fertilization of a ripe female ovum (egg).

Vas Deferens (Ductus Deferens)

The **vas deferens** are two long, thin ducts that originate in the base of the testis and extend up and around the bladder and into the prostate gland. There, they merge with the urethra. Each vas deferens is responsible for transporting mature sperm from the epididymis to the urethra. Each vas deferens joins the ejaculatory duct of the seminal vesicles just prior to entering the prostate gland.

The smooth muscle tissue of the vas deferens contracts during ejaculation, moving sperm as it does so. The sperm mix with secretions of the seminal vesicles, prostate gland, and Cowper's glands to form the milky-white fluid released through ejaculation. Each ejaculate contains about 1 teaspoon of fluid.

During a **vasectomy,** the vas deferens are located, a piece is cut out of each, and the end is tied or burned off. This prevents sperm from mixing in the ejaculate. We will discuss this method of male sterilization more fully in Chapter 14.

What Do You Know?

After drawing and labeling the male sexual anatomy, you will be able to identify what is accurate and inaccurate about your knowledge of the male anatomy.

Before completing this chapter on male anatomy, take a few minutes to see how much you know or don't know about the male sexual anatomy. Take a sheet of paper and draw from memory the internal and external male sexual anatomy. If possible, get a friend of the opposite sex to team up with you to do the drawing. This will be more fun and will show which sex has the most knowledge of the male anatomy. Once you have drawn the anatomy, label the following parts: penis, bladder, testicles, Cowper's glands, ureter, scrotum, urethra, vas deferens, seminal vesicles, epididymis, ampulla, corona, glans penis, and prostate gland.

When you have finished, compare your drawing to the one in this chapter. Are you surprised by how little or how much you know? How comfortable were you drawing this sexual anatomy? Ask one of your friends to do this activity. Does your friend's drawing indicate that he or she has good knowledge of the male anatomy? How comfortable was your friend drawing the sexual anatomy?

Seminal Vesicles

The **seminal vesicles** are two saclike glandular structures located behind the urinary bladder. Each gland is about 2 inches long and tapers into a short duct that joins with the vas deferens to form the ejaculatory duct. The seminal vesicles produce an alkaline fluid that is high in the sugar fructose. The alkalinity helps neutralize the acidity of the urethra, protecting sperm as they pass through it. The fructose provides energy the sperm need to reach their ultimate destination, a mature female egg, or ova. Seminal vesicle fluid contributes 60 to 70 percent of the total amount of fluid ejaculated.

Seminal vesicles Small structures connected to vas deferens, which release fluids that nourish and buffer sperm as they are ejaculated

Prostate Gland

The **prostate gland** is about the size and shape of a chestnut. The prostate produces several enzymes that play a role in activating sperm. These enzymes are released in a milky-white alkaline fluid that mixes with seminal vesicle fluid and sperm to make up about 30 percent of the total fluid ejaculated.

The prostate is located immediately in front of the rectum, enabling digital (by finger) examination to detect any changes in shape and size. A routine prostate examination is recommended for all men over 40 years of age as part of their preventive health checkups. Some men find stimulation of the prostate (through digital penetration or receptive anal intercourse) sexually arousing. Others find any contact with the prostate uncomfortable.

Prostate gland A chestnut-sized gland connected to neck of the bladder and vas deferens, which secretes alkaline fluid and enzymes that are part of ejaculatory fluid

Cowper's Glands

The **Cowper's glands,** also known as the *bulbourethral glands,* are ducts that secrete a thick, clear mucus during the plateau stage of sexual arousal, prior to ejaculation. This alkaline, preejaculatory fluid provides an additional buffer for sperm against the acidic environment of the urethra as the sperm make their way out of the body.

Advocates of birth control have long speculated that enough live sperm can be present in preejaculatory fluid to cause an unintended pregnancy. This has not been proven, however, in scientific studies of preejaculatory fluid. Two studies intended to determine the ability of preejaculatory fluid to transmit HIV found that the preejaculate was free of spermatozoa (Ilaria et al., 1992; Pudney, Oneta, Mayer,

Cowper's glands Bulbourethral glands, located below seminal vesicles, which produce preejaculatory fluid that lubricate vas deferens and urethra and protect sperm that are being ejaculated

Seage, & Anderson, 1992). Some sperm may remain in the urethra following ejaculation. The two variables that contribute to the presence or absence of live sperm within the urethra are *time* (sperm live 3 to 5 days) and *urination* (urination flushes the urethra and the acidity kills sperm). If live sperm are present in the urethra before a man urinates, they possibly could get mixed into the preejaculatory fluid secreted by the Cowper's glands and thus increase the risk of pregnancy.

Diseases and Disabilities Related to Male Sexual Anatomy

The most common disorders of the male sexual anatomy are benign prostatic enlargement, prostatitis, prostate cancer, urethritis, urethral strictures and trauma, phimosis and balanitis, hydrocele, Peyronie's disease, testicular cancer, gynecomastia, and male breast cancer.

Benign Prostatic Enlargement (BPH)

BPH is a noncancerous enlargement of the prostate gland. Because the prostate gland surrounds the urethra, any prostatic swelling, irritation, or infection can obstruct the flow of urine. Men with BPH usually have problems with urination, such as a weak, hesitant, or interrupted stream of urine or an urgency to urinate, more frequent urination (especially at night), and leaking or dripping. In extreme cases, urination is impossible.

Cystoscopy Direct visual examination of interior of urethra, urinary bladder, and kidneys by inserting a cystoscope (optical viewing tube) into the urethra

The risk for BPH increases with age. BPH occurs in about 10 percent of men by the age of 40, more than 50 percent of men by age 60, and close to 90 percent of men in their 70s and 80s (American Cancer Society [ACS], 2003a; Coley, Barry, Fleming, & Mulley, 1997). The cause of BPH is unknown. Diagnosis is usually made by a rectal exam or measurement of urine flow using a flow meter. In some cases **cystoscopy** is used to diagnose BPH. The urethra is anesthetized, and a cystoscope is inserted into the urethra. The instrument has a light and camera lens that allow the physician to observe the inside of the urethra and the bladder.

Treatment of BPH depends on the size of the enlargement and the extent of complications. Up to one-third of all cases clear up spontaneously. Drugs can be used to help shrink a mildly enlarged prostate gland. Balloon dilation—a new treatment similar to what is used to open clogged coronary arteries—stretches the urethra and facilitates the passage of urine, alleviating the condition until the prostate can shrink. If no spontaneous shrinkage occurs, surgery is performed to remove the enlarged part of the prostate pressing against the urethra.

Prostatitis

Prostatitis Inflammation and irritation of the prostate gland

Prostatitis is an inflammation of the prostate gland. The symptoms of prostatitis are lower back and pelvic pain, a sensation of heat and tenderness in the area, a thin discharge from the penis, and swelling in the genital area. The two types of prostatitis are infectious and congestive.

- *Infectious prostatitis* is caused by bacterial or viral infection. Treatment usually involves taking antibiotics.
- *Congestive prostatitis* is associated with failure to ejaculate prostatic fluid. Prostate secretions are produced in response to a man's sexual behavior patterns. Reducing the frequency of sexual activity disrupts the pattern of production and removal of prostatic fluid. If prostatic fluid is not ejaculated, it begins to decompose and build up, causing congestion. Congestive prostatitis usually responds to warm baths and prostate massage (ACS, 2003d).

Prostate Cancer

Prostate cancer has become the most common type of cancer among men, and it is the second leading cause of cancer deaths in males (lung cancer is number one) (ACS, 2003c, 2003e). In 2003, it was estimated that in that year approximately 220,900 men in the United States would develop prostate cancer, and approximately 28,900 would die from the disease (ACS, 2003c). The lifetime risk for clinical prostate cancer among men in the United States is approximately 10 percent; approximately 3 percent die of this disease. Prostate cancer mortality increased an average of 1 percent per year between 1973 and 1990. Since 1990, the prostate cancer death rate in the United States has fallen an average of 1.1 percent annually, the decrease totaling 6.7 percent from 1991 to 1995 (ACS, 2003d; Dennis & Resnick, 2000).

These changes in incidence are consistent with the introduction of a successful screening test that detects slower-growing tumors and with an effect of lead time bias due to the early detection of prostate cancer beginning in the late 1980s and early 1990s (Hankey, Feuer, Clegg, Fever, Midthune, & Fay, 1999). Prostate cancer is a very slow-growing cancer. The early warning signs of prostate cancer are frequent or difficult urination, blood in the urine, painful ejaculation, and lower back pain.

Risk Factors   Major risk factors are age, family history, race, and possibly dietary fat.

Age. The risk of acquiring prostate cancer increases after age 50, and greater than 70% of all prostate cancers are diagnosed in men over the age of 65. Prostate cancer is rare in men under 50 years of age (ACS, 2003d).

Race. Between 1995 and 1999, the rate of prostate cancer in African American men was 60 percent higher than that of white men. Much of this disparity is attributed to an increase in early diagnosis through stepped-up screening using the PSA blood test among African American men (ACS, 2003b). Despite this increase in early diagnosis, African American men are still more likely to be diagnosed at an advanced stage and are twice as likely to die of prostate cancer than white men (ACS, 2003d). Late-stage diagnosis of cancer is usually attributed to lack of access to health care and preventive health services.

Diet. Men who eat a lot of red meat and diary products have a lot of fat in their diet and appear to have a greater chance of developing prostate cancer. No one is sure which of these factors is responsible for increasing risk, but men with diets high in meat and dairy products tend also to consume less fruits and vegetables. Nutrients such as lycopenes (found in high levels in some fruits and vegetables, such as tomatoes, grapefruit, and watermelon), vitamin E, and the mineral selenium may lower prostate cancer risk (ACS, 2003d; Herbert, Hurley, Olendzki, Teas, Ma, & Hampl, 1998).

Family History. Having a father or brother with prostate cancer doubles a man's risk of developing this disease. The risk is even higher for men with several affected relatives, particularly if their relatives were young at the time of diagnosis. These data imply a genetically inherited risk for prostate cancer. Research has linked the BRCA1 or BRCA2 genes with breast, ovarian, and a small percentage of prostate cancers (ACS, 2003d).

Early Detection and Diagnosis of Prostate Cancer   The prostate gland, as previously described in this chapter, is a chestnut-sized gland located immediately in front of the rectum. Although several other cell types are found in the prostate, over 99 percent of prostate cancers develop from the glandular cells. Glandular cells make the seminal fluid that is secreted by the prostate. Because of its location, the prostate gland can be reached through digital examination.

Early detection is potentially important because the survival rate of patients diagnosed in early-stage disease is much higher than that of patients diagnosed with late-stage disease (Mettlin, Jones, & Murphy, 1993; ACS, 2003d). The main screening tests in use today for the early detection of prostate cancer are digital rectal examination (DRE), measurement of the serum concentration of prostate-specific antigen (PSA), and transrectal ultrasound (ACS, 2003d; Catalona, Richie, Ahmann, Angier, & Holman, 1994; Coley et al., 1997).

Digital Rectal Examination (DRE). DRE involves the insertion of a gloved, lubricated finger into the rectum and the palpation of the prostate gland (see Figure 3.6). DRE is used to identify any abnormalities, including nodules or changes in size and shape that may indicate the presence of cancer. The use of DRE as a screening tool for early detection is limited because it can't always pick up the presence of small tumors and those deep within the prostate gland (ACS, 2003d; Catalona et al., 1994).

Prostate-Specific Antigen (PSA). PSA is an antigen normally produced by the prostate gland. Healthy men have levels of PSA of 4 nanograms per milliliter of blood. Men with prostate cancer usually have PSA levels above 4 (ACS, 2003d; Catalona et al., 1994). If a man's level is above 4 but less than 10, he has about a 25 percent chance of having prostate cancer. If it goes above 10, his chance of having prostate cancer is over 67 percent and increases further as the PSA level rises (ACS, 2003d).

Many factors other than prostate cancer can influence PSA levels. It increases with enlargement of the prostate (called *benign prostatic hyperplasia,* or BPH), a common condition in older men. It can also increase with prostatitis. Because PSA elevations are not specific for prostate cancer, the PSA test has a high false-positive rate when used as a screening tool. On initial screening, 8 to 15 percent of men will have a PSA greater than 4 nanograms/milliliter, and only 1.5 to 4.1 per-

Figure 3.6 *Digital Rectal Examination* A digital rectal examination is a routine examination performed in a clinician's office.

cent will have a positive biopsy (ACS, 2003d; Mettlin, Murphy, Babaian, Natarajan, Nemeto, & Nemeto, 1997).

The combined use of DRE and PSA can yield higher results than either test alone. The PSA assay detects about one-third of diagnosed cancers in asymptomatic men that are missed by DRE, whereas DRE detects about 20 percent of those missed with PSA. In studies employing both DRE and PSA, about 25 percent of screened men require further assessment, but no more than 4 percent will be diagnosed with cancer (ACS, 2003d; Catalona et al., 1994).

Transrectal Ultrasound (TRUS). TRUS uses sound waves to make an image of the prostate on a video screen. When performing TRUS, the health care provider inserts a small probe into the rectum, and sound waves enter the prostate. This creates sound echoes that are picked up by the probe and turned into a picture on a computer monitor. TRUS is not recommended as an initial screening test because of its expense and intrusive nature, but it can be employed to confirm results detected by the PAS or DRE examinations (ACS, 2003d).

The Prostate Biopsy. After a man has a positive PSA, DRE, and/or positive TRUS screening test, a core needle biopsy is the main method used to diagnose prostate cancer. A *biopsy* is a procedure in which a sample of tissue is removed and then examined under a microscope. During a core needle biopsy, the physician inserts a narrow needle through the wall of the rectum into several areas of the prostate gland and removes cylinders of tissue about 1/2 inch long and 1/16 inch across. These samples are examined in the laboratory for cancerous changes. Anywhere from 6 to 13 samples are taken to get a representative sample of the gland that will show how much of the gland is affected by the cancer (ACS, 2003d).

Prostate Cancer Stages   Prostate cancer, like other forms of the disease, is reported by stage. Treatment options vary according to the stage of the disease.

Stage I: The cancer has not spread to lymph nodes or elsewhere in your body. Less than 5 percent of the tissue was cancerous.

Stage II: The cancer has not spread to the lymph nodes or elsewhere in any of these cases, and more than 5 percent of the tissue contained cancer.

Stage III: The cancer has begun to spread outside the prostate and may have spread to the seminal vesicles, but it has not spread to the lymph nodes or elsewhere in the body.

Stage IV: The cancer has spread to tissues next to the prostate (other than the seminal vesicles), such as the bladder's external sphincter (muscles that help control urination), the rectum, and/or the wall of the pelvis, and/or it has spread to the lymph nodes or to other, more distant sites in the body (ACS, 2003d).

Treatment   Prostate cancer treatment varies according to several factors:

- The man's age and expected life span
- The man's feelings about the side effects associated with each treatment
- Any other serious health conditions
- The stage and grade of the cancer
- The likelihood that each type of treatment will be curative

Treatment options include surgical removal of the prostate, radiation, radiation "seed" implantation, hormone therapy, chemotherapy, and cryotherapy. Each has its own pros and cons and needs to be evaluated in relation to the factors discussed earlier. Some of the treatments can result in urinary incontinence and impotence and therefore may be unacceptable (ACS, 2003e).

Urethritis

Urethritis Inflammation and irritation of urethra

Dysuria Burning upon urination

Discharge Draining of pus from the urethra

Urethritis is the inflammation and irritation of the urethra. The two most common symptoms of urethritis are **dysuria** and **discharge.** Urethritis can be caused by a variety of things, including mild injury, exposure to irritants, and infection. The urethra can incur mild injury from too vigorous masturbation or other sexual activity. The tissue is temporarily damaged and becomes sensitive to the passage of urine. The urethra also can become irritated from exposure to harsh soaps or other personal hygiene products. Mild injury and irritation usually resolve within a day or two without any special treatment.

Urethral infections can be sexually transmitted or nonsexually transmitted. (We cover sexually transmitted infections in great detail in Chapter 15.) Nonsexually transmitted urethritis is usually associated with poor personal hygiene and infection with micro-organisms. Daily washing or bathing of the genitals will remove most micro-organisms capable of causing urethritis. Uncircumcised men who do not practice normal daily hygiene have a slightly higher risk for infectious urethritis. Infectious urethritis is treated with antibiotics and responds rapidly to treatment.

Urethral Strictures

A *urethral stricture* is a scar anywhere along the urethra. The scar can be congenital (present at birth) or the result of an injury, untreated urethral infection, or multiple cases of urethritis (Swanson & Forrest, 1984). The scar can cause urinary hesitancy, decreased force and caliber of urine stream, postvoid dribbling, and excessive nighttime urination. Strictures are treated surgically either by dilating the urethra or surgically removing the stricture (Swanson & Forrest, 1984).

Urethral Trauma

Trauma to the urethra can cause damage to the urethral walls or, in extreme cases, severing of the urethra. In milder trauma, ice and rest can reduce swelling and prevent further trauma. In more severe trauma, a catheter is often inserted and left in place until surgical repair and antibiotic treatment is completed (Swanson & Forrest, 1984).

Phimosis and Balanitis

Phimosis A tight foreskin that cannot be retracted fully

Balanitis Inflammation of the glans penis

Phimosis is a condition of uncircumcised men who have a tight foreskin that is not fully retractable. **Balanitis** is an inflammation of the glans penis. By adolescence, more than 95 percent of all uncircumcised males have fully retractable

healthy sex hints 3.2
Preventing Urethral Trauma

Many cases of urethral trauma can be prevented by using risk-reducing protective devices. Protective plastic cups that fit securely in athletic supporters provide excellent protection against most sports-related trauma. Newer bicycle seats are designed with a protective groove or gap along the middle of the surface that comes in contact with the urethra.

Other ways to avoid trauma are to always read user manuals and understand safe ways to operate equipment and machinery that can cause blunt force to the lower body.

Do you routinely use these strategies?

foreskins. Although it was once thought that all newborn males had fully re-tractable foreskins, studies in the 1960s and 1970s showed that fewer than half of newborn males had fully retractable foreskins.

Newborns and young, uncircumcised boys often have some degree of tight-ness in their foreskins. A tight foreskin usually is not a problem in prepubescent boys. As long as the urethral opening and urine flow remain unobstructed, this condition has no negative health risks. Phimosis that occurs in a young man who has gone through the physiological changes and growth of puberty can be cor-rected with a variety of treatments ranging from topical steroids to surgery de-signed to loosen the foreskin and separate it from the glans.

Phimosis also can be caused by infection as a possible complication of urethri-tis. The discharge associated with urethritis can get trapped under the foreskin, causing balanitis and inflammation of the foreskin, which results in increased tightness and difficulty retracting the skin. Because both conditions are associated with the infectious urethritis, antibiotic treatment of this infection usually reduces swelling and alleviates balanitis and phimosis. In rare instances, emergency cir-cumcision is done to relieve the swelling and pain associated with infectious phi-mosis (AAP, 1999).

Hydrocele

A **hydrocele** is an accumulation of fluid in any saclike cavity or duct. Hydroceles are commonly found in the scrotum. Fluid accumulates in the *tunica vaginalis,* a small, closed sac that covers most of the testes. The condition is caused by an in-flammation of the testis or epididymis or obstruction in blood or lymphatic fluid within the spermatic cord.

Hydrocele Accumulation of fluid in any sac, cavity, or duct

A hydrocele can develop as a result of congenital malformation or from injury during any period in a man's life. Hydroceles usually require surgical repair. In some cases the sac may be aspirated and the fluid removed. This usually is con-sidered a temporary treatment because in most cases the sac will refill with fluid. A hydrocele is distinguished from the small, solid lump associated with testicular cancer; hydroceles are larger, fluid-filled sacs.

Peyronie's Disease

Peyronie's disease is similar to Dupuytren's contracture, a deformity of the hand in which there is a contracture of fingers toward the palm, often resulting in func-tional disability. Peyronie's disease is a condition in which collagen plaques form on the shaft of the penis and interfere with erection and sexual intercourse. The condition usually manifests itself through a curve in the penis. The curve can range from a slight bend to an angle severe enough to make intercourse impossi-ble. Treatment involves collagenase injections and/or surgery.

Emotional Wellness

Issues related to men's sexual health can provoke strong emotions. A diagnosis of testicular cancer, for instance, can conjur images ranging from death to disformity. High-level emotional well-being can make the difference between facing the chal-lenge of cancer and working with health care providers to ensure that everything possible is done, or turning your back to the problem and hoping it will go away by itself. High-level emotional wellness involves recognizing, accepting, and working with our emotions. It involves asking for help when needed and taking responsibil-ity for your feelings.

Testicular Cancer

Testicular cancer is a relatively rare form of cancer, representing less than 2 percent of all cancers). Although fairly uncommon, it is the leading cancer killer of men under 35 years of age. Most cases of testicular cancer affect men between the ages of 15 and 40 years (ACS, 2003c; Landis, Murray, Boldon, & Wingo, 1999).

Risk Factors   The major risk factor for testicular cancer is cryptorchidism (undescended testicle). About 14 percent of the cases of testicular cancer are attributed to cryptorchidism (ACS, 2003d). Most of these cases occur in the undescended, testicle but 25 percent occur in the normally descended testicle. Some experts believe that performing surgery to lower the testicle prior to the onset of puberty can reduce the risk of developing some tumors in the testicle (ACS, 2003d).

Family history can also increase risk. Research indicates that a history of testicular cancer in one brother can increase risk in other male siblings. Cancer in one testicle slightly increases the risk for cancer in the other testicle. Certain occupations (mining, oil and gas workers, food- and beverage-processing workers, janitors, and utility workers) have an increased risk for testicular cancer.

Lastly, the incidence of testicular cancer among white American men is five times that of African American men and double the risk of Asian American men (ACS, 2003d).

Symptoms   Ninety percent of all men with testicular cancer have a painless or uncomfortable lump in the testicle or testicular enlargement or swelling. The remaining 10 percent notice no specific problem in their testicles but often report a sensation of heaviness or aching in the lower abdomen or scrotum. In rare cases, men with certain testicular tumors notice breast tenderness or swelling caused by an overproduction and release of the hormone human chorionic gonadotropin (HCG).

healthy sex hints 3.3

Testicular Self-Exam

How do I do this examination?

Roll each testicle between your thumb and first three fingers until you have felt the entire surface (see illustration). The testicles should feel round and smooth, like hard-boiled eggs. These are the things to be on the lookout for:

Lumps
Irregularities
A change in the size of the testicle
Pain in the testicle
A dragging or heavy sensation

How often do I have to do this exam?

Do it at least once a month. It helps to pick a regular day of the month—the date of your birthday, the first of the month, the first Sunday, or some other day that's easy for you to remember. You can do the exam more often if you like.

Testicular self-exam should be performed monthly while in the shower.

Many conditions can mimic the signs and symptoms of testicular cancer. The most common are injury and orchitis, both of which often cause pain and swelling that can be mistaken for testicular cancer symptoms. These can easily be ruled out by a physician through examination and testing.

Testicular Cancer Stages   There are three stages of testicular cancer:

Stage 0: Preinvasive cancer of the testicular germ cells is present.
Stage 1: No cancer has spread to the lymph nodes or distant organs.
Stage 2: The cancer has spread to regional lymph nodes.
Stage 3: The cancer has spread to nonregional lymph nodes.

Early Detection   Testicular self-examination is recommended for the early detection of the condition because there are no acceptable blood or other screening tests available for testicular cancer. The American Cancer Society (2003d) does not believe that, for men with average testicular cancer risk, any medical evidence suggests that monthly examination is any more effective than simple awareness and prompt medical evaluation. The authors, however, believe that performing monthly testicular examinations is a relatively noninvasive, easy-to-perform procedure that can be combined with awareness and prompt medical evaluation, regardless of one's personal risk. (See Healthy Sex Hints 3.3 for instructions regarding how to perform this procedure.)

Diagnosis and Treatment   Most cases of testicular cancer are diagnosed through a combination of medical history (to rule out injury, preexistent medical conditions, and so forth), blood tests (to look for proteins and enzymes associated with the disease), ultrasound (to rule out fluid buildup and other conditions), and biopsy (to detect the presence of cancer growth) (Schmidt, Mettlin, Natarajan, Mench, McGinnis, & Piver, 1986; ACS, 2003d).

Treatment of early-stage testicular cancer typically consists of removing the cancerous tumor and administering chemotherapy. The chemotherapy is usually a prophylactic treatment to reduce the likelihood that the cancer has spread beyond the local lymph nodes. More rigorous combinations of surgery, chemotherapy, and radiation treatment might be indicated for later-stage testicular cancer.

The long-term survival rates for early-stage testicular cancer treatment are excellent. Most men treated for testicular cancer have no loss of fertility, sexual desire, or sexual response (ACS, 2003e).

Gynecomastia

Gynecomastia, the abnormal swelling or enlargement of one or both of a man's breasts, is usually temporary and benign. If it occurs around the time of puberty, it usually is the result of a temporary hormonal imbalance. If it occurs later in life, it may be attributable to a tumor of the testis or pituitary, taking medications that contain estrogen or other steroids, or liver failure associated with cirrhosis or other causes. In cases where gynecomastia does not resolve spontaneously, corrective surgery may be necessary, especially if it is contributing to psychological stress and illness.

Gynecomastia Enlargement of one or both breasts in men

Male Breast Cancer

Breast cancer is primarily a disease occurring in women; however, men can have it, too. Male breast cancer accounts for less than 1 percent of the overall incidence and mortality of breast cancer. Even though men are at low risk of developing breast cancer, they should be aware of risk factors, especially family history, and report any changes in their breasts to a physician. Early detection improves the chances for successful treatment.

Your responses to the Personal Assessment, Thought Questions, and Test Yourself! quiz questions can be logged online in your Virtual Workbook at **http://health.wadsworth.com/blonna1.**

Personal Assessment

3.1 Body Image: Males

Body image refers to our evaluation and perception of our body, specific body parts, and their functioning. It includes the messages (positive and negative) that we tell ourselves about our bodies, our self-esteem, and our behaviors and choices as a result. The following inventory will help males assess their body image.

Rate each body part listed below using the following scale: extremely satisfied = 5; satisfied = 4; neutral = 3; dissatisfied = 2; extremely dissatisfied = 1.

1. eyes _____	2. ears _____	3. nose _____
4. hair _____	5. teeth _____	6. mouth _____
7. weight _____	8. face _____	9. shoulders _____
10. chest _____	11. arms _____	12. calves _____
13. hands _____	14. height _____	15. stomach _____
16. buttocks _____	17. hips _____	18. thighs _____
19. feet _____	20. sex organs _____	21. overall body _____

Scoring:

105–80	Very positive body image	20–40	Negative body image
60–80	Positive body image	0–20	Very negative body image
40–60	Ambivalent about your body		

Rate each item below, using the following scale: very comfortable = 5; comfortable = 4; neutral = 3; uncomfortable = 2; very uncomfortable = 1.

_____ 22. looking at my nude body in the mirror

_____ 23. performing self-examinations of my nude body

_____ 24. being nude when I am alone

_____ 25. being nude when I am with my lover

_____ 26. being nude when I am around my kids

_____ 27. sunbathing in the nude

_____ 28. swimming in the nude

_____ 29. walking around the house nude

Scoring:

32–40	Very comfortable with nudity	12–16	Uncomfortable with nudity
21–32	Comfortable with nudity	0–12	Very uncomfortable with nudity
16–21	Ambivalent about nudity		

Complete the following sentences:

30. The thing I like best about my body is _____

31. The thing I dislike most about my body is _____

Thought Questions

1. Describe the nature of penile erectile tissue. How does it facilitate erection?

2. Discuss the pros and cons of circumcision.

3. What are the major functions of the scrotum?

4. What two major processes occur within the testicles? Where do they occur in the testicles?

5. Describe the route of the ejaculate from the testes to expulsion from the end of the penis.

6. What is the role of testosterone in male sexuality?

7. Describe how you can reduce your risks for all of the sexual disorders discussed in the chapter.

Test Yourself!

1. The shaft of the penis consists of two cylinders of _____ tissue.
   a. spongy
   b. mucous
   c. muscle
   d. connective

2. Erection of the penis is caused by
   a. bony tissue within the penis.
   b. cartilage that moves into place during sexual arousal.
   c. engorgement of spongy tissue.
   d. muscle tension in the penis.

3. The most recent recommendations regarding circumcision of newborn males is
   a. circumcision should be performed on all males for health reasons.
   b. circumcision is not recommended under any circumstances.
   c. circumcision should only be performed to save the life of the child.
   d. circumcision is considered elective surgery.

4. Which of the following is *not* a part of male sexual anatomy?
   a. Seminal vesicles
   b. Cervix
   c. Urethra
   d. Prostate gland

5. The two primary functions of the testes are
   a. hormone and sperm production.
   b. sperm and egg production.
   c. hormone and lubricant production.
   d. sperm and pheromone production.

6. The vas deferens and urethra
   a. meet at the cervix.
   b. merge at the prostate gland.
   c. are shared by male and female sexual anatomy.
   d. contain miles of tiny passageways.

7. Which of the following best describes the significance of prostate cancer?
   a. It is relatively uncommon in men.
   b. It is the number one cause of death in men.
   c. It is the second leading cause of cancer death in men.
   d. It is the most common cause of cancer in men but is rarely fatal.

8. Which of the following best describes the significance of testicular cancer?
   a. It accounts for about 2 percent of cancers in men.
   b. It is the number one type of cancer in men.
   c. It is the second leading cause of cancer death in men.
   d. It is the leading cause of cancer in men but is rarely fatal.

9. The American Cancer Society recommends that a digital rectal exam (DRE) be performed
   a. annually for men over 40.
   b. every 5 years for men over 50.
   c. only when symptoms are present.
   d. every 5 years for men over 21.

10. Testicular self-exam (TSE) should be performed
    a. every year by a qualified physician.
    b. monthly by all men.
    c. every 5 years after the age or 50.
    d. annually for men over 40.

Media Menu

You can link to the following online tools by visiting
http://health.wadsworth.com/blonna1.

Animation

Male Reproductive System
Male Reproductive Function
Ejaculation Pathway

InfoTrac Activity

Sutter, P. (2001, June 11). Mirror, mirror why am I bald? Did I have the strength to go where no razor had gone before? *Maclean's,* pp. 10–12.

Web Resources

Male Health Center

www.malehealthcenter.com

The first center in the United States specializing in male health. The center takes a holistic approach to health and covers impotence, prostate disorders, sexually transmitted diseases, vasectomy, cancer screening, and wellness.

Men's Health Network

www.menshealthnetwork.org

An information and educational organization that recognizes men's health as a specific societal concern and is committed to promoting issues affecting men's health. See "Library" and "Men's Links" for 54 pages of links to magazines and journals, books, organizations, miscellaneous resources, and men's health resources.

Men's Web Health Page

www.menweb.org/mensheal.htm

This is the health page for Men's Web, an organization that provides information and services on a variety of men's topics. The health page features information and links on a host of topics covered in this chapter.

American Cancer Society

www.cancer.org

The home page for the definitive source of information about cancer for men.

American Medical Association's Patient Education Page

www.ama-assn.org/ama/pub/category/3158.html

This is the home page for the AMA's patient education section. In it you will find information on a variety of health issues. The following address is a link to their report on circumcision: www.ama-assn.org/ama/pub/article/2036-2382.html.

Discovery Health Channel Prostate Cancer Assessment

http://health.discovery.com/tools/hra/prostate/prostate_pg1.html

This link is a questionnaire, provided by the online Discovery Channel, to help give you an idea about your individual risk for prostate cancer based on proven medical and scientific evidence. It will provide you with an overall summary of your risk factors and how they compare to those for the general population. It is an approximation of your risk; the results should not be interpreted as an absolute risk value. Rather, you should use your individualized results to assess those factors that you can modify to minimize your risk of developing prostate cancer.

References

AIDS Weekly Staff. (2002, September 30). *AIDS Weekly,* pp. 4–6.

American Academy of Pediatrics. (1999, March). Task Force on Circumcision report. *Pediatrics, 103* (3), 686–693.

American Cancer Society. (2003a). Can prostate cancer be found early? [Online]. Available: www.cancer.org/docroot/CRI/content/CRI_2_4_3X_Can_prostate_cancer_be_found_early_36.asp.

American Cancer Society. (2003b). Cancer facts and figures for African Americans 2003 [Online]. Available: www.cancer.org/downloads/STT/861403.pdf.

American Cancer Society. (2003c). Cancer facts and figures 2003 [Online]. Available: www.cancer.org/downloads/STT/CAFF2003PWSecured.pdf.

American Cancer Society. (2003d). Cancer prevention and early detection: Facts and figures 2003 [Online]. Available: www.cancer.org/downloads/STT/CPED2003PWSecured.pdf.

American Cancer Society. (2003e). Making treatment decisions [Online]. Available: www.cancer.org/docroot/ETO/ETO_1.asp.

American Medical Association. (2003). *Neonatal circumcision* [Online]. Council on Scientific Affairs Report #10. Available: www.ama-assn.org/ama/pub/article/2036-2382.html.

Catalona, W. J., Richie, J. P., Ahmann, F. R., Angier, N., & Holman, J. R. (1994). Comparison of digital rectal examination and serum prostate specific antigen in the early detection of prostate cancer: Results of a multicenter clinical trial of 6,630 men. *Journal of Urology, 151,* 1283–1290.

Coley, C. M., Barry, M. J., Fleming, C., & Mulley, A. G. (1997). Early detection of prostate cancer. I. Prior probability and effectiveness of tests. *Annuals of Internal Medicine, 126,* 394–406.

Dennis, L. K., & Resnick, M. I. (2000). Analysis of recent trends in prostate cancer incidence and mortality. *Prostate, 42,* 247–252.

Hankey, B. F., Feuer, E. J., Clegg, L. X., Fever, E. J., Midthune, D. N., & Fay, M. P. 1999). Cancer surveillance series: Interpreting trends in prostate cancer—part I: Evidence of the effects of screening in recent prostate cancer incidence, mortality, and survival rates. *Journal of the National Cancer Institute, 91,* 1017–1024.

Harding, R., & Golombok, S. E. (2002, August). Test–retest reliability of penile dimensions in a sample of men. *Archives of Sexual Behavior, 31* (4), 351–358.

Herbert, J. R., Hurley, T. G., Olendzki, B. C., Teas, J., Ma, Y., & Hampl, J. S. (1998). Nutritional and socioeconomic factors in relation to prostate cancer mortality: A cross-national study. *Journal of the National Cancer Institute, 90* (21), 1631–1647.

How, A. C. S. W., Ong, C. C. P., Jacobsen, A., & Joseph, V. T. (2003). Carbon dioxide laser circumcisions for children [Online]. Available: http://link.springer-nv.com/link/service/journals/00383/contents/02/00894/s00894/s00383-002-089.

Ilaria, G., Jacobs, J. L., Plosky, B., Koll, B., MacLow, C., Armstrong, D., & Schlegal, P. N. (1992). Detection of HIV-1DNA sequences in pre-ejaculatory fluid. *Lancet, 340* (8833), 1469.

Landis, S. H., Murray, T., Boldon, S., & Wingo, P. A. (1999). Cancer statistics, 1999. *CA: A Cancer Journal for Clinicians, 49,* 8–31.

Masters, M. H., Johnson, V. E., & Kolodny, R. (1996). *Human sexuality* (6th ed.). New York: HarperCollins.

Mettlin, C., Jones, G. W., & Murphy, G. P. (1993). Trends in prostate cancer care in the United States, 1974–1990: Observations from the patients care evaluation studies of the American College of Surgeons Commission on Cancer. *CA: A Cancer Journal for Clinicians, 43,* 83–91.

Mettlin, C. J., Murphy, G. P., Babaian, R. J., Natarajan, N., Nemeto, D., & Nemeto, L. (1997). Observations on the early detection of prostate cancer from the American Cancer Society National Prostate Cancer Detection Project. *Cancer, 80,* 1814–1817.

Peleg, D., & Steiner, A. (1998, September 15). The Gomco circumcision: Common problems and solutions. *American Family Physician, 58* (4), 891–899.

Pudney, J., Oneta, M., Mayer, K., Seage, G., & Anderson, D. (1992). Pre-ejaculatory fluid as a potential vector for the transmission of HIV-1. *Lancet, 340* (8833), 1470.

Schmidt, J. D., Mettlin, C. J., Natarajan, N., Mench, H. R., McGinnis, L. S., & Piver, S. (1986). Trends in patterns of care for prostate cancer, 1974–1983: Results of surveys by the American College of Surgeons. *Journal of Urology, 136,* 416–421.

Swanson, J. M., & Forrest, K. A. (1984). *Men's reproductive health.* New York: Springer.

chapter *four*
Sexual Identity

Student Learning Objectives

After reading this chapter, students will be able to

- Identify the components of sexual identity and appreciate its complexity.
- Describe the components of gender development.
- Evaluate the impact of biological, psychological, sociological, and cultural factors on gender development.
- Evaluate the impact of biological, psychological, sociological, and cultural factors on sexual orientation.
- Analyze the similarities and differences in the development of a variety of sexual orientations.
- Understand the challenges of "coming out."
- Discuss the more common forms of gender incongruities.

Test your understanding of these objectives by taking the end-of-chapter quiz, available online at **http://health.wadsworth.com/blonna1.**

activity teaser: *What would it be like to change sexes for a day? See the Personal Exploration Activity on page 109.*

case study 4.1

Emily

Emily, 23, is white.

In these past 6 years, I haven't hooked up with a man, but I still feel uneasy about identifying as either lesbian or bisexual. "Lesbian" speaks to the fact that I date women, but naming myself as a lesbian does not mean that I am closed off to the potential of being with a man. "Bisexual," although allowing for fluidity, isn't really me. I pursue sexual and romantic relationships with women, not men. Queer—that's the word that says me best. "Queer" is like the antilabel label for me, a way to say "I'm here and I'm different" but at the same time not demand that I make any promises about what choices I might make in the future. "Queer" connects me to a political community that is inclusive of many different expressions of gender and sexuality. I identify as a queer femme, and what attracts me the most are alternative forms of masculinity, butch women, and female-to-male transgendered people.

Of course, many LGBT (lesbian, gay, bisexual, transgendered) people find the term queer offensive because the term has been derogatory. For this reason, I am deliberate about which label I use depending on whom I'm talking to. When I talk to someone who does not have much experience or knowledge of the LGBT community, I usually identify as a lesbian because that label is easier for them to understand. Because I am a queer femme, most people assume that I am straight. I identify as queer or femme with other queers and with straights who are both supportive of and sophisticated in their understanding of queer identity. Being queer celebrates my gender and sexuality in all its fabulousness and lets me feel comfortable being myself.

Biological/anatomical sex Categorizing individuals based primarily on their reproductive organs, chromosome makeup, and hormone levels; traditionally, one sex is labeled male and the other female

Secondary sex characteristics Physical traits that develop during puberty and signal sexual maturity; examples are developed breasts, armpit and pubic hair, and coarse facial hair

Gender identity One's personal perception and sense of being male, female, or blended

Gender role The ways we express our gender identity—including appearance, clothing, movement, and life choices

A basic philosophical question about sexuality is, Why are we the sexual beings we are? Some find a spiritual or religious answer to the question, looking toward their Supreme Being for the answer. Others turn to science and claim factual answers. Some question why, after decades of argument and research, scientists and theorists in the 21st century are still embroiled in the "nature versus nurture" controversy. Still others do not even appreciate why the question is being asked in the first place.

We are using the term *sexual identity* in a comprehensive way, to include the various factors that affect how we see ourselves. Individual sexual health requires that we appreciate the impact biology has on our being. The experiences one has in life, occurring in varied social and cultural contexts, help frame how we see ourselves. Sexual identity becomes a part of who we are as whole people: we have physical bodies, we show them to the world in a variety of ways, and we form romantic attachments with others. Ideally, our healthy sexual identities leave us comfortable with our bodies, expressing ourselves in ways that are true to who we "are."

Our sexual identities develop from the interaction of several variables:

1. **Biological/anatomical sex** focuses on the anatomical parts associated most closely with reproductive capabilities and sexual arousal, specifically internal and external reproductive organs. The term *natal sex* has been used to describe that part of identity connected to what is visible at birth (Bockting, 1999). Included as well are the influences of the endocrine system hormones, as reflected in **secondary sex characteristics** and the process of sexual differentiation in the brain.

2. **Gender identity,** the private sense of maleness or femaleness, and **gender role,** the exhibited and shared behaviors that reinforce gender, bring sexual identity beyond the physical domain. In the scheme of things, how we see and express ourselves is expected to correlate with our anatomy. Therapists who provide services to those with sexual identity concerns have preferred the term *social sex role,* which goes beyond *gender role*—the outward presentation

of gender—to include culturally defined sexual stereotypes and what the individual adopts from a spectrum of masculinity to femininity (Bockting, 1999).

3. **Sexual orientation** defines romantic and erotic attachments in choice of partners. One can be drawn to male partners, or to female partners, or be receptive to both men and women.

The question of why we are the sexual beings we are has no simple answer. Sexuality is complex, and our understanding of it continually grows. A number of questions have been, and are continuing to be, researched:

- What factors contribute to the individuals we are? Can those factors be controlled? Altered?
- At what point, if any, is our sexual identity fixed? Is this locked in our genes?
- Are parents and other caregivers the principal forces in shaping our sexuality?
- How powerful are the actual experiences we have in determining how we see ourselves, and how we make decisions?

In this chapter, we will explore the various dimensions of sexual identity, keeping in mind the following principles:

1. The research that has been conducted to date is not conclusive or definitive. Ongoing research from biologists, psychologists, sociologists, anthropologists, sexologists, the medical community, and others supports a variety of positions. Most likely, the persons we are result from an interaction among a variety of forces.

2. The culture has forced a dichotomous view of sexual identity. A person is supposed to be either male or female, heterosexual or homosexual, masculine or feminine. In working toward a healthy sexual identity, we might, instead, think of issues along various continua.

3. The premise that sexuality "just is" and that by some magical age one has evolved into a healthy, self-accepting, sexual being is false. The culture has defined rather narrowly what is deemed "acceptable," with an obvious preference for people to be heterosexual, attractive, able-bodied, and young. When we fall outside that norm—which for many is the reality—self-acceptance and acceptance or tolerance from others may be difficult to attain.

Sexual orientation One's propensity for romantic and erotic attachments. *Heterosexuality* refers to attaching to a partner with different anatomy; *homosexuality* refers to a same-sex partner; *bisexuality* refers to attaching to both men and women.

Arthur Tilley/GettyImages

Being better educated and respectful of people with diverse sexual identities promotes greater sexual health.

To be sexually healthy, we have to become introspective, examine our past, look for explanations and answers, and work through aspects of our sexual identity that are uncomfortable for us. To promote greater sexual health, society, too, has to become better educated and respectful of people with diverse sexual identities.

Intellectual Wellness

It is often said that "knowledge is power." In the area of sexual identity, it is helpful to know that theorists do not agree on why we are who we are. Parents should recognize where they can and cannot influence the sexual development of their children. Also, the individual should know where to turn for more information.

The Internet offers myriad opportunities to click on to useful information. Prior to personal computers, however, groups still found ways to connect. Support groups are available for gay and lesbian youth. Boutiques provide clothing to transgendered men and women. Some hospitals conduct sex reassignment surgery. And most large bookstores today have sexuality sections where individuals can learn more about themselves and people they hold dear and care about.

Continua of Sexuality

Sandra Bem (1995), Charlene Muehlenhard (2000), and others have challenged the approach to sexuality that limits the individual to dichotomous choices about his or her sexuality. You are either "male" or "female." You are either "masculine" or "feminine." You are either "heterosexual" or "homosexual." Needless to say, the culture at large seems to have mandated the dichotomy while simultaneously confusing issues of physical sexuality, gender identity, and sexual orientation. Greater sexual health may come from viewing identity along the continua described in this chapter.

Self-acceptance, as well as a more sophisticated and accurate assessment of others' sexuality, benefits from the recognition that three continua influence our sexual identity (see Figure 4.1). For each variable, the individual can place him- or herself at any point along the continuum. Permutations of the intersections are many. As a result, the tremendous diversity within sexuality becomes apparent.

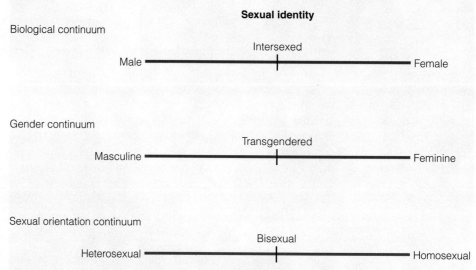

Figure 4.1 *Conceptualization of Sexual Identity* Identities can be fluid and form at various intersections.

For example, in the traditional model of female sexuality, the female has female reproductive organs—clitoris, vagina, uterus, and so on—and female secondary sex characteristics such as developed breasts, broader hips, and narrow waist. To be viewed as an attractive female, the culture further prescribes an acceptable presentation of those characteristics. The female identifies herself as female, adopts the prescribed female role, enjoys feminine things, and behaves in feminine ways. She sees herself as heterosexual, making herself available to males in the culture. This person assumes positions at the extremes of the three continua.

Above and beyond fundamental questions regarding "feminine things and feminine ways" is the basic reality that this description defines only certain females in the culture. Relying on a broader model of sexual identity, someone who is female can possess female reproductive structures but appear more "masculine" to others. A female could enjoy male clothing and be attracted to women. She could have both male and female reproductive structures and enjoy relating to both men and women sexually. The possibilities and realities are numerous.

The *biological continuum* of identity is often thought to be separated clearly into "male and female," yet some individuals have reproductive structures from both. The term *hermaphrodite* has been used when the gonads of both sexes are present and *pseudohermaprodite* when gestational hormone imbalances have caused the external genitalia to be ambiguous and different from the internal structures (Sherwood, 2004). Today, such individuals have embraced the preferred label of **intersexual** and, as will be discussed later, have become vocal in their concerns about medical and psychological interventions and practices. Some individuals experience hormone fluctuations that affect secondary sex characteristics, such as a female having male patterned facial hair (a moustache and beard). A male may have soft features and developed breasts. How the individual then goes on to define himself/herself and what label is taken or what cosmetic "corrections" get made is a matter of increasingly personal choice.

> **Intersexual** An individual possessing some degree of both male and female internal or external reproductive structures; the preferred term, replacing earlier labels of *hermaphrodite* and *pseudohermaphrodite*

The *gender identity* continuum offers numerous points for placement. It is predicated on the cultural ability to distinguish female traits from male traits. Individuals who consider themselves **androgynous** make choices about how they look and act without adhering to sexual stereotypes. Earlier literature defined androgyny in positive terms, in which the individual adopted the healthier traits of both male and female. For example, a woman would not be afraid to voice her opinions, and a man would not hesitate to express his emotions. Clothing, and more significantly one's occupation, would be chosen without gender restrictions. In essence, each would freely choose characteristics and behaviors that best suit his or her personality, not the cultural stereotypes.

> **Androgynous** Expressing characteristics and traits considered stereotypically male and female

Woodhill and Samuels (2003) propose that individuals may be "positively androgynous" or "negatively androgynous" by incorporating desirable or undesirable characteristics. Gender-based characteristics can be positive or negative. The positively androgynous person may demonstrate high levels of compassion, a positive female quality, along with high levels of independence, a positive male quality. In contrast, the negatively androgynous person would demonstrate high levels of submissiveness, a negative female quality, and selfishness, a negative male quality. Their research findings identify positive androgyny as the developmental ideal, associated with higher scores on indicators of mental health and well-being; such individuals have the potential to live a more fulfilled life.

As discussed later in this chapter, those identifying as **transgendered** also place themselves at varying points on the gender identity continuum. For some, their physical appearance is of primary concern. For others the core gender identity is under question, and at some point hormonal and surgical interventions may be sought to become more authentic.

> **Transgendered** The preferred term to describe individuals whose gender identity and gender role encompass both masculine and feminine qualities

Heterosexuality Forming sexual relationships with members of the other sex

Homosexuality Forming sexual relationships with members of the same sex

Bisexuality Forming sexual relationships with both men and women

Placement along the *sexual orientation* continuum allows for erotic connections to males, females, or both. Exclusive **heterosexuality** involves erotic relationships with members of the other sex; males would connect with females and females with males. Exclusive **homosexuality** involves erotic relationships between members of the same sex—that is, males with males and females with females. **Bisexuality** is reflected by erotic connections in which the individual relates to both males and females.

Figure 4.1 is intended to provide a visual model for understanding sexual identity. Individuals may place themselves at different points along each continuum, and those points may vary at different times in their lives. The continua can also intersect at various points, resulting in a great diversity of sexual identities.

Biological Sex

Some researchers perceive that "biology is destiny"; biological influences are the strongest influences over our sexuality. At issue are not only one's anatomical parts but also the need to examine influences of hormones on the brain, particularly during gestation and puberty. For many years, the prevailing wisdom held that "nurturing could override nature" (Money & Ehrhardt, 1972).

In 1972, John Money and Anke Ehrhardt wrote of the case of identical twin boys, in which, because of damage to one infant's penis during a circumcision repair, the child received sex reassignment surgery and was reared as a girl. Through strict feminine gender role experiences, the girl was thought to have a secure gender identity. For many years, sexologists relied on this case to highlight that biology was *not* destiny—nurturing behaviors and socialization could override biological beginnings.

Milton Diamond and H. Keith Sigmundson reported that this boy whose identity was changed in early childhood was not well adjusted, as had been previously described in academic circles (Diamond, 1982; Diamond & Sigmundson, 1997). The child struggled with identity issues, rejected playing with dolls, and attempted to urinate in a standing position. A suicide attempt in adolescence led to learning the truth, a cessation of female hormone treatments, and later extensive surgery to restore his masculinity. John Colapinto (2000) published *As Nature Made Him: The Boy Who Was Raised as a Girl*, bringing the story of David Reimer to the public at large. After an emotionally troubled childhood, Reimer found happiness and married. He later committed suicide in 2004. Diamond and Sigmundson have publicly argued for great restraint in treating intersexed children as well as conducting sex-changing surgery in early childhood. Although they recognize that a child must be raised as either a boy or girl, they recommend limiting that nurturing to hair length, clothing, and name and strongly advise against any irreversible surgical intervention (Diamond, Sigmundson, & Reimer, 2002). Reimer's case gives support to those who argue that the brain has a fixed sexual identity resulting from genetic and gestational influences.

The biological dimension of sexuality leads toward a more dichotomous approach, yet in reality—like the other dimensions to be reviewed—one can evolve in varying ways. The process of **sexual differentiation** embraces the term *different*. Males are different from females. If this is true, in what ways and how significant are the differences?

Sexual differentiation The processes by which the embryo/fetus develops into a male or a female; internal and external genitalia develop in distinct ways, as does the brain

Sexual Differentiation

The moment of conception marks our beginning. The union of a sperm and an ovum represents the chromosomal level of development.

Chromosomal Level

Sperm and ova are known as **gametes,** each of which carries 23 individual chromosomes. Together they become the 23 chromosome pairs carrying the complex array of genes that define us. One of those pairs, the sex chromosomes, determine our biological sex. If a Y-bearing sperm fertilizes the ovum, the species presumably develops as a male, with the gender chromosomes designated as XY; if the X-bearing sperm fertilizes the ovum, the species develops as female, with the gender chromosomes designated as XX (Figure 4.2). The genetic material within the gender chromosomes then acts to shape the organism in a way that is consistent with that differentiation.

Many factors influence identity. Chromosomes represent the beginning of a process that unfolds over many years, hopefully leading toward a clear identity.

Gametes The reproductive cells—sperm and ova

In Utero Development

During the second and third months of pregnancy, the **gonads,** the primary reproductive organs, develop. We refer to the two testicles as male reproductive organs and two ovaries as female. Because these structures evolve from the same embryonic tissue, they are called **homologous structures.** If the embryo follows a male pattern of development, the Y chromosome causes the testicles to produce testosterone, helping shape the structures that will develop. Specifically, the presence of the TDF gene—testis-determining factor—allows for male sexual differentiation. Without it, the fetus develops along female lines, regardless of chromosomes.

Estrogen and testosterone continue to play important roles in sexual development in utero as well as appearance and sexuality after birth. During development, the ratio of the two hormones will produce a child who is anatomically matched to the chromosomes and gonads. If the embryo is chromosomally XX, the ovaries will produce estrogen, which in turn will cause tissue to evolve into the internal and external reproductive organs associated with the female. If the embryo is chromosomally XY, testosterone will direct the tissue to developing into the internal and external reproductive structures of the male. Figure 4.3 shows the sexual differentiation of internal and external structures.

Hormones circulate throughout the developing fetus, affecting the brain, too, through a process referred to as *neural encoding.* Questions arise as to how the male brain may be different from the female brain. Researchers continue to debate whether the brain becomes encoded to later respond to the environment in a biologically predetermined way or whether the forces of socialization cannot be

Gonads The primary endocrine glands in men (testes) and women (ovaries) that influence sexuality

Homologous structures Body parts that develop from the same embryonic tissue (for example, the female clitoris and the male penis)

Figure 4.2 *Genetic Sex*

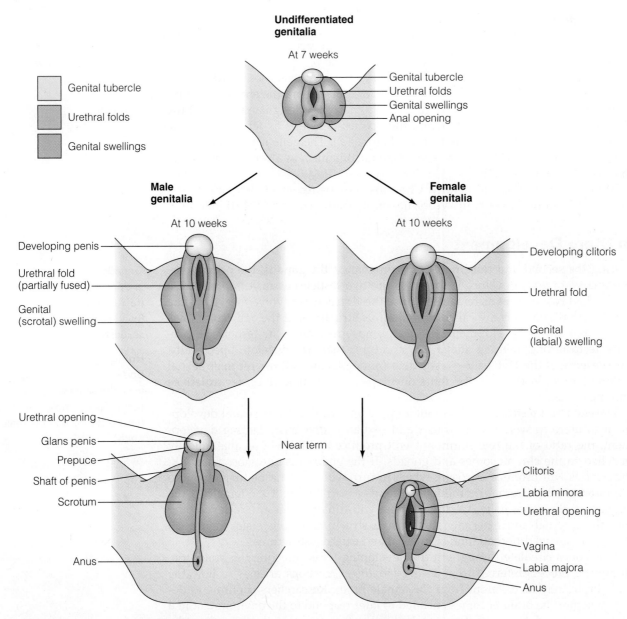

Figure 4.3 *Differentiation of Internal and External Reproductive Structures*

separated from identity. Although it has been reported that gonadal steroid hormones affect sexual differentiation of the brain in laboratory animals, the same case cannot be made for humans (Coleman, Gooren, & Ross, 1989; Hines & Collaer, 1993). Researchers continue to examine the role of hormones on the brain during both gestation and puberty, working toward a better understanding of differences in male and female brains.

Questions continue, however, as development progresses in the areas of gender identity, gender role expression, and sexual orientation. The pituitary gland in the brain and the hypothalamus interact to regulate the sex hormones estrogen and testosterone. One might ask whether the brain is set up to respond to the environment in a particular way, so that perhaps gender identity and sexual orientation evolve in a predetermined fashion.

Anthropologists, however, argue that gender identity, gender role, and sexual expression are not strictly a function of biology. Their studies of non-Western cultures challenge commonly held assumptions about the universality of sexual impulses, the importance of sexuality in human life, the private status of behavior, or its assumed reproductive nature (Vance, 1988).

Birth

Traditionally, the next level of differentiation—gender assignment—is thought to occur at birth. Physicians, nurse midwives, and parents look at the external genitals of the baby and proclaim, "It's a girl!" or "It's a boy!" In today's high-tech world of prenatal screening, many couples know the sex of the offspring months before the baby is born. Chorionic villus sampling and amniocentesis—two prenatal screening techniques discussed in greater detail in Chapter 13—provide data about chromosomal abnormalities. In the second trimester of the pregnancy, prospective parents can be informed, if they are interested, as to whether the fetus is male or female. Sonograms have become routine in obstetrical practice, and they can yield pictures revealing the external genitalia. Thus, parents may be well aware of their child's gender before birth. In essence, they have time to begin gender socialization earlier than they could previously. Whether knowing the gender of the offspring prior to birth has any relevant impact on the development of sexual identity has yet to be researched.

Childhood

As soon as a baby begins to interact with the environment, the gender scripting and gender role learning begin. (We examine psychosexual development in greater detail in Chapter 5.) Early childhood experiences play a pivotal role in a child's learning what being male or female means in a given culture. The classic work of Margaret Mead (1935) conveys the concept that social scripts and gender roles are culture-specific.

Apart from primitive cultures, today's world is vastly connected through technology, and though cultural distinctions remain, men and women can have a clearer understanding of how people in other cultures may learn to be. As a result, the argument that males and females must behave in any one prescribed manner is becoming difficult to make. Reality stands testament to the wide differences in behavior.

Feminists in the United States during the late 1960s and 1970s argued that girls and women were oppressed by the stereotypical and limited scripts they were to learn and the roles they were to play. Sandra Bem (1993) proposed three lenses that frame our understanding of gender:

1. **Androcentrism,** defined as male centeredness
2. **Gender polarization,** the belief that males and females are fundamentally different and have mutually exclusive scripts for being male or female
3. **Biological essentialism,** which explains that androcentrism and gender polarization result from the fundamental biological differences in nature between males and females; when the individual attempts to carve out an identity that may be comfortable, deviation from society's script becomes problematic.

Sex role stereotyping—in which girls were to be pretty, nurturing, and domestic to the exclusion of being independent and earning a meaningful wage—is now thought to be damaging to women's overall health and survival. As an outgrowth of criticizing the female role, male health has been questioned in its relationship

Androcentrism A position of viewing the world with the male at its center

Gender polarization The belief that males and females are fundamentally different, with mutually exclusive gender scripts

Biological essentialism The position that biology is destiny and our biology explains our nature

Toys, games, and ideas of fun all affect our sexual development.

to rigid, stereotyped roles. Furthermore, it has been argued that stereotypes, by the mere fact that they are exaggerated, are inaccurate and ignore the cultural context in which people live (Brody, 1997).

Dressing children and teaching them about life are roles of the parents and the culture; television, schools, and other institutions play a big part in how children learn about themselves. By 24 months of age, a child is usually able to distinguish between males and females, and by 3 years of age, he or she has developed a gender identity, a clear understanding of being male or female.

Children today do not experience the rigidity in gender role learning that those of previous generations did. It could be argued that the culture has changed somewhat in its tradition of "color-coding" babies—that is, boys wear blue, and girls wear pink. Girls now wear blue, but can boys wear pink? The answer is still no. This may reflect the unspoken parental fear that putting a boy baby in pink clothes will feminize him. The color pink is purported to "sissify" boys, yet girls seem to have the ability to develop normally in spite of wearing blue clothes.

Boys and girls today can make freer choices for play and toys. Boys and girls can play with kitchen sets. Both can play with blocks and Legos. Broader questions remain as to why children are drawn to certain types of toys and what kinds of play are fun versus what kinds of play are needed to reinforce established gender roles. The women's movement in the early 1970s called into question stereotyped gender roles and forced gender play. The prevailing wisdom was that both boys and girls would benefit from broader choices based on interest and skill. Even though children in schools, for example, are no longer pushed to play in the "boys' corner" or the "girls' corner," evidence of gender preferences remains. Activities such as jumping rope, playing with dolls, and dressing up are more stereotypically female, whereas playing with toy guns, playing Star Wars, climbing trees, and so forth, are more stereotypically male.

Regardless, examining play activity patterns in children remains only one piece of a complicated puzzle for identity development. A *persistent* preference for "gender-inappropriate" play or dress may be connected to various states of **gender dysphoria,** whereas greater gender role flexibility may be considered a sign of health.

Gender dysphoria The condition in which one's anatomy is inconsistent with one's gender identity

case study 4.2

The Flower Boy

The flower boy is white and was 4 at the time.

When my sister was planning her wedding, she asked us if our 4-year-old son could be the flower boy. He would walk down the aisle just before the bride and throw rose petals along the path as he went. Though neither of us had ever seen or heard of a flower "boy," we thought that it was a wonderful idea. When we asked our son, he was excited about his important job.

It never occurred to us that there would be a problem until we started mentioning, in casual discussions, that our son was going to be the flower boy at the upcoming wedding. Reactions we got from family members and friends (not all, luckily) ranged from astonishment to disgust: "Boys don't throw flowers." "That is a girl's job." "How can you do that to your son? You will humiliate him." "You'll confuse him," and so on. Frankly, we could not believe the reactions people had. After all, we argued, we weren't planning to put him in a dress, and since when were flowers the sole purview of girls? Remember, we are talking about a 4-year-old—a boy who happens to love picking flowers for his mommy and daddy.

In the face of scandal, we became even more committed to seeing this through. The day came, and our son, along with everyone else in the wedding party, was very excited and very nervous. As he came down the aisle, dressed in his tuxedo, a basket of rose petals in his hand, spontaneous "oohs" and "aahs" could be heard from those assembled. People saw not a radical, gender-bending experiment but an adorable 4-year-old spreading beauty and love. We were so proud of him!

Critical Thinking

When parents want to encourage role flexibility, what strategies and responses might be made to those who voice strong, negative reactions?

Use your Virtual Workbook to explore your answer to this question at **http://health.wadsworth.com/blonna1.**

Dress-up dolls remain very popular with girls, with Barbie clearly dominating the market. Increasingly, the doll has been criticized for negatively impacting the self-perception of young girls. Barbie seems obsessed with clothes and has features that distort the female form. Yet, for close to 40 years, Barbie continues to be popular, with numerous versions available. In 1998, the manufacturer announced its plans to make Barbie's proportions more realistic; Barbie added a few pounds yet remained quite thin.

Childhood also is the time when affectional patterns develop, and the basis for whom we find sexually attractive, what behaviors interest us, and with whom we want to romantically attach become set. Our sexual orientation defines whether the object of our attachment is male or female, or whether one becomes receptive to both males and females. In reflecting on their early childhoods, adults may remember being attracted to others in a particular pattern ("I always knew I was attracted to men"). Still, the concept of sexual orientation doesn't really take hold until adolescence and later.

John Money, internationally renowned researcher and clinician, coined the term *lovemaps* to refer to the patterns that develop in the brain, dictating what sexual behaviors will become arousing and pleasurable). His research highlights that lovemaps are formed in early childhood, underlying the power of this phase of development (Money, 1999).

Peter Cade/GettyImages

Barbie has remained very popular despite criticisms about the unrealistic standard she sets.

Adolescence

Puberty, marked by surges in estrogen and testosterone, represents another passage in gender development. Secondary sex characteristics develop in both males and females, and sexuality becomes eroticized. For boys, the surge in testosterone prompts an increase in body hair, specifically armpit and pubic hair. The pitch of the voice lowers, the male reaches adult height, muscles develop, and the genitals, both penis and testicles, increase to their adult size. For females, the hips broaden, breasts develop, hair grows on the mons pubis and in the armpits, and the uterus and ovaries begin to function to allow for menstruation and ovulation. For some adolescents, hormones also have the undesirable impact of producing acne.

Heredity also plays a key role in how we end up. To some extent, our adult physical selves reflect the genetic material passed down. If members of your family tend to be hairy, your hairy chest is more likely to reflect your heritage than to make a comment on your masculinity. If you descend from large-breasted women, your large chest reflects that heritage rather than an unusually high estrogen level.

This phase of development is extremely powerful in its impact on self-esteem. Because of the many changes happening to the body, adolescents explore and play with appearance. A sense that we are acceptable as potential partners arises at this time: "Am I pretty?" "Am I thin enough?" "Are my breasts big enough?" "Are my muscles big?" Is my penis big enough?" "Am I too tall?" "Am I too short?" "Am I OK?"

Physical Wellness

As we age, particularly at puberty, our physical selves become a statement of gender. Heredity and hormones play a significant role in size, structure, and, to some extent, shape. Once we've matured, we make decisions about appearance—what clothes to wear, how to cut our hair, what we accentuate, what we hide.

In the past several years, males and females alike have been using steroids as a way to increase muscle mass. The evidence is clear that steroids used in this way can be dangerous. Women bodybuilders, for example, may have the desired large muscles but will notice diminished breast size, changes in the menstrual cycle, and more masculine contours to the face, not to mention increased facial hair. Males who use steroids may be excited by the size and strength of their muscles but unprepared for what is commonly called "roid rage," a pronounced and intense level of anger.

Illness and disability may also influence the physical aspects of our identity. When cancer treatment results in the loss of a breast, testicle, prostate, ovary, or uterus, the repercussions are physical as well as psychological. Surgery and chemotherapy can alter hormone functioning, which in turn can affect physical appearance and sexual functioning. Disability may affect movement, which in turn may affect how we see ourselves and how others react to us.

Our physical body becomes the machine through which we express our sexuality, and taking care of it, in whatever condition it is, is essential.

sex in society 4.1

Body Image as a Lifelong Concern

The concept of "body image" refers to how one views one's body. It is a matter of self-perception, formed over years of looking in the mirror, receiving a myriad of comments both critical and complimentary from others, comparing oneself to friends and models in magazines, and experimenting with looks. Who hasn't looked back at old photographs and cringed with the thought "How could I have cut my hair like that!" or "Whatever possessed me to wear that outfit?" What is fashionable in one decade can be passé in the next.

Changes in what is seen as desirable can certainly have an impact on a person's health, in all its dimensions. It has been documented that a desire to be thin has led to elementary-aged girls going on diets. Although the research on eating disorders indicates greater rates among white, middle- and upper-class women, clinicians and researchers are seeing eating disorders in both males and females, regardless of race and ethnicity (Woodside et al., 2001). A person can have a "bad hair day," want to hide his or her head under a hat, and generally feel self-conscious. Individuals with body dysmorphic disorder (BDD), however, have a clinical diagnosis, and they see themselves as ugly, often becoming obsessive about one particular part of their body. Their disordered thinking about appearance can disrupt all aspects of their everyday lives, with some becoming housebound.

Increasingly, high school and college students seem interested in body adornment in the form of tattoos and body piercings. The need to make sure that tattoo and piercing parlors operate under sanitary conditions is of paramount concern for the prevention of infection, both bacterial and viral (for example, HIV).

Concern for appearance and positive body image is very entrenched in the American culture. The process of aging causes adults to reevaluate their acceptability as sexual partners. For example, with menopause comes a drop in estrogen levels, which may cause the development of coarse facial hair. Although the adrenal glands continue to produce estrogen, the amount in the body may not be at a level to suppress facial hair. Because estrogen and testosterone are present in both genders, their balance becomes important to external appearance. An older male may find that his breasts are growing as a result of aging or treatment for cancer. Some female cancer patients are given estrogen-inhibiting medications, and male cancer patients have been given testosterone-inhibiting medications. Although we take the medications to stay healthy, the resulting side effects do not always impact positively on our sexuality.

To find the right balance between attending to appearance and taking care of oneself versus getting caught up in the momentum of ever-increasing options for improving appearance remains a challenge.

Adolescence is the time when sexual experimentation takes place for many teens. Social norms support the development of a heterosexual orientation—choosing a partner of the opposite sex. Males choose females, and vice versa. For teens who begin to struggle with confusing feelings, the social supports are less obvious. Gay and lesbian youth may find groups that help them clarify their orientation. On the other hand, in reflection, many gay and lesbian adults report "playing the game" during their junior high and high school years. They feigned crushes and dated opposite-sex partners to fit in with their peers.

Developing a clear sexual orientation may not happen during adolescence. For those who know that they are lesbian, gay, or bisexual, being able to be open with others may or may not occur during adolescence. In an ideal world, individuals would be free to explore what makes them comfortable and happy. In reality, those who do not fit the norm, in whatever way, may find themselves lying, keeping secrets, and holding off from being who they are.

Adulthood

In the past, theorists would argue that, by the end of adolescence, one would be moving on to adulthood and therefore should embrace the tasks of adulthood. One's initial adult sexual identity should be complete. In reality, though, we all continue to struggle with questions of who we are, how we want to present ourselves, and what types of partners are most attractive to us. A key piece in adult happiness is having a clear sense of one's sexual orientation. As shown in Figure 4.4, the process of "arriving" at one's sexual identity is a journey that involves many sources of input.

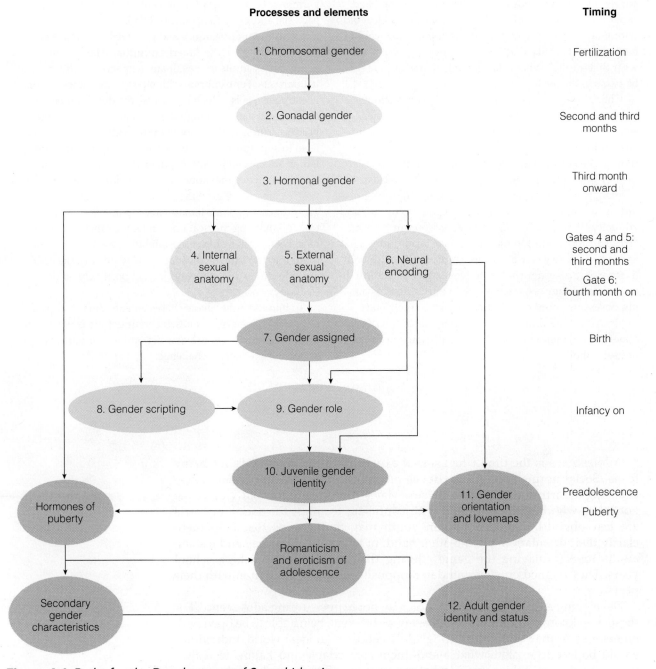

Figure 4.4 *Paths for the Development of Sexual Identity*

Source: Becoming a Sexual Person, 2nd Edition, by Robert T. Francouer (Boston: Allyn & Bacon, 1991) p. 74. Based on the work of John Money. Reprinted with permission.

All the Things I Would Never Do
If I Were the Opposite Sex

The goal of this activity is to inspire you not only to look at behaviors of the opposite sex that annoy you but to identify your own behaviors that hinder your relationships with the opposite sex.

Imagine that you have the ability to change what really irritates you about the opposite sex. All you have to do is make your wish list, and everything you wanted would be granted.

Take a minute and make a list of all the things that the opposite sex does that you really wish they would never do again. After you have finished making your list, show your list to your best same-sex friend and see whether he or she has the same wishes or can add to your list. Then be very brave and show it to your best opposite-sex friend. How does he or she react to your list? Ask this best opposite-sex friend if he or she could make any changes in the behavior of your sex, what would they be? Notice all the behaviors on your friend's list that you presently do. Are you willing to make those changes?

For example:

If I were a female I would never

- lead a guy on sexually.
- wear so much makeup.
- always expect the guy to pay for everything.

If I were a male, I would never

- scratch my genitals in public.
- expect sex because I pay for dinner.
- talk with the guys about my sexual experiences.

Sexual Orientation

In attempting to explain sexual orientation, theorists have often focused their efforts on explaining why some people identify as homosexual or bisexual. There is thought to be no need to explain heterosexuality, as that is the norm. That is what is expected. The strongest arguments for heterosexuality lie in the reproductive aspects of heterosexual behavior. Without heterosexuals, the argument goes, no children would be born. The species would die.

Some individuals look to their religious doctrines, citing passages that condemn behavior between same-sex individuals. There is the oft-quoted "If God wanted there to be homosexuals, he would have created Adam and Steve, not Adam and Eve." Still others perceive homosexuals as having a form of mental illness. And history is replete with violence, gay bashing, arrests, and even death for those thought to be homosexual. Consequently, homosexuals themselves have found their sexuality framed as a form of mental illness, a sin, or a form of illegal behavior.

Although we appreciate the strength of various convictions, we take the position that sexual health requires accepting our sexual orientation and that individuals who are comfortable with themselves are less likely to feel threatened by people who have orientations that are different from their own. The gay and lesbian rights movement has often pointed out, "We are everywhere. We are your children, your brothers and sisters, your parents, your friends." The issue is whether an individual can be open about his or her sexuality, and whether you are willing to know that aspect of those with whom you are close.

Theories of Sexual Orientation

Theories on sexual orientation abound, following different tracks. Biological theorists have looked toward genetic, hormonal, and structural differences in the brain to explain homosexuality. Social theorists emphasize learning as a key factor in determining orientation. Wiederman (2001), in his critique of research on orientation, elaborates on the difficulties inherent in studying orientation. While the question of causality may be the primary focus, the experimental research that would be needed to systematically identify key factors cannot be conducted. It is unethical, for example, to manipulate genetic material in an attempt to identify difference. It would be just as unethical and impossible to manipulate the behavior of parents, or experiment with childhood experiences, in order to assess the impact on later interpersonal attachments. Consequently, a lot of the research on orientation ends up being speculative and correlational; for example, researchers will survey and interview adults about their past to identify related variables (Wiederman, 2001).

Biological Theories   Studies of sexual orientation among identical twins and fraternal twins show varying rates of being gay or lesbian, yet the rates are not 100 percent. In one study of gay men, with an admittedly small sample, 52 percent of the twins had a gay twin; among lesbians, the rate was 48 percent (Bailey & Pillard, 1991; Bailey, Pillard, Neal, & Agyei, 1993). If the explanation for orientation were totally a genetic one, twins, particularly identical twins, would have to have the same sexual orientation. That is not always the case.

Research on hormonal influences during gestation has been conducted more carefully with rats than humans. Theorists look to the period of time when sexual differentiation occurs in the brain and the hypothalamus develops, arguing that hormonal imbalances may cause homosexuality as well as gender dysphoria (Ellis & Ames, 1987; Ellis, Ames, Peckham, & Burke, 1988). The hormonal imbalances may be a result of medications, steroid use, or high stress levels. A problem with the research in this area is the basic difficulty of carefully monitoring hormone levels in a large enough sample of pregnant women throughout their pregnancies and then being able to follow, in a longitudinal study, the development of their offspring. That kind of research has not been conducted.

Theorists also have looked to hormonal differences after birth, particularly from a "deficiency" perspective. This approach—which holds that gay men lack adequate testosterone and lesbian women lack adequate estrogen—smacks a bit of old stereotypes that gay men are effeminate and lesbian women are mannish. Most of the research in the area has been done on males, which also becomes a problem. The work conducted on males has not found any differences based on orientation (Banks & Gartrell, 1995). At one time, treatment for male homosexuality involved testosterone therapy. Rather than changing orientation, that therapy just made patients "hornier and hairier."

The most publicized research on anatomical brain differences came from the work of Simon LeVay (1991), who dissected the brains of a small sample of gay men and compared them to the brains of straight men and women. He found structural differences in a section of the hypothalamus of the gay men. The research has been roundly criticized for sample size, absence of lesbian women in the sample, and the complicating factor that the gay men had died of AIDS. The research sparked a lot of discussion but offered limited findings.

Psychological and Learning Theories In looking to psychological theories, particularly psychoanalytic and learning theories, explanations of sexual orientation again have limited uses. In his *Three Essays on the Theory of Sexuality*, published in the early part of the 20th century, Freud spoke of the child as having an undifferentiated sexuality and having to learn appropriate responses as he or she ages. Part of that learning would be to identify with the parent of the same sex, and to seek out a partner of the opposite sex. To be homosexual then could be construed as inappropriate identification. The female child, for example, would identify with her father and seek out women as partners.

For years, the field of mental health, led by psychiatrists, psychoanalysts, and psychologists, considered homosexuality a form of mental illness. Not until 1973 did the American Psychiatric Association remove homosexuality from its *Diagnostic and Statistical Manual of Mental Disorders* (DSM). Even with its removal, some professionals, as well as the lay population, still view homosexuality as a disorder.

Very popular for years was the notion that homosexuality in males resulted from a weak or absent father and a strong, domineering, overly intimate mother. In short, parental ways of interacting with their children and between themselves were responsible for the homosexuality of their children. In cases where such a relationship between the parents was found, however, the household also had heterosexual children. It becomes quizzical, to say the least, that the nature of the parental relationship would explain only homosexuality and not heterosexuality. Nonetheless, parents of gays and lesbians often struggle to understand their role in their child's homosexuality.

Another notion has been that homosexuals were seduced into their lifestyle by an older adult. This myth is particularly destructive, for it sets up gay and lesbian adults as seducers, likely to seek out children and adolescents for their personal pleasure. As a result, professions where adults have contact with children (teacher, coach, and so on) become particularly risky places to "come out."

Learning theory as applied to sexual orientation can go in a variety of directions. A basic tenet is that the rewards and punishments associated with various behaviors and experiences channel sexual orientation in a certain direction. For example, negative reactions to heterosexual experiences could encourage later homosexual experiences. This line of thinking is supported by sex histories of lesbians who were sexually abused by their fathers in childhood. In contrast, positive childhood experiences could explain later homosexuality. This idea is exemplified by the adolescent male who had enjoyed oral sex with an older male cousin and develops into a gay adult whose partners are men.

One study extensively interviewed and compared responses from close to 1,000 gay and lesbian adults with those from a sample group of approximately 500 heterosexual males and females (Bell, Weinberg, & Hammersmith, 1981). The interviewees were asked about their child and adolescent years. The results showed no patterns of family dysfunction, no prevalence of positive or negative sexual experiences to explain orientation, and, most important, no predetermination of orientation before adolescence.

Researchers have also had difficulty obtaining samples of adults to study. A common practice has been to seek out volunteers for convenience samples, advertising in publications targeted to the gay, lesbian, and bisexual community. Individuals are asked to recall childhood and adolescent experiences, which are then used to frame a developmental picture. The costs and sample size involved in following very young children over time become prohibitive. The results of such research, however, may be tainted by selective memories and inaccuracies (Wiederman, 2001).

At the risk of oversimplification in describing various theories, it should become obvious that no one theory explains it all. Homosexual, bisexual, and heterosexual children can and do have the same biological parents, grow up in the same households, and end up differently along the continuum of sexual orientation.

Labels and Categories

Alfred Kinsey's work on male and female sexuality continues to provide a reference point for work on sexual orientation (Kinsey, Pomeroy, & Martin, 1948; Kinsey, Pomeroy, Martin, & Gebhard, 1953). Along with his colleagues, he developed a 7-point scale that categorized sexual experience, shown in Figure 4.5.

After interviewing more than 10,000 people, Kinsey found it useful to categorize behaviors on a continuum based on sexual experience with same-sex and other-sex partners. If one's behavior was exclusively with a member of the other sex, that person was referred to as a "Kinsey 0." A person whose behavior was exclusively with members of his or her own sex was labeled a "Kinsey 6." All other positions between 1 and 5 represented interest in both men and women.

Because the culture often seems to want to classify or label people regarding orientation, only Kinsey 0's would fit the definition of heterosexual. Individuals categorized as Kinsey 6's would be homosexual, and those falling within categories 1 through 5 would be bisexual or ambisexual.

Later researchers and theorists, as well as groups holding to one or more political positions, have objected to classifying individuals based only on their behavior, as well as questioning the need to classify and label at all. Fred Klein pointed out the limitations of using behavior as the sole variable for labeling. Common sense dictates that *what we do* is only a part of *who we are* and what identity we have. Klein proposed that orientation be assessed on seven factors (Klein, 1978; Klein, Sepekoff, & Wolf, 1985):

1. *Sexual attraction:* To whom do we find ourselves attracted? Who turns us on? Do we respond only to women? Only to men? To both?
2. *Sexual behavior:* When you've engaged in sexual behavior, who have been your partners?
3. *Sexual fantasies:* When you fantasize or masturbate, what sex/gender is your partner?

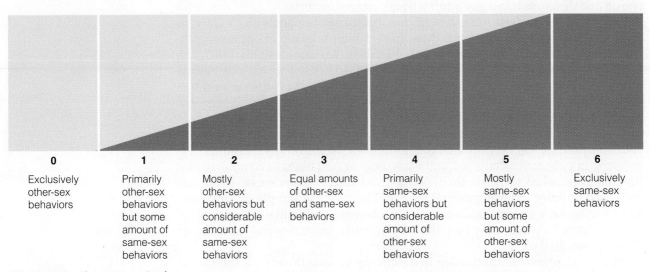

0	1	2	3	4	5	6
Exclusively other-sex behaviors	Primarily other-sex behaviors but some amount of same-sex behaviors	Mostly other-sex behaviors but considerable amount of same-sex behaviors	Equal amounts of other-sex and same-sex behaviors	Primarily same-sex behaviors but considerable amount of other-sex behaviors	Mostly same-sex behaviors but some amount of other-sex behaviors	Exclusively same-sex behaviors

Figure 4.5 *The Kinsey Scale*

4. *Emotional or affectional preference:* To whom do you connect on an emotional level? With whom do you "fall in love"?

5. *Social preference:* With whom do you prefer to socialize? With whom do you "go out"?

6. *Lifestyle:* In your community, with whom do you spend most of your time? Are your friends primarily lesbian or gay? Bisexual? Heterosexual?

7. *Self-identification:* How do *you* label yourself? Where do you place yourself on the Kinsey grid?

The American Academy of Pediatrics has prepared a statement on homosexuality and adolescence, identifying four stages of identity formation (Ryan & Futterman, 2001). First, there is "Sensitization," where a feeling of being different is experienced by prepubertal children and adolescents. The second stage, "Sexual Identity Confusion," is marked by a self-awareness of same-gender attraction yet confusion reconciling oneself with what are negative societal stereotypes. The third stage, "Sexual Identity Assumption," is the process of acknowledgment and social and sexual exploration of one's identity. Delving into the gay and lesbian community is more common in late adolescence. Finally, the fourth stage, "Integration and Commitment," represents the individual's ability to incorporate being gay or lesbian into positive self-acceptance, and sharing that part of oneself with others. This stage, if and when reached, typically occurs in adulthood.

Important to consider is not only *what you have done* but *what you would like to be doing and with whom.* Another important aspect in sorting this out is whether you find yourself enjoying the behavior. Some women and men, for example, claim to have been happily married, followed the heterosexual script, and had children. Later, they met someone of the same sex, fell in love, enjoyed lovemaking to an extent they hadn't before, and "came out." They don't feel the need to negate all of their past, nor do they claim that the sexual part of their relationship was dissatisfying but, rather, that they have discovered an identity and a lifestyle that feel right.

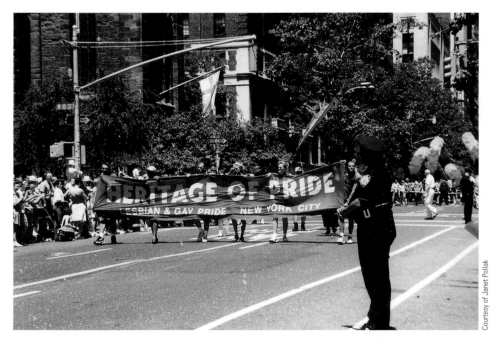

Gay Pride parades take place in many cities across the United States.

case study 4.3

Marcus's Story

Marcus, 32, identifies as African American.

Critical Thinking

Do you think that the images presented in the media today make it easier for students to be open about their sexual orientation?

Use your Virtual Workbook to explore your answer to this question at **http://health.wadsworth.com/blonna1.**

Growing up the son of a professional football player, I was pretty sure that being attracted to other guys wasn't something I was ever going to talk about to anyone. For as long as I could remember, there was something there that I couldn't define. When I was a kid, there were no gay characters on sitcoms—no Ellen DeGeneres coming out on television. No show like Will and Grace, *no* Queer Eye for the Straight Guy. *No one ever said that being attracted to guys was an OK thing for a guy. The only talking I ever heard about homosexuality was the constant tossing around of the word fag that was just used as a general, all-purpose term for anyone you were mad at. My older brother used to call me a fag all the time, not because I was unlike other guys in any way—that whole sissy-boy thing is pretty much a myth—but because he was my older brother and that's what older brothers do—torment their younger brothers.*

Going off to college, I admitted to myself that I was gay and that I would always be attracted to men. But, as a second-semester freshman, I swore that I would never act on it. I wouldn't think about guys. I wouldn't fantasize about guys. I wouldn't date guys. I would search out the perfect best friend, and the two of us would embark on a completely chaste relationship that would be mutually satisfying. Of course, no such guy existed, and several attempts to pin my flagging hopes on various friends of mine ended up in disaster. I had told myself that I would never do anything for which I would be ashamed.

After almost a full year of repressing all feelings of attraction for anyone, I came to realize that perhaps I could be happy and sexually active, and not end up living alone for the rest of my life. My feelings of self-hatred and shame, however, had run far too deep, and I started having anxiety attacks.

Over the next two and a half years, I saw a therapist whose office was about a block off campus. I went not because I was sick but because I wanted to feel better about myself. Over those two and a half years, I talked to the therapist about how I felt and who I was.

Coming out is a long and hard process for many people, and my story is probably not all that unusual. Many of us still hear and see messages of hatred and spend some time hating ourselves. I'd hope that the positive images seen these days and supportive statements from various celebrities, magazines, books, and movies might make it much easier for gay people who are younger than I am. Some friends—whom I thought would never understand or accept me—have. Now, instead of admitting that I'm gay—as if it were something to be ashamed of—I can say with comfort and confidence that I'm a gay man. And when people get to know me, they'll learn other things about me as well.

It seems safe to say that society at large presumes people are heterosexual until proven otherwise. And then, if someone's gay or lesbian orientation becomes known, it is not unusual to hear someone remark, "Oh, I didn't know that person was gay." At one time in history, gays and lesbians were called "the invisible minority." The 1969 Stonewall Uprising in New York City, during which a police raid of a gay bar was met with resistance, has been credited as the event that began the gay and lesbian rights movement. That movement has led to more individuals feeling freer to be open about their sexual orientation, although many still report that to "come out" would leave them vulnerable to harassment, violence, and loss of jobs, housing, friendships, and family members. Some states (such as New Jersey) have included sexual orientation, along with race, creed, gender, ethnicity, military and veteran's status, and disability, as a basis for which one's civil rights must be protected.

sex in society 4.2

Dealing with the Categories

Audre Lorde, a feminist writer, highlighted our culture's need to categorize and stigmatize individuals around issues of race, sex, class, and sexual orientation. "As a forty-nine-year-old Black lesbian feminist socialist mother of two, including one boy, and a member of an interracial couple, I usually find myself a part of some group defined as other, deviant, inferior, or just plain wrong" (Lorde, 2001, p. 588). She speaks to the constant drain of energy it takes to respond to a world that oppresses individuals for a variety of qualities—sex, race, social class, ethnicity, and sexual orientation—and challenges the culture to redefine the way it deals with difference.

For sexual health, it is necessary to realize that issues of race and ethnicity cannot be separated from the ways the individual functions in his or her community. The Families of Color Network is a coalition of Asian–Pacific Islanders, Latinos, African Americans, Arab Americans, Native Americans, Caucasians, and biracial individuals who come together as an activist and advocacy group around LGBT issues.

Nila Marrone (2001), in an article for *The SIECUS Report*, identifies issues in the Latino culture, for example, that make dealing with LGBT concerns more difficult:

- Very strong family ties are more common and all family problems must be solved internally by its members.
- The family name and image must be protected.
- Traditions are highly valued, and change is generally not welcome.
- Respect for elders is highly prized.
- There is no tradition for forming or joining support groups.
- Privacy is highly prized.
- Limited economic resources are a serious obstacle to joining civic or support groups.
- Most Latinos are Catholic.

Other racial and cultural groups may share some of these values and characteristics, adding others that are unique to them. Overall, the LGBT community must address its diversity on race, class, ethnicity, religion, politics, and other issues as it works to build the connections stemming from sexuality.

Source: Adapted from N. Marron (April/May 2001), "Advice to Latino Parents of GLBT Children," *SIECUS Report, 29* (4).

How Many?

The subject of sexual orientation has often led to a need to document "how many." How many people are heterosexual? How many are lesbian and gay? How many are bisexual? As researchers attempt to count, a number of problems arise. What criterion will be used? How easily assessed is a sample, and can it be determined to be generalizable to the population at large?

Kinsey reported that 37 percent of males and 13 percent of females had engaged in adult same-sex behavior to the point of orgasm. He estimated that 2 percent of males and 1 percent of females could be categorized as Kinsey 6's (Kinsey et al., 1948, 1953). A limitation of Kinsey's work, particularly as it pertains to the Heterosexual-Homosexual Rating Scale, is that behavior is emphasized without attending to the other factors that Klein identified.

When the National Health and Social Life Survey (NHSLS) results were reported (Laumann, Gagnon, Michael, & Michaels, 1994), the researchers addressed the difficulty they, or others, have in "counting" homosexuals. A primary problem lies with the definition of *homosexual*. They point out that people change their behavior during their lifetime, that patterns of sexual desire and identification vary, and that, because of oppression, it can be difficult to get respondents both to identify themselves and honestly respond to questions (Michael, Gagnon, Laumann, & Kolata, 1994). As a result, a definitive picture of homosexuality in the United States becomes difficult to paint.

The NHSLS examined issues of attraction by asking respondents, "In general, are you sexually attracted to … only women, mostly women, both men and women, mostly men, only men?" Appeal was measured by "How would you rate this activity: having sex with someone of the same sex … very appealing, somewhat appealing, not appealing, not at all appealing?" For self-identification, they asked, "Do you think of yourself as heterosexual, homosexual, bisexual, something else?" Figure 4.6 presents some of the findings.

The NHSLS researchers have claimed that their research represented a scientifically accurate survey of sex in the United States, representing nearly all adult U.S. men and women (Michael et al., 1994). Although the researchers are not above criticism, they were able to interview and survey a wider range of people than other studies to date. For what it's worth "toward the count," they found that more people find others of the same gender sexually attractive than have homosexual sex.

Approximately 5.5 percent of women found the idea of having sex with another woman very appealing or appealing, with 4 percent reporting that they were sexually attracted to women. Less than 2 percent had had sex with a woman during the past year, yet slightly more than 4 percent reported having sex with a woman at some time in their lives.

About 6 percent of the men in the NHSLS study reported being attracted to other men, with 2 percent saying they had had sex with a man in the past year. By comparison to females, 9 percent reported having had sex with a man at least once since puberty. When respondents were asked to label themselves, only 1.4 percent of women thought of themselves as homosexual or bisexual, and 2.8 percent of men identified themselves as homosexual or bisexual.

healthy sex hints 4.1
Advice on Coming Out

The decision to be open about one's homosexuality is a personal one, one that heterosexuals don't have to confront. It is almost as if lesbian and gay individuals have to explain to the world that they are not heterosexual, rather than "the world" having considered that possibility.

The risks a person takes for being open about sexual orientation depend on a variety of factors including age, geography, employment, and financial solvency, among others. Although civil rights protections are gradually being extended to people at the local and state levels, no constitutional amendment guarantees civil rights protection regardless of sexual orientation.

The following guidelines are adapted from the brochure *Be Yourself** (Sauerman, 1998):

1. *Are you sure about your sexual orientation?* Don't raise the issue unless you're able to respond with confidence to the question "Are you sure?" Confusion on your part will increase your parents' confusion and decrease their confidence in your judgment.

2. *Are you comfortable with your gay sexuality?* If you're wrestling with guilt and periods of depression, you'll be better off waiting to tell your parents. Coming out to them may require tremendous energy on your part; it will require a reserve of positive self-image.

3. *Do you have support?* In the event your parents' reaction devastates you, there should be someone or a group that you can confidently turn to for emotional support and strength. Maintaining your sense of self-worth is critical.

4. *Are you knowledgeable about homosexuality?* Your parents will probably respond based on a lifetime of information from a homophobic society. If you've done some serious reading on the subject, you'll be able to assist them by sharing reliable information and research.

5. *What's the emotional climate at home?* If you have the choice of when to tell, consider the timing. Choose a time when they're not dealing with such matters as the death of a close friend, pending surgery, or the loss of a job.

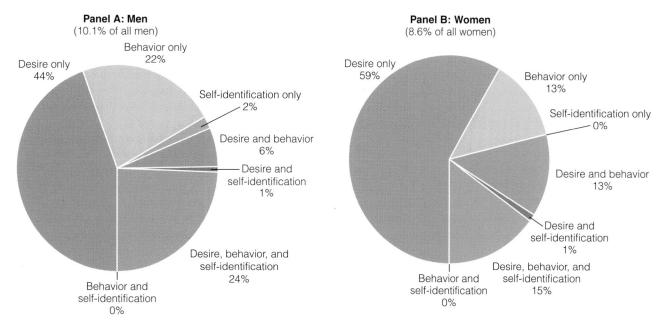

Figure 4.6 *Interrelationship of Three Aspects of Same-Gender Sexuality: Desire, Behavior, and Self*

Source: Sex in America: A Definitive Survey, by R. Michael, J. Gagnon, and E. Laumann. Copyright © 1994 by CSG Enterprises, Inc. Little, Brown, and Company. Reprinted with permission.

6. *Can you be patient?* Your parents will require time to deal with this information if they haven't considered it prior to your sharing. The process may last from six months to two years.

7. *What's your motive for coming out now?* Hopefully, it is because you love them and are uncomfortable with the distance you feel. Never come out in anger or during an argument, using your sexuality as a weapon.

8. *Do you have available resources?* Homosexuality is a subject most non-gay people know little about. Have available at least one of the following: a book addressed to parents, a contact for the local or national Parents and Friends of Lesbians and Gays, the name of a nongay counselor who can deal fairly with the issue.

9. *Are you financially dependent on your parents?* If you suspect they are capable of withdrawing college finances or forcing you out of the house, you may choose to wait until they do not have this weapon to hold over you.

10. *What is your general relationship with your parents?* If you've gotten along well and have always known their love—and shared your love for them in return—chances are they'll be able to deal with the issue in a positive way.

11. *What is their moral societal view?* If they tend to see social issues in clear terms of good/bad or holy/sinful, you may anticipate that they will have serious problems dealing with your sexuality. If, however, they've evidenced a degree of flexibility when dealing with other changing societal matters, you may be able to anticipate a willingness to work this through with you.

12. *Is this your decision?* Not everyone should come out to their parents. Don't be pressured into it if you're not sure you'll be better off by doing so—no matter what their response.

*Be Yourself highlights the process that most parents go through when told that their child is gay. The stages include shock, denial, guilt, expression of feelings, personal decision making, and true acceptance. It highlights that each family is unique, and offers suggestions of resources and support.

Source: Read This Before Coming Out to Your Parents by T. H. Sauerman, PFLAG Philadelphia, 1998. For ordering information: PFLAG Philadelphia, P.O. Box 176, Titusville, NJ 08560-0176; vrb@pupgg.princeton.edu.

Social and Environmental/Occupational Wellness

Social health depends on making connections with others. We learn to do that by first making connections with our families, and then making friends and expanding our social groups. Once children interact in schools, turn on a television set, or take a trip to a shopping mall, they become exposed to the various ways that males and females appear and act. Comments of approval and disapproval shape our behaviors; they also can be the basis for whether we feel good or bad about ourselves.

The process to a clear and comfortable sexual identity is not always easy. For those who are gay, lesbian, bisexual, or transgendered, relationships with others may add risk in a way that heterosexuals don't experience: being thrown out of one's home, losing a job, or losing friends. Although people do not segregate themselves socially based on sexuality, at times the ability to join a community of others like yourself becomes critical to one's health. That community may be on the Internet, at a conference or gathering, in a therapeutic support group, and in the home. Urban areas offer more social opportunities than small towns regarding sexual identity, with such cities as New York City and San Francisco, in particular, being known for their tolerance.

On an individual basis, we all must find a place to call home—a place that feels safe and secure and where we can be ourselves. The homes we grew up in may or may not have been places like this. Health and positive growth require that children be loved and nurtured and allowed to develop in their own unique way.

Some children live in environments that are threatening to their sexual development. Taunts and abuse from schoolmates, threats of, and real, violence from strangers, and, for some, self-abuse and suicide can result from identity issues. No longer should a child who is transgendered be mistaken as schizophrenic. No longer should a child be institutionalized in a mental hospital where shock treatments or other forms of aversive therapy are used to change sexual orientation. The medical community is better informed—though not necessarily better prepared—to deal with these issues. Laws at the federal, state, and local levels have been slow to protect the civil rights of gay, lesbian, and transgendered individuals.

Creating environments where people can be who they are helps reduce the power of sexual difference and allows society to be enriched with citizens who can safely develop to their full potential. People learn that sexual identity is only one piece of a person's being and that a person can form working relationships and even friendships that allow for differences. Tolerant, respectful, and safe environments improve the opportunities for everyone.

Atypical Paths of Development

As the influences affecting sexual identity come into play, the question persists as to whether one is developing "normally." Regardless of one's definition of *normal*, what, if anything, is to be "done" when development varies? After birth, questions such as "Is the child happy with him- or herself? "and "Are the parents happy with the child?" may be secondary to concerns expressed from family, physicians, and other outside observers.

Every year children are born who are not genetically, anatomically, or hormonally consistent with one sex or the other. Some situations are immediately apparent, as in ambiguous external genitalia. In other situations the chromosomal makeup may be abnormal, yet the impact of the genetic mosaic may not be obvious until childhood or adolescence. Table 4.1 charts the more common of variations.

Table 4.1 Atypical Chromosomal and Hormonal Patterns in Prenatal Development

Syndrome	Chromosomal Sex	Gonads	Internal Reproductive	External Reproductive	Secondary Sex Characteristics	Gender Identity
Klinefelter syndrome	Male, XXY	Testes	Normal male	Small penis and testes	Female secondary sex characteristics develop at puberty	Male
Turner syndrome	Female, XO	Nonfunctioning or absent ovaries	Normal female except for ovaries	Underdeveloped genitals	No breast development or menstruation at puberty	Female
Androgen insensitivity syndrome	Male, XY	Testes, but body unable to utilize testosterone	Shallow vagina, lacking normal male structures	Labia	Female secondary sex characteristics develop at puberty; no menstruation	Female
Congenital adrenal hyperplasia	Female, XX	Ovaries	Normal female	Ambiguous, tending toward male appearance; enlarged clitoris may be mistaken for penis	Female secondary sex characteristics develop at puberty	Usually male
DHT deficiency	Male, XY	Undescended testes	Partially formed, but no prostate	Ambiguous until puberty when penis enlarges and testes descend	Male secondary sex characteristics develop at puberty	Female until puberty when male identity taken

healthy sex hints 4.2
Support in Faith Communities

Spiritual health needs get met in many ways, and having a sense of community is one of them. One of the challenges of considering yourself "religious" and part of the LGBT community is to be able to reconcile religious teachings with your lifestyle. The Internet has enabled groups within various religious communities to provide support and resources. Here is a sample of sites organized by Lambda Families (E. Schroeder, personal communication, September 3, 2002):

Soulfource: Activism to Stop Spiritual Violence:
   www.soulforce.org
Baptist: Association of Welcoming and Affirming Baptists:
   www.wabaptists.org
Catholic: Dignity: **www.dignityusa.org**
Episcopalian: Integrity: **www.integrityusa.org**
Evangelical: Evangelicals Concerned: **www.ecinc.org**

Jewish: The World Congress of GLBT Jews:
   www.glbtjews.org
Lutheran: Lutherans Concerned: **www.lcna.org**
Methodist: Reconciling Ministries Network:
   www.rmnetwork.org
Metropolitan Community Churches: **www.ufmcc.com**
Mormon: Affirmation: **www.affirmation.org**
Presbyterian: More Light: **www.mlp.org**
Quaker: Friends for Lesbian, Gay, Bisexual, Transgender, and Queer Concerns: **www.quaker.org/flgbtqc**
Seventh-Day Adventists: Kinship International:
   www.sdakinship.org
Unitarian Universalist: Interweave:
   www.interweave.uua.org
United Church of Christ: Coalition for LGBT Concerns:
   www.ucccoalition.org

U.S. culture traditionally has looked at atypical patterns as problems, and the medical community has become involved where possible to "fix" the child. The terms used to describe ambiguities are clinical. *Pseudohermaphrodism* describes the conditions in which the child is genetically one sex, with mixed external and internal structures. Genetic females whose genitals are masculinized because of an accumulation of androgens from the adrenal glands are referred to as having *congenital adrenal hyperplasia* (CAH), also called *adrenogenital syndrome*. A condition with parallel outcomes—*androgen insensitivity syndrome*—is found in a genetic male whose body does not respond to the testosterone it produces, leading to female external genitalia. Adult individuals with these conditions have recently become more visible and political. They are asking to be referred to as intersexuals and demanding their civil rights.

The Intersex Society of North America (ISNA) is a support, education, and advocacy group founded by and for individuals who are intersexual. The organization opposes the predominant model of treatment that recommends emergency sex reassignment for infants, followed by hormonal treatments and gender role learning that reinforces that assignment. As a result of sharing their experiences, the intersexuals involved with ISNA (1995) claim that these early interventions, considered a form of genital mutilation, have impaired them in many ways.

The ISNA (1995) has recommended a new model of treatment that avoids harmful or unnecessary surgery, requires family therapy by well-trained mental health professionals, and asks that intersexual individuals be empowered to decide on treatment after fully understanding their status. For the overall health of the individual, the organization argues against genital surgery that is primarily rooted in cosmetic concerns.

Other atypical patterns of development that fall along the gender identity continuum may not receive attention or any intervention until the child is older. Broad questions remain as to how strongly a child must identify with gender-appropriate appearance and roles and, indeed, what the list of "appropriateness" contains. Bartlett, Vasey, and Burkowski (2001) reviewed the research as to whether gender identity disorder in children (a classified disorder at the time of their research) should be viewed as a form of mental illness. Of importance was looking at whether there was distress, disability, an increased risk of loss of freedom, pain, or death, and whether a child's behavior was an individual problem or just in conflict with society. These researchers recommend that children who experience discomfort with the culturally prescribed role yet not with their biological sex should not be viewed in psychiatric terms.

A movement away from enforcing rigid gender role stereotypes is under way. Girls can have short hair; males can have long hair. When the girl wants a military-type crew cut or the male not only wants long hair but wants to set it in curls, those choices move them away from stereotypes. Similarly, parents may not worry when little girls play aggressively, wear pants, climb trees, and are interested in sports.

It seems safe to say, however, that the girl "tomboy" is more easily accepted than the "sissy boy." The boy who wants to play with dolls, is interested in female clothing, and doesn't like sports may become subjected to questions about both his gender identity and sexual orientation.

Individuals whose gender identity and gender role encompass both masculinity and femininity are referring to themselves as transgendered. The terms *transvestite* and *transsexual* have become too simplistic to cover the range of trans identities. The range of issues for these individuals varies. Being transgendered often gets confused with orientation issues, although being gay, bisexual, or heterosexual falls along another continuum. Some people cross-dress in private, finding the process sexually arousing. Others cross-dress for entertainment and are known for their skills at impersonation. Barbra Streisand is frequently a subject of impersonation. During her HBO concert in 1996, she joked that New York City is such a comfortable place for her to walk around; there were so many Barbra impersonators that she could pass without notice!

The essence of being transgendered is that one's gender identity falls somewhere away from the extremes of masculine or feminine. A person may desire to dress as the other sex does, move as the "other" sex does, and be treated as though one were a member of the other sex. The Society for the Second Self, referred to as Tri-Ess, is a chapter-based organization with members across the United States. It produces a quarterly journal filled with essays, information, and resources. The group focuses on providing support, serenity, and service (SSS) to the heterosexual cross-dresser and his/her family (Boyd, 2002).

Increasingly, college students are "coming out," so to speak, as transgendered, with campus organizations addressing LGBT issues. The concept of "transitioning" has been used by some who are exploring new ways of looking and being. A rejection of mutually exclusive categories of male and female is replaced with a perspective of fluidity and blended self-definitions. Transgendered communities share such concerns as coming out, violence, self-esteem, and access to health care along with their gay, lesbian, and bisexual peers (Maurer, 1999). At the same time, there are unique concerns, such as what physician to use to get comprehensive health care and perhaps hormone treatments.

As mentioned earlier, *gender dysphoria* is the condition in which one's anatomy is inconsistent with one's gender identity. Someone who believes he or she is trapped in the wrong body suffers greatly and may even attempt genital mutilation to remove that which emphasizes the "mistake." Even though there are more male-to-female transsexuals, female-to-male transsexuals do receive treatment. More often, however, it is the male-to-female transsexual who seeks treatment and is given sex reassignment surgery (Abramowitz, 1986).

Sex reassignment surgery, along with the array of psychiatric, hormonal, and subsequent cosmetic surgeries, represents a long and painful process. Transsexuals first must be thoroughly evaluated to ensure that gender dysphoria is the correct diagnosis. Cross-dressing is encouraged, followed by hormonal interventions to feminize male-to-female transsexuals or, conversely, masculinize female-to-male transsexuals. Changes in body hair, changes in the face, and fat deposits all move these individuals in their desired direction. These interventions are reversible if necessary and, for some, represent the extent of treatment that is both comfortable and affordable.

Surgical interventions are more complicated. The male-to-female transsexual will have the testicles and penis removed, and the skin of the penis is used to construct a vagina that can respond to sexual stimulation. A female-to-male

Courtesy of Donald R. Laub, M.D.

Surgery is used to create authentic-appearing genitalia.

transsexual will have a complete hysterectomy and a double mastectomy and will have a penis constructed. Because the clitoris is small and behind the penis, it can be left to improve sexual response.

The personal adjustments required of transgendered individuals are many. Some have lost friends, family, and jobs as they attempt to find personal happiness. The following lyrics from the Broadway musical *La Cage aux Folles* (music and lyrics by Jerry Herman, 1983), are sung by one of the main characters, a gay, effeminate, often cross-dressed man who demands to be accepted. Read the words and think of how they can apply to us all.

I Am What I Am

I am what I am. I am my own special creation.
So come take a look, Give me the hook or the ovation.
It's my world that I want to have a little pride in
My world and it's not a place I have to hide in.
Life's not worth a damn 'til you can say
"Hey world, I am what I am."
I am what I am. I don't want praise. I don't want pity.
I bang my own drum. Some think it's noise. I think it's pretty.
And so what—if I love each feather and each spangle
Why not try and see things from a different angle?
Your life is a sham 'til you can shout out loud
"I am what I am!"
I am what I am and what I am needs no excuses
I deal my own deck . . . sometimes the ace, sometimes the deuces.
There's one life, and there's no return and no deposit
One life, so it's time to open up your closet
Life's not worth a damn 'til you can say
"Hey world, I am what I am!"

Source: "I Am What I Am," Music and Lyric by Jerry Herman. © 1983 Jerry Herman. All Rights Controlled by Jerryco Music Co. Exclusive Agent: Edwin H. Morris & Company A Division of MPL Communications, Inc. All Rights Reserved.

Emotional Wellness

The cornerstone of emotional well-being is positive sexual self-esteem. Feeling good about ourselves and accepting who we are is vital to health. What is unique about emotional health is that it derives from the other dimensions of health. Feeling good about yourself may result from others liking you, or feeling good about yourself may depend on your liking your body, or a combination of these.

All of us need to have realistic expectations about who we are. As the lyrics from "I Am Who I Am" highlight, though, "Life is not worth a damn until you can shout 'I am who I am.'" In essence, we all need to accept ourselves.

The road to positive self-acceptance is longer for some than others. If you cannot be open about who you are, secrecy and oppression take their toll. Support groups and mental health professionals trained in the area of sexuality can be extremely helpful to those who are struggling with identity issues, seeking acceptance of their orientation, and figuring out how to negotiate environments that prove to be hostile. The use of resources available in books, journals, and online can greatly add to positive sexual self-esteem (Sexuality Information and Education Council of the U.S. [SIECUS], 2001).

Because our emotional health is also connected to others' behavior, we must focus attention on the need to reduce the hostility and discrimination faced by those who are perceived as "different." Improving the mental health of others and their ability to accept difference are critical factors in reducing oppression and permitting variations in lifestyle to coexist.

Your responses to the Personal Assessment, Thought Questions, and Test Yourself! quiz questions can be logged online in your Virtual Workbook at **http://health.wadsworth.com/blonna1.**

Personal Assessment

4.1 Messages About Gender

Our present thoughts and feelings concerning what being a man or a woman means have evolved over the years. A myriad of people and sources have contributed to our development. The purpose of this assessment is to trace the origin of many of the assumptions we all have about gender by examining the messages we received as children.

1. Describe in writing one specific message you received about expected male/female behavior during the following phases in your life that are applicable:
   a. Preschool
   b. Elementary school
   c. Junior high/middle school
   d. High school
   e. College
   f. Young adult (20s)
   g. Adulthood (30s–40s)
   h. Older adulthood

2. Describe the source of the message (parents, family, friends, and so forth) and the context (where/when it was delivered).

3. Describe the immediate impact of the message on your gender identity/role.

4. Describe the long-term impact of the message.

Thought Questions

1. How do biological identity, gender identity, and sexual orientation relate in the overall model of sexual identity?

2. How do biological and psychological factors interact to influence gender development?

3. What are some of the issues related to the process of "coming out" for lesbian, gay, and bisexual people?

4. Describe the various patterns of development and their impact on the identity of the individual.

Test Yourself!

1. Which term refers to one's psychological sense of being male or female?
   a. Gender role
   b. Sexual identity
   c. Gender identity
   d. Sexual preference

2. All but which are examples of sexual orientation?
   a. Transgendered
   b. Heterosexual
   c. Gay
   d. Lesbian

3. Which of the following body parts are considered *homologous* structures?
   a. Penis/vagina
   b. Uterus/prostate
   c. Clitoris/penis
   d. Testicles/uterus

4. Of the various aspects of sexual identity formation, which comes first?
   a. Chromosomal gender
   b. Gender role
   c. Secondary sex characteristics
   d. Sexual orientation

5. Adolescents are most likely to confront all but which aspect of sexual identity formation?
   a. Secondary sex characteristics
   b. Sexual orientation
   c. Gender role
   d. Gonadal development

6. Kinsey developed a continuum related to sexual identity that
   a. examines how adults valued their sexual behavior.
   b. categorizes how adults organized their sexual fantasies.
   c. categorizes how adults engaged in same-sex and opposite-sex behaviors.
   d. examined how adults identified themselves.

7. Before a young adult decides to "come out," it is recommended that he or she do all but which of the following?
   a. Join a college LGBT club.
   b. Be comfortable with labeling sexual orientation.
   c. Be sure there are financial and emotional supports in place.
   d. Assess the emotional climate in his or her home.

8. New research on the treatment of intersexed children recommends
   a. immediate postpartum surgery to create normal genitalia.
   b. delayed or no surgical intervention until adolescence or later.
   c. having young children switch gender roles to understand their situation.
   d. hormonal treatments to correct all imbalances.

9. Theories on the development of sexual orientation
   a. point to biological determinants as key.
   b. identify social determinants as key.
   c. identify parental dynamics as key.
   d. do not concur nor fully explain the development of orientation.

10. Body image issues for adolescents
    a. have developed primarily around weight issues.
    b. are more common among boys than girls.
    c. have been connected to a variety of unhealthy practices and interventions among teens.
    d. have little impact on emotional and social health.

Media Menu

You can link to the following online tools by visiting
http://health.wadsworth.com/blonna1.

Face to Face Video

Jennifer, Scott, and David speak about their sexual identity.

Animation

Kinsey Continuum

Film

Sexual Orientation

 InfoTrac Activity

Knight, J. L., & Giuliano, T. A. (2003, September). Blood, sweat, and jeers: The impact of the media's heterosexist portrayals on perceptions of male and female athletes. *Journal of Sport Behavior, 26* (3), 272.

 Web Resources

Intersex Society of North America (ISNA)

www.isna.org

A peer support, education, and advocacy group established for intersexuals, individuals born with anatomy or physiology different from cultural ideals of male and female.

Available at this site are facts and commonly asked questions, as well as the capacity to ask your own questions as well, a library to order books on the subject of transgender, and current information on a variety of health issues.

National Lesbian and Gay Health Association (NLGHA)

www.nlgha.org

Based in Washington, DC, this organization is dedicated to improving the quality of health care through education, advocacy, policy development, and facilitation of health care delivery.

Kinsey Institute for Research in Sex, Gender, and Reproduction

www.indiana.edu/~kinsey/

Supports interdisciplinary research, scholarship, and study in the field of human sexuality, gender, and reproduction. The site lists professional organizations, articles, reference resources, and a new link to Kinsey Institute Sexuality Research Information Service.

National Gay and Lesbian Task Force (NGLTF)

www.ngltf.org

A well-established national organization that advocates for gay and lesbian issues, along with providing information and support.

Parents, Families, and Friends of Lesbians and Gays (PFLAG)

www.pflag.org

A national, nonprofit organization supporting parents, families, and friends of lesbians and gays. The site provides resources, literature to assist in coping and to educate society to work to end discrimination and secure equal civil rights.

Renaissance Transgender Association

www.ren.org

Provides comprehensive education and support to transgendered persons and those close to them. The association offers programs and resources for cross dressers, transvestites, and transsexuals. The site offers articles from the International Congress on Sex and Gender.

National Association of Lesbian, Gay, Bisexual, and Transgender Community Centers (NALGBTCC)

www.lgbtcenters.org

Coordinates information on community centers across the United States that serve the LGBT community.

References

Abramowitz, S. (1986). Psychosocial outcomes of sex reassignment surgery. *Journal of Consulting and Clinical Psychology, 54,* 183–189.

Bailey, J. M., & Pillard, C. (1991). A genetic study of male sexual orientation. *Archives of General Psychiatry, 48,* 1089–1096.

Bailey, J. M., Pillard, C., Neal, M. C., & Agyei, Y. (1993). Heritable factors influence sexual orientation in women. *Archives of General Psychiatry, 50,* 217–223.

Banks, A., & Gartrell, N. K. (1995). Hormones and "sexual orientation": A questionable link. *Journal of Homosexuality, 28,* 247–268.

Barlett, N. H., Vasey, P., & Bukowski, W. (2000, December). Is gender identity disorder in children a mental disorder? *Sex Roles: A Journal of Research.*

Bell, A., Weinberg, M., & Hammersmith, S. (1981). *Sexual preference.* Bloomington: Indiana University Press.

Bem, S. (1993). *The lenses of gender: Transforming the debate on sexual inequality.* New Haven, CT: Yale University Press.

Bem, S. (1995, April). *Dismantling gender polarization: Shall we turn the volume down* or *shall we turn the volume up?* Keynote address, 1995 Eastern Region Annual Conference, Society for the Scientific Study of Sexuality, West Atlantic City, NJ.

Bockting, W. O. (1999, October/November). From construction to context: Gender through the eyes of the transgendered. *SIECUS Report, 28* (1), 3–7.

Boyd, R. (2002, Fall). What do you say to a college class? *The Mirror, 27*(3), 54–56.

Brody, L. (1997, Summer). Gender and emotion: Beyond stereotypes. *Journal of Social Issues, 53* (2), 369.

Colapinto, J. (2000). *As nature made him: The boy who was raised as a girl.* New York: HarperCollins.

Coleman, E., Gooren, L., & Ross, M. (1989). Theories of gender transpositions: A critique and suggestions for further research. *Journal of Sex Research, 26* (4), 525–538.

Diamond, M. (1982). Sexual identity, monozygotic twins reared in discordant sex roles and a BBC follow up. *Archives of Sexual Behavior, 11* (2), 181–186.

Diamond, D., & Sigmundson, H. K. (1997, March). Sex reassignment at birth: Long-term review and clinical implications. *Archives of Pediatrics and Adolescent Medicine, 51,* 298–304.

Diamond, M., Sigmundson, H. K., & Reimer, D. (2002, November 9). *Sexual and gender identities: The significance of the John/Joan case.* Paper presented at the annual meeting of the Society for the Scientific Study of Sexuality, Montreal.

Ellis, L., & Ames, M.A. (1987). Neurohormonal function and sexual orientation: A theory of homosexuality-heterosexuality. *Psychological Bulletin, 101,* 233–258.

Ellis, L., Ames, M. A., Peckham, W., & Burke, D. (1988). Sexual orientation of human offspring may be altered by severe maternal stress during pregnancy. *Journal of Sex Research, 25,* 152–157.

Hines, M., & Collaer, M. L. (1993). Gonadal hormones and sex differences. *Annual Review of Sex Research, 4,* 1–48.

Intersex Society of North America. (1995). *Recommendations for treatment: Intersex infants and children.* San Francisco: Author.

Kinsey, A., Pomeroy, W., & Martin, C. (1948). *Sexual behavior in the human female.* Philadelphia: Saunders.

Kinsey, A., Pomeroy, W., Martin, C., & Gebhard, P. (1953). *Sexual behavior in the human female.* Philadelphia: Saunders.

Klein, F. (1978). *The bisexual option.* New York: Arbor House.

Klein, F., Sepekoff, B., & Wolf, T. J. (1985). Sexual orientations: A multivariable dynamic process. In F. Klein & T. J. Wolf (Eds.), *Bisexualities: Theory and research.* New York: Haworth.

Laumann, E., Gagnon, J., Michael, R., & Michaels, S. (1994). *The social organization of sexuality: Sexual practices in the United States.* Chicago: University of Chicago Press.

LeVay, S. (1991). A difference in hypothalamic structure between heterosexual and homosexual men. *Science, 253,* 1034–1037.

Lorde, A. (2001). Age, race, class, and sex: Women redefining difference. In P. S. Rothenberg (Ed.), *Race, class, and gender in the United States: An integrated study* (5th ed., pp. 588–594). New York: Freeman.

Marrone, N. (2001, April/May). Advice to Latino parents of GLBT children. *SIECUS Report, 29* (4).

Maurer, L. (1999, October/November). Transgressing sex and gender: Deconstruction zone ahead? *SIECUS Report, 28* (1).

Mead, M. (1935). *Sex and temperament in three primitive societies*. New York: Morrow.

Michael, R., Gagnon, J., Laumann, E., & Kolata, G. (1994). *Sex in America*. Boston: Little, Brown.

Money, J. (1999). *The lovemap guidebook: A definitive statement*. New York: Continuum.

Money, J., & Ehrhardt, A. (1972). *Man and woman, boy and girl*. Baltimore, MD: Johns Hopkins University Press.

Muehlenhard, C. (2000, May). Categories and sexuality. *Journal of Sex Research, 37* (2), 101–107.

Ryan, C., & Futterman, D. (2001, April/May). Social and developmental challenges for lesbian, gay, and bisexual youth. *SIECUS Report, 29*(4).

Sauerman, T. H. (1998). *Read this before coming out to your parents*. Philadelphia: PFLAG Philadelphia.

Sexuality Information and Education Council of the U.S. (2001, April/May). Lesbian, gay, bisexual, and transgender sexuality and related issues: Annotated bibliography and website directory. *SIECUS Report Supplement, 29*(4).

Vance, C. (1988). Anthropology rediscovers sexuality: A theoretical comment. *Social Science Medicine, 33* (8), 875–884

Wiederman, M. W. (2001). Orientation: What determines sexual attraction to men or women? In *Understanding sexual research* (pp. 74–81). Belmont, CA: Wadsworth/Thomson Learning.

Woodhill, B. M., & Samuels, C. A. (2003, June). Positive and negative androgyny and their relationship with psychological health and well-being." *Sex Roles: A Journal of Research*.

Woodside, D., Blake, M., Woodside, D. B., Garfinkel, P. E., Kin, E., Goering, P., Kaplan, A. S., Goldbloom, D. S., & Kennedy, S. H. (2001, April). Comparisons of men with full or partial eating disorders, men without eating disorders, and women with eating disorders, in the community. *American Journal of Psychiatry, 158*, 570.

chapter *five*

Child *and* Adolescent Sexuality

Student Learning Objectives

After reading this chapter, students will be able to

- Compare and contrast a variety of theories of personality from birth through adolescence.

- Describe how the key aspects from various psychological theories impact sexual development.

- Discuss the effects of parenting practices such as bonding, toilet training, and nudity on healthy sexual development.

- Compare the biological consequences of puberty with the psychosocial aspects of adolescence.

- Describe the findings of a variety of studies concerning adolescent sexual behavior.

- Compare the adolescent sexual behavior of people in the United States with those from other cultures.

- Evaluate the positive and negative aspects of sexual activity during adolescence.

Test your understanding of these objectives by taking the end-of-chapter quiz, available online at **http://health.wadsworth.com/blonna1.**

activity teaser: *How do you decide what sexual behavior is right for you? Find out with the Personal Exploration Activity on page 150.*

case study 5.1

Rebecca and Jake

Rebecca, 24, and Jake, 25, are white.

Critical Thinking

How do parents develop parenting strategies that bridge the gaps among how they each were raised, what they have learned to be healthy for their child, and what they are each comfortable with as parents?

Use your Virtual Workbook to explore your answer to this question at **http://health.wadsworth.com/blonna1.**

Rebecca and Jake became parents for the first time in their mid-20s. They both were so excited at the birth of Adam yet nervous at the same time about how to be good parents.

REBECCA: I grew up in a very puritanical household. My parents rarely touched or showed any kind of physical affection toward each other or my brother and me. I know they loved each other and us, but it just wasn't their way to express it physically, in public. Nudity also was not tolerated, and sex was never discussed. Being with Jake has taught me that the physical expression of affection and love is a natural and positive thing.

JAKE: I come from a very physical, touchy family. Our whole family loves to hug and kiss, and visitors rarely get in or out of the house without a big hug hello and good-bye. When Rebecca and I got together, differences in our attitudes about touch had to be worked out between us. I love being naked, and for me touch does not always mean "I want some sex." I felt it was really important that Rebecca commit to breastfeeding Adam . . . she knew the health benefits, but the reality of if at all seemed to scare her a bit.

We often just sit and look at Adam, our precious little baby. We want him to grow up healthy and comfortable with his sexuality. We've been taking turns getting up to change and feed Adam. When it's Rebecca's turn, she gets up, goes into Adam's room, and nurses him while rocking in the chair in his room. When it's my turn, I bring Adam into our bed and then put him back in his crib after nursing. We both love the skin–skin contact we share with the baby and each other.

REBECCA: Despite how tired we both are, we know that this phase of being parents is only the beginning. There will be so many more challenges down the line. What we know for sure is that we will work together to help Adam navigate through the sexual challenges of childhood and the teen years.

As you sit here reading, you may want to ask yourself, "How did I get to be the sexual person that I am?" You look a particular way and have your own unique thoughts, feelings, attractions, and needs. Despite what is often a cultural desire to protect children from things sexual, the reality is that profound aspects of sexual development occur in childhood and adolescence. How you are as an adult stems from the varied influences and experiences you have had "growing up." And as we explore adult issues in Chapter 6, you may want to question when, if ever, development *stops*.

Psychosexual development is the process of becoming a sexual person. The term traditionally refers to the psychological aspects of sexual development. As we've mentioned throughout this text, though, to completely separate the psychological from the physical, intellectual, emotional, social, spiritual, and environmental facets of our sexuality is not possible. Most discussions of psychosexual development present it as an outgrowth of personality, with great emphasis placed on the first years of life. Although the classic personality theorists remain important as a foundation, current theorists and critics have examined the interplay of biological, psychological, social, and cultural influences on the overall development of sexuality. In addition, debates continue as to what is truly "healthy" for children and teens.

Personality is the entire collection of one's thoughts, attitudes, values, beliefs, perceptions, and behaviors. Our personalities define how we see ourselves independently and within our environment. Personality is constantly evolving and is

Psychosexual development The blending of sexual aspects of one's development with other psychological factors

Personality The collection of values, attitudes, and behavior that make us who we are cumulative in nature. Your personality today is the sum total of all of the things you have experienced until this point in your life. Various theories have been proposed to explain how personality develops.

Traditional Theories of Personality

Behaviorism: John Watson

Behaviorism, developed by John Watson (1970), proposes that personality develops as a result of responses to general and specific stimuli. Behaviorists believe that at birth we are blank slates with no predetermined attributes. Our personalities evolve as the result of myriad interactions between stimuli (people, places, events, situations, images) and the responses they evoke. Responses can be either positive or negative and vary in strength. The more powerful the response, the more likely we will either embrace (positive response) or reject (negative response) whatever stimulus prompted it.

Let's use masturbation to explain how this stimulus-response model works. Imagine that when you were an infant, your mother caught you fondling yourself while lying on the rug in the living room in front of your grandmother. Your mother was upset and smacked your hand, saying, "Bad girl. Little ladies don't touch themselves down there." This negative reinforcement (slapping the hand away and saying "bad girl") in response to a stimulus (touching yourself) begins to shape how you feel toward masturbation. The specific context (in the living room, in a public setting, in front of Grandma) also contributes to shaping the behavior.

If this response is repeated over time, in similar and different contexts, it can either extinguish (get rid of) the behavior of masturbation or drive it underground and surround it with shame and guilt. The person then might practice the behavior in private and associate it with negative feelings.

Other personality theories stress developmental stages and tasks. These theories propose that personality develops in stages that build upon each other.

> **Behaviorism** A stimulus-response theory of personality development grounded in the belief that human personality evolves as a result of the interaction between exposure to stimuli and the responses that this exposure evokes in the person. Watson is credited with the theory, expanded later by Skinner.

Humanism: Abraham Maslow

Abraham Maslow (1970) was one of the most influential humanists. The premise of **humanism** is that human beings are motivated by a desire for personal growth. Maslow believed that all humans are unique and are capable of growth and reaching their utmost potential in all facets of their lives. Humans are essentially good and are capable of making choices about the direction their lives will take. Maslow believed that all people are capable of reaching their highest potential if they progress through a series of stages of development that meet various basic human needs. Figure 5.1 presents Maslow's hierarchy of needs. As you can see, they reflect the physical, social, intellectual, emotional, spiritual, and environmental domains that characterize present-day wellness theory.

Before people can develop loving, intimate relationships, they must meet their most fundamental needs for survival and safety that form the basis of the pyramid. To get to the top, one has to pass through all of the previous levels, successfully meeting the needs of each stage before proceeding to the next. The top of Maslow's pyramid, self-actualization, represents the pinnacle of human development. People reaching the top are said to be fully self-actualized.

Maslow also believed that, as we work our way up this pyramid, we often encounter "peak experiences"—moments that crystallize what it means to be fully alive, to **transcend** mere existence. He felt that these peak experiences help us feel connected to the world around us, to be one with our universe.

> **Humanism** A theory of personality development proposing that human personality development is shaped by innate desire and need for maximizing personal growth

> **Transcend** To rise above or extend beyond ordinary limits

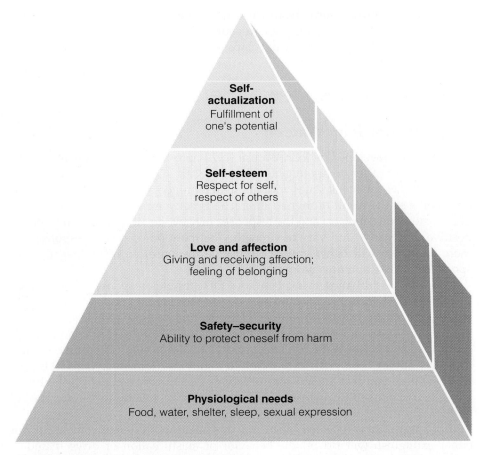

Figure 5.1 *Maslow's Hierarchy of Needs*

The following are characteristics of individuals who achieve self-actualization through transcendence:

1. Transcenders have more "peak" or creative experiences than others.
2. Transcenders are more responsive to beauty and more holistic in their perceptions of humanity and the world.
3. Transcenders are innovators who are attracted to the unknown, embrace change, and see themselves as the instruments of their transcendence.
4. Transcenders can fuse work and play. They are less attracted by the rewards of money and more motivated by the satisfaction of being true to whom they really are and serving others.
5. Transcenders are more likely to accept others with unconditional positive regard.

Psychoanalytic Theory: Sigmund Freud

Freudian **psychoanalytic theory** purports that personality develops as a result of a struggle between conscious and unconscious forces in our lives (Hall, 1954). These forces are directed by our **ego** (the rational, thinking mind), **superego** (the conscience), and **id** (the pleasure-seeking life force). The ego is conscious and based in reality, interweaving sensory perceptions with thoughts and memories. The superego, which is partially unconscious, is judgmental; it factors in our beliefs about right and wrong.

Psychoanalytic theory Also known as Freudian theory (after its founder, Sigmund Freud), describes personality development as outgrowth of interaction of id (pleasure-seeking, guilt-free), superego (the conscience, influenced by society and parents), and ego (rational, analytical mind driven by logical thinking)

Ego Rational, analytical facet of human mind, according to Freudian theory

Superego The conscience, influenced by society and family, according to Freudian theory

Freud called the fuel of this life force "libidinal energy." The id does not distinguish between right and wrong, good and evil. Whatever brings pleasure is good. The superego (in concert with the ego) is supposed to keep the id in check.

Freud believed that the transference of libidinal energy has direct consequences for our psychosexual development. He outlined stages of development, each with a set of needs to be satisfied:

Oral stage. The first, or oral, stage lasts from birth to the second year of life. During the oral stage, stimulation of the mouth through sucking, biting, and swallowing is the main source of erotic satisfaction. Inadequate satisfaction during the oral stage, according to Freud, would produce an "oral personality"— someone preoccupied with mouth habits such as overeating or smoking.

Anal stage. During the second, anal phase, from ages 2 to 3, libidinal energy shifts to the anus. During this stage, the child derives pleasure from anal stimulation and being in control of defecation. This provides the child's first real opportunity to assert some independence from parental control. This stage coincides with toilet training. Freud believed it is the holding back or letting go of bowel movements (personal control) that produces physical and psychological pleasure for the child. Rushing a child through toilet training (thereby limiting the ability to derive anal pleasure) or making too big a fuss over soiling the diapers or making a mess could result in fixation at this stage. People who are fixated at this stage are either anal-expulsive (dirty, extravagant, wasteful) or anal-retentive (excessively clean, neat, cheap, and compulsive).

Phallic stage. The third phase of development is the phallic stage, between the third and fourth years. During this time, libidinal energy shifts to the genitals, and the child derives erotic pleasure through fondling and exhibitionism. Freud also believed that during this time the child develops a sexual attachment to the opposite-sex parent and becomes fearful of the parent of the same sex. Named the **Oedipal complex** (after the Greek legend in which Oedipus killed his father and married his mother), this attachment, if handled calmly and without undue concern or punishment, gradually subsides as the child moves into the next stage, latency. Psychoanalytic theorists focus on the dynamics of this phase in their attempts to explain sexual orientation.

Latency stage. Freud believed that sexuality goes into a period of latency extending from age 5 until **puberty.** At this time, the child becomes more focused on nonsexual interests such as intellectual and social issues. Modern observance of young children and preadolescents clarifies the difficulties with accepting such a concept. Sexual exploration, sex games, and, for some, mature sexual involvement makes latency an archaic idea.

Genital stage. At puberty, genital sexuality reemerges, and the adolescent becomes sexually attracted to members of the opposite sex, a prerequisite for marriage and childrearing. Freud placed marriage as the culmination of normal psychosexual development.

Freud's theory is valued more for its place in history than its current usefulness. His work brought the importance of sexuality to an understanding of personality development, yet serious questions about his methods and biases have diminished the value of his work for contemporary analysis of sexual development. From a modern perspective, Freud was sexist and heterosexist, not understanding female sexual response or the healthy development of homosexuality and bisexuality.

Eight Stages of Development: Erik Erikson

Erik Erikson (1978) constructed a model of personality development that views it as the result of a struggle between opposing forces that present themselves in a series of stages that occur throughout our lives. Figure 5.2 shows Erikson's eight

Id Pleasure-seeking, guilt-free facet of human mind, according to Freudian theory

Oedipal complex A psychoanalytical term (named after Oedipus in Shakespeare's play) that describes the internal struggle that 3- to 4-year-olds face as they begin to identify more with their opposite-sex parent

Puberty Biological transition from childhood to young adulthood

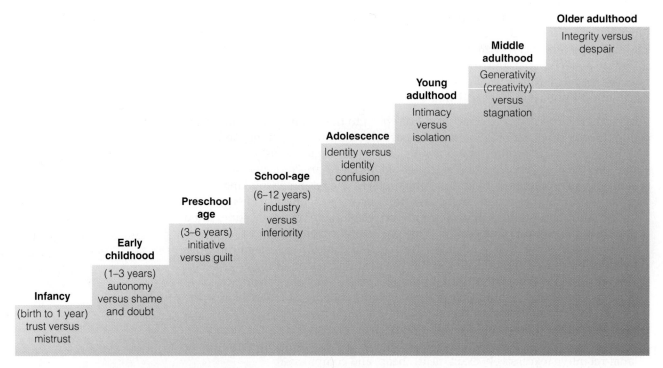

Figure 5.2 *Erikson's Developmental Stages and Conflicts*

stages of development. Instead of the struggle between the libidinal-driven id and the ego/superego, Erikson viewed development as a conflict between opposing psychosocial forces and qualities. According to Erikson, to continue to grow, we must resolve these crises.

Healthy personality development results from accomplishing the developmental tasks required for the stage and then moving on to the next one. In a sense, positive attributes win out over negative attributes, and the personality development moves to the next level. Inadequate task resolution results in thwarted development in that particular area. This leaves the person with a lack of certain skills and attributes that will be needed later in life.

For example, if, as an infant, one never successfully develops a sense of trust in oneself and others, the person will grow up with a stronger sense of mistrust. This stays with the person throughout life, limiting the ability to trust others, develop sustained loving relationships, and maximize the individual's potential as an adult. The inability to trust another person makes it difficult to develop intimate relationships based on faith and sharing deeply personal emotions.

Modern Theory

It is important to understand that certain theorists provided the basis from which contemporary work has evolved. Today, some question the very foundations of traditional personality theory. **Feminist theory,** for example, posits that personality and identity are socially constructed. What is "correct development" for boys is different from what is deemed "correct development" for girls. Judith Lorber (2001) writes, "I am arguing that bodies differ in many ways physiologically, but they are completely transformed by social practices to fit into the salient categories of a society, the most pervasive of which are 'female' and 'male' and 'women' and 'men'" (p. 48). Feminist scholars challenge the culture to reexamine

Feminist theory Theories that argue that personality and identity are socially constructed. What is "correct development" for boys is different from what is deemed "correct development" for girls.

the power structure, encouraging broader developmental choices for both boys and girls.

As feminism worked to increase options for girls, others brought to light the need to reexamine how boys are raised, and the limitations placed on their development as well. Michael Gurian (1996), in *The Wonder of Boys*, writes:

> It requires pretty effective blinders these days to think as I did in the early 1980's—that boys are boys and girls are girls predominantly because of environmental forces. It is more accurate to say that much of who we are is determined by body chemicals, brain differences, hormones, and by society's efforts to honor this biology through its socializing forces. (p. 5)

Gurian is a firm believer that boys are hard-wired to be a particular way but can be raised to be confident, caring contributors to the culture at large.

The new area of research called **Queer theory** has expanded the scholarship that examines the development of sexual orientation. In particular, those identified with this movement challenge heterosexuality as the only valid "end point" of psychosexual development. They argue for a more fluid understanding of gender and orientation, and the role that power and politics play in development (Butler, 1999).

In 2002, Judith Levine raised the ire of many with her book *Harmful to Minors: The Perils of Protecting Children from Sex*. She writes that sex is and should be a positive and wonderful part of children's lives, and that cultural attempts to protect them from information and experiences was harmful to their health and development. She was both critical of conservatives who promoted abstinence-until-marriage ideology and curricula, as well as those who were advocating comprehensive sexuality education, which in her view was doing too little, too late.

Bookstores today are filled with shelves of books on parenting. Write parenting on the search line of a browser, and numerous references and selections for purchase will appear. Is there one book that is the ultimate guide for the development of sexually healthy children? Our response is no. Professionals do not agree. Theorists do not agree. Even family members do not agree. That said, it is important to understand that both scholarship and clinical practice have much to offer for better parenting. The realities and complexities of sexual development, however, do not lend themselves to easy guidelines and rules.

Early Development

Five common themes related to early sexuality transcend all of the theories about sexual development: bonding, other expressions of physical intimacy, self-exploration and masturbation, nudity, and toilet training. Even though theorists might differ in their interpretation and significance, most would agree that they exert a tremendous impact on sexual development. These critical sexual development issues surface during infancy and childhood and remain throughout life. How our caregivers initially handle these issues strongly influences the direction our development takes.

The major task of infancy, according to Erikson, is to develop a sense of trust. For trust to win out over mistrust is essential to continuing healthy psychological development in all of us.

Bonding

One of the earliest behaviors that helps foster trust and satisfies our most primal physiological needs is bonding. **Bonding** is a process of developing a close physical and psychological relationship with one's primary caregiver. Bonding be-

Queer theory Theories that look to explain sexual orientation and sexual identity without relying on heterosexuality as the norm

Bonding The close physical emotional attachment between infants and their primary caregiver(s)

Bonding can take many forms. Here a mom plays in the pool with her child.

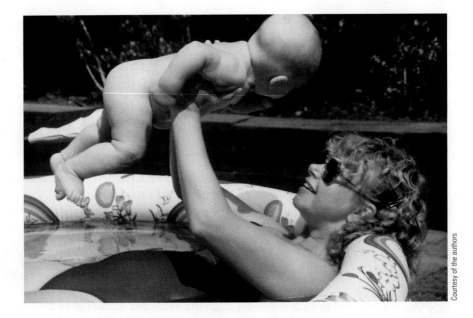

Courtesy of the authors

tween mother and child begins almost immediately as the newborn and mother are brought together to share the first moments of life. Bonding continues as mother and child are brought together during feeding, diaper changing, and simple things such as smiling, talking to the child, and acknowledging the child when approaching him or her.

Fathers also fulfill a bonding role. They are often present at the birth of the baby and develop strong, close physical bonds with their children, sharing in their care and feeding. The increased use of the word *parenting* rather than *mothering* and *fathering* reflects social changes around the raising of children. Parents increasingly divide child-rearing responsibilities to fit with their work schedules and time at home.

During the bonding process, infants learn to associate the mother and father with fulfilling the most basic needs for sustaining life. Trust in the world as a whole begins by trusting in mothers and fathers. Infants respond positively to touch. **Thriving**—a term pediatricians use to describe physical and psychological growth—is enhanced by touch and bonding. Failure to thrive has been noted in infants who, among other things, have been deprived of sufficient physical nurturing during infancy. As children, these infants often lack the cognitive and motor abilities of their peers.

Thriving Pattern of normal weight gain, neuromuscular development, and other developmental attributes of infants

Other Forms of Physical Intimacy

In addition to bonding as a contributor to the development of sensuality and sexuality, other forms of touch play an important part. Beyond the basic need of touch for infants to thrive, touch is related to the development of sensuality. Our entire skin surface is capable of acting as an erogenous zone. It is sensitive to touch in all of its manifestations. Babies love to be held, stroked, and rocked. Although we can't interview them, we can tell this from the cooing sounds they make, their facial expressions, and their continued responsiveness to our stroking and hugging them. Our ability or inability to respond positively to physical intimacy is believed to be rooted in the time our parents spent touching and stroking us as infants (Montague, 1986).

How we touch babies varies from generalized hugging and stroking to infant massage and baby exercise. Infant massage strokes are similar to those used with adults, but much gentler. Care must be taken to avoid sharp movements. Infants generally won't last through an entire full-body massage; they begin to wriggle and laugh. Beyond the closeness and benefits from touch that massage affords, research has identified additional health benefits that result from the effect massage has on the body. Infant massage has been found to help babies adjust their circadian rhythms and move toward better sleeping habits, as well as promote better health and development (Ferber, Laudon, Kuint, Weller, & Zisapel, 2002; Globus, 2002).

Unfortunately, many parents feel awkward or uncomfortable expressing themselves through touch and physical contact. Some of us have grown up in households where touch was withheld or minimized. Sometimes parents worry that their feelings (or their child's) are sexual, not sensual. Even though infants are capable of experiencing erotic pleasure, sensual pleasure shared with your child and sexual desire are different. Mature, parental sensual pleasure associated with hugging and stroking one's child is vastly different from sexually desiring that child. There is no intention of genital sexual contact, nor is there any desire to experience such behavior.

An aversion to touch is a learned behavior. As such, you can unlearn it and not make the same mistakes with your own children. In sharing the joys of touch with them, you can relearn the joys of physical closeness and sensuality.

Grandparents can lavish love and attention on their grandchildren, bringing extra sources of affection.

Michael Newman/PhotoEdit, Inc.

Spiritual and Emotional Wellness

Although we are not always cognizant of it as infants and children, we begin to develop a sense of connectedness or disconnectedness during this stage. Probably the earliest manifestation of spirituality is the bonding with primary caregivers. This is a powerful connection not only to other human beings but also to the world as a whole. Developing a sense of trust in ourselves, others, and the world as a whole begins with the skin-to-skin nurturing we receive from our parents in times of need. Parents and caregivers often describe the feeling of bonding and nurturing of an infant as one of the most profoundly spiritual feelings they have ever experienced. Many rediscover a sense of awe and faith in the power of love by connecting with and nurturing our children.

Infant and childhood emotional development forms the foundation for much of our adult emotional makeup. Basic personality constructs such as self-esteem, trust, happiness, and optimism begin to take shape during infancy and childhood. As Maslow and other developmental theorists point out, the ability to fully self-actualize as adults requires people to meet basic emotional needs early in life. It's harder to love others as adults if a person was not loved as an infant and if pieces of one's emotional development were left scattered on the floor of childhood and **adolescence.** Nurturing infants, children, and adolescents, attending to their needs, and providing a safe haven and outlet for their desires are all essential for their continuing emotional development and healthy sexuality.

Adolescence Time period representing the psychosocial transition from childhood to young adulthood

Self-Exploration and Masturbation

All infants discover the joys of genital pleasure inadvertently. They discover what it feels like to have their genitals rub against things in their immediate environment (crib, blanket, toys, diaper, clothing, their mother and father). If allowed to do so, infants between 6 and 12 months of age will touch their genitals. They will learn that they are capable of initiating the same pleasurable feelings they felt when rubbing against objects.

Masturbation Individual or mutual stimulation of genitalia by hand or using other objects

Sexologists have long debated whether this behavior should be considered **masturbation,** a form of "sexual" behavior. Although it is definitely sensual and erotic, it lacks the associated sexual connotations that older children and adults have concerning genital pleasuring. These associations are learned later. This genital play should be evaluated exactly for what it is—play (Kaplan, 1974). It feels good, and children become frustrated if their hands are kept away from their genitals.

Infant self-exploration and masturbation also lay the foundation for developing a broad continuum of sexual feelings and behaviors. Masturbation is a normal developmental act, one of the earliest forms of sexual activity. Most children discover masturbation quite innocently as a physical, not sexual, act.

Boys' penile erections often occur as sexual reflexes in response to a variety of stimuli ranging from self-touching to breastfeeding. Girls experience clitoral erection and lubrication under similar circumstances.

These earliest attempts at self-exploration teach us about our body and the potential it has for providing pleasure. Conversely, the body has the potential for negatively influencing sexual development if parents overreact to their children's attempts at self-stimulation. Adults who punish children for masturbating may be denying them valuable opportunities for learning about self-pleasuring and setting the stage for negative attitudes (shame, guilt, fear) about sex. Parents who say nothing about masturbation send negative messages through their omission. Children learn that these omissions represent areas that are off-limits for discussion.

Yelling at a child, slapping his or her hand away, admonishing the child for doing something "dirty"—these adult responses to masturbation convey strong negative messages. Negatively reinforcing a behavior that is pleasurable—self-exploration—creates a confusing mixed message. If it is more related to the timing of these acts (little Billy always seems to play with his penis when Grandma is sitting next to him), gently moving the child to a crib or playpen in another room might help. When children become verbal, caregivers might explain to them that playing with themselves under private conditions (such as in their own rooms) is OK but it is not all right in more public settings where it might offend others (such as Grandma or the neighbors).

Self-exploration, again, is normal. It cannot be carried to excess and is self-limiting if children are left alone. Adults should view it like other forms of play. It is amusing for a while, and then the child moves on to something else. If left alone, children will not sit in their rooms all day and play with themselves. Parents who cannot accept their children's self-exploration might discuss the matter with a counselor, priest, rabbi, minister, pediatrician, or sex therapist to get help in dealing with their feelings. Exploring their sexual fears and concerns will reassure them that this self-touching behavior will not misguide their children's sexual development.

Nudity

Infants and children are nudists at heart. Most infants and young children are perfectly comfortable lying and running around the house naked. They do not associate nudity with morality. To be naked to them is simply to be without clothes. Parents and other caregivers (and, later, society at large) teach infants and children that nudity has sexual overtones.

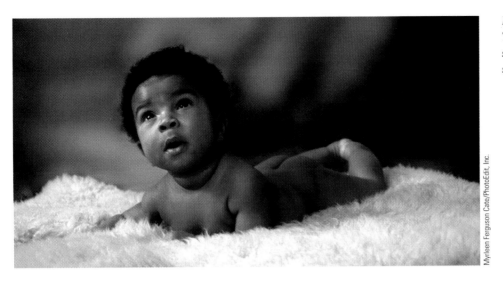

Myrleen Ferguson Cate/PhotoEdit, Inc.

Babies are sensual creatures. They like to be nude and feel softness and textures of things such as sheepskin throws.

Our culture, however, associates nudity with sexuality. In contrast, Scandinavian cultures have nude beaches that cater to families. Being naked with one's family is considered normal and healthy.

Unlike some other cultures that accept nudity as part of life and don't make a big deal about it one way or another, U.S. culture frowns upon most public displays of nakedness. We owe this to our Puritan heritage. When they came to America, the Puritans enacted many laws that attempted to curtail public displays of nakedness and sexual behavior. To this day, laws dating back to the early 1800s still are on the books concerning things such as proper swimming attire. The rigid views concerning sex and nudity grew out of Victorian England in the 19th century. In that formal, rigid culture, visions of naked flesh were linked to uncontrolled sexual desire and giving into the will of the devil. In an almost comical adherence to covering their exposed limbs, the Victorians went to extremes such as putting "skirts" onto the legs of pianos and chairs lest they offend and tempt their owners to engage in lewd behavior.

Even though most states allow private displays of nudity in nudist colonies, this behavior is the exception rather than the rule. Community opposition to nude beaches, clubs, and public displays of nudity is still strong. Women seem to bear a heavier burden than men in our culture. Men are almost always allowed to go topless in public, whereas female toplessness is considered lewd and almost always against the law.

Given our puritanical heritage and history of opposition to nudity, most Americans, not surprisingly, feel more comfortable with their clothes on than off. This collective discomfort with nudity affects our comfort level with our own bodies and our ability to relax and be sensual and sexual with others.

Understanding nudity and how we deal with it with our infants and children has many facets. How we handle nudity plays a big part in the kind of foundation we lay for our children's psychosexual development. Many parents fear being nude with their children. Their fears range from their baby "having an accident" (unintentional urination/defecation) to transmitting the wrong message about sex. In actuality, letting your child be naked or being nude with your child is perfectly normal and healthy.

Bonding is enhanced by nudity. The warmth and close, physical contact that can be achieved from skin-to-skin contact is unparalleled. Even partial nudity, torso to torso, conveys a special closeness that cannot be achieved any other way. Allowing your children to be nude while establishing reasonable parameters for family nudity seems to be a prudent, middle-of-the-road approach to this issue.

case study 5.2

The Family Bath

Cara and Charles are in their early 30s; she identifies as biracial and he as African American.

Critical Thinking

What are your views on family nudity? Do you think that parents and children "should" be comfortable seeing each other without clothes? Is it more appropriate to cover up at some point for healthy development?

Use your Virtual Workbook to explore your answers to these questions at **http://health.wadsworth.com/blonna1.**

Cara and Charles loved being naked and seldom wore a lot of clothes around the house when the children, Aisha and Rakeen, were little. As a couple, they had a ritual of bathing together as much as possible. Once the kids outgrew their infant tubs, each parent took turns being responsible for giving the kids a bath. Because the children were only 2 years apart, sometimes both kids were bathed together. On other occasions one parent or the other would get into the tub with the kids. Getting the whole family into the tub was just too crowded.

As a family, all four were able to enjoy being in water together when they visited the grandparents in South Carolina. Next to a small swimming pool was a tiny hot tub that fit four very comfortably. The freedom of being naked in the water, however, was replaced with the need to be in a bathing suit. Nonetheless, all four could enjoy the family time together in the water.

When Cara and Charles added a new addition to their home, they purposely spent the extra money so that a large bathtub could be installed. The ritual of bathing as a couple could now be continued without overlapping legs and arms. Even the faucet was out of the way! What was missing, however, was the family nudity. The kids, now 11 and 13, had no interest in getting in the water naked with their parents. While getting changed in front of the kids and being naked is still a pattern at home, Cara and Charles seem to be getting more unsolicited feedback about their own bodies. "Ewww . . . you have so much hair there! Am I going to get hair like that?" Or, "Mom, why do you have so many stretch marks over there? Do all moms get those?" The kids seem to have moved to greater body awareness, self-consciousness, and a general need *not* to see their parents naked. The family bath will have to be relegated to memory.

Sol Gordon, renowned sexuality educator, believes that parents are taking on a relaxed attitude about nudity (Gordon & Gordon, 1983). Furthermore, Gordon believes that being nude with your child creates many "teachable moments"—those points in time when a child's curiosity about sexuality is given a natural outlet. Children will want to know why "Mommy doesn't have a penis" or why "Daddy's penis is bigger than Junior's." These spontaneous questions provide opportunities to ask questions and explore basic sexual information and issues. In a way, it helps parents become more "askable." Capitalizing on teachable moments is a way to take advantage of children's natural curiosity and is preferable to forcing discussions about the "birds and the bees" at inopportune times. Children naturally grow out of the desire to be nude around their parents. As they move into middle childhood and prepubescence, they become more independent and develop a personal sense of modesty. This is usually accompanied by their desire for more privacy and for other family members to be more fully clothed around the house.

Skin-to-skin contact is something babies and adults enjoy.

Lawrence Manning/CORBIS

Toilet Training

The mastery of toilet training is essential in completing the developmental tasks of toddlers, as well as building a solid foundation for sexual health and positive psychosexual development. Toilet training is empowering for children. Along with mastering bowel control, they gain a measure of self-control, self-esteem, and independence. Wearing "big boy pants" is how one friend's son refers to his newfound freedom from diapers.

If parents or caregivers handle toilet training properly and do not rush their children, they develop a sense of pride in accomplishing something important to them. Toilet training is messy and involves a lot of time and work. Parents need to understand this and be careful not to punish their children or criticize them too harshly for the inevitable "mistakes" and soiled underpants they will encounter. Splitting the labor can help. When moms and dads (or other combinations of caregivers) work together, they each get a break from changing diapers and cleaning up messes.

Parents also need to accept that each child progresses through this stage on a different time schedule. When children are ready to give up diapers, they will. Adults can't rush the process or predict how long it will take. Trying to rush the child to fit someone else's time line (for example, the day care center will take only toilet-trained children) may not be the best strategy. Following these simple guidelines, your children can develop those all-important feelings of self-control and self-esteem (Gordon & Gordon, 1983).

Other Early Tasks

Another major developmental task of early childhood is learning to walk. Children who are helped with, but not overly protected from, the bumps and falls that are a normal part of learning to walk develop a sense of control over their environment. They learn about the literal "bumps and bruises" that are a normal part of achieving anything meaningful in life.

As children become more autonomous, they need to be able to explore their environment safely. To develop a sense of self-control and self-esteem, they need to have hazard-free environments and the freedom to explore them autonomously. Children whose exploratory play is restricted or unsafe may even become fearful of being alone or taking a risk later in life. Children who are overly protected and shielded from even the most minor stumbles have a harder time becoming autonomous.

Parents have to realize that boys and girls alike need to develop this sense of autonomy, and they are equally able to sustain the normal bumps and bruises inherent in developing autonomy. Traditional parents may feel a need to protect their daughters out of some ill-conceived notion of their frailty. Realize that the skills essential for developing autonomy are also critical for healthy sexual development. Although they are not overtly sexual in nature, these skills help build self-esteem and self-confidence that will influence the child's, and later the adolescent's, ability to make good sexual decisions and minimize unnecessary risk taking.

Development in Early Childhood

Self-exploration continues during early childhood (ages 3 to 5) and often extends to playmates. The more mobile child now begins to interact with other children more frequently. Games such as "doctor" and "nurse" typically provide opportunities for sex play and exploration. The availability of playmates often influences the nature of play. Same-gender versus opposite-gender exploration is a function of who is available to play with rather than representing any adult sexual orientation (such as heterosexual or homosexual).

Children continue to gain freedom and begin to be exposed to a variety of people and experiences as they further explore their environment. The major task at this stage corresponds to Erikson's developmental initiative versus guilt (refer to Figure 5.2). Children's actions are more purposeful as they evaluate their own competencies and initiate behaviors consistent with these limits. Children's likes and dislikes at this stage are more firmly established, and their behavior is more purposeful. They know what they want and use their greater mobility and freedom to pursue these desires. When this pursuit puts conflicts with how significant others want them to behave, they begin to feel guilt.

Children at this level struggle with their overwhelming preoccupation with self as they are increasingly exposed to other youngsters in a variety of play and social situations. They find themselves in situations with other youngsters that force them to share, take turns, and accommodate others. This socialization is a vital and necessary developmental step that will prepare children for the kinds of social interactions necessary for their future success in school.

As we pointed out in Chapter 4, gender identity is already strongly established by this stage. Little boys and girls know what being masculine and feminine means, and they continue to explore and refine these roles. The more freedom they are given to explore behaviors and roles, the greater opportunity they will

healthy sex hints 5.1
Becoming an Askable Parent

Becoming an askable parent is a lifelong process. A neon sign doesn't suddenly appear during adolescence signaling approachability. Being an askable parent is a reward earned after years of sending subtle messages about the desire to listen and willingness to help. The following are guidelines on how to be an askable parent:

1. *Start early.* Body language and nonverbal behaviors concerning bonding, nudity, and toilet training send messages about approachability.
2. *Don't worry about giving too much information.* Scientific evidence doesn't indicate that too much information too soon will overstimulate children. If a child is getting too much information, he or she will simply get bored, tune you out, and change the subject.
3. *Communicate even if you're not entirely comfortable about the topic.* If you are uncomfortable with a specific sexual issue, you can still address it openly and honestly with your children. The child might respond positively to your admission that you have difficulty talking about an issue.
4. *Admit your ignorance.* You don't know it all. Even the best teachers don't know everything about their sub-

ject. If your child asks a question you can't answer, admit it and offer to look it up. Better yet, look it up together.

5. *Realize that less is better.* Concise, simple answers that address the question at hand are better than long-winded answers.
6. *Don't worry about offering information that children can't understand.* If you make a mistake by being too technical, children will extract what they need or understand, and the rest will go over their head.
7. *Don't be afraid to make mistakes.* Everyone makes honest mistakes. Handle these as you would any other mistakes: Admit you were wrong, and try to correct the mistake, if possible.
8. *Relate your values.* Children want to know how you feel about sexual matters. Take every opportunity to share relevant values with them.
9. *Have a sense of humor.* Lighten up. Sexuality education gives rise to opportunities to laugh and learn at the same time. Children feel less inhibited about an adult's talking about sexual matters if sex isn't always portrayed as a deadly serious topic.

have in moving toward a more flexible gender identity. For instance, little girls who are allowed to play with boys and engage in active, physical play and sports might find that they enjoy this type of activity. Little boys who are allowed to play house and with dolls might find this an enjoyable addition to or replacement of more traditional roughhouse activities.

Development in Childhood

Children continue to explore and mimic gender role behaviors and scripts they learn from their parents and the culture. "Playing house" is a common script for 5- to 7-year-olds. The boys play the "daddies," and the girls play the "mommies." Often these games include kissing, hugging, cuddling, and lying on each other. Children at this age talk about people they love and will marry someday. Children often have a "special friend" to whom they are attracted and for whom they have loving feelings. Elementary school children exchange valentines and other symbols of endearment.

   Children at this age also begin to develop their own language and sense of sexual humor. Jokes about bodily functions are common. These children have a great deal of interest in sounds and smells associated with bodily functioning. Children of this age are amused by riddles and rhymes that often are crude and sexually coarse.

healthy sex hints 5.2
Education for Children

Most parents and professional educators feel that children need to talk about sexuality issues in the home. Having the resources with which to do that in an informed way has been possible for many years. In addition, so much more is accessible over the Internet. Here is a brief list of helpful books for both parents and children.

   Two by Deborah Roffman, published by Perseus Publishing:

Sex and Sensibility: The Thinking Parent's Guide to Talking Sense About Sex (2001)
But How'd I Get in There in the First Place? Talking to Your Young Child About Sex (2002)

Two by Debra Haffner, along with her daughter Alyssa Haffner Tartaglione, published by Newmarket Press:

From Diapers to Dating (1999)
Beyond the Big Talk: Every Parent's Guide to Raising Sexually Healthy Teens, from Middle School to College (2001)

Two by Robie Harris, published by Candlewick Press:

It's Perfectly Normal: Changing Bodies, Growing Up, Sex and Sexual Health (1994)
It's So Amazing! A Book About Eggs, Sperm, Birth, Babies, and Families (1999)

Robert Hatcher, Shannon Colestock, Erika Pluhar, and Christian Thrasher have a book designed for older adolescents and young college students:

Sexual Etiquette 101 and More (Bridging the Gap Communications, 2001)

   These books are honest and forthright about sexuality information. Contacting the Sexuality Information and Education Council of the U.S. (SIECUS) or Planned Parenthood Federation of America will link parents to a wide array of books and pamphlets that address how to promote sexual health. Books and pamphlets have also been developed to help families learn and talk about adoption, gay, lesbian, bisexual and transgendered youth, intersexuality, sexual assault, disability, and other related topics.

By 8 or 9 years of age, children begin to become more segregated in their play. Boys tend to play with other boys, and girls with their girlfriends. Although they still have the same interest in the opposite gender, the socialization process begins to segregate them more and more. Formal activities such as team sports and school-based extracurricular activities are often segregated, sometimes formally but usually informally. Little girls who might have played touch football with the guys last season may try out for cheerleading this year. Boys who played sandlot baseball with the neighborhood boys and girls may sign up for Little League, while their female counterparts sign up for softball. Leagues in some towns encourage mixed-gender participation.

In addition to cultural influences that help shape boys and girls and influence which direction they might take regarding sports, economic and political factors play a big part. Often, funding for girls' sports and recreational activities does not equal that earmarked for boys. Consequently, girls haven't always been offered the same opportunities as boys to compete in youth sports. To attempt to rectify that, Title IX of the Civil Rights Act was passed to ensure parity in funding. The law refers to all benefits and activities available in schools. Most of the controversy regarding Title IX revolves around sports and athletic programs. Title IX has been instrumental in getting more girls and women involved in sports and athletic activities.

Development in Preadolescence

Many of the books available for children and teenagers reinforce the idea that children develop at their own pace. A new term, *tweens*, refers to children roughly between 10 and 12 who, although not teenagers, are confronting issues not commonly associated with young children.

Studies show that although segregation of the sexes is more pronounced during this time, feelings of desire and affection are strong. Most boys and girls of this age view relationships with other preadolescents as important and something they desire. Children in this age range are learning how to interact with members of the same and opposite sexes they find desirable. They are learning the scripts and rehearsing the behaviors necessary to make the transition from childhood to young adulthood. Adults may find some of the behavior amusing, yet the fact that we use the term *social skill* literally means that skill development is crucial.

Sixth-grade dances are good examples of this learning process. The room is filled with 11- and 12-year-olds who want to mix and mingle with girls and boys they are attracted to. What usually happens, though, is that boys line up along one wall and the girls the other. They horse around and act goofy but rarely cross the line and ask someone to dance. This is a transition, a rite of passage in American culture. The next year or the year after that, they will begin to cross the line and ask each other to dance. Some will even bring partners to the dance. For now, it is a stepping stone, an opportunity to try out another script.

Hedgepeth and Helmich (1996), as they developed materials for sexuality educators, have noted that young adolescents between the ages of 12 and 14 are dealing with the following developmental issues:

1. They're worried about their bodies.
2. They're engaged in a search for identity, including sexual orientation identity.
3. They are very centered on the self yet influenced by peer attitudes.

4. They intellectually understand that behavior has consequences but don't necessarily think the consequences will happen to them.
5. They're fearful of asking questions of adults that may make them appear uninformed.

Negative Influences

In today's world, children are exposed to sexual content in much more direct ways than their parents' and grandparents' generations. A parent who may be preparing dinner in a kitchen with the evening news on the television may inadvertently be exposing a child to stories of sexual abuse, abduction, and murder. Some children have interacted online with pedophiles, while some of those interested in children get picked up due to FBI sting operations. While the rates of reported cases of child sexual abuse have been declining ("Reports of Child Sexual Abuse," 2001), the raw numbers of children sexually abused in 1997 were estimated at 223,000. Beyond that are the numbers of cases that never make it into the databases of police departments, social service agencies, and schools.

In an attempt to teach children such skills as "Yell no!" and "Reach out to an adult you can trust," some schools began putting sexual abuse prevention programs into place during the 1980s. The thought was that teaching "good touch versus bad touch" would empower children to protect themselves. Those programs along with drug and HIV/AIDS prevention programs often took precedence over time devoted to more positive developmental lessons.

Increasingly, children also spend time online, checking out Web sites, going into chat rooms, and "IM-ing" (instant-messaging) their peers. As a result, some children have found unsolicited pornography attached to their e-mails. There are constant challenges to promoting sexual health in children. It is our position that parents must talk with their children and be aware of the myriad influences on their sexual development.

Intellectual Wellness

Individuals begin to learn about sexuality from the day of birth. Infants and children learn symbolically. They learn about what feels good through direct physical exploration. They learn about what is taboo by the reactions of significant others.

Children continue to grow as they become more verbal and are able to communicate by asking questions and seeking clarification. Development takes shape according to the answers received and the nonverbal messages attached to the information. If children grow up in a household where sexual questions are allowed and teachable moments are capitalized, the natural curiosity about sex is satisfied.

This learning continues through childhood and adolescence. What differs is the sheer quantity of information to which people are exposed and the sources from which it is derived. Infants and young children receive sexual information mostly from parents and other caregivers. By the time of adolescence, sexual information flows in torrents from sources ranging from parents to mass media to the Internet.

Today, more than ever before, many excellent sources of information about sexuality are available—books, recordings, educational television shows, Web sites, and more. Unfortunately, many poor sources of information and negative gender roles also bombard us daily. The ability to process all of this information and make sense of it is aided by our ever-growing intellectual development and rests on a foundation of "askable parents" and a school environment and curriculum that encourage questions and make information readily available.

Development in Adolescence

Adolescence denotes a period of years (roughly between 12 and 18). The major task associated with adolescence is to develop a self-identity (Erikson, 1978). Adolescence can be a time of great excitement and joy as individuals literally move from childhood to adulthood. During adolescence, both the body and the mind change and grow. They outgrow not only their old clothes but often their old ideas as well, and sometimes their old friends, as they struggle to come to grips with who they are and where they are going.

Experts have come to understand that the promotion of good health behaviors at this stage has a critical impact on adult lifestyles (Hatcher & Scarpa, 2002). Consequently, health programs directed at teens often focus on adolescent risk-taking behaviors with particular attention to tobacco and alcohol use, exercise and nutrition, sleep, accident reduction, and sexuality. Set up within the Centers for Disease Control (CDC), the Youth Risk Behavior Surveillance System has surveyed adolescents across the United States for the risk-taking behaviors felt to contribute to social problems, death, and disability (CDC, 2003). Its rich database has provided information from representative samples taken between 1991 and 2001 from students sampled from 50 states along with more intensive analysis of urban youth (CDC, 2003). Unfortunately, those surveys, discussed later, ask only eight questions about sexual behavior, with the questions having a strong focus on participation in sexual intercourse related to alcohol, condom use, and frequency within a designated time frame (CDC, 2003).

Puberty is the time of myriad physiological events that characterize adolescence. It is a time of profound physiological change as the body matures and becomes "reproductively ready" with fully adult genitalia, a reproductive system, and hormones coursing through the bloodstream, sending messages to the brain of arriving sexually.

Psychosocial readiness for sexual activity with another person takes a while to catch up to **reproductive readiness.** Adolescents become caught in a state of confusion as the body sends the mind messages about sex that the adolescent may not be ready to handle psychosocially.

Reproductive readiness
Pubertal development resulting in full growth of genitalia and onset of fertility

The media likes to exploit this confusion and report about the problems and the failures associated with adolescence. We hear about teenage drug and alcohol misuse, HIV disease, teen pregnancy, satanic cults, and defiant behavior. Movies glorify adolescent rebelliousness and juvenile delinquency. In contrast, however, many teenagers navigate adolescence in a healthy, productive way with both peer and adult support systems providing guidance.

Michael Carrera, a respected adolescent sexuality expert, works to help teenagers emerge from adolescence as young adults who are strong, competent, and whole. Along with the Children's Aid Society, Carrera (2003) has developed a model for working with youth that has had demonstrable positive results on adolescent health. His program includes getting participants involved with work and money management, educational support that includes tutoring and test preparation designed to move students toward college, a family life/sex education program, involvement in the arts, and participation and development of lifetime individual sports. Simultaneously, students have access to comprehensive medical care including reproductive health care and mental health counseling. Students in his program, some 5,000 over 19 years, have shown lower pregnancy rates, delayed onset of intercourse, better sexual health behaviors, and higher graduation rates.

Physical, Psychological, and Social Wellness

Child and adolescent health is positively impacted by participation in exercise and organized sports. Historically, organized sports were seen as important for boys' development, yet of little interest to most girls. Title IX of the 1972 Education Amendments Act outlawed discrimination in secondary and postsecondary educational institutions receiving federal funding. Its impact on reducing gender discrimination in sports has been significant.

In 1971, 1 in 27 girls participated in high school sports compared to 1 in 2 boys. By 2001, the ratio for girls was almost the same as for boys, with 1 in 2.5 girls participating compared to the 1 in 2 ratio for boys (Lopiano, 2001). Participation in sports helps teens learn about teamwork, goal setting, and the pursuit of excellence. Physical activity can enhance self-esteem and improve body image. Research has also shown that teenage female athletes are less likely to get pregnant, delay their first sexual intercourse, and report that they had not had sexual intercourse compared to nonathletes (Lopiano, 2001).

Figure 5.3 highlights the physiological changes associated with puberty. In general, these can be grouped into changes associated with primary and secondary sex characteristics.

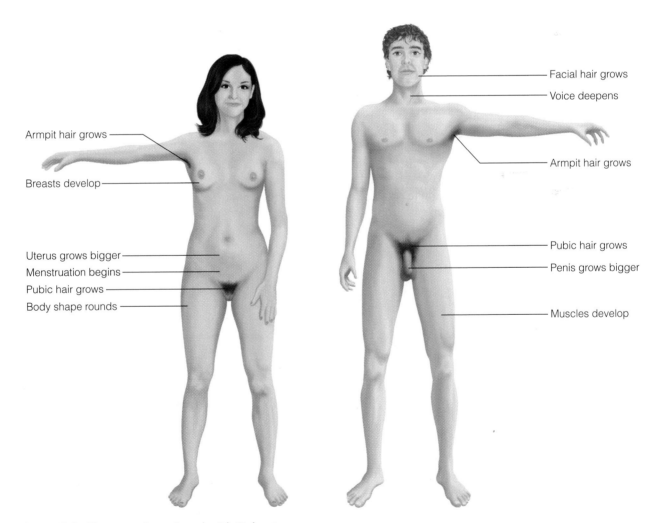

Figure 5.3 *Changes Associated with Puberty*

Primary Sex Characteristics

Primary sex characteristics
Growth of the sex organs

Primary sex characteristics are associated with the full growth and development of the sex organs. A boy's penis and testicles grow and reach full adult size by the end of puberty. The testes begin to produce sperm and androgens, and first ejaculation signals the onset of reproductive readiness.

In girls, the major internal (vagina, ovaries, uterus, and fallopian tubes) and external (labia, mons, clitoris) sexual structures reach maturity. First menstruation is the sign that puberty has arrived.

Secondary Sex Characteristics

Secondary sex characteristics Nongenital changes associated with puberty; include growth of pubic, facial, and underarm hair, breast development, increases in height and weight

Secondary sex characteristics are nongenital changes associated with puberty. Boys and girls both experience a growth spurt and begin to attain their subsequent adult height. They both grow pubic, underarm, and body hair. Although boys characteristically grow significantly more facial hair than girls do, this generally represents a continuum with a range of possibilities for boys and girls, from relatively hairless to very hairy.

Body contours begin to develop. Girls naturally deposit more fat on their hips and breasts than boys do, but, as with facial and body hair, there is a wide continuum of growth possibilities for both boys and girls. The voice box in boys enlarges, creating a deeper, more resonating sound. The transition period involved in this change causes a squeaky quality to boys' voices.

Gonads The primary endocrine glands in men (testes) and women (ovaries) that influence sexuality

By the end of puberty, the body has reached a stage of reproductive readiness with two major components: mature reproductive anatomy and hormonally influenced sexual desire. The sex organs are fully developed and capable of procreating as well as recreating. Not only are parts such as the penis and vagina fully mature and capable of responding to sexual desire, but ovaries and testes are also fully able to produce viable ova and sperm, respectively. This is often the time when a young girl discovers that her clitoris is capable of providing sexual pleasure.

Androgens A group of naturally occurring steroid hormones produced by both men and women

Testosterone The most notable androgen, recognized for fueling sexual desire and aggressiveness in males

In nature's eyes, humans are able and ready to propagate the species. Nature gives a boost in that our **gonads** (testes and ovaries), which have long been silent, now begin to produce hormones that stimulate sexual desire. **Androgens,** primarily **testosterone,** stimulate sexual receptor centers in the brain, which trigger feelings of

Shaving is an exciting rite of passage for teens.

Suza Scalora/GettyImages

Tony Freeman/PhotoEdit, Inc.

sexual desire. All of the cold showers in the world will not quell this sexual desire because, to a certain extent, it is fueled by hormones circulating in the bloodstream.

Most books and support materials for parents, preadolescents, and adolescents will reinforce the concept that maturation proceeds at its own unique pace, and barring evidence of medical problems, children will indeed grow into healthy adults. Pediatricians, many of whom have expanded their practices to address the health care needs of infants, children, and adolescents, need to be sensitive to physical growth along with the other aspects of sexual development. Family practitioners, nurse practitioners, physician's assistants, nurses, and other professionals as well need to be educated and comfortable with the realities of teen health to best meet the health needs of their patients. Ideally, information about the physical body should be able to be discussed along with concerns about sexual orientation, sexual decision making, protection from infection and unintended pregnancy, and so forth. To facilitate such conversations, however, the provider must be comfortable with such topics and able to create a safe space to talk with the teen patient.

In the physical realm, the Sexual Maturity Rating scale, sometimes referred to as the Tanner Scale (American Nurses Association, 1999), can be used to measure levels of physical maturity. The scale, as represented in Table 5.1, has five stages that allow for charting growth of pubic hair, breast development, and

Table 5.1 Sexual Maturity Rating Scale for Girls and Boys

Female		SMR	*Male*		
Breast	**Pubic Hair**		**Testes and Scrotum**	**Penis**	**Pubic Hair**
No development	No pubic hair	1	Testicular volume: <1.5 ml	Childlike	None
Breast bud, areola widens	Long, slightly pigmented, straight hair along labia	2	Testicular volume: 1.6–6 ml; scrotum: reddened, thinner, larger	No change	Light, downy hair laterally
Breast larger, more elevation. Extends beyond areolar parameter.	Increased in quantity, darker, more curly and coarser; present in typical female triangle	3	Testicular volume: 6–12 ml; scrotum: great enlargement	Increased length	Extended across pubis
Breast larger and more elevation. Areola and papilla form a mound projecting from the breast contour.	Hair more dense, curled, and adult in distribution but in a smaller quantity	4	Testicular volume: 12–20 ml; scrotum: further enlargement and darkening	Increased length and circumference	More abundant with curling
Breast adult appearance. Areola and breast in same plane, with papilla projecting above areola.	Abundant, adult-type pattern; hair extends to medial aspect of thigh.	5	Testicular volume: >20 ml; scrotum: adult appearance	Adult appearance	Adult quantity and distribution with hair present on inner thighs

Source: American Nurses Association (1999).

size and color of the penis and scrotum. Because the scale has no ages connected to it, health practitioners cannot make assumptions based on age, sex, or racial and ethnic background. Furthermore, a thorough physical exam is required which may or may not occur; some teens resist the physical inspection needed.

Ironically, sexuality educators have shared anecdotal reports with us of teens and young adults increasingly shaving their pubic hair. The motivation for such shaving has been explained, especially for young females, as a response to the trend for small underwear. Just as females would shave so that pubic hair would not show when wearing a bathing suit, shaving is seen as necessary when wearing bikini and thong underwear. Another explanation for both male and female shaving is connected to attitudes toward oral sex, with the presence of pubic hair thought to be "dirty." Consequently, examining teens relative to pubic hair growth may become less important for assessing their maturation.

Adolescence has a profound impact on sexuality for the rest of our lives. Often our body image and initial impressions about our masculinity and femininity that were formed at this time color how we view ourselves for the rest of our lives. Old labels and images such as "I'm not a good dancer" or "I'm shy" or "I'm not very good-looking" influence our self-concept and stay with us for years to come.

Body Image Issues

Both boys and girls at some point during the preteen and teen years become obsessed with physical appearance. So many changes are happening to the body, and peer comparisons become constant. Standing out for being "too fat" or "too short" or "too pimply" can leave children feeling self-conscious and sometimes the brunt of other's teasing.

Research has indicated that teens are becoming increasingly overweight, partly due to lack of exercise as well as increased consumption of high-calorie foods. Although states mandate that students have regular physical education classes, other programs often interfere with regular, daily exercise. There are barriers to participation in organized sports such as costs, lack of transportation, competing time commitments, competitive pressures, and lack of facilities (American Psychological Association, 2002). Early in 2003, a family in New York City attempted to sue McDonald's for contributing to the gross obesity of their children. The case was thrown out of court, but public articles began to appear in newspapers and pieces on television about the amounts of "junk" and fast food consumed by adolescents. The federal government in 2003 convened professionals to address the rise in obesity overall, with plans to address childhood and adolescent diet and exercise patterns. And the food industry, in response, has increased its efforts to improve the nutritional quality of its foods, which will entail reducing the fat, sugar, and salt content.

Another public health concern has been the growing numbers of teens who get depressed because of their appearance. The depression with looks can result in disordered eating, with an unrealistic expectation of normal body weight. The majority of teens with eating disorders are female, although boys are becoming vulnerable to body pressures as well (American Psychological Association, 2002).

Adolescent Sexual Behavior

What has improved significantly in recent years has been the recognition that asking teens "what behaviors they engage in" is necessary to understanding their needs and how to provide for better health. Close examination of various survey instruments will highlight a range of questions, some more specific than others.

For example, the National Survey of Adolescent Males surveyed males about the variety of genital experiences they had with females beyond sexual intercourse (Gates & Sonenstein, 2000). The importance of using clear language was evident in the phrasing of questions. For example, males were asked to answer yes or no to whether "a female touched your penis until you ejaculated or 'came.'" The Youth Risk Behavior Survey, in contrast, asks participants only about sexual intercourse (CDC, 2003). The questions focus on partner frequency, use of condoms and other forms of birth control, and alcohol and drug use, yet they cannot provide the depth of information needed to understand youth sexual behavior. The Henry J. Kaiser Family Foundation (Henry J. Kaiser Family Foundation, Hoff, Greene, & Davis, 2003) issued a report on teen sexual activity that focused on sexual intercourse, partners and relationships, abstinence, contraceptive use, pregnancy and sexually transmitted diseases, sex and substance abuse, and sexual pressure and dating violence.

Overall, different groups have studied selected samples of adolescents and various aspects of their adolescent sexual behavior. A full understanding is often limited by access to a broad group of subjects, along with limitations on what types of questions get asked. The government will more often fund studies related to teen pregnancy and sexually transmitted diseases. Data on masturbation, oral sexual behaviors, and anal sexual behaviors are more limited; some types of questions are deemed too sensitive to ask youth (A. Levine, personal communication, October 2003).

Masturbation   Conscious, erotic self-stimulation is thought to be among the most common expressions of adolescent sexual behavior, particularly for males. Kinsey and his associates discovered that the rate of masturbation was different for boys and girls (Kinsey, Pomeroy, & Martin, 1948). Among boys in that early study, the level of masturbation increased from 21 percent of 12-year-old boys to 82 percent of 15-year-old boys. Among girls, the level of masturbation increased from 12 percent of 12-year-old girls to 20 percent of 15-year-old girls. By the end of adolescence, more than 90 percent of the boys and about 35 percent of the girls had masturbated.

Other studies since Kinsey have shown that the level of masturbation for boys across adolescence is relatively unchanged, but the rate among girls has risen. By the time they reach the end of adolescence, approximately 75 percent of all girls reported having masturbated (Sorenson, 1983; Sarrel & Sarrel, 1984). The gender differences have been supported in later research, with 33 percent of girls by age 15 reporting that they had masturbated, compared to 58 percent of boys at that age (Baldwin & Baldwin, 1997).

Sexual Intercourse   Despite public health messages and the goals of the "abstinence until marriage" education efforts, adolescents do engage in sexual intercourse. National headlines were made, however, when the Henry J. Kaiser Foundation released its report in 2003 showing a decline in the rates of high school students grades 9 through 12 who had had intercourse over the past decade. In 1991, the rate was 54 percent compared to 46 percent in 2001 (Kaiser Family Foundation et al., 2003). Of concern to health providers and educators was the accompanying finding that for those who reported being sexually active, there was an increase in the use of condoms; substantial numbers of teen girls still became pregnant, with an estimated 4 million teens getting a sexually transmitted infection each year nonetheless.

As Laumann, Gagnon, Michael, and Michaels (1994) point out from the National Social Health and Life Survey (NSHLS), first sexual intercourse, especially for women, has traditionally been a symbol for loss of innocence, transition to adulthood, and assumption of responsibility for procreation for the next genera-

personal exploration activity

What Is Right for You?

It is easy to avoid openly examining our beliefs and values concerning sexual activity. Often our sexual behavior is dictated by the moment, not by our values and rational decisions. The goal of this activity is to help you clarify the sexual behavior that is comfortable and acceptable for you and to identify a plan for making sure you can stick to your sexual values.

Take a few minutes to really examine what you believe and respond to the following questions honestly and openly. You do not need to share this with anyone; however, you might enjoy discussing it with a close friend.

What would be some good reasons or advantages for you to choose to have premarital sex? (If you are married, substitute *extramarital* for *premarital* in each question.) *Example:* "It's fun."

What would be some good reasons or disadvantages for you to choose not to have premarital sex? *Example:* "I could get hurt."

What are some guidelines you need to follow if you choose to have premarital sex? *Example:* "Be honest with my partner about my motives for having sex."

What are some guidelines you need to follow if you choose not to have premarital sex? *Example:* "Don't drink too much."

List the reasons you might choose to have premarital sex in two columns, reasons that would make you feel guilty versus guilt-free reasons.

How can you tell when a premarital sexual relationship becomes unhealthy or harmful to yourself?

tion. The popular belief about the widespread level of premarital sexual intercourse is that this is a fairly recent phenomenon that is linked to social decay, a decrease in family values and the like. As Laumann et al. demonstrated, the drop in average age of first intercourse, and the increased level of adolescent sexual intercourse, has been at a fairly steady level for decades. Various studies have shown a general trend related to a decline in the average age of first intercourse and an increase in the number of sexual partners of adolescents.

By age 19, 20 percent of the girls and 45 percent of the boys in the Kinsey study had had intercourse. Thirty years later, Sorenson (1983) reported a 25 percent increase (from 20 to 45 percent) in the percentage of female adolescents having intercourse and a 14 percent increase (45 to 59 percent) among males. Using data from 1971 and 1976, Zelnick, Kanter, and Ford (1981) confirmed Sorenson's findings and added that the increases for whites was two times greater than for blacks.

Nearly another 10 years later, Forrest and Singh (1990) and Sonenstein, Pleck, and Hu (1989) reported another increase in the level of adolescent intercourse. Citing data from the National Study of Family Growth, Forrest and Singh demonstrated that the proportion of 15- to 19-year-old females having intercourse rose steadily in the 1970s and 1980s. In 1970, 28 percent of white and 45 percent of nonwhite girls were nonvirgins. By 1988, 52 percent of white and 65 percent of nonwhite girls had experienced sexual intercourse. By 1988, 25 percent of all 15-year-olds and 75 percent of all 19-year-old girls had experienced intercourse (Forrest & Singh, 1990).

The National Survey of Adolescent Males (NSAM) reported that approximately 30 percent of its 15-year-old subjects had experienced intercourse. By age 19, 86 percent of all the subjects had lost their virginity (Laumann et al., 1994).

150

The Youth Risk Behavior Survey. The Youth Risk Behavior Survey (YRBS) has yielded a large database for studying adolescent behavior. Federal funding and support have been instrumental to this research effort; the typical sexuality researcher seldom can get access to so many diverse students across the United States. Although the latest survey was administered in 2003, the analysis of data has not been published.

The survey instrument examines sexual activity comparing results by sex, race, age, and ethnicity. The data become invaluable to those determining policy to promote the sexual health of adolescents. Unfortunately, the section of the survey related to sexual behavior is limited to eight questions related to sexual intercourse (CDC, 2003). Discussion of oral and anal behaviors, along with greater sensitivity to the behaviors, and gay, lesbian, and bisexual youth are missing. The findings are further limited in that only students who attend high schools are surveyed.

The findings reported for 2001 showed that 46 percent of high school students had experienced sexual intercourse, 14 percent had had four or more sex partners, and 42 percent of sexually active high school students had not used a condom at the time of their last intercourse (CDC, 2003).

Analysis of 10 years of YRBS data, as presented in Table 5.2, reveals patterns among the youth surveyed. The prevalence of sexual experience, as defined by having had sexual intercourse, decreased 16 percent among high school students. The prevalence of multiple sex partners decreased 24 percent, yet the overall prevalence of current sexual activity did not change. Furthermore, the prevalence of alcohol or drug use before the last act of sexual intercourse among those defining themselves as sexually active increased 18 percent (CDC, 2003).

Number of Partners The information gathered from the NSHLS provided three interesting findings related to the number of sex partners adolescents have by age 18:

- As the average age for the onset of intercourse drops, the average number of teenage partners increases.
- Females from the oldest age cohorts had fewer partners before age 18 than women from the youngest cohorts.
- Females are catching up to males.

Concerning the first point, as teens are beginning to have sex at a younger age, they also are experiencing more partners. This finding is in contrast with teens over 50 years ago. At that time, teens who experienced first intercourse early (before 18 years of age) had fewer partners because they tended to marry their first sex partner. Often their first teenage encounter was as man and wife. Teens today rarely have first intercourse on their wedding night. Most of them have already had intercourse prior to this event (Laumann et al., 1994).

Laumann and colleagues also found differences among the age cohorts regarding the number of partners before age 18. The females from earlier generations (born between 1933 and 1942) were much less likely to have had five or more partners by age 18 than the youngest cohort (born between 1963 and 1967). This relates to the last finding—that females are catching up to males in terms of overall number of sexual partners. The number of sex partners for males and females by age 18 is less variable for the youngest cohorts than for the oldest.

The Youth Risk Behavior Survey data for 2001 found that 11.4 percent of females and 17.2 percent of males had had more than four sex partners during their lifetime. When grade in school is factored in, 9th graders reported 9.6 percent compared to 12th graders reporting 21.6 percent of students having had more than four partners. Over the 10-year period during which YRSB data have been reported, the percentage of students having more than four partners has gone down from 18.7 to 14.2 percent, a "trend" viewed positively by public health officials (CDC, 2000).

Table 5.2 Percentage of High School Students Who Reported Sexual Risk Behaviors, by Sex, Grade, Race/Ethnicity, and Survey Year

Characteristic	Ever Had Sexual Intercourse %	(95% CI*)	≥4 Sex Partners During Lifetime %	(95% CI)	Currently Sexually Active† %	(95% CI)	Condom Use During Last Sexual Intercourse§ %	(95% CI)	Alcohol Drug Use Before Last Sexual Intercourse§ %	(95% CI)
Sex										
Female										
1991	50.8	(±4.0)	13.8	(±1.8)	38.2	(±3.4)	38.0	(±4.3)	16.8	(±3.2)
1993	50.2	(±2.5)	15.0	(±1.9)	37.5	(±1.8)	46.0	(±2.8)	16.6	(±2.2)
1995	52.1	(±5.0)	14.4	(±3.5)	40.4	(±4.2)	48.6	(±5.2)	16.8	(±3.0)
1997	47.7	(±3.7)	14.1	(±2.0)	36.5	(±2.7)	50.8	(±3.0)	18.5	(±3.0)
1999	47.7	(±4.1)	13.1	(±2.2)	36.3	(±4.1)	50.7	(±5.8)	18.6	(±3.4)
2001	42.9	(±2.8)¶	11.4	(±1.5)	33.4	(±2.5)	51.3	(±3.4)¶**	20.7	(±2.7)
Male										
1991	57.4	(±4.1)	23.4	(±3.0)	36.8	(±3.4)	54.5	(±3.8)	26.3	(±3.3)
1993	55.6	(±3.5)	22.3	(±2.7)	37.5	(±3.0)	59.2	(±3.8)	25.7	(±3.0)
1995	54.0	(±4.7)	20.9	(±2.6)	35.5	(±3.5)	60.5	(±4.3)	32.8	(±4.1)
1997	48.8	(±3.4)	17.6	(±1.5)	33.4	(±2.6)	62.5	(±2.8)	30.5	(±2.8)
1999	52.2	(±4.0)	19.3	(±3.6)	36.2	(±3.9)	65.5	(±4.3)	31.2	(±4.0)
2001	48.5	(±2.7)¶	17.2	(±1.6)¶	33.4	(±2.3)	65.1	(±2.7)¶	30.9	(±2.9)¶
Grade										
9										
1991	39.0	(±5.0)	12.5	(±2.9)	22.4	(±3.9)	53.3	(±6.2)	20.9	(±6.9)
1993	37.7	(±4.2)	10.9	(±2.0)	24.8	(±3.2)	61.6	(±5.7)	22.4	(±3.9)
1995	36.9	(±5.9)	12.9	(±3.0)	23.6	(±4.0)	62.9	(±5.5)	29.7	(±5.7)
1997	38.0	(±3.8)	12.2	(±2.5)	24.2	(±3.3)	58.8	(±5.6)	33.2	(±8.3)
1999	38.6	(±6.1)	11.8	(±2.3)	26.6	(±5.7)	66.6	(±7.8)	25.6	(±5.2)
2001	34.4	(±3.6)	9.6	(±1.6)	22.7	(±3.1)	67.5	(±3.3)¶	24.0	(±4.4)**
10										
1991	48.2	(±5.7)	15.1	(±2.8)	33.2	(±4.6)	46.3	(±4.7)	22.3	(±4.9)
1993	46.1	(±3.6)	15.9	(±2.0)	30.1	(±3.0)	54.7	(±4.5)	24.2	(±4.2)
1995	48.0	(±5.1)	15.6	(±2.0)	33.7	(±3.1)	59.7	(±4.6)	28.6	(±5.9)
1997	42.5	(±4.3)	13.8	(±2.7)	29.2	(±2.9)	58.9	(±3.6)	22.9	(±3.3)
1999	46.8	(±5.6)	15.6	(±5.0)	33.0	(±5.2)	62.6	(±6.1)	23.1	(±4.2)
2001	40.8	(±3.0)¶	12.6	(±1.8)	29.7	(±2.9)	60.1	(±4.5)¶**	27.7	(±3.1)
11										
1991	62.4	(±3.2)	22.1	(±3.6)	43.3	(±3.6)	48.7	(±5.8)	22.2	(±3.5)
1993	57.5	(±3.5)	19.9	(±3.1)	40.0	(±3.6)	55.3	(±3.0)	22.0	(±2.6)
1995	58.6	(±5.0)	19.0	(±3.7)	42.4	(±4.4)	52.3	(±6.2)	24.3	(±3.1)
1997	49.7	(±5.2)	16.7	(±2.9)	37.8	(±4.8)	60.1	(±5.2)	23.1	(±4.1)
1999	52.5	(±3.8)	17.3	(±4.1)	37.5	(±3.4)	59.2	(±4.8)	28.6	(±5.8)
2001	51.9	(±2.9)¶**	15.2	(±1.5)¶	38.1	(±2.6)	58.9	(±4.0)¶	24.7	(±2.9)¶
12										
1991	66.7	(±4.4)	25.0	(±4.0)	50.6	(±4.5)	41.4	(±3.6)	20.8	(±3.7)
1993	68.3	(±4.6)	27.0	(±3.6)	53.0	(±3.9)	46.5	(±4.0)	19.1	(±3.3)
1995	66.4	(±4.0)	22.9	(±3.5)	49.7	(±3.9)	49.5	(±4.4)	20.3	(±3.6)
1997	60.9	(±6.5)	20.6	(±3.5)	46.0	(±5.0)	52.4	(±3.5)	23.3	(±1.8)
1999	64.9	(±4.9)	20.6	(±2.8)	50.6	(±5.1)	47.9	(±5.7)	22.0	(±3.8)
2001	60.5	(±4.0)¶	21.6	(±2.4)¶	47.9	(±4.0)	49.3	(±3.1)¶**	25.4	(±2.6)¶

Table 5.2 *(continued)*

Characteristic	Ever Had Sexual Intercourse		≥4 Sex Partners During Lifetime		Currently Sexually Active[†]		Condom Use During Last Sexual Intercourse[§]		Alcohol Drug Use Before Last Sexual Intercourse[§]	
	%	(95% CI*)	%	(95% CI)	%	(95% CI)	%	(95% CI)	%	(95% CI)
Race/Ethnicity[††]										
Black										
1991	81.4	(±3.2)	43.1	(±3.5)	59.3	(±3.8)	48.0	(±3.8)	13.7	(±2.9)
1993	79.7	(±3.2)	42.7	(±3.8)	59.1	(±4.4)	56.5	(±3.8)	12.2	(±3.5)
1995	73.4	(±4.5)	35.6	(±4.4)	54.2	(±4.7)	66.1	(±4.8)	19.2	(±4.6)
1997	72.6	(±2.8)	38.5	(±3.6)	53.6	(±3.2)	64.0	(±2.8)	18.1	(±3.1)
1999	71.2	(±8.2)	34.4	(±10.3)	53.0	(±8.9)	70.0	(±5.4)	18.1	(±7.9)
2001	60.8	(±6.6)[¶]	26.6	(±3.7)[¶]	45.6	(±5.4)[¶]	67.1	(±3.5)[¶**]	17.8	(±2.6)[¶]
Hispanic										
1991	53.1	(±3.5)	16.8	(±2.6)	37.0	(±3.6)	37.4	(±6.2)	17.8	(±4.2)
1993	56.0	(±4.1)	18.6	(±3.1)	39.4	(±3.7)	46.1	(±4.4)	18.2	(±4.8)
1995	57.6	(±8.6)	17.6	(±3.7)	39.3	(±7.1)	44.4	(±11.1)	24.9	(±5.2)
1997	52.2	(±3.6)	15.5	(±2.4)	35.4	(±3.9)	48.3	(±5.6)	25.3	(±5.3)
1999	54.1	(±4.8)	16.6	(±3.6)	36.3	(±4.0)	55.2	(±6.8)	22.5	(±4.0)
2001	48.4	(±4.5)	14.9	(±1.7)	35.9	(±3.2)	53.5	(±5.1)	24.1	(±2.8)[¶]
White										
1991	50.0	(±3.2)	14.7	(±1.8)	33.9	(±2.8)	46.5	(±4.6)	25.3	(±3.7)
1993	48.4	(±2.8)	14.3	(±2.1)	34.0	(±2.1)	52.3	(±3.9)	24.4	(±2.7)
1995	48.9	(±5.0)	14.2	(±2.4)	34.8	(±3.9)	52.5	(±4.0)	26.6	(±3.1)
1997	43.6	(±4.2)	11.6	(±1.5)	32.0	(±3.1)	55.8	(±2.0)	26.0	(±2.5)
1999	45.1	(±3.9)	12.4	(±2.1)	33.0	(±3.3)	55.0	(±5.1)	27.4	(±4.8)
2001	43.2	(±2.5)[¶]	12.0	(±1.4)[¶]	31.3	(±2.2)	56.8	(±3.0)[¶]	27.8	(±2.2)
Total										
1991	**54.1**	**(±3.5)**	**18.7**	**(±2.1)**	**37.4**	**(±3.1)**	**46.2**	**(±3.3)**	**21.6**	**(±2.9)**
1993	**53.0**	**(±2.7)**	**18.7**	**(±2.0)**	**37.5**	**(±2.1)**	**52.8**	**(±2.7)**	**21.3**	**(±2.0)**
1995	**53.1**	**(±4.5)**	**17.8**	**(±2.6)**	**37.9**	**(±3.4)**	**54.4**	**(±3.5)**	**24.8**	**(±2.8)**
1997	**48.4**	**(±3.1)**	**16.0**	**(±1.4)**	**34.8**	**(±2.2)**	**56.8**	**(±1.6)**	**24.7**	**(±1.8)**
1999	**49.9**	**(±3.7)**	**16.2**	**(±2.6)**	**36.3**	**(±3.5)**	**58.0**	**(±4.2)**	**24.8**	**(±3.0)**
2001	**45.6**	**(±2.3)[¶]**	**14.2**	**(±1.2)**	**33.4**	**(±2.0)**	**57.9**	**(±2.2)[¶**]**	**25.6**	**(±1.7)[¶]**

* Confidence interval
[†] Sexual intercourse during the 3 months preceding the survey
[§] Among students who are currently sexually active
[¶] Significant linear effect ($p < .05$)
** Significant quadratic effect ($p < .05$)
[††] Numbers of students in racial/ethnic groups other than white, black, or Hispanic were too small for meaningful analysis.
Source: Centers for Disease Control [Online]. Available: www.cdc.gov/mmwr/preview/mmwrhtml/mm5138a2.htm.

Laumann et al. examined what motivated men and women to initiate first intercourse. Table 5.3 summarizes the reasons for first intercourse by sex. For those who wanted to engage in sexual intercourse, affection for one's partner was ranked first among women and second among men, while curiosity and readiness for sex were ranked first for men and second for women. For those who had not wanted to engage in sexual intercourse but were not forced, affection for one's partner was ranked first for women followed closely by peer pressure and curiosity/readiness for sex. Males reported their reasons as curiosity/readiness for sex first, followed by peer pressure. Contrary to popular belief, only a small percentage of males and females (4 percent and 3 percent, respectively) reported peer pressure as the underlying motivation for first intercourse.

Table 5.3 Reasons for Having First Intercourse by Sex

	Wanted First Intercourse (%)		Not Wanted but Not Forced (%)	
	Men	Women	Men	Women
Attributed reasons				
Affection for partner	24.9	47.5	9.9	38.5
Peer pressure	4.2	3.3	28.6	24.6
Curiosity/readiness for sex	50.6	24.3	50.5	24.9
Pregnancy	0.5	0.6	0.0	0.0
Physical pleasure	12.2	2.8	6.6	2.1
Under the influence of alcohol or drugs	0.7	0.3	3.3	7.2
Wedding night	6.9	21.1	1.1	2.7

Source: E. O. Laumann et al., *The Social Organization of Sexuality: Sexual Practices in the United States,* © 1994, University of Chicago Press. Reprinted with permission.

Data from the National Survey for Family Growth (NSFG), an ongoing study of women's and family health, reported a higher incidence of involuntary first intercourse. According to the study, approximately 8 percent of the 53,793 females ages 15 to 44 reported that their first intercourse was forced (categorized as either "rape" or "not voluntary") (Abma, Chandra, Mosher, Peterson, & Puccini, 1997).

First Sex Among Lesbian/Gay Youth   Sexual behavior patterns in gay and lesbian youth are more complex because of the added dimension of coming to terms with a sexual identity that is different from their heterosexual peers. Despite increased attention to gay and lesbian issues in the media, widespread acceptance still seems problematic for mainstream America. Sexual behavior seems to be the fourth step in a five-step coming-out process that involves these stages:

1. Fear and suspicion that one's sexual desires and attraction are different (although still not clearly defined)
2. Labeling of those feelings as homoerotic (sexual feelings for someone of the same sex)
3. Defining oneself as gay or lesbian
4. Having one's first gay love affair
5. Becoming involved in the gay or lesbian subculture (Herdt & Boxer, 1992; Troiden, 1988)

Having sexual feelings for someone of the same sex (homoerotic feelings) almost always precedes sexual activity by several years among gay and lesbian people. Gay and lesbian youth today recognize feelings for same-sex partners and act on them earlier than their peers of 20 years ago (Savin-Williams & Rodriguez, 1993).

Oral Sex   The popular media created quite a stir in 2002 when reports started circulating that teenagers were engaging in oral sex with a very casual attitude. During the Monica Lewinsky scandal, President Bill Clinton testified before a congressional committee, "I did not have sex with that woman." He did admit, however, to having experienced oral sex. It is not known just how influential that statement became, yet increasingly reports surface of boys in particular getting "blow jobs" from girls with whom they're not particularly involved. The Henry J.

sex in society 5.1

Other Cultures, Other Ways

Over the years, researchers have studied societies that recognize and celebrate the onset of puberty in adolescent boys and girls. Ford and Beach (1951) found that more than 70 societies celebrated the onset of puberty in girls and more than 65 that in boys. In a sample of 192 societies, Schlegel and Barry (1979, 1980) found that

80 had no rites of passage,
17 had ceremonies for boys only,
39 had rites for girls only, and
46 had ceremonies for both sexes.

Larger societies, with intensive agricultural and manufacturing bases, and those with more complex forms of social organizations, tended not to have initiation rites.

Of the societies celebrating puberty in girls, these celebrations usually coincide with the onset of first menses and are directly related to the sexual significance of menstruation. Schlegel and Barry found that first menses signified fertility and the tribe's continued existence.

These ceremonies often included seclusion of the young women, prohibiting any contact with men. In many instances, the ceremonies included instruction from older women in matters pertaining to sex and marriage. In some cultures, the young women were "deflowered" or subjected to piercing, tattooing, or genital adornment or mutilation. Frequently, the occasion was also marked by a feast or celebration.

Schlegel and Barry found that segregation from males at this time is usually based on avoiding contact with menstrual flow, which is feared because of its supposed ability to weaken a hunter's abilities or contaminate the tribe's meat sources.

For boys, unlike with girls' first menses, no clear demarcation indicates that puberty has begun. Generally, boys are given the rites when evidence is sufficient (usually secondary sex characteristics) that they have reached puberty. Boys' ceremonies are similar to girls' in that they

usually include some form of seclusion, instruction, and ritualistic physical sacrifice (often circumcision).

The Sexual Culture of Mangaia

In the 1950s, anthropologist Donald Marshall studied the sexual attitudes and activities of the people of Mangaia, the southernmost island in the Polynesian Cook chain. There, he found, the people were exposed to sexuality from early childhood. They listened to folk stories that included detailed accounts of sex acts and sexual anatomy, and they watched sensual ritual dances.

As adolescents, males underwent *superincision*, a surgical procedure in which the tissue at the end of the penis was cut and folded back, which exposed the glans. They were taught how to stimulate a woman's genitals and breasts with the mouth, how to bring female partners to orgasm, and how to control the timing of ejaculation. Mangaian girls were taught to be responsive and to participate actively during sexual activity.

In a practice called "night-crawling," a young male would sneak into the home of a young woman with the intent to have sexual intercourse. Because most homes had a single sleeping area, this act tended to be more public than private, though the other family members feigned sleep. The parents approved of night-crawling and listened for their daughter's laughter—a sign that she was happy with her partner. The parents encouraged their children to have more than one sexual partner before marriage, to find the most sexually compatible mate.

After marriage, couples in Mangaia continued to engage in sex more often than most Western countries. The emphasis, though, shifted from the number of orgasms during a single session to a goal of copulation every night. Throughout life, the emphasis for males and females alike was on pleasing the partner (Marshall, 1971).

Kaiser Family Foundation (2003), along with *Seventeen* magazine, reports that 23 percent of students in grades 7 through 12 have had oral sex. By 11th and 12th grades, that number increased to 42 percent (Billhartz, 2003). Anecdotally, teachers and counselors who talk with teens are learning that oral sex is "not sex." Probing further, the reports of casual oral sex seem more commonly to involve girls performing fellatio than boys performing cunnilingus.

Patterns in oral sexual behavior among adolescents have mimicked the changes of adults in the United States. In general, changes in cultural acceptance of nongenital sexual behavior have led to increasing levels of all forms of oral sex among adults (Wilson & Medora, 1999). This pattern holds true for adolescents. Between 40 and 50 percent of all teenagers have engaged in oral sex by the time they finish puberty (Young, 1986; Newman & Udry, 1988).

Cultural Attitudes About Adolescent Sexuality

How does U.S. society view adolescent sexuality? It seems to view adolescent sexual behavior in general, and intercourse in particular, as a "problem" that will lead to negative outcomes (such as unintended pregnancy, sexually transmitted diseases including HIV, and sexual abuse, among others). A surprising finding of the NHSLS study was that, even though increasing numbers of study subjects reported engaging in intercourse by age 18 and having more partners, almost 80 percent of the respondents still think that teen sex is always or almost always wrong. These views are inconsistent with their own behavior. No wonder adolescents get mixed messages about sex!

Many other cultures view this matter entirely differently and celebrate this time in a young person's sexual life. Indeed, in some Pacific Island cultures, adolescent sexual behavior is encouraged, not merely tolerated. This is not to say that these cultures advocate promiscuity. Most have rules pertaining to adolescent sex.

The United States has a conservative sexual history. American culture evolved from devoutly religious, puritanical ancestors who escaped persecution for their views in Europe by coming to this country. The American patriarchal culture emphasized the family and historically has viewed sex as something that occurs within the context of a marriage, with the primary function being procreation. A strong history, institutionalized formally in law and enforced informally through cultural taboos and parenting styles, perpetuated this view. The United States is still a country where sex education is not universally taught in every school. Even when it is, it is mostly a course in reproductive anatomy (Forrest & Silverman, 1989). In some states, nonprocreative sexual acts, including oral sex and anal intercourse between consenting adults (whether heterosexual or homosexual), is considered sodomy and is illegal.

Besides having a moral tradition that prohibits adolescent sexual education and experimentation, U.S. culture, like that of many industrialized societies, prolongs adolescent and young adult dependency. To succeed, adolescents, in most cases, need to further their education. For most of them, this means remaining indebted to their parents and pursuing additional training and education while either living at home or remaining financially obligated to their parents. In a sense, what this does is delay the transition from childhood to adulthood, and delaying with it adult privileges such as sexual experimentation. In many other cultures, adolescents are encouraged to begin to separate from their parents earlier, and this separation is often institutionalized in a formal rite of passage.

Education and Sexual Development

It has been argued that adolescents in the United States experience "retarded sexual development" (Martinson, 1982). Although statistics can be cited regarding specific sexual behaviors and such consequences as unintended pregnancies and rates of sexually transmitted disease, the knowledge base ranks poorly compared to other developed nations. They know significantly less about sexuality and place less value on issues such as consistent use of contraceptives and prevention of pregnancy than adolescents from other developed countries.

In a multinational study of teenage pregnancy and sexuality, U.S. youth scored the lowest of five similar industrialized nations (Canada, Sweden, France, England, and the Netherlands) on tests of knowledge and attitudes concerning sexuality

case study 5.3

Paul and Rich: Tumultuous Adolescence

Rich and Paul, both 42, are white.

Paul and Rich met as adults and compared their experiences of going through puberty and adolescence. Even though Paul is gay and Rich is heterosexual, their adolescent years had many similarities, and both had a tremendous amount of curiosity and guilt about their sexual desires.

Rich's adolescence was a fairly typical experience for a straight, lower-middle-class young man growing up in urban America. His parents were high school graduates who worked in factories as piecework tailors. Although both were loving and attentive parents, neither was skilled at communicating openly with Rich about the issues he would face as an adolescent. Neither knew about the key developmental components of puberty and adolescence and weren't comfortable talking with Rich about these issues. Consequently, Rich's adolescence was a hit-or-miss, trial-and-error experience for which he was totally unprepared.

Rich remembers experiencing things such as wet dreams, his first "true love," masturbation, his first ejaculation, and how puzzled he was trying to figure out how male and female genitalia come together during sexual intercourse. He remembers agonizing about his first ejaculation, feeling as if perhaps he had injured himself or something had gone wrong because all of a sudden this liquid was coming out of the end of his penis. Rich had to be content with asking his friends or older brother about some of these things. Based on the responses he received, he knew that some of the answers were not the "right" ones. It took Rich several years to get over much of the guilt and shame he had about his sexual feelings and behavior during adolescence. He spent the better part of his 20s looking for the answers to unresolved questions and issues from his adolescence.

The major difference between Paul and Rich is in sexual orientation. Paul just never felt any sexual desire toward females. He played along when his friends talked about "getting laid" and carrying on with girls in general. Inside, however, Paul was troubled because he felt attracted to some of the boys in his class. In addition, Paul's church had a stated position against masturbation, which created much confusion and guilt in Paul whenever he engaged in that activity. He did not dare to discuss his sexual feelings with anyone connected with his church. Furthermore, as the only son of immigrant parents who did not discuss things of a sexual nature with him, he began to feel isolated. All through his adolescence, Paul agonized over who or what he was. He tried dating girls but found it unsatisfactory. He suspected he was gay but didn't want to admit it and believed he had no one in whom he could confide or trust while exploring this facet of himself.

Paul coped with adolescence by suppressing most of his sexual feelings. He denied that they existed and spent most of his time immersed in studying. Not until he entered college as a pre-med student did he finally give in to his urges to explore this part of himself. Later, in medical school and a steady relationship with another male student, Paul was able to work through some of the pain and confusion that had marred his adolescence.

Critical Thinking

If Rich and Paul were adolescents today, how might their stories be different?

Use your Virtual Workbook to explore your answer to this question at **http://health.wadsworth.com/blonna1.**

---

and conception (Dryfoos, 1985). Lack of basic information concerning sexual anatomy and physiology, contraception, and pregnancy were cited among other findings as indicators of what international experts would consider arrested sexual development.

As discussed in Chapter 1, the Sexuality Information and Education Council of the U.S. (SIECUS) has developed guidelines for comprehensive sexuality education.

Access to the Truth

For 20 years, the Network for Family Life Education, based at the Rutgers University Center for Applied Psychology, has provided resources, advocacy, training, and technical assistance in support of age-appropriate, balanced comprehensive sexuality education in New Jersey and now nationwide. In 1994, the network asked young people if they would read a newsletter about sexuality and health written by teens, for teens. The response was an immediate and electric "*Yes!*" The National Teen-to-Teen Sexuality Education Program was thus established, and today it has five thriving components:

- *SEX, ETC.*, the award-winning newsletter written by teens, for teens, a free resource produced three times each year by a multiethnic board of New Jersey high school students (circulation began with 30,000 copies in 1994 and in 2003 has risen to 2.1 million copies)
- Discussion Guides designed to help adults spark lively discussions about vital health topics in each issue of *SEX, ETC.*, including a newly published teaching manual
- *The Roadmap: A Teen Guide to Changing Your School's Sex Ed*, a book to teach teens to become advocates for effective sexuality education
- Youth Media Outlets such as a monthly column on MTV.com and feature articles in *Teen People* magazine
- A Web site—www.sexetc.org—launched in 1999, that offers teens more than 300 articles written by their peers, weekly feature stories, reader polls, quizzes, opportunities to get involved, and honest and expert answers to frequently asked questions through the Ask the Experts feature

The Ask the Experts section of the Web site takes in questions from teens all over the world, and a panel of 12 experts, including health educators, physicians, social workers, psychologists, and other professionals, responds to over 350 questions a week. Each question is given a private, confidential, and individual response that is edited carefully by the experts and returned to the teen in about 3 to 5 days. The Web site averages 350,000 teen users each month, and in 2002, it individually answered more than 18,000 teen questions.

The average age for teens writing to the site is about 15 years old, but it ranges from 13 to 21. The kinds of questions teens send to the SEX, ETC. Web site reflect their general ignorance and naiveté about most sexuality issues. The site receives a substantial percentage of questions about body image, penis size, breast size, and whether or not to shave pubic hair. In addition, the majority of questions are about what behaviors are risky for pregnancy, how to make sex more pleasurable and less painful, and how to access birth control, gynecological care, and STI testing.

The site's experts always offer honest and completely straightforward answers to all questions sent in. They also provide information about negotiating and communicating with partners, reducing risk, delaying sexual involvement, and finding alternatives to high-risk behaviors. It is clear that teens are not getting the vital health information they need at home or at school.

The popularity of Web sites that offer information about sexuality shows how greatly teens (and adults) need honest and accurate information that they can access when they need it. Many Web sites feature FAQs and Ask the Experts sections, including www.teenwire.com, www.gurl.com, and www.puberty.org. Most teens are not comfortable asking parents their most intimate questions (although the SEX, ETC. Web site encourages them to try), and most teachers in schools are ill equipped or forbidden to respond to questions about contraception, abortion, sexual response, body image, growth and puberty, safer sex, and many other topics.

Having a place where teens can find information, resources, and answers to their most pressing questions is a service that has been needed for a long time. Although the Internet can have all kinds of negative and potentially dangerous possibilities, being a source of honest, accurate information about health and sexuality is one of its best uses, especially for teens.

Source: Elizabeth Casparian, New Jersey Network for Family Life Education (2003).

At the same time, the U.S. government continues to fund abstinence-based curricula that do not cover such topics as birth control methods, sexual orientation concerns, and sexual decision-making skill development, to name a few.

Education Online

Government leaders, state and local departments of education, not-for profit agencies devoted to health, educators, and parents have debated just what children and teens need to know about sexuality for over 100 years (Moran, 2000). Unintended pregnancies and sexual infections, whether syphilis concerns from the early 1900s or HIV/AIDS concerns in the late 1900s and early parts of this century, remain the driving forces behind the debate. Unfortunately, what has often won out are moralistic policies focused on heterosexual marriage as a solution, rather than health policies that focus on the health and welfare of children.

As the Internet becomes increasingly available, children and youth are connecting with good sources to answer their myriad questions. Sex in Society 5.2 highlights the work of one such source that provides reliable information to teens.

Consequences of Teen Risk-Taking Behaviors

Of the estimated 11 million unmarried adolescent females who are having intercourse, reports indicate that between 900,000 and 1 million become pregnant each year. The majority of these pregnancies are unplanned, with one-fourth of unintended pregnancies ending in abortion (CDC, 2000) and one-tenth in stillbirth or spontaneous abortion/miscarriage (McGrew & Shore, 1991).

The teens who maintain their pregnancies are more likely to have pregnancy-related problems than women who delay childbearing until they are in their 20s. Adolescents are more likely to suffer from toxemia, hemorrhaging, and miscarriages than women who delay pregnancy. In addition, teen mothers are more likely to drop out of school, need public assistance, receive poor prenatal care, have low-birthweight babies, and a higher infant mortality rate (CDC, 2000). These unmarried, teenage mothers face a harder future than their peers who delay bearing children until they are older and married. Although keeping pregnant teens out of public school is illegal, most (approximately 80 percent) wind up dropping out and do not return (White & DeBlassie, 1992). Because of the twin burdens of the lack of a high school degree and the need for child care, these teens earn less, have less schooling, work in blue-collar professions and in general have a lower standard of living than their peers who delay marriage and childbirth.

Most of the negative health outcomes associated with teenage pregnancy are believed to be caused by **biological immaturity,** women having children before their bodies are physiologically ready for them. Some evidence suggests that teenagers, given adequate prenatal care and proper nutrition, may have as good or better pregnancy outcomes than women who are older (Trussel, 1988).

Unfortunately, obtaining adequate prenatal health care is the exception rather than the norm for most teens who get pregnant. Many are not under the care of a physician, midwife, or other health care provider for all three trimesters of pregnancy. As a result, routine testing and screening is delayed or is not done. When routine trimester examinations are not done, close monitoring of the size, weight, positioning, and vital signs of the fetus is not possible. In addition, these visits provide an opportunity for the health care provider to assess the health of the pregnant teen and talk about critical issues such as nutrition, substance use, and plans for delaying future pregnancies and adequately caring for their child if the pregnancy is going to be carried to full term.

Biological immaturity The incomplete anatomical and physiological development associated with early adolescence or preadolescence

Approximately 95 percent of unmarried teenage mothers keep their babies (Steven-Simon & White, 1991). Most of them continue to live at home and rear their babies with the help of their parents or grandparents while they try to cope with the realities of parenthood.

Other teens who become pregnant decide they aren't ready to become mothers and decide to use foster care or place their babies for adoption. Foster care is designed to provide temporary help for mothers or parents who feel they can't take care of their child now but will be able to do it in the near future. Under foster care, mothers still have legal rights to their children, have formal visitation privileges, and are actively involved with their children. Women who place their children for adoption permanently give over their rights as parents to another person or family.

Foster care and adoption offer viable options for teen mothers who are unable to cope with the demands of being a parent. Regardless of which of these options for coping with an unintended pregnancy is chosen, carrying the pregnancy to term and following through with giving up the baby can be extremely stressful. Many pregnant teens choose to terminate their pregnancies rather than be forced to choose between keeping their children, putting them in foster care, or placing them for adoption. Increasingly, however, states are mandating that minors not be able to secure abortions without parental consent. Parental consent laws remain another area of controversy among politicians, health care providers, and reproductive rights activists.

Good communication between teens and their parents, along with growing up in a supportive family, is clearly a healthy ideal. Nonetheless, many teens cannot share their pregnancies with their parents and get the guidance and help they need to manage their situations. The news too frequently reports cases where babies have been abandoned and killed.

Other negative health consequences are associated with adolescent sexual activity. Adolescents have higher rates than all other age groups of syphilis, gonorrhea, and pelvic inflammatory disease (PID). Adolescents also engage in sexual behavior that has high risk for HIV/AIDS (Jemmott, Jemmott, & Fong, 1992). Although the number of 13- to 19-year-olds reporting being infected with HIV is small (3,130 from 1981 through June 1998), many more young people are thought to be infected with HIV (CDC, 1998). In addition, since one in five of all people diagnosed with AIDS is between 20 and 29 years of age (101,368 cases from 1981 through June 1998), and the incubation period for AIDS can last several years, many, if not most, of these people became infected when they were teenagers.

Dealing with Adolescent Sexuality

Some people believe that the best way to deal with adolescent sexuality is to be honest with young people. If parents think their adolescent children would be better off to delay sexual intercourse or other forms of sexual activities with a partner, the best way for them to deal with it is to tell their children this and explain why. The healthy way to do this is to admit honestly to young people that sex is a powerful force in their lives and that, as parents, you would prefer them to redirect that sexual energy from sexual intercourse into other, less risky sexual outlets, such as hugging, kissing, and masturbation. To deny the power of adolescent sexual urges or, worse, not mention it and hope the subject will never come up is unhealthy and dishonest.

Trivializing adolescent sexual desire with simplistic advice such as "When you feel horny, take a cold shower" contributes to the mixed messages adolescents are already receiving about their sexuality. These mixed messages can be a real source of stress. On the one hand, their bodies are telling them, "Yes, yes, yes," and on the other hand, adult society is telling them, "No, no, no." Media—music stars, television, movies—that target adolescents are telling them it is OK and a normal part of teenage rebelliousness to give into, even glorify, their sexual urges, yet parents tell them to take a cold shower and the urges will disappear.

To further complicate matters, federally funded abstinence-only sex education curricula purport to reduce the incidence of unintended pregnancy and sexual intercourse. Parents can help their children by learning about and supporting comprehensive sexuality education programs in their local school districts.

Gay adolescents face an even tougher problem. Not only do they have to deal with the mixed messages and pressures associated with this part of their lives, but they also face a wall of silence concerning their own emerging preferences. Gay adolescents usually learn early on that discussing their attraction to same-gender partners is taboo. Few social supports and people are available to turn to for these adolescents whose school guidance counselors and other community helpers are often either misinformed about how to help these young people or homophobic and a threat to the very youth they are being paid to care for. Many school districts forbid teaching that homosexuality is an acceptable lifestyle. Local chapters of Parents and Friends of Lesbians and Gays (PFLAG) and other gay and lesbian organizations are excellent places to find help and information about resources.

The murder of Matthew Shephard brought the issues of violence against LGBT teens and young adults to the public consciousness. Helping teens and adolescents learn to accept themselves and develop tolerance and respect for the sexuality of others remains an ongoing challenge to schools and agencies working with youth.

Parents can be a great source of support and information.

Healthier Teens

One of the national health objectives for Healthy People 2010, a federal government plan to improve the health of Americans, is to improve the health of youth by sustaining the decrease in their rates of pregnancy, birth, and gonorrhea and reducing rates of HIV and other STD infections. The U.S. teen birthrate remains one of the highest among developed nations along with rates of STD infection. Child Trends, a nonprofit, nonpartisan research center that studies children and families, reviewed more than 150 research studies to identify the factors that contribute to improving adolescent reproductive health. Sound public policy and programming require that a holistic approach be taken, looking at the adolescent, the adolescent's family, the role of peers, the teenager's partners, the school context, and the neighborhood and community context (Manlove, Terry-Humen, Papillo, Franzetta, Williams, & Ryan, 2002). Some of the key summary findings are as follows:

1. Males are more likely than females to initiate sexual activity at an earlier age, yet for both sexes, earlier onset of puberty and an older appearance are associated with teens becoming involved in sexual activity. Adolescents who are engaged in positive activities such as sports and school and who are confident in their ability to delay activity are more likely to do so.
2. Adolescents with close family ties and good communication engage in more positive reproductive behaviors, whereas those whose mothers were teens at the time of their birth and have sexually active teen siblings are more likely to engage in risky behaviors.

3. Teens are influenced by their friends, and when their peer group engages in risky behaviors, they are more likely to do so themselves.
4. Adolescents who have experienced coercive sex and those who have much older sexual partners appear to be at greater risk for multiple partners, lack of contraception, and pregnancy.
5. There is variability in the types of sexuality programs offered in schools, with some programs associated with reduced sexual activity and increased contraceptive use and other programs associated with delayed sexual activity. It is difficult, however, to separate the school from the community context.
6. Higher rates of sexual activity, pregnancy, and birth are associated with higher rates of poverty.

Overall, Manlove et al.'s (2002) analysis shows that the best programs focus on early childhood development, combine sexuality education for older children with community service activities, and send nurses to visit with teenage mothers.

Beginning with the Adolescent Family Life Act in 1981, the federal government funded programs designed to prevent teen pregnancy through the promotion of chastity and self-discipline. An attachment to the Welfare Reform Act in 1996 provided $50 million annually to state programs that would teach "abstinence-only until marriage"; those states that accept federal funds were required to match the federal grants with state funds (three state dollars to every four federal dollars). The Special Projects of Regional and National Significance—Community Based Abstinence Education (SPRANS-CBAE) in 2001 provided funding for subsequent years to continue the educational efforts for abstinence-only-until-marriage programs (Kreinin, 2003).

Despite research findings on effective educational programs, statistical data on teen sexual activity, reports of dating violence and harassment related to sexuality, undesirable outcomes of unwanted pregnancy and infection, realities of teen parenting, and other pertinent issues, controversy still persists in the United States surrounding the design and implementation of comprehensive programs to meet the sexual health needs of adolescents.

Your responses to the Personal Assessment, Thought Questions, and Test Yourself! quiz questions can be logged online in your Virtual Workbook at **http://health.wadsworth.com/blonna1.**

Personal Assessment

5.1 Rites of Passage

U.S. culture has been criticized for lacking traditional rites of passage that help adolescents make a smoother transition from childhood to adulthood. The purpose of this assessment is to help you explore rites of passage in our culture and others by reflecting on your own experiences. This assessment will enable you to understand why adolescence is often troubling for youth in the United States.

1. Read Sex in Society 5.1, "Other Cultures, Other Ways," in this chapter.

2. Describe, in writing, your own thoughts and feelings about this reading.

3. How do you think these rites of passage would be accepted in the United States?

4. List and describe any cultural rituals that you have experienced while growing up that could be considered rites of passage, and explain how they differ from the examples in the reading.

Thought Questions

1. Describe the different psychological theories and their contributions to the understanding of healthy sexual development.

2. How do bonding, nudity, and toilet training practices affect the development of healthy sexuality?

3. What are the effects of masturbation on childhood and later adult health?

4. What are some of the key developmental issues that young adolescents confront?

5. What are the pros and cons of sexual activity during adolescence?

Test Yourself!

1. Maslow identified characteristics of those who achieve self-actualization through "transcendence." Someone who is a transcender would most likely
   a. focus on the financial rewards of work.
   b. embrace change and creativity.
   c. prefer what is familiar, tried, and true.
   d. be judgmental of others.

2. Modern personality theorists
   a. widely support the Freudian perspective that libidinal energy is the basis for sexuality.
   b. agree that biology is the primary influence on sexual development.
   c. increasingly examine social and environmental influences that help frame ideas of what is normal and expected.
   d. reject all earlier theories of development as being antiquated and irrelevant.

3. Masturbation in young children
   a. is statistically rare.
   b. should be encouraged by parents and teachers.
   c. is normal and usually self-limiting.
   d. can lead to other forms of interpersonal sexual activity.

4. A primary developmental task of adolescence is
   a. to form a sense of identity.
   b. to create close, intimate relationships with members of the opposite sex.
   c. to achieve positive self-esteem through experimentation.
   d. to separate from parents and live independently.

5. All but which of the following are considered secondary sex characteristics in males?
   a. Increased muscle development
   b. Pubic hair
   c. Facial hair
   d. Higher voice

6. The term used to describe the biological transition from childhood to adulthood is
   a. *puberty.*
   b. *transcendence.*
   c. *adolescence.*
   d. *maturation.*

7. Most research on adolescent sexual behavior has revealed
   a. little interpersonal sexual activity until the last years of high school.
   b. drastic differences in the experiences of boys and girls.
   c. increasing rates of sexual experimentation as teens age.
   d. greater experimentation among gay and lesbian students than heterosexual students.

8. Today, teens who want detailed answers to their questions about sexuality
   a. can go online to Internet sites and receive quality information.
   b. will find that the majority of school programs talk about sexuality issues in an honest, comprehensive manner.
   c. will initiate conversations with their parents
   d. complain that no resources are available to them.

9. Which statement about nudity is most accurate?
   a. All cultures react to public nudity in the same way, expecting adults to be dressed.
   b. Families are encouraged to be nude as much as possible in order to teach positive messages about the body.
   c. Young children seem to enjoy nudity and develop a sense of personal modesty as they age.
   d. Most children get upset seeing their parents naked.

10. Becoming an "askable parent" for your child's sexuality questions requires
   a. always being serious when discussing sexuality.
   b. not discussing anything that makes you uncomfortable.
   c. being careful not to make mistakes with information.
   d. letting your child know your values on a subject.

Media Menu

You can link to the following online tools by visiting
http://health.wadsworth.com/blonna1.

Film

Perceiving Gender Roles
Teen Slang for Having Sex
Adolescent Body Image
Adolescent Sexual Risk Taking

 InfoTrac Activity

Shelby, L. (2003, February–March). Youth first: An integrated sexuality education program for pre-adolescents. *SIECUS Reports*, 31 (3), 31.

 Web Resources

Here are sites where teens can write and get honest answers to their sexual health questions:

www.teenwire.com
www.sexetc.org
www.goaskalice.columbia.edu
www.gurl.com
www.puberty.org

The following resources are of additional value to adolescents and adults:

Advocates for Youth

www.advocatesforyouth.org

Creates programs and promotes policies that help young people make informed and responsible decisions about their sexual and reproductive health with the purpose of preventing pregnancy and sexually transmitted diseases, including HIV. Large selection of links as well as links to minority youth sites. One section, which changes monthly, addresses contemporary issues that affect society and the way in which we live.

Coalition for Positive Sexuality

www.positive.org

A grassroots volunteer group started in 1992 to respond to the health crisis among Chicago teenagers. Teens receive information needed to make healthy decisions about sex, condom availability, and sex education. This site has FAQs with links to answers, national Web links, and information on sexuality, health issues, and birth control.

References

Abma, J. C., Chandra, A., Mosher, W. D., Peterson, L., & Puccini, L. (1997). Fertility, family planning, and women's health: New data from the National Survey of Family Growth. *National Center for Health Statistics, Vital Health Statistics, 23*, 19.

American Nurses Association. (1999). Sexual maturity rating scale [Online]. Available: www.nursingworld.org/mods/archive/mod4/ceah2.htm.

American Psychological Association. (2002). *Developing adolescents: Reference for professionals.* Washington, DC: National and Child Health Bureau, Health Resources and Services Administration, and the U.S. Department of Health and Human Services.

Baldwin, J. D., & Baldwin, J. I. (1997). Gender differences in sexual interest. *Archives of Sexual Behavior, 26*(2), 181–210.

Billhartz, C. (2003, February 25). Teens don't realize risk of their oral sex practices. *CDC News Updates.*

Butler, J. (1999). *Gender trouble: Feminism and the subversion of identity.* New York: Routledge.

Carrera, M. (2003, October). *The Children's Aid Society—Carrera Adolescent Sexuality and Pregnancy Prevention Program.* Paper presented at the Network for Family Life Education's 20th Anniversary Conference, "20 Years of Great Sex(Ed): Lessons from the Past, Plans for the Future."

Centers for Disease Control and Prevention. (1998, June 2). AIDS information [Online]. Available: www.cdc.gov/nchstp/hiv_aids/stats/cumulati.htm.

Centers for Disease Control and Prevention. (2002, September 27). Trends in sexual risk behaviors among high school students—U.S., 1991–2001. *Morbidity and Mortality Weekly Report, 51*(38), 856–859.

Centers for Disease Control and Prevention. (2003, July). *Why is an awareness of sexual behavior important?* [Online]. National Center for Chronic Disease Prevention and Health Promotion. Available: www.cdc.gov/nccdphp/dash/sexualbehaviors/index.htm.

Centers for Disease Control, U.S. Department of Health and Human Services. (2000, July). *Health, United States, 2000.* DHHS Publication No. 00-1232. Washington, DC: U.S. Government Printing Office.

Dryfoos, J. (1985). What the United States can learn about prevention of teenage pregnancy from other countries. *SIECUS Report, 14*(2), 1–7.

Erikson, E. (1978). *Childhood and society* (2nd ed.). New York: Norton.

Ferber, S. G., Laudon, M., Kuint, J., Weller, A., & Zisapel, N. (2002, December). Massage therapy by mothers enhances the adjustment of circadian rhythms to the nocturnal period in full-term infants. *Journal of Developmental & Behavioral Pediatrics, 23*(6), 410.

Ford, C. S., & Beach, F. A. (1951). *Patterns of sexual behavior.* New York: Harper.

Forrest, J. D., & Silverman, J. (1989). What public school teachers teach about preventing pregnancy, AIDS, and sexually transmitted diseases. *Family Planning Perspectives, 21*, 65–72.

Forrest, J. D., & Singh, S. (1990). The sexual and reproductive behavior of American women 1982–1988. *Family Planning Perspectives, 22*, 206–214.

Gates, G. J., & Sonenstein, F. L. (2000, November/December). Heterosexual genital sexual activity among adolescent males: 1988 and 1995. *Family Planning Perspectives, 32*(6).

Globus, S. K. (2002, Spring). Touch me, I'm yours: The benefits of infant massage. *Special Delivery, 25*(1), 8.

Gordon, S., & Gordon, J. (1983). *Raising a child conservatively in a sexually permissive world.* New York: Simon & Schuster.

Gurian, M. (1996). *The wonder of boys.* New York: Putnam.

Hall, C. S. (1954). *A primer of Freudian psychotherapy.* New York: Mentor.

Hatcher, J. L., & Scarpa, J. (2002, July). *Encouraging teens to adopt a safe, healthy lifestyle: A foundation for improving adult behaviors.* Child Trends Research Brief. Washington, DC: Child Trends.

Hedgepeth, E., & Lemich, J. (1996). *Teaching about sexuality and HIV.* New York: New York University Press.

Henry J. Kaiser Family Foundation. (2003). *Teen sexual health fact sheet* [Online]. Available: www.kff.org.

Henry J. Kaiser Family Foundation, Hoff, T., Greene, L., & Davis, J. (2003). *National Survey of Adolescents and Young Adults: Sexual health, knowledge, attitudes, and experiences* [Online]. Publication No. 3218. Available: www.kfg.org.

Herdt, T. G., & Boxer, A. (1992). Introduction: Culture, history, and life course of gay men. In G. Herdt (Ed.), *Gay culture in America: Essays from the field.* Boston: Beacon.

Jemmott, J. B., Jemmott, L., & Fong, G. T. (1992). Reductions in HIV risk-associated sexual behaviors among black male adolescents: Effects of an AIDS prevention intervention. *American Journal of Public Health, 82*(3), 372–377.

Kaplan, H. S. (1974). *The new sex therapy.* New York: Brunner/Mazel.

Kinsey, A. C., Pomeroy, W. B., & Martin, C.E . (1948). *Sexual behavior in the human male.* Philadelphia: Saunders.

Kreinin, T. (2003, May). Letter from the president of the Sexuality Information and Education Council of the U.S. to SIECUS membership.

Laumann, E. O., Gagnon, J. H., Michael, R. T., & Michaels, S. (1994). *The social organization of sexuality: Sexual practices in the United States.* Chicago: University of Chicago Press.

Levine, J. (2002). *Harmful to minors: The perils of protecting children from Sex.* Minneapolis: University of Minnesota Press.

Lopiano, C. (2001). *Equity in women's sports: A health and fairness perspective* [Online]. Available: www.womenssportsfoundation.org.

Lorber, J. (2001). The social construction of gender. In P. S. Rothenberg (Ed.), *Race, class, gender in the United States* (pp. 47–56). New York: Freeman.

Manlove, J., Terry-Humen, E., Papillo, A., Franzetta, K., Williams, S., & Ryan, S. (2002, May). *Preventing teenage pregnancy, childbearing, and sexually transmitted diseases: What the research shows.* Child Trends Research Brief. Washington, DC: Child Trends.

Marshall, D. (1971). Sexual behavior on Mangaia. In D. Marshall & R. Suggs (Eds.), *Human sexual behavior: Variations in the ethnographic spectrum.* Englewood Cliffs, NJ: Prentice Hall.

Martinson, F. M. (1982). Against sexual retardation. *SIECUS Report, 10*(3), 3.41.

Maslow, A. (1970). *Motivation and personality* (2nd ed.). New York: Harper & Row.

McGrew, M., & Shore, W. (1991). The problem of teenage pregnancy. *Journal of Family Practice, 31,* 17–25.

Montague A. (1986). *Touching* (3rd ed.). New York: Columbia University Press.

Moran, J. (2000). *Teaching sex: The shaping of adolescents in the 20th century.* Cambridge, MA: Harvard University Press.

Newman, S., & Udry, J. (1988). Oral sex in adolescent populations. *Archives of Sexual Behavior, 14,* 41–16.

Reports of child sexual abuse. (2001, January). *Juvenile Justice Bulletin.*

Sarrel, L., & Sarrel, P. (1984). *Sexual turning points: The seven signs of adult sexuality.* New York: Macmillan.

Savin-Williams, R., & Rodriguez, R.G. (1993). A developmental, clinical perspective on lesbian, gay male, and bisexual youth. In T. P. Gullets et al. (Eds.), *Adolescent sexuality.* Newbury Park, CA: Sage.

Schlegel, A., & Barry, H. (1979). Adolescent initiation ceremonies: Cross-cultural codes. *Ethnology, 18,* 199–210.

Schlegel, A., & Barry, H. (1980). The evolutionary significance of adolescent initiation ceremonies. *American Ethnologist, 7,* 696–715.

Sonenstein, F. L., Pleck, J. H., & Hu, L. C. (1989). Sexual activity, condom use, and AIDS awareness among adolescent males. *Family Planning Perspectives, 2*(14), 152–158.

Sorenson, R. (1983). *Adolescent sexuality in contemporary America.* New York: World, 1983.

Steven-Simon, C., & White, M. (1991). Adolescent pregnancy. *Pediatric Annals, 20,* 322–331.

Troiden, R. (1988). *Gay and lesbian identity: A sociological analysis.* New York: General Hall.

Trussel, J. (1988). Teenage pregnancy in the United States. *Family Planning Perspectives, 20,* 262–272.

Watson, J. *Behaviorism* (1970). New York: Norton.

White, S., & DeBlassie, R. (1992). Adolescent sexual behavior. *Adolescence, 27,* 183–191.

Wilson, S. M., & Medora, N. P. (1999). Gender comparisons of college students: Attitudes towards sexual behavior. *Adolescence, 25,* 615–627.

Young, S. M. (1986). Attitudes and behavior of college students to oral-genital sexuality. *Archives of Sexual Behavior, 9,* 61–67.

Zelnick, M., Kanter, J., & Ford, K. (1981). *Sex and pregnancy in adolescence.* Beverly Hills, CA: Sage.

chapter six

Adult Sexuality

Student Learning Objectives

After reading this chapter, students will be able to

- Describe the typical developmental tasks associated with young adulthood through older adulthood.
- Relate the findings of a variety of studies concerning the sexual behavior of college students and young adults.
- Assess a variety of living arrangements of the college years and young adulthood.
- Examine the major developmental tasks associated with adulthood.
- Assess a variety of sexual lifestyles in adulthood.
- Explain the impact of aging on sexual response and behavior.
- Describe the developmental course of long-term straight, gay, and bisexual relationships.
- Identify the major areas of discord and stress in marital and long-term intimate relationships.
- Discuss the effects of divorce and widowhood on adult sexuality.

*Test your understanding of these objectives by taking the end-of-chapter quiz, available online at **http://health.wadsworth.com/blonna1**.*

activity teaser: *What do you really need to have a successful relationship? Find out with the Personal Exploration Activity on page 177.*

case study 6.1

Maria, aka Supermom

Maria, 35, identifies as white, Italian American.

Maria has been married for 15 years and has three children, ages 12, 10, and 7. Married as soon as she finished at the local community college with an associate's degree, she worked full-time for a year at an accounting office. As soon as she started having her kids, however, the idea of continuing to work and pay for day care made no financial sense. She and her husband decided she should stay home with the kids, and she could bring in some money doing child care in her home.

Once the kids were in school all day, Maria realized that she wanted to finish her own education and earn her bachelor's degree in accounting. All along she's taken primary responsibility for the child rearing, cooking, cleaning, and chauffeuring the kids to appointments, activities, and play dates. She was an officer with the PTA, den mother for the Cub Scouts, Sunday school teacher, and all-around busy stay-at-home mom. The change of going back to school has markedly increased her stress but, in an odd way, also energized her.

Maria is finding that her relationships with her kids and husband are changing. She seems to have less time to give each the attention they want. Maria heads off for her own classes as soon as the kids are on their way. She carries a cell phone for emergencies and has been lucky that the kids have stayed well and she hasn't been beeped in the middle of her classes. Dinners aren't quite as nutritious as they had been, with more drive-through pickup meals than she'd like. She likes to get up at 5:30 A.M to enjoy the quiet of the morning before all the chaos sets in. That has been a good time for her to study while running the wash.

She and her husband find that they have to schedule "dates" now in order to be together as a couple. At the end of the week, it takes purposeful planning to keep the romance alive. It hasn't been easy, juggling the demands of motherhood, housework, and school, but everyone is adjusting. Maria feels she's making a successful passage into another phase of her life.

Critical Thinking

Can you identify some strategies Maria and her family could develop to reduce her workload and stress levels?

Use your Virtual Workbook to explore your answer to this question at **http://health.wadsworth.com/blonna1.**

Intimacy A gradual process of sharing one's innermost feelings with another

The primary task we face as young adults, according to Erik Erikson (1978), is the development of **intimacy**—forming committed, intimate, loving relationships. We begin to move away from the adolescent focus on ourselves toward exploring mutually satisfying relationships. This stage emphasizes commitment, both in intimate relationships and in work.

This is an exciting time of life. We meet new friends, explore intimate, loving relationships, and test the waters for work and career possibilities. This is the first time many college students are living apart from their parents. It is a time of unparalleled freedom. Students who have mastered the developmental tasks of adolescence and childhood enter this period in their lives ready and eager to sample all that life has to offer. Maria's life, as described in Case Study 6.1, highlights the many demands of adulthood, some of which compete for time and attention.

Forming Friendships

New adult friendships form the basis of intimate relationships for many college students. Intimacy grows out of friendships as we become more trusting and comfortable with each other. In his book *Friendship*, Joel Block (1980) contends that humans are "wired" with a basic desire for contact with others. Our friend-

Friendships fill a special place in our lives.

ships, Block believes, are what make us whole. He says that friends enrich our existence and bond with us to form a conspiracy against the world. We like one another, understand each other, share interests, and have similar lifestyles or problems in life.

Although college literally throws people together (dorm pairings, class scheduling, and so on), what is it that draws friends together? Many friendships grow out of meeting people who share similar interests and experiences. We meet fellow students who have the same major, take the same classes, and join the same organizations. These similarities provide the initial attraction. If the attraction is strong enough, it provides the basis for spending more time together. As the friendship progresses, the friends share more time and experiences, reinforcing their commonality, deepening their bonds, and enriching their lives. Many people form their deepest friendships in college during young adulthood.

Friendship is a unique bond. Although it is fraught with entanglements that also characterize romantic relationships—competition, jealousy, and betrayal—it offers what Block calls "psychological space." Friendships are more open-ended than relationships with family, mates, or lovers. Unlike these other, more intimate relationships, our friendships provide separate lives that allow time off and away from entanglements. Consequently, friends develop a greater tolerance for growth and change. We are most truly ourselves with our friends.

Dating and Intimate Relationships

Whereas friendships may be casual, intimacy by definition is deeply personal and trusting. Intimate relationships are characterized by sharing deep personal information. Intimacy grows out of friendship and usually is nurtured through dating. We'll cover intimacy in detail in Chapter 10, "Intimate Relationships."

Every society has some rituals or norms for pairing and courtship. Although the "rules" for dating and courtship vary from culture (and subculture) to cul-

Dating provides an opportunity to get to know each other.

Jacobs Stock Photography/GettyImages

ture, every society has traditions that it passes along from one generation to the next. Adults who came of age in the late 1960s and early 1970s in the United States vividly remember the differences between the rigid rules of the 1950s and the more liberated late 1960s and early 1970s. Prior to the cultural revolution of the 1960s, a young woman would not even consider asking a man out for a date. Men were expected to ask women out, pay for the evening's activities, and be responsible for picking up and dropping off their dates. Women were expected to wait for men to call them, even if a woman was interested and wanted to initiate contact. The popular media played out these and other traditional dating scenarios, and mothers and fathers passed them on to their daughters and sons. Everyone was assumed to be heterosexual, and sex was not a part of the evening's activities.

The face of dating today looks dramatically different. As will be discussed in this chapter, it may be more comfortable for students to use the terms *hooking up* and *seeing someone* rather than *date* (Crawford & Popp, 2003). Regardless of the term used, the behavior involved reflects greater role flexibility. A woman can initiate a date, pick up her date, and pay for herself. Straight, gay, and bisexual men and women have their own clubs, organizations, and dating services that make finding a partner easier and safer. In the past, bars and clubs for gay and lesbian women were disguised and subject to harassment from bullies and the police. Today they are more accepted and open, with directories available identifying various facilities, particularly in urban areas.

Although the rituals and rules of dating change over time, the purpose of dating hasn't changed much. Dating is a mechanism for developing intimate relationships. Intimate relationships, in turn, influence both sexual behavior and living patterns.

Emotional and Social Wellness

The emotional dimension of wellness requires that we acknowledge the full range of emotions associated with our changing roles and responsibilities. Most of the major developmental tasks associated with the adult stages of our lives are part of social wellness: forming intimate relationships, committing ourselves to others and to our work, being productive—in relationships, work, and so on. Understanding our emotional responses and developing interpersonal social skills become critical as we navigate the challenges associated with adulthood.

The social legacy we develop and leave behind can be one of a caring child, loving partner, and/or devoted parent. We can move through the stages of our relationships eagerly anticipating the changes and tasks that await us. We can also move through life and relationships with a self-centeredness that obscures all propensities for caring, sharing, and nurturing. Adulthood and old age may be viewed as opportunities for continued growth, reflection, and self-acceptance; for some, this stage of life may be marked by bitterness and regret. Overall health is enhanced by positive attitudes and a willingness to remain socially engaged.

College Sexual Standards

Many people equate intimacy with sexual activity and love, yet they are three separate entities. A person can be intimate and sexual with another person but not love that person. One can be in love, but with limited sexual involvement. And a person can be sexual with another but neither love nor be intimate with that person. In a survey of more than 10,000 adults, most respondents agreed that the best possible combination of all three would be to be sexual with someone toward whom you feel both intimate and loving (Blumstein & Schwartz, 1983).

Research on college sexual mores has often focused on students' attitudes toward "premarital sex," defined as premarital intercourse, and "double standards" for males and females, specifically looking at how males and females engage in the same behaviors but are judged differently. Sexual standards may have been prefaced with such adjectives as *permissive* or *traditional*. Primary concern was when behaviors took place relative to marriage or a commitment to marry.

In our discussions with students about acceptable dating behaviors, invariably the word *slut* will enter the conversation. Males anecdotally report not being interested in a woman who has had too many partners; females express their concern that they wouldn't want to be considered a slut by having engaged in sex too quickly or with too many males. At the same time, there is an expressed view that promiscuity by either sex is less than desirable.

A review of the research confirms that sexual attitudes may have become more egalitarian in recent years, yet there are still differences for males and females. Females may be judged for having had sex at an early age, having had many partners in the past, and for having sex outside a committed relationship. Males may also judge behaviors differently when seeking dating partners as opposed to long-term partners (Crawford & Popp, 2003).

Because of sampling issues, it is more difficult to assess lesbian, bisexual, and gay student mores. The process of "coming out," finding a partner, and being free to date openly is of paramount concern to the gay, lesbian, and bisexual community of students. Although working toward committed relationships may be a goal, judging behaviors as "premarital" obviously doesn't work. Like their heterosexual peers, however, gay, lesbian, and bisexual individuals may judge a potential partner's past sexual history.

All students, irrespective of sexual orientation, however, need to assess their personal levels of interest, sexual involvement, and commitment as they form pairs with others. Engaging in behavior that is consistent with one's personal values and feeling comfortable in sexual situations continue as challenges during college years.

Hooking Up

The term **hooking up** has increasingly been used to describe a variety of sexual interactions that take place on a casual basis, often with alcohol part of the picture. Students may refer to having "hooked up" with someone over a weekend, yet the specifics of that interaction may be unclear. Two individuals may have met at a party or bar and engaged in some form of sexual behavior without the need for commitment (Lambert, Kahn, & Apple, 2003). *Hooking up* may be defined as "a sexual encounter between two people who may or may not know each other well, but who usually are *not* seriously dating" (Lambert et al., 2003, p. 129). When asked about experiences with hooking up, researchers found college students citing the occurrence of petting below the waist, oral sex, and sexual intercourse as part of the behaviors included in the definition (Paul, McManus, & Hayes, 2000).

Hooking up A sexual encounter between two people who may or may not know each other well and are not seriously dating

In addition to the term not being specific, males and females who hook up may have differing expectations of what sexual behaviors they want to engage in. Alcohol further complicates the situation, which may lead to participation in sexual behaviors that are not desired. Students may have "bad hooking-up experiences," where the next day they regret the behavior and do not care to even talk with the sexual partner. At the most negative would be cases where the interaction involved force and qualified as sexual assault. One study found that college students thought their peers were more comfortable with hooking up than they themselves were. Men were more comfortable with hooking-up behaviors than women, yet men were less comfortable than women believed them to be, and women were less comfortable than men believed them to be. Overall, although it may appear that hooking up is the norm for college campuses, peer pressure and misperceptions of comfort may be part of the picture (Lambert et al., 2003).

Students have also described having "friends with benefits." In those situations, a comfortable friendship exists with consensual sexual activity. There is no apparent expectation that the two will see themselves or be viewed by others as a couple.

Research on Adult Behavior

The National Health and Social Life Survey (NHSLS) conducted by Laumann, Gagnon, Michael, and Michaels (1994) remains a critical source of data for understanding adult sexual behavior. Their research relied on random sampling, well-constructed survey instruments, and interviews. Controversy about the "need" to study adult sexual behavior—even for its public health value—led to congressional opponents effectively stopping National Institute of Health funding for the initial survey designed in the late 1980s (Laumann & Michael, 2001). The researchers were able, however, to secure funding from seven foundations: The Robert Wood Johnson Foundation, the Henry J. Kaiser Family Foundation, the Rockefeller Foundation, the Andrew Mellon Foundation, the New York Community Trust, the John D. and Catherine T. MacArthur Foundation, and the American Foundation for AIDS Research. Although it would be exciting and valuable to have periodic, government-sponsored, comprehensive studies of adult sexual behavior, such efforts have not been widely funded.

Nonetheless, various efforts have been made to provide more information about adult sexual behavior since Kinsey's detailed work in the mid–20th century. Students may find great personal value in reading qualitative research, where issues are explored in greater depth. Carol Ellison and Bernie Zilbergeld have each discussed female and male sexuality in depth from their experiences as clinical practitioners and psychologists. Both *Women's Sexualities* (Ellison, 2000) and *The New Male Sexuality* (Zilbergeld, 1999) provide students the opportunity to understand that their own personal behaviors and needs are "normal" and part of the spectrum of human sexual behavior.

Laumann and colleagues (1994) reported in *The Social Organization of Sexuality* that the sexual behavior of most American adults was rather conventional. Although popular culture would lead to the opposite conclusion, the actual data collected point to most reporting a limited number of sexual partners with a somewhat limited repertoire of sexual activities. A significant finding was that the critical factors that frame our sexual lives are gender, age, and marital status, with only modest differences in behavior when such characteristics as race/ethnicity, educational level, or religious affiliation are taken into account (Laumann & Michael, 2001).

Sexual Partners

Laumann and colleagues studied the number of sexual partners their subjects had, providing comparisons by gender, age, marital status, education, religion, and race/ethnicity. Table 6.1 shows the number of sexual partners during the past 12 months and since age 18.

The researchers discovered that most people interviewed reported a modest number of partners over the course of their lifetime. Married and cohabiting couples reported being faithful to their partners. Those who reported having had more than one partner during the past 12 months were not married or living with anyone, and they were mostly young and male. The researchers did discover that the more educated people were, the more partners they had had over their lifetime. An important explanation for that finding was that many who pursue a college education delay marriage; sexual relationships develop, yet individuals are more likely to be somewhat older before committing to one partner (Michael, Gagnon, Laumann, & Kolata, 1994, p. 104).

Looking at those between ages 18 and 24, 57 percent of subjects reported having had only one partner in the past 12 months, compared to 9 percent who had had five or more partners during that time. Another study specific to college students found that the total number of sex partners for both the previous year and total lifetime had increased for college men and women (Reinisch, 1992). The average number of total sexual partners for college women was 5.6 compared to 11.2 partners reported by males.

Sexual Behavior Among College Students

The trends we discussed in Chapter 5 regarding adolescent sexual behavior seem to continue into the college years. Specifically, evidence suggests increasing levels of sexual activity among college students over the past two decades, and women seem to be catching up to men in terms of the number of partners, level of sexual activity, and activities engaged in. Data concerning the sexual behavior of college students are difficult to extract from large-scale studies. Often, data on college students are reported in studies of adolescent or teenage sexual behavior because the teen years extend into the first year or two of college. College students are also merged into studies of adult sexual behavior.

In one study, similar percentages of male and female college students were found for the following behaviors: vaginal intercourse (68 percent for men and women), masturbation (men 78 percent, women 71 percent), performing oral sex (60 percent men, 68 percent women), receiving oral sex (64 percent men, 71 percent women), anal intercourse (6 percent men, 10 percent women), and using pornography (58 percent men, 37 percent women) (Person, 1989).

The frequency of sexual activity for men and women aged 18 to 29 is compared within Table 6.2. From these data, women aged 18 to 29 seem to enjoy a slightly higher level of sexual activity. Table 6.2 illustrates the percentages of men and women engaging in various levels of sexual activity over a 12-month period.

Other interesting findings from Laumann et al. regarding the sexual behavior of 18- to 29-year-olds were related to masturbation and oral sex. Those behaviors are presented in Tables 6.3, 6.4, and 6.5 later in this chapter.

Approximately 41 percent of the men and 64 percent of the women reported that they currently did not masturbate. Of those who masturbated, approximately 30 percent of the men and only 10 percent of the women did so at least once a week.

Men and women in the 18- to 24-year-old age group were similar in their levels of both active and receptive oral sex. Approximately 72 percent of the men and 70

Table 6.1 Number of Sex Partners in Past 12 Months and Since Age 18

	Sex Partners Past 12 Months				Sex Partners Since Age 18					
	0	1	2–4	5+	0	1	2–4	5–10	10–20	21+
Total	12%	71%	14%	3%	3%	26%	30%	22%	11%	
Gender:										
Men	10	67	18	5	3	20	21	23	16	
Women	14	75	10	2	3	31	36	20	6	
Age:										
18–24	11	57	24	9	8	32	34	15	8	
25–29	6	72	17	6	2	25	31	22	10	
30–34	9	73	16	2	3	21	29	25	11	
35–39	10	77	11	2	2	19	30	25	14	
40–44	11	75	13	1	1	22	28	24	14	
45–49	15	75	9	1	2	26	24	25	10	
50–54	15	79	5	0	2	34	28	18	9	
55–59	32	65	4	0	1	40	28	15	8	
Marital status:										
Never married, noncohabiting	25	38	28	9	12	15	29	21	12	
Never married, cohabiting	1	75	20	5	0	25	37	16	10	
Married	2	94	4	1	0	37	28	19	9	
Divorced, separated, widowed, noncohabiting	31	41	26	3	0	11	33	29	15	
Divorced, separated, widowed, cohabiting	1	80	15	3	0	0	32	44	12	
Education:										
Less than high school	16	67	15	3	4	27	36	19	9	
High school graduate or equivalent	11	74	13	3	3	30	29	20	10	
Some college/vocational	11	71	14	4	2	24	29	23	12	
Finished college	12	69	15	4	2	24	26	24	11	13
Master's/advanced degree	13	74	10	3	4	25	26	23	10	13
Current religion:										
None	11	68	13	7	3	16	29	20	16	16
Mainline Protestant	11	73	13	2	2	23	31	23	12	8
Conservative Protestant	13	70	14	3	3	30	30	20	10	7
Catholic	12	71	13	3	4	27	29	23	8	9
Jewish	3	75	18	3	0	24	13	30	17	17
Other religion	15	70	12	3	3	42	20	16	8	13
Race/ethnicity:										
White	12	73	12	3	3	26	29	22	11	9
Black	13	60	21	6	2	18	34	24	11	11
Hispanic	11	69	17	2	4	35	27	17	8	9
Asian	15	77	8	0	6	46	25	14	6	3
Native American	12	76	10	2	5	28	35	23	5	5

Note: Row percentages total 100 percent.

Source: From *Sex in America* by Robert Michael, et al. Copyright © 1994 by CSG Enterprises, Inc., Edward O. Laumann, Robert T. Michael, and Gina Kolata. By permission of Little, Brown, and Company, Inc.

Table 6.2 Frequency of Sexual Intercourse During Past 12 Months and Since Age 18

Master Status Variables	Not at All	Frequency of Sex in the Past Year (%)			
		A Few Times per Year	A Few Times per Month	Two to Three Times a Week	Four or More Times a Week
Men					
Total population	9.8	17.6	35.5	29.5	7.7
Age:					
18–29	21.4	35.9	54.9	64.2	23.8
30–44	23.2	46.2	119.1	93.2	18.3
45–59	36.2	64.1	120.0	67.2	12.3
Marital status:					
Never married, not cohabitating	22.0	26.2	25.4	18.8	7.6
Never married, cohabitating	0.0	8.5	35.6	37.3	18.6
Married	1.3	12.8	42.5	36.1	7.3
Divorced/separated/ widow, not cohabitating	23.8	22.5	28.5	20.5	4.6
Divorced/separated/ widow, cohabitating	0.0	8.3	36.1	44.4	11.1
Education:					
HS graduate equivalent	10.1	15.1	34.4	31.7	8.7
Finished college	9.0	15.8	43.9	25.8	5.4
Women					
Total population	13.6	16.1	37.2	26.3	6.7
Age:					
18–29	15.7	26.4	69.6	65.6	22.7
30–44	33.5	47.8	118.5	82.3	17.8
45–59	76.2	59.2	110.6	46.2	7.7
Marital status:					
Never married, not cohabitating	30.2	23.5	26.0	13.3	7.0
Never married, cohabitating	1.4	6.9	31.9	43.1	16.7
Married	3.0	11.9	46.5	31.9	6.6
Divorced/separated/ widow, not cohabitating	34.3	23.2	21.9	16.8	3.7
Divorced/separated/ widow, cohabitating	0.0	9.4	39.6	39.6	11.3
Education:					
HS graduate equivalent	10.8	15.9	37.7	29.6	6.0
Finished college	12.5	18.3	33.5	29.7	6.1

Source: The Social Organization of Sexuality: Sexual Practices in the United States, by E. Laumann et al. (Chicago: University of Chicago Press, 1994). Used with permission.

percent of the women reported ever performing oral sex on their partners. Of this group, 28 percent of the men and 19 percent of the women reported performing oral sex during their last sexual encounter with their partners. Similar percentages for men (75 percent ever and 29 percent last encounter) and women (75 percent ever and 24 percent last encounter) were reported for receiving oral sex.

Living Arrangements of College Students

Living arrangements of college students vary, determined by personal finances, whether they are commuting or living on campus, whether living with a friend or romantic partner, and so forth. At some universities, the majority of undergraduates live in either dormitories or apartments. Other institutions have minimal housing for full-time students, are more accommodating to the commuting student, and have sizeable populations who attend school part-time. Whereas the married undergraduate student used to be the exception years ago, today many students are both married and older, some with young children. Consequently, more colleges are finding the need to include day care facilities on campus. The National Coalition for Campus Childcare has surveyed campuses to determine the availability of child care for their students and employees. At the majority of institutions, students participate in the centers in a variety of ways from student teachers, paid work/study students, unpaid student observers, researchers, and other roles. As more nontraditional students are drawn to undergraduate and graduate education, the need for such facilities grows (Thomas, 2000).

Single

Many college students are single and live off-campus, either at home with their parents or in shared living environments. In 1991, the overwhelming majority of young adults lived at home. Decades ago, the majority of men and women in this age group were married and out of their parents' houses. The current pattern where young adults remain living with parents has been tied to trends in delaying marriage, increasing percentage of never-marrieds, high cost of housing, and the need for more people to continue education.

The U.S. Bureau of the Census (2002) reports that there is a substantial increase in the proportion of "young, never-married" adults. For example, in the past three decades, the proportion of women who have never married doubled for those ages 20 to 24 and more than tripled for women ages 30 to 34 (Fields, 2001). Additionally, the median age of marriage has been pushed back to 25 years for women and 27 for men (U.S. Bureau of the Census, 2002). It must be noted, however, that the census bureau does not ask how many of the "never-marrieds" have that status due to being gay or lesbian and therefore are unable to marry.

Cohabiting

According to the U.S. Bureau of the Census (2002), about 6.3 million people in the United States cohabited in 1998. Of those, approximately half were under 25 years of age. No accurate numbers have been forthcoming regarding the actual number of college students who cohabit. **Cohabitation** is distinguished from having roommates of the opposite gender by the nature of the sexual interaction between cohabiters. *Cohabiters* are lovers who live together but are not married. They initially describe their relationship as intimate and affectionate but not necessarily as leading to marriage.

Cohabitation Living together without being married

Relationship Contract: How Much Am I Willing to Compromise?

The goal of this activity is to help you decide what you really need to have a healthy, happy, and supportive long-term relationship.

The following questions could be made into a relationship contract by which you and your future long-term partner agree to abide. Answer the questions as if you could have your ideal in the relationship. If you are in a relationship now, ask your partner to do the same and then compare your answers. This should cause a lively debate.

Freedom

Will we still maintain our outside friendships? Do we have the freedom to make new friends? Are we free to spend time with our same and opposite-sex friends without our partner? In what types of activities can we participate? Will we participate in sexual relationships outside this one?

Money

How will we make sure money is not a problem for our relationship? Will we have a budget, and, if so, what do we do if one does not follow the budget? Will we keep our own money or have a joint bank account? What will be our financial priorities?

Chores

How will we divide our responsibilities so that neither of us feels overwhelmed or taken advantage of?
Who will do the laundry, pay the bills, clean the house, take care of the yard, shop for groceries, cook, buy gifts for our families, run the errands?

Free Time

Will we spend all of our free time together? What types of activities will we do to keep the relationship from becoming boring? Will we spend most of our free time with friends, family, or alone?

Children

Will we have children? How many? What lengths are we willing to go to if one of us is infertile?

Married

For comparison, students may want to interview parents and grandparents who attended college about attitudes toward being a married student during their time in school. Generations ago, to be married was often thought incompatible with formal education, particularly for women. Some institutions of higher learning in the early to mid–20th century either strongly discouraged or outright forbid undergraduates to be married.

Today, most undergraduates who plan on marriage wait until they finish school. Data show that for undergraduate students surveyed during 1999–2000, 21.6 percent were married, with 76.8 percent reporting "not married." Within the unmarried group, however, can be individuals committed to a partner and possibly living with that partner (National Center for Education Statistics, 2000).

sex in society 6.1

Cohabitation Facts

- An estimated 6.3 million Americans were in cohabitation relationships as of March 1998. That is up from about 5.3 million as recently as 1995.
- The age breakdown is as follows:

  15.5 percent of men and 22.1 percent of women under 15 to 24;
  38.7 percent of men and 37.2 percent of women 25 to 35;
  21.8 percent of men and 23.1 percent of women 35 to 44;
  23.9 percent of men and 17.5 percent of women over 45

- 4.2 percent of the female (approximately 134,000) and 1.7 percent of the men (approximately 55,000) cohabiters are students.
- 37 percent of college-educated women had lived in a cohabitating relationship, and that number is rising.
- Most cohabitations are short-lived, and the couple either separates or marries.

Source: U.S. Bureau of the Census, "Current Population Survey," Center for Demography and Ecology (University of Wisconsin, Madison, 1998).

Adult Sexual Behavior

We will extend the discussion of sexuality during the college and young adult years into adulthood and old age. The phrase "use it or lose it" is often bantered about to express the idea that overall sexual health and activity connect to ongoing patterns established in life. The data from the NHSLS study continue to provide a portrait of adult behavior.

Laumann and Youm (2001) developed a model to explain the factors that influence a person's mode of sexual expression. Figure 6.1 shows the determinants of sexual expression.

There are three areas where individual attributes are key. First, *individual preferences* for specific sexual activities and level of sexual interest must be considered. Great variability exists from person to person as to what they want to do and how strong their drive is to engage in a specific activity. Those preferences may be different when a college student has moved from one partner to another, changed after a negative experience, and so forth. Second, *physical health* becomes important; a person may or may not be able to participate in activities due to impaired physical and/or mental health. Depression and erectile dysfunction, for example,

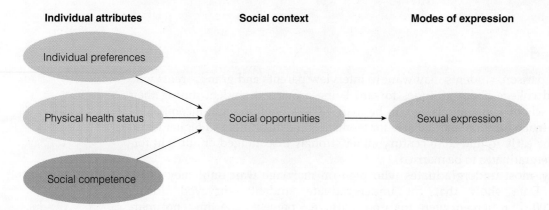

Figure 6.1 *Model of Determinants of Sexual Expression*

Source: E. O. Laumann and Y. Youm, "Sexual Expression in America," in Laumann and Michael, *Sex, Love, and Health in America* (2001), p. 111.

are two conditions that are known to interfere with sexual activity. *Social competence* as a third factor refers to the skills and resources needed to initiate and maintain social relationships. Individuals have to be able to communicate with a partner as well as be able to compete effectively for the attention of a potential partner. Social competence would seem to be a learned set of behaviors yet certainly can be influenced by how one is feeling about her- or himself at a set period of time.

Finally, the model posits that the three individual attributes jointly affect the *social opportunities* individuals confront when attempting to establish sexual relationships: who do you meet, where do you go, what are your social networks, how does geographic context affect socializing, and so on. All together, the four factors then affect what modes of sexual expression will result (Laumann & Youm, 2001).

In 2003, books, magazine articles, and popular television programs began to highlight what were being termed "sexless or no-sex marriages." Within relationships in which time was consumed by dual careers, children, and fatigue, the frequency of sexual activity was reported to be diminished. Therapists were providing advice, couples were going public with their concerns, and issues once thought private were making their way into popular discourse. As in many areas of sexuality, the power of the media can obscure and/or highlight what may or may not be going on in the privacy of the bedroom.

Physical and Intellectual Wellness

As we move through adulthood, we continue to be responsible for maintaining and enhancing our physical well-being. The experiences we've had earlier on may "catch up," making physical health no longer something to be taken for granted. The choices we made, behaviors we adopted, and lifestyles we lived will either enhance or undermine our sexuality. Abusing our bodies and letting our physical well-being decline will have a negative impact on our sexuality. Everything from body image to sexual response to overall energy level may decline. This will impact negatively on our social relationships with lovers, spouses, employers, and others. Better body image, sexual response, and energy level will help us meet the demands of our ever-changing sexuality. This state of wellness will not only enhance our personal functioning but also positively influence our relationships.

The ability to gather information, critically analyze it, and make good decisions are hallmarks of high-level mental functioning. Rational thinking and logical reasoning can help us understand the nature of our ever-changing sexuality as we pass through young adulthood into adulthood and old age. Having reasonable expectations about our sexuality, based on solid information, can guide us in decision making. It also can help us avoid unrealistic expectations about relationships and sexuality that are likely to lead to personal unhappiness and dissatisfaction with partners. It is important to determine the personal value of the information to which we're exposed—what relates to us, what can constructively impact our sexual health.

Masturbation in Adulthood

Adult masturbation is often viewed as a second-class sexual experience and is inversely related to the availability of a steady partner (Laumann et al., 1994). The common belief is that masturbation is primarily motivated by the relief of sexual tension. This belief grows out of a Western cultural viewpoint that masturbation is juvenile sexual behavior, almost preintercourse in its development. We join Laumann et al. in taking issue with this notion. In Chapter 7, we provide a detailed overview of masturbation throughout the life cycle.

Laumann et al. have examined masturbation in light of its relational context. They believe that masturbation, like all forms of sexual expression, is driven by a variety of social and biological factors throughout the life cycle and can have complementary, supplementary, or independent status with reference to partnered sex. This means that masturbation can enhance partnered sexual activity. It also can be an additional source of sexual expression within the context of the relationship, and last, it can serve as a solitary source of sexual pleasure independent of partnered sex.

Table 6.3 illustrates the frequency of masturbatory behavior by age and other selected demographic variables. Results shown here are not segregated by sexual orientation. Laumann et al. emphasize one of the key findings of the table: The level of masturbation is not related to relationship status. Although the table does show a decline in the level of masturbatory behavior among married people, it does not show a similar pattern among those who are single but cohabit. This group tended to be younger overall than the married sample.

Rather than reinforce the stereotype that masturbation is a substitute for partnered sex, this finding shows that this isn't necessarily so. The frequency of individual masturbation is as likely to be a function of social factors and a

Table 6.3 Frequency of Masturbation

| Master Status | Frequency (%) | | | |
| | Not at All | | Once a Week | |
	Men	Women	Men	Women
Total population	36.7	58.3	26.7	7.6
Age:				
18–24	41.2	64.4	29.2	9.4
25–29	28.9	58.3	32.7	9.9
30–34	27.6	51.1	34.6	8.6
35–39	38.5	52.3	20.8	6.6
40–44	34.5	49.8	28.7	8.7
45–49	35.2	55.6	27.2	8.6
50–54	52.5	71.8	13.9	2.3
55–59	51.7	77.6	10.3	2.4
Marital status:				
Never married, not cohabitating	31.8	51.8	41.3	12.3
Never married, cohabitating	15.8	54.9	36.8	12.7
Married	42.6	62.9	16.5	4.7
Divorced/separated/widow, not cohabitating	30.2	52.7	34.9	9.6
Divorced/separated/widow, cohabitating	41.2	50.9	17.6	12.7
Education:				
HS graduate equivalent	45.1	68.4	20.0	5.6
Finished college	24.2	47.7	33.2	10.2
Master's/advanced degree	18.6	41.2	33.6	13.7

Source: The Social Organization of Sexuality: Sexual Practices in the United States, by E. Laumann et al. (Chicago: University of Chicago Press, 1994). Used with permission.

variety of reasons as it is the availability of alternative outlets. Table 6.4 gives some of the reasons for masturbation, cited by gender.

Sexual Intercourse Among Adults

Table 6.2, presented earlier, shows the frequency of sexual intercourse in the past year. Laumann et al. summarize the three main levels of sexual activities for adults: About 35 percent have sex with a partner two or more times per week, about 35 percent have partnered sex one to a few times per month, and the remaining 30 percent have partnered sex only a few times a year. These rates were fairly consistent across all racial, ethnic, and religious groups. About 7 to 8 percent of the respondents had partnered sex four or more times a week, and about 10 percent reported having had no sex at all during the previous year. This response, the researchers point out, paints quite a different picture of adult sexual behavior than the one portrayed in the popular media. The sexual activity of most Americans is much more modest than the frequency and expectations created by the media.

An additional finding concerning partnered sexual activity related to the number of sex partners during the past year. As Table 6.1 points out, the number of different sex partners in the past year declines with age. In general, the largest percentage of respondents in each age cohort reported only one sex partner during the past year. Two moderating factors seem to be marital and cohabiting status. Young, single, noncohabiting men and women were much more likely than all other groups to report two or more different partners during the previous year.

Adult Oral Sex Activity

Table 6.5 illustrates the frequency of oral sexual activity among adults. The table does not segregate by sexual orientation. Straight and gay men and lesbian and heterosexual women are lumped together. The proportion of men reporting having had oral sex performed on them during their lives was similar to that of women reporting ever having had cunnilingus performed on them—roughly 75 percent. This percentage drops dramatically, however (about 50 percent), when oral sexual behavior is reported as latest sexual experience. Laumann et al. interpret this response as meaning that, although the majority of American men and women have experienced oral sex, it isn't as much a staple in their sexual repertoire as vaginal intercourse and kissing.

Laumann et al. view the increased frequency of oral sex as one of the basic changes in U.S. sexual behavior during the past century. They reported that the current incidence is probably an outgrowth of a trend that began in the 1920s. Kinsey and his colleagues publicized oral sex in the late 1940s, and it has continued to work its way into the fabric of American sexual behavior. The impeachment proceedings of President Clinton in the late 1990s provided daily grist for a discussion of oral sex—was oral sex really "sex"? In 2003, the U.S. Supreme Court ruled that oral and anal sexual behavior were not criminal. Specifically, the high court struck down Texas's Homosexual Conduct law that made oral and anal sex between homosexuals criminal activity (Lambda Legal Defense Fund, 2003). The

Table 6.4 Reasons for Masturbation

Reasons for Masturbation	Gender of Respondent (%)	
	Men	Women
To relax	26	32
To relieve sex tension	73	63
Partner unavailable	32	32
Partner doesn't want sex	16	6
Boredom	11	5
Physical pleasure	40	42
Go to sleep	16	12
Fear of AIDS/STD	7	5
Other	5	5

Source: *The Social Organization of Sexuality: Sexual Practices in the United States,* by E. Laumann et al. (Chicago: University of Chicago Press, 1994). Used with permission.

Table 6.5 Frequency of Oral Sex

Master Status Variables	Men	Women	Occurrence of Active Oral Receptive Sex (%)				Occurrence of Oral Sex (%)			
			Men		Women		Men		Women	
	Mean Frequency of Sex per Month		Life	Last Event	Life	Last Event	Life	Last Event	Life	Last Event
Total population	6.5	6.3	76.6	26.8	67.7	18.8	78.7	27.5	73.1	19.9
Age:										
18–24	7.2	7.4	72.4	27.7	69.1	19.1	74.2	28.9	74.7	24.2
25–29	7.6	7.5	84.8	32.0	76.2	23.8	84.8	33.7	79.8	24.3
30–34	6.7	6.8	78.9	29.6	76.6	19.1	78.9	32.2	83.1	22.3
35–39	6.6	6.1	82.3	30.4	71.3	21.0	87.5	29.8	73.7	23.3
40–44	5.9	5.5	84.0	31.2	72.7	16.9	85.7	28.9	76.8	12.6
45–49	6.2	5.5	73.4	21.2	65.2	21.6	77.4	22.1	72.7	18.3
50–54	5.5	4.6	60.0	16.1	48.5	11.7	66.0	13.8	59.4	12.6
55–59	4.4	3.5	58.4	9.9	38.9	5.5	58.0	14.1	44.3	6.9
Marital status:										
Never married, not cohabiting	5.6	5.3	66.7	28.9	59.4	21.0	70.3	32.8	67.7	26.8
Never married, cohabiting	8.6	8.8	85.7	30.2	72.2	21.5	89.3	34.0	76.4	22.7
Married	6.9	6.5	79.9	25.2	70.7	16.9	80.4	23.0	73.9	16.9
Divorced/separated/ widow, not cohabiting	5.4	5.1	81.5	30.1	64.1	25.4	88.1	34.5	73.1	24.2
Divorced/separated/ widow, cohabiting	8.0	7.6	80.0	29.7	79.6	16.3	80.0	37.8	85.2	20.4
Education:										
Less than high school	6.5	6.3	59.2	16.4	41.1	10.1	60.7	16.4	49.6	13.2
High school graduate or equivalent	6.9	6.3	75.3	30.1	59.6	16.4	76.6	25.3	67.1	18.5
Some college/ vocation	6.6	6.3	80.0	31.1	78.2	20.7	84.0	31.0	81.6	22.2
Finished college	6.0	6.4	83.7	23.7	78.9	22.9	84.6	31.1	83.1	20.7
Master's/advanced degree	6.1	5.1	80.5	20.6	79.0	28.8	81.4	30.4	81.9	27.0

Source: The Social Organization of Sexuality: Sexual Practices in the United States, by E. Laumann et al. (Chicago: University of Chicago Press, 1994). Used with permission.

ruling was seen as a great victory for the gay and lesbian community, where members could have been punished for engaging in the same behaviors practiced by heterosexuals.

Adult Anal Sexual Activity

Unlike oral sex, anal sex has yet to make a serious entry into the basic fabric of American sexual behavior. The overall level of heterosexual anal intercourse in the past year was around 9 percent. Only 2 percent of those ever having anal intercourse reported engaging in this activity at their last sexual encounter. As with other forms of sexual activity reported in the NHSLS, anal intercourse seems to be reported across all categories of respondents and is not limited to certain racial, ethnic, or religious groups.

Some evidence indicates that a small segment of adolescent and college women view heterosexual anal intercourse as an acceptable alternative to vaginal penetration. We, too, have received similar anecdotal reports from students engaged in internships in family planning agencies and from other health care providers serving young women.

Adult Relationships

One of the major developmental tasks of adulthood is the continuation and deepening of the commitment to relationships that began in young adulthood. For most Americans, this means a commitment to marriage and a family. For many, the commitment to someone else does not involve marriage but, instead, cohabitation. This is also a period frequently marked by divorce or the death of a spouse. In the remaining part of this chapter, we'll examine the changing nature of adult relationships.

Singlehood

A significant percentage of Americans are choosing to remain single for life. Reasons for remaining single include changes in sexual standards, greater financial independence for women, changing economic times, and shifting conceptions of marriage. Sometimes, postponing marriage results in an inadvertent slide into permanent singlehood (Cavanaugh, 1993). As people postpone marriage, they often realize that they can live satisfying lives being single. There is less urgency to marry, especially if they feel no desire to have children.

Regardless of the reasons, most people who chose to remain single for life in one study reported that they were quite happy. Contrary to popular beliefs, most singles are not lonely, and they develop alternative social patterns based on friendships and nonmarital love relationships. The satisfaction that singles derive from these relationships and their careers is more than adequate for their happiness (Phillis & Stein, 1983).

Dating and Single Adults   The two most stressful issues for single people are how to handle dating and others' expectations that they should marry (Cavanaugh, 1993). The United States is a "couples-oriented" society that puts a premium on adults interacting socially as part of a heterosexual couple. The prevailing assumption is that everyone expects to get married someday. This view puts inordinate pressure on single people, especially when friends and associates are continually trying to "fix them up." Singles typically find themselves having to defend their position. Old friendships also tend to disappear when a friend marries and starts a family.

Gay single people find themselves in a double-bind. People are continually trying to fix them up with members of the opposite sex so they can "find someone" and settle down. When gay singles finally do "find someone," they may not feel comfortable sharing their relationship with their straight friends.

Cohabitation   Unmarried adult couples who live together are not much different from married couples. They share, argue, quarrel, make decisions about money, sex, household labor, and so on. The reasons for adults living together but not marrying are many and varied. Generally speaking, three forms of cohabitation are casual or temporary involvement, preparation or testing for marriage, and a substitute for or alternative to marriage.

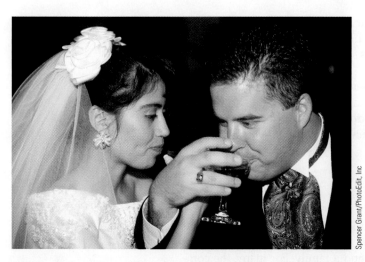

Weddings are important rituals that symbolize hope and lifelong commitment.

Monogamy Married to only one person at a time

Marriage

The vast majority of Americans want to marry, although they are postponing it longer than in the past. The median age at first marriage has been rising for the past three decades. Even though it is an integral part of most cultures, marriage takes many forms and assumes many different purposes throughout the world. In the United States, most people take the following issues for granted concerning marriage: a legal bond, having children, permanence, heterosexuality, sexual exclusivity, emotional exclusivity, and **monogamy** (Berry & Williams, 1987).

U.S. culture also expects more from marriage than many other cultures do. Historically, marriages were intended to provide a stable economic unit in which to rear children. Today, people expect marriage to fulfill their social, emotional, financial, and sexual needs. When people marry, they find that many of these expectations are unrealistic and cannot be fully realized. This discovery can lead to frustration, disillusionment, separation, and divorce. They also find that marriage is hard work. Even under the best of circumstances and with a good match in a partner, successful marriage requires continual assessment, communication, commitment, and willingness to change.

The Developmental Course of Marriage   Berry and Williams (1987) propose a developmental model of marriage across adulthood, shown in Figure 6.2. In the early, honeymoon phase, marriage is at its most intense. The two spend considerable time together, talking, sharing interests and leisure, establishing their roles within the relationship, arguing, and making up. As the honeymoon phase begins to wind down and the couple settles into a routine, the intensity of the honeymoon phase diminishes and, along with it, marital satisfaction. A big reason for

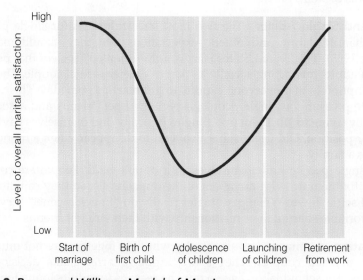

Figure 6.2 *Berry and Williams Model of Marriage*

Source: "Assessing the Relationship Between Quality of Life and Marital and Income Satisfaction: A Path Analytic Approach," by R. E. Berry and E. Williams, *Journal of Marriage and the Family, 47*(1987), 107–116. Copyrighted 1987 by the National Council on Family Relations, 3989 Central Avenue NE, Suite 550, Minneapolis, MN 55421. Reprinted with permission.

sex in society 6.2

Learning by Laughing at the Movies

Laughter is one human behavior that is shared by people all over the world. It represents a positive emotion, with the power to reduce stress, relieve pain, and encourage healing. Laughter stimulates the heart, alters the rhythms of breathing, and positively impacts the immune system (Hales, 2003). We can laugh at a joke. We can laugh at a situation watched on television or on the big screen. The power of creating laughter, along with making people feel good, is that wonderful lessons about life can be transmitted in a nonthreatening manner.

Many movies have been made with central themes on the institution of marriage. Some of the recent selections listed here illustrate how film can tackle various crises and sexual themes with humor, reality, and diversity.

La Cage aux Folles (1978) is a French-made film, later turned into a Broadway musical, that humorously deals with a gay couple whose son, much to their chagrin, is planning a marriage to a woman. The woman is the daughter of a conservative minister of morality for the government. Through the meeting of the parents and ensuing charades, humor is used to illustrate basic parental concern for children's happiness. Students may be more familiar with the American version of the film entitled *The Birdcage*, starring Robin Williams.

The Wedding Banquet (1997) shows the culture clash and secrecy involved when the parents of a rich Taiwanese family visit their son in New York City, not knowing he is gay and living with his partner. To help a female tenant who is an immigrant in need of a green card, a fictitious marriage is arranged. The film uses humor to address issues of love, marriage, homosexuality, and cultural traditions.

Meet the Parents (2000) focuses on the introduction of the male character to his fiancée's somewhat unwelcoming parents. The father, in particular, is very uncomfortable that his possible future son-in-law is a male nurse. The macho father views the female-identified profession negatively, not to mention the overall clumsiness of the man.

Monsoon Wedding (2001) looks at the marriage rituals among upper-middle-class Indians. Although the culture subscribes to arranged marriages, the influences of Western culture on the values of family members add to the culture clash.

Far from Heaven (2002) is not a comedy but rather an intense look at the breakup of an upper-class family as the wife learns of her husband's homosexuality. Although a "period piece," it teaches how oppressive and secretive being gay yet trying to live the heterosexual life was in the 1950s.

My Big Fat Greek Wedding (2002) depicts culture clash at its finest. A Greek American woman, hoping to break free from her overbearing family, falls in love with an upper-class non-Greek male. The differences in the families are extreme, from the Greeks being joyous and involved in every aspect of each other's lives, to the stereotypical WASP family, being overwhelmed by the outgoing, involved way of the soon-to-be in-laws.

Overall, this sampling of films highlights the cultural variations around weddings. What is as important, however, is that the themes of love, family, and working through conflict are underscored. Whether the couples live "happily ever after" is a question better left to fairy tales.

---

this outcome is the birth of children. Children result in less time available for the mate and the relationship.

Marital happiness reaches its lowest point during the midlife phase of the relationship, which also coincides with adolescence of the couple's children. A myriad of problems—ranging from financial issues to coping with teenagers to changing roles for husband and wife—contribute to the unrest.

Happiness begins to rebound when the children leave home as adults. This frees up time and money, and the couple has rediscovered privacy to reestablish the things in their relationship that provide pleasure, as well as investigate new things together.

Marital happiness continues to rise in the later adult years and carries over into retirement. Depending on a number of factors ranging from health to retirement income, the couple continues to enjoy their freedom and in some cases relationships with their children's families and their grandchildren.

Rob & Sas/CORBIS

More than half of all married couples report being extremely sexually satisfied with their sexual relationship.

Obviously, not all couples fit the Berry and Williams model. Other variables, such as physical illness, children living at home into their 30s, and loss of jobs, can strain the relationship. In some cases, children growing up and leaving the nest magnify problems in the relationship that lead to divorce. Not all relationships flourish in retirement. Sometimes work serves as a buffer between a couple and their problems.

Sexual Satisfaction and Happiness   Sexual satisfaction and happiness in marital and other partnered relationships have two dimensions: physical satisfaction and emotional happiness (Laumann et al., 1994). The relationship between the two is complex. Highly satisfying physical relationships usually bring with them high emotional happiness. High levels of emotional satisfaction, however, don't necessarily indicate high levels of physical satisfaction.

Overall, a fairly high proportion of men (47 percent) and women (41 percent) described their partnership as extremely physically pleasurable. Satisfaction seems to vary with age. Among men, the level of physical satisfaction was high to begin with and increased with age. Among women however, high levels of physical satisfaction dropped significantly after age 55. Findings are similar regarding emotional satisfaction. Laumann et al. account for this by explaining that men in their 50s and older are more likely than similar-aged women to acquire new sex partners after divorce.

Sources of Marital Problems   The potential sources of trouble over the life span of a marriage range from loss of initial sexual passion to economic instability in retirement. Many relationships are doomed from the

healthy sex hints 6.1

Lessons from Happy Marriages

In a happy marriage:

1. The partners find their prime source of joy in each other but maintain separate identities.
2. They are generous and giving out of love, not because they expect repayment or are keeping score.
3. The partners enjoy a healthy and vigorous sexual relationship.
4. The partners "fight" in a constructive way, airing feelings and frustrations without attacking or blaming the other.
5. The partners communicate with each other openly and honestly.
6. The partners trust each other.
7. Both talk about their future together. They have mutual goals.
8. The best marriages tend to be ones in which the partners are similar in these ways:
   - ethnicity
   - locality (geography; urban or rural)
   - maturity (emotional and social)
   - goals and ideals
   - intelligence levels
   - amount of education
   - economic level and financial resources
   - social strata
   - value system
   - religious beliefs

sex in society 6.3

Midlife Crisis or Middle-Age Myth?

You have heard the story before. A happy, successful 45-year-old businessman quits his job, leaves his wife and kids, and runs off to Tahiti with his 25-year-old secretary. Or, perhaps it is the 40-year-old mother of two facing the "empty nest" who jumps into her convertible BMW with her 25-year-old tennis instructor and heads west into the sunset in a torrid blaze of passionate sex.

These and other "midlife crises" that have been popularized by the print and film media make interesting stories and pose a romantic solution to many of the difficult issues that appear during middle age. In real life, however, relatively few people experience such catastrophic, radical changes. New information fueled by long-term research on aging is showing that middle age is the very best time of life. It is a developmental stage unlike most others, because it is not tied particularly to changes in the body, such as early childhood, adolescence, and old age. Midlife is characterized more by psychological adaptations and is reality based.

By midlife, many of the stressful questions that faced us as young adults are answered, such as, Will anyone ever love me? Will this marriage work out? Will I ever find a job? What kind of lifestyle can I afford to lead? By midlife, most people have found love. If they are married, they are more likely to stay married (the overwhelming majority of divorces occur within the first 6 to 8 years of marriage). They have settled into a job and have a pretty good idea of where they are headed (most professionals who are going to "make it" have made it by this time). They have a good sense of their earning capacity and therefore can gauge the kind of lifestyle they can expect.

Although the myth of midlife is that this period is characterized by unrest, discomfort, dissatisfaction, and upheaval, the reality is that it is a comfortable, satisfying time. It is a time to enjoy the rewards of 10 to 20 years of scuffling. It is a time to push a little easier at work, to get off a little early to watch your kid's Little League game. It is a time to focus on vacations and social gatherings, to take a class to learn how to paint or improve your backhand. It is a time to lighten up a little.

Midlife is a period of gradual adjustment, not tumultuous change. It gradually unfolds and is based on several adjustments to reality. For most people it is based in reality, not fantasy. Those most likely to experience a true crisis (about 5 percent) are people who generally have experienced similar crises in all developmental stages of their lives. Their lives are based on unrealistic (therefore unrealized) notions and expectations. One of the major criticisms of earlier studies of midlife is that they were based on small numbers of case studies of atypical populations (mostly affluent, professional, and white). In the recent cross-sectional studies of more representative samples of Americans, researchers found that the average person's midlife adjustment is based on reality. People gradually adjust their expectations to fit the reality of their lives. By the time they settle into midlife, they have learned to make the best of what they have and are not constantly longing for things that are beyond their reach.

Source: R. Blonna, *Coping with Stress in a Changing World* (3rd ed.) (Dubuque, IA: McGraw-Hill, forthcoming), p. 537.

---

start because they are based on an ideal that never can be fulfilled. Many expectations are unrealistic as a result of immature or romantic perceptions. The continuing intensity and bliss of romantic love cannot be expected to continue throughout marriage. Bliss turns to boredom and aggravation, passion to comfort, and happiness to times of sadness. This does not mean that love is dead. Romantic love should be expected to transform into mature love.

Furthermore, communication problems can sabotage a relationship. These problems may be rooted in a lack of assertiveness in which one or both members of the couple are unable to stand up for themselves. Communication problems also can arise when the partners are unable to express positive and constructive thoughts and feelings. Many people grow up in an environment where communication revolves around problems and the expression of negative emotions. Relationships can wither from a lack of expressions of recognition, caring, tenderness, and compassion.

Communication problems can be summarized as stemming from a lack of communication skills, the lack of desire to communicate, or both. The easier problem to remedy is the skill-based one. If one or both members of the relationship do not know how to communicate clearly and effectively or don't know how to fight fairly, they can learn—assuming they have the desire. If either or both don't have the desire to work things out, no amount of skill will improve the situation.

Loss of desire to talk and work things out is a warning sign of a deteriorating relationship. Sometimes a vicious cycle begins in which a lack of skill in communicating leads to a deteriorating relationship, which feeds a loss of desire. Low levels of desire keep the cycle going by not having the interest in talking about problems in the relationship. In the last case, one or both members may want to try to communicate in general but think the problem is too difficult to talk about. Or they may want to try to communicate more effectively but lack the energy and commitment necessary to work out their problems.

Couples who want to resolve their problems but don't know where to start can benefit tremendously from couple's counseling. Sometimes, problems that seemed insurmountable before counseling seem workable after seeing a therapist.

Another factor, money—or, more precisely, what money means to each partner—is a major source of stress in long-term relationships. If the two differ in their perceptions and values surrounding money, this difference could create problems within the relationship. For instance, one partner may view money as relatively unimportant, only a means to obtain the things necessary for survival. The other, however, perceives money as important—a ticket to a better life, higher status, more luxuries, and so on. This couple is in trouble because their core values concerning money are the opposite. Often this variance is reflected in how much they spend and what they buy. If one partner perceives that the other is spending too much and making unnecessary purchases, it is bound to lead to problems. As described in Case Study 6.2, couples can develop a plan to override their differences.

Or one person may view credit as a fundamental economic necessity and have no problem with outstanding balances on credit cards, loans, and home equity lines. Meanwhile, the other may not be comfortable even with a mortgage or a car loan, preferring to delay all purchases until they can be paid for in cash. The problem is compounded by today's easy access to credit and aggressive marketing.

healthy sex hints 6.2
Fighting Fairly

- Use *I* rather than *you*. Instead of saying, "You're insensitive," say, "I feel hurt when you ignore me."
- Don't argue without good reason. Think before you speak.
- Don't fight in front of other people, including your children. The issue involves only the two of you.
- Don't make personal attacks—name-calling, put-downs—that you will regret later.
- Be specific. Don't generalize.

- Focus on only the issue that precipitated the argument.
- Learn to use active listening skills so your partner will know he or she is being heard.
- If you cannot agree after a "fair fight," agree to disagree or to renew the discussion later.
- Take responsibility for your own behavior. Avoid blaming.
- Obviously, do not resort to physical attacks or any form of violence.

case study 6.2

Tom and Suzanne: Dealing with Finances

Tom and Suzanne, both age 30, are white.

Tom and Suzanne have an interesting way of dealing with family finances. They met at age 27 in graduate business school, where they were pursuing their MBAs. Both had lived by themselves for a few years and had several years of work experience behind them. Each had savings and checking accounts.

In discussing marriage, both were concerned about financial independence and protecting their savings, income, and spending patterns. Tom was a saver. He had banked well over $20,000 in savings before he met Suzanne, and he wanted to preserve this money. He was disciplined and always paid cash, even for his personal automobiles.

Suzanne was a spender. She believed in buying with credit cards, and catalog shopping was a favorite pastime. Saving was something people did once they turned 50 and began to think about retirement. For as long as she could remember, she had outstanding balances on her credit accounts yet eventually would pay them off.

Being so different concerning money but so alike in a number of other ways, Tom and Suzanne decided that after they were married, they would have three separate accounts: his, hers, and ours. The "ours" account would be used for all joint bills (rent, food, joint vacations, and child rearing (if it came up). Suzanne had wanted other expenses covered from this account, such as car purchases and retirement savings, but Tom, knowing she was a spender and he'd wind up contributing more than she, did not accept this arrangement. After reviewing salaries and projected earnings, they decided that each would contribute two weeks take-home salary to the joint account, with the other two weeks kept separately. With basic expenses covered, each could then spend and/or save without guilt or explanation.

Despite some stress, things have worked out okay for Tom and Suzanne. He's still a saver and has over $20,000 in his bank account. She's still a spender and has a $15,000 car loan and credit card debts exceeding $3,000. Tom considered helping her out with some payments but decided against it, as he thought she'd never learn if he were to bail her out. Some of their friends think they're a little eccentric and that their marriage seems more like a business than a loving partnership. In any case, for the time being it seems to work for them.

Critical Thinking

Some would argue that married couples who maintain separate checking accounts demonstrate a lack of trust in their relationships. Others might argue that it is wise for two people with different approaches to managing money to keep some of their finances separate. What is your view on money management within a marriage?

Use your Virtual Workbook to explore your answer to this question at **http://health.wadsworth.com/blonna1.**

The perception of money affects everything from long-term planning to daily quality of life. It also involves the perception of gender roles as couples decide if one or both partners will work, whose job is more important, if one of them is to leave a career to take care of the children, and so forth. If one partner has a traditional gender role concerning money and the other doesn't, this could be a major source of marital discord. Couples need to discuss these issues and develop creative approaches to deal with their own money and the "couple's" money.

Unrealistic expectations about sex within the marriage also can lead to dissatisfaction. The partners might have differing expectations about the frequency of sex, use of protection, level of desire, and a host of other variables. These differing and unrealistic expectations about sex can be a sign of sexual incompatibility. Often, couples who cohabit in preparation for marriage do so in an effort to gauge sexual compatibility before they enter into a marital relationship. Unfortunately no evidence is available to suggest that couples who do this are more likely to stay together and have marital satisfaction than noncohabiters (Masters, Johnson, & Kolodny, 1992).

Once people leave the single life and pair off in either cohabiting or marital relationships, sex changes. It no longer is as frantic or as segmented from the rest of one's life as it was when the couple lived separately. Although sexual pleasure is not sacrificed, sex becomes integrated into the ebb and flow of the couple's life. It is balanced with other needs and responsibilities—an important developmental task in this stage of the relationship. If a partner is unable or unwilling to communicate about sexual concerns and problems, the problems can worsen and become a source of stress within the relationship. Partners who cannot adjust become sexually dissatisfied and may turn to extramarital sex or divorce.

As we've reported, the frequency of sexual intercourse declines as relationships age. Sexual activity peaks within the first year of marriage and then begins to drop off. The frequency of sexual relations is highly correlated with marital satisfaction. In one study, 9 of 10 married couples who were having sex three or more times a week reported satisfaction with their relationships (Blumstein & Schwartz, 1983). Conversely, only half of couples having sex one to four times a month were satisfied with their relationships. A more recent study found a similar relationship between the frequency of marital sex and level of satisfaction with the relationship (Laumann et al., 1994).

Many factors affect the level of sexual activity within a relationship. Work and other responsibilities affect the level of energy people have. Sexual desire may change in response to stress. Sometimes people have common sexual dysfunctions (such as situational erectile dysfunction in men) that lessen sexual frequency and pleasure.

Parenting and Relational Satisfaction   Children can be a major source of stress within a committed adult relationship. Whether married or cohabiting, straight or gay, children change a couple's established patterns of interaction. As we've seen from the Berry and Williams analysis of marital happiness and adult developmental phases, satisfaction within a marriage reaches its lowest point about the time the children reach adolescence. Even though this seems to indicate that adolescents are responsible for their parents' stress, the demands of parenting pose formidable stressors at all stages of child development.

Parenting requires a tremendous amount of time and effort. The specific demands change with the child's stage of development, but the responsibility remains. Newborns require constant supervision. Even when they are sleeping, parents learn to sleep lightly, ready to react to their children's cries for help in the night. Young children need help with everything from getting washed and dressed to cutting the food on their plates. Older children need parents to spend time helping them with everything from doing their homework to getting them safely to and from friends' houses. Parents of young adolescents spend countless hours carpooling their kids all over the place, and parents of older teens stay up all hours of the night waiting for the safe return of their teenager and the family car.

Children decrease up to half the amount of time parents have to share activities with each other (Cavanaugh, 1993). This can disrupt everything from a couple's sexual relationship to the time they spend pursuing hobbies or other activities. In addition to the stress associated with the sheer time demands of children, children's needs are unpredictable. From early-morning feedings of babies, to car-pooling, to waiting for an adolescent to return home from a date, children pose unpredictable demands on the time, temperament, financial resources, and parents' sexual desire.

Divorce   Not all marriages progress completely through the Berry and Williams phases described earlier in the chapter. More than half of all first marriages end in divorce. Raw numbers are misleading when interpreting divorce statistics. The divorce *rate*, which examines numbers of divorces in relation to numbers of marriages, rose steadily for 20 years, reaching a high of 5.3 divorces per 1,000 Americans in 1981, then began declining. In 2000, there were a reported 4.7 divorces for every 1,000 people (Hughes, 2003).

Most people marry with the hope that the relationship will last forever. Divorce, therefore, often represents a loss of this hope. This often is accompanied by the loss of economic status (particularly for low- and middle-income women), lifestyle, security of familiarity, friends, and sometimes children. The psychological effects of divorce can be compared with those of the grieving process associated with death of a loved one. First, shock sets in ("Is this really happening to me?"), followed by disorganization ("Everything feels topsy-turvy"). Volatile emotions, then guilt ("It's my fault") usually follow. Loneliness, too, often accompanies divorce. Finally, after several months to a year, these feelings are replaced by a sense of relief and acceptance.

The grieving process leads to healing, a cleansing of wounds, that allows divorced people to move on with their lives. If, after a year or so, the divorced person hasn't gotten over the divorce and begun to accept what has happened, counseling and psychotherapy may be helpful.

Approximately three in four divorced persons remarry, most within 3 years after their divorce. Although most remarried people report that their second marriage is better than their first, the likelihood that this marriage also will end in divorce is greater than that among first marriages. No one knows why this is so for sure, but some of the reasons given are less willingness to stay in the second marriage when they are embittered, closer scrutiny of the second marriage, financial problems (such as alimony and child support), and the trauma of divorce being less threatening after having experienced it once.

Long-Term Gay, Lesbian, and Bisexual Relationships

Most research regarding relationships has related to married heterosexuals, with far less written regarding long-term gay, lesbian, and bisexual relationships. In fact, the prevailing stereotype has been that such relationships were unlikely to even exist. In practice, gay and lesbian couples have increasingly had commitment ceremonies, where vows are shared, friends and family may be present, and some of the rituals of traditional marriages are repeated. In August 2002, the *New York Times* decided to begin publishing reports of commitment ceremonies in its Sunday Styles section. What had been the "Wedding" section became the "Weddings/Celebrations" section, with the backgrounds of gay and lesbian couples written up in the same manner as those of heterosexual couples. The newspaper required that couples celebrate their commitment in a public ceremony and/or enter into a legally recognized civil union (which at that time was in Vermont) or register their **domestic partnership** in those places allowing registration (*New York Times*, 2002). The significance of that editorial decision is reflected in the fact that the *New York Times* has national distribution, is considered a mainstream newspaper, and is a powerful force in public opinion. At the same time, the biographies of any couples reported tend to reflect high-level positions of employment, education at highly ranked universities, and be the children of parents who also wield levels of power and influence in their respective lives.

On a national level, gay and lesbian activists have been working to change legislation that would enable them to marry. When Hawaii changed its laws to allow for gay and lesbian marriage, federal legislation in the form of the Defense of Marriage Act was initiated. That law passed in 1996 ensuring that if a same-sex couple married in one state, their marriage did not have to be recognized in any other. It also defined marriage as being between a man and a woman. In 2003, Massachusetts legalized gay and lesbian marriage, furthering the national controversy.

Domestic partnerships
Registered relationships between gay and lesbian couples

The politics surrounding marriage for lesbian and gay couples relate on one level to principles of fairness, constitutional protections, and recognition of loving, committed relationships. On another level, the politics are rooted in the economic protections of legal marriage. Health insurance, pensions, inheritance, and the like, are "rights" that come within marriage and affect daily living. As of 2003, 10 states and the District of Columbia provide benefits for domestic partners of public employees. Hawaii, California, and New Jersey have the broadest domestic partnership laws, with Vermont endorsing civil unions (Cahill & Slater, 2003, p. 6).

Religious conservatives maintain that marriage must be seen as a union between a man and a woman. Nonetheless, the Netherlands in 2000 became the first nation to make same-sex marriage legal, followed by Belgium in 2003 and the provinces of Ontario and British Columbia in Canada in 2003. Other countries have provisions for gay and lesbian couples to varying degrees (Cahill & Slater, 2003, p. 7).

Because of the controversies related to marriage, legislation has been more successful thus far in the area of registered domestic partnerships and civil unions. Urban governments, some universities, and some corporations have extended health and pension benefits to the partners of their employees.

A prospective study of 65 gay and 47 lesbian long-term relationships found that the duration of the relationship was a predictor of satisfaction (Kurdek, 1989). Gay and lesbian subjects in relationships of longer than an 8-year duration reported greater satisfaction than relationships of shorter duration. Furthermore, lesbian couples reported higher levels of relationship satisfaction than gay men (Kurdek, 1989).

Another study found that as homosexuals aged, those in close, committed relationships were the happiest (Lipman, 1986). Variables related to happiness in relationships, such as commitment, companionship, intimacy, and fulfillment of needs, were the same for homosexual and heterosexual couples.

The stereotypical picture of old age for gay men and women is one of unhappiness and loneliness. In actuality, it is quite the opposite. As a rule, homosexual men and women may be better prepared for the demands and challenges of old age than many traditional heterosexual couples. Because of stereotypical male and female gender roles, traditional heterosexual marriages are more likely to be built on dependency. In traditional heterosexual relationships, husbands rely on wives for certain activities, and wives are more dependent on husbands for other activities.

In the absence of social norms for gay male or female relationship roles, gay and lesbian relationships are, of necessity, more egalitarian. Each partner has been socialized to be self-reliant. The lack of hard-and-fast gender role stereotypes forces homosexual men and women to communicate more effectively and to be more flexible and creative in meeting relationship needs. Gay men and women are more willing to communicate, experiment, and be more attentive to detail in their sexual behavior (Kurdek, 1993).

Research on long-term relationships for those identifying as bisexual has, by definition, needed to examine adult relationship patterns along with assumptions held about sexual orientation. If a bisexual woman, for example, has a long-term committed relationship with another woman, has she moved to a lesbian identity, or does she maintain her identification within that relationship, choosing to be monogamous and not be involved with men?

Weinberg, Williams, and Pryor (2001) have conducted longitudinal research with a group of adults from the San Francisco area. Beginning in 1983, surveying again in 1988 and then in 1996, the researchers were able to collect data that describe how changing life commitments such as marriage and parenthood affect sexuality. They also analyzed how age-linked social roles changed commitments and how individuals have been affected by various sexual identity movements such as queer politics. As individuals got older, changes were found in sexual involvement, the direction of sexual behavior, ties to the bisexual community, and the stability of sexual identity. Specifically, as people got older, their levels of sexual activity declined, citing reasons such as reduced energy levels, menopause-related concerns, fear of AIDS, and partner availability.

Weinberg and colleagues also found that there was a move toward monogamy with a sexual drift in the direction of heterosexuality. Part of that drift was explained by some participants as owing to having moved away from San Francisco, where people were more likely to be "out" and available. Fear of AIDS sometimes led people to choose heterosexual monogamy, thinking that option left them safe from infection. At the same time, more than one-fifth of the study group had become exclusively homosexual in their sexual behavior, feeling sex and relationships were easier with same-sex partners.

In contrast to lesbian and gay older adults, aging bisexuals do not have the same social networks and political groups for affirmation. Generational differences and newer political approaches have not created a bisexual community, whereas gay and lesbian communities are more visible. Nonetheless, participants were very clear about their identities as bisexual, able to look at their sexual history and sustained dual attraction (Weinberg et al., 2001).

Stages in Homosexual Relationships   In one of the most extensive, long-term prospective studies of male homosexuals to date, McWhirter and Mattison (1984) followed 156 gay couples for more than 20 years. The subjects were gay couples who had been together approximately 9 years before enrolling in the study. The researchers found that gay relationships, like those of their heterosexual counterparts, went through a series of stages.

Stage 1: Blending. This stage characterizes the first year of the relationship. As with heterosexual couples, this year has the highest levels of sexual activity, strong love and passion, and a merging of personal interests.

Stage 2: Nesting. Nesting takes place during years 2 to 3, emphasizing relationship building and starting a home together. Ambivalence, problems, and doubts about the relationship are most likely to begin to surface at this stage.

Stage 3: Maintaining. The third stage is characterized by a decline in passion and frequency of sexual activity, with an emphasis on conflict resolution and re-assertion of some of the individuality subverted during the initial stages of the relationship.

Stage 4: Building. The building stage occupies years 6 through 10 and is marked by increased personal productivity and independence but also enhanced collaboration and developing sense of trust and dependability between the partners.

Stage 5: Releasing. From years 11 to 20, this stage is characterized by merging of money and other assets and beginning to take each other for granted. Sexual activity drops off noticeably in this stage.

Stage 6: Renewing. The last stage extends beyond 20 years together and is marked by personal security and a restored sense of partnership based on remembering shared experiences and good times together.

Because of better planning throughout their relationship, homosexual men and women may be better prepared for dealing with losses such as the death of their partner and retirement. Many homosexuals have planned for their own financial support and have consciously developed supportive social networks. They also may be better prepared to cope with hardship, having lived a life of adversity as a member of a stigmatized group. This combination of attitude, social and financial resources, and self-reliance may help gay men and women cope with the demands of aging.

Sexuality in Older Adults

In Erik Erikson's (1978) final stage, old age, our major developmental task is to maintain integrity in the face of death. This last stage begins in older adulthood with the growing awareness of the nearness of death. This is a time for facing our mortality and accepting the worth and uniqueness of our lives.

Maintaining integrity entails evaluating our lives and accomplishments. In a sense, we are verifying our existence and seeking its meaning. We do this by looking back at where we've been, what we've accomplished, whom we have touched (Erikson, 1978). This process often involves reminiscing with family, friends, and others.

One problem with discussing "old age" is the need to define it. College students may think old begins in the 60s and 70s, whereas 70-year-olds may view those in their 80s and 90s as being "old." When widows and widowers reenter the social scene, they need to acclimate to what may seem to be new dating rules. In particular, at what point should couples be sexual with each other? Will dating lead to love, commitment, and possible remarriage? How does one's family react to the new partner?

Particular attention and educational programs have been developed for older adults who must learn to practice safer sex. HIV/AIDS rates among older adults are not uncommon (D. Joslin, February 2003, personal interview), yet many are not prepared to integrate condom use, for example, into their social and sexual lives ("The Elderly and HIV" Conference, 2000).

Sexual Response and Aging

Sex doesn't necessarily get better or worse as we age; it just gets different. Many myths have arisen in regard to sexual response and aging. The following three are common ones that usually surface during classroom discussions in our classes:

Once you start to get old (over age 50), you lose interest in sex.
Older people aren't sexually attracted to each other.
Older people can't perform sexually or have orgasms.

healthy sex hints 6.4

Changes in Sexual Response Associated with Aging

Women

The following changes are associated with sexual response in women who have gone through menopause:

1. The vagina is less elastic and not able to expand as much.
2. Physiological responses to sexual stimuli take more time.
3. Vaginal lubrication takes longer and may be less effective in reducing vaginal irritation.
4. The clitoris is smaller but not less responsive.
5. The intensity of orgasmic contractions diminishes slightly.
6. The ability to have multiple orgasms does not change.

Men

The following physiological changes have been observed in men older than age 55:

1. Arousal takes longer and may require manual stimulation of the penis.
2. Erections tend to be less firm.
3. Less semen is ejaculated.
4. There is less need to ejaculate to enjoy sexual activity.
5. The intensity of orgasmic contractions is slightly diminished.
6. More time is necessary to get another erection.

case study 6.3

Happy Harry

Harry, 78, is white.

Harry is living in an apartment at a newly developed senior residence. The residence is private and costs approximately $5,000 a month. Harry doesn't mind the cost because his meals are free, the staff takes care of most of his needs, and his pension, fortunately, provided nicely for his retirement. Harry's children no longer need his financial support, so he's enjoying life without worrying about taking care of anyone else.

Harry had been happily married to June, but when she passed away 5 years earlier, he decided he could no longer live in their house by himself. Little did he know how much in demand he would be once he arrived at the residence! The ratio of ladies to gentlemen is 4:1, and Harry is very popular. He knows he's not the best-looking guy, but he is agile and loves to dance, go out to movies, and generally have a good time. He's decided not to commit to any one woman, although he's had plenty of offers. At this point, being a free man with a lot of attention is just fine.

As for sex . . . well, he does have one or two special ladies with whom he spends the night. He feels a bit like a teenager again, sneaking around the residence hoping that one doesn't see him enter the room of the other.

Critical Thinking

The ratio of men to women in many adult residences is such that "partner sharing" may become necessary for heterosexual individuals. How do you think you would react to such an arrangement? Would sharing a partner be acceptable if the alternative meant being unattached?

Use your Virtual Workbook to explore your answers to these questions at **http://health.wadsworth.com/blonna1.**

Physiologically, most men and women change very little during their 30s and early 40s. The most noticeable changes in sexual response in women are associated with menopause. They begin to experience a syndrome called the **female climacteric** between 45 and 55 years of age, as a result of a drop in levels of estrogen production associated with menopause. Common symptoms are hot flashes, irritability, inability to concentrate, and declines in sexual desire. The climacteric ends with menopause, which is the cessation of ovulation and loss of fertility. About one-fourth of women experience menopause before age 45, half from 45 to 50, and the remaining fourth after the age of 50 (Kart, 1994).

The changes in sexual physiology among most men in their 40s and 50s are less noticeable. Although sperm production slows down after age 40, it continues into the 80s and 90s. Similarly, though male sexual hormone levels decline gradually after age 55, most men have no noticeable drop-off in sexual desire. About 5 percent of men older than 60 experience the **male climacteric,** which produces symptoms similar to those of menopause. Men, however, do not lose their fertility as a result of the climacteric as women do when they experience menopause.

These physiological changes, in men and women, which basically revolve around the sexual response slowing and the intensity of response lessening slightly, are more than offset by greater comfort about sexuality, no fear of pregnancy, familiarity with one's partner, and extending the sex act.

Changing Relationships

Older age is often affected by the changing nature of relationships and family life as the commitment to relationships that began in young adulthood continues and deepens. For many, this is a period marked by divorce or the death of a mate or

Female climacteric A syndrome experienced by women between about 45 and 55 years of age as a result of declining levels of estrogen production associated with menopause

Male climacteric A syndrome experienced by about 5 percent of men in their 40s and 50s, characterized by diminished interest in sex, loss of appetite, fatigue, and inability to concentrate

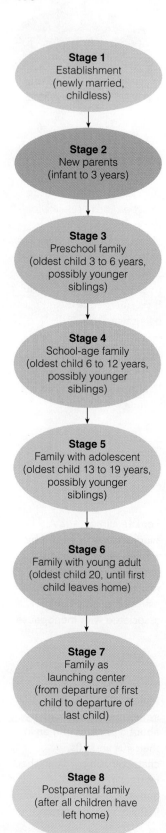

Stage 1
Establishment
(newly married,
childless)

Stage 2
New parents
(infant to 3 years)

Stage 3
Preschool family
(oldest child 3 to 6 years,
possibly younger
siblings)

Stage 4
School-age family
(oldest child 6 to 12 years,
possibly younger
siblings)

Stage 5
Family with adolescent
(oldest child 13 to 19 years,
possibly younger
siblings)

Stage 6
Family with young adult
(oldest child 20, until first
child leaves home)

Stage 7
Family as
launching center
(from departure of first
child to departure of
last child)

Stage 8
Postparental family
(after all children have
left home)

Figure 6.3 *Duvall's Family Life Cycle*

lover. The case study featuring Harry illustrates that loss of a partner need not mean loss of a social and sexual life.

Duvall (1977) developed an often-cited eight-stage theory of the family life cycle given in Figure 6.3. Stage 8, the postparental years, generally coincides with late adulthood and old age. Many events blend during this time: menopause and other physiological changes of aging, retirement, older children leaving the nest, and grandchildren, to name just a few. Although often characterized negatively as a time of loss and failed health, it also is a dynamic period in which newfound freedom, psychological and social stability, and wisdom can be a springboard to greater happiness for couples.

Duvall's model admittedly assumes that "family life" includes children. Obviously there are adults, coupled or single, who have never had children. Some older adults also have no contact with their children and extended family.

Most older couples today have grown old together. The average couple can expect at least 15 years of living together after the last child leaves. This is quite different from the turn of the century, when death affected half of all marriages before the last child left the house (Kart, 1994).

Studies have revealed mixed findings concerning marital satisfaction and happiness in the older years. In general, most of those who remain married report high levels of marital satisfaction in their older years, but divorce among older people has doubled since 1960 and is predicted to be more prevalent in future populations over age 65 (Kart, 1994).

Marital Satisfaction and Aging

As married couples reach midadulthood, happiness that was at an all-time low in their early 40s begins to rebound when the adult children leave home (Berry & Williams, 1987). Children's moving out frees up time and money. The couple finds they have the time, money, and privacy to reestablish the things in their relationship that provide pleasure, as well as investigate new things together.

Marital happiness continues to rise in the later adult years and carries over into retirement. Depending on a number of factors ranging from health to retirement income, the couple continue to enjoy their freedom and, in some cases, relationships with their children's families and grandchildren (Cavanaugh, 1993).

Most of us know couples who have celebrated their 50th, or golden, wedding anniversary. We marvel at their longevity and wonder about the secret to their success. Researchers have studied this issue, and the findings are inconsistent. Part of the problem lies with defining happiness. Older couples differ from younger ones in their standards for happiness. They share a history that includes memories of the Great Depression, world wars, and more traditional roles for marriage and marital satisfaction. Their marital happiness and contentment may be based on a different set of standards than those of younger married people.

A long-term study of 17 happily married couples found that the most significant factor related to marital satisfaction was their ability to adapt to change and "roll with the punches" (Weishaus & Field, 1988). These couples had the ability to adapt to changing circumstances that normally might be interpreted as stressful and potentially damaging to the relationship. They might view a serious illness, for instance, as an opportunity for caring and closeness rather than anger and alienation.

Divorce in Older Couples

In many cases, marital dissatisfaction in older adulthood is not related to any age-specific cause but, rather, resurfaces after years of being subordinated by issues related to child rearing. With the children grown and out of the house, old tensions and discontent surface and become a source of stress. Dependency is a key issue in the level of marital satisfaction in older couples. The extent of dependence of one mate on the other seems to be related to the strength of the relationship and its ability to last. When dependence is mutual and the level is relatively equal for both partners, relationships are strong and close. When dependence is not equal and one partner's needs are much greater than the other's, marital conflict is much more likely (Cavanaugh, 1993). When dependence is not equal or mutual, one partner may perceive normal developmental issues such as retirement and relocation as threatening, and, therefore, they become a source of resentment, discontent, and stress. Other issues that dampen marital happiness in old age include health problems, caring for sick parents and children, and financial problems.

Divorce is particularly distressing to older adults because of the long time invested in another's personal and practical life. In general, the longer the marriage, the greater is the trauma. In many cases, an elderly person's identity is closely wrapped up in being another person's husband or wife. Loss of this status often results in loss of economic status and lifestyle, friends (who often choose sides), and self-concept (Cavanaugh, 1993).

Divorce carries a much greater stigma for elderly people than for young people. Because of this, many elderly people underreport their status as divorced when filling out forms, applying for services, and the like (Kart, 1994). Divorce in an elderly person, particularly a woman, also may account for much greater loss than for a younger adult because of retirement, the empty nest, and relocation of family. Whereas younger divorced persons still have a job to report to, children to care for and interact with, and friends and family in the vicinity, elderly people often face the loss of these important connections.

Widowhood

Although a person can become widowed at any time during a marriage, it is much more likely later in life. **Widowhood** is more common for women; more than half of all women over age 65 are widows, whereas just 15 percent of men are widowers at that age. The two main reasons are that men have a shorter average life expectancy than women and women tend to marry men older than themselves. Consequently, most married women in the United States can expect to live between 10 and 12 years as a widow if they choose not to remarry (Cavanaugh, 1993).

Widowhood can be stressful in a number of ways besides ending a partnership. U.S. society does not have well-defined social roles for widowed people. Therefore, they often are left alone by family and friends who don't know how to respond to them. Widowed individuals also may feel awkward as single people trying to fit into their previously coupled world.

Men are generally older than women when they become widowed. Men are thought to be less able to cope with the death of their wife than women are by the loss of their husband. This outcome may be a result of the way men are reared; the wife's having been the husband's only close confidant; the lack of experience of most men in cooking, cleaning, doing the laundry, and so forth; and the tendency of men to be more socially isolated than women (Cavanaugh, 1993).

Women may be able to cope better because they have more extensive social networks and are better equipped to live alone, as most are able to maintain a household and take care of themselves. At the same time, women's widowhood behavior patterns seem to be more variable than men's.

Widowhood The period of time between loss of spouse and remarriage

Not all women find widowhood equally stressful or stressful at all. In studying more than 300 widows in Chicago, Lopata (1973) found six different behavior patterns in women after the deaths of their husbands:

1. "Liberated wives" were able to grieve the loss of their spouse and move on to live full productive lives.
2. "Merry widows" went on to live lives of fun, dating, and various forms of entertainment.
3. "Working widows" continued their career or took a new job.
4. "Widows' widows" continued to live alone, were independent, and enjoyed the company of primarily other widows.
5. "Traditional widows" moved in with their children and took an active role in the lives of their grandchildren.
6. "Grieving widows" were unable to work through their loss and willingly isolated themselves from others.

The death of a loved one can lead to feelings of helplessness, hopelessness, and a sense of emptiness that can precipitate a variety of physical and mental illnesses. Cohen and Syme (1985) studied 4,500 adults over age 45 who had lost a spouse to premature death. Their study became known as the "broken heart" study because they found that nearly 40 percent of the surviving spouses died of heart problems during the 6 months following the death of their spouse. The percentage of deaths dropped steadily after this time and returned to that of the control group after 5 years. Other studies have confirmed these findings and have indicated that one of the factors mediating a return to normal risk of death is remarriage of the surviving spouse (Hafen, Frandsen, Karren, & Hooker, 1992).

healthy sex hints 6.5

Dealing with Grief and Loss

The death of a loved one ranks at the top of life's most stressful events. The loss can impact all dimensions of our health—we may lose our appetite, feel depressed, experience a sense of emptiness in our home, not be able to concentrate, and so forth. How individuals grieve varies, with some able to cry openly while others bury themselves in tasks. Individual reactions to loss may also depend on whether a death was sudden or the culmination of a long and painful illness.

The loss of one's partner can be devastating. Individuals who have lived decades as part of a couple may struggle to understand how to find joy in life and live independently. Some may need to find a new partner quickly; others may feel that the lost love could never be replaced.

Grieving for a lost partner can be compounded by the relationship having been secret. It may be difficult to openly grieve and attend a funeral, for example, if your partner had never shared your existence with too many others. Long after the death of the famous aviator Charles Lindbergh, and shortly after the death of Senator Strom Thurmond, the facts of their secret "other" families came to light. Those descendents who had long been recognized as family were suddenly confronted with learning that the father they had loved had a past with which they were unfamiliar.

Whatever the circumstances, however, individuals must work through their grief. The following guidelines may prove beneficial:

- Accept your feelings, and understand that such emotions as anger, guilt, and relief are normal.
- Accept help from others, who may bring food, provide emotional comfort, and listen to you talk about your loss.
- Although grief can be private, you don't have to pretend to be strong and hold in your feelings.
- Give yourself time—grieving can be a long process. There is no set timetable for working through grief. There may be good days and bad days.
- Seek professional help if you remain intensely distressed for more than 6 months.

Source: Adapted from Hales (2003, p. 615).

Grief and Loss in Nontraditional Long-Term Relationships

In a study of grief and loss among those in **nontraditional relationships** (extramarital affairs, cohabitation, and homosexual relationships), the normal stages of grief were compounded by the nontraditional nature of the relationships studied (Doka, 1987). In homosexual and other relationships, conflicting needs compound the healing process of grief. A need to declare and demonstrate sorrow and affection for the loved one is tempered by a need to maintain secrecy and fear that the relationship will be disclosed. Some hospitals, for instance, restrict access to "husbands or wives" or "immediate family." The need for social support, and to grieve with the other mourners, is countered by a sense of social isolation and distancing. These compounding factors are minimized for homosexual couples who are not maintaining a secret relationship. Being active in the gay community has helped gay couples develop social support networks that enable them to cope more effectively with a variety of issues associated with aging (Quam & Whitford, 1992).

Nontraditional relationships Any relationships other than a monogamous, legal marriage between a man and a woman

Spiritual Wellness

Adulthood and old age are potentially a time of great spiritual awakening and renewal. For most people this is a time of developing intimate, loving relationships, making permanent (sacramental) commitments, having children, caring for sick and dying parents, and coming to terms with our own mortality. We are forced to examine these issues, all of which have a spiritual dimension. Understanding the meaning of these events, coping with them and their universality, help us develop a sense of connectedness with something other than ourselves. If we allow ourselves to look beyond the self and gain strength through connecting with others, we can enhance our spirituality, which can help us lead more satisfying and productive lives.

Your responses to the Personal Assessment, Thought Questions, and Test Yourself! quiz questions can be logged online in your Virtual Workbook at **http://health.wadsworth.com/blonna1.**

Personal Assessment

6.1 Relationship Contract

Relationships are fluid, yet many couples move toward commitment. Traditionally, heterosexual couples will marry. Until the institution of marriage is extended to gay and lesbian couples, commitment ceremonies remain an emerging ritual that parallels weddings. How couples structure their commitment varies tremendously, regardless of sexual orientation.

The purpose of this assessment is to help you examine the nature of your intimate relationships. A secondary purpose is to help you realize that you have the ability to structure your relationships any way you want.

Fill out the following relationship contract. There are no right or wrong answers. Just jot down your thoughts and feelings regarding the various categories. You may wish to ask your instructor for the opportunity to go over your contract with other students in a small group.

Name
Should the wife take on the husband's last name?
Should the husband take on the wife's last name?
If the partners are same sex, will either or both change last names?
Should both take on a hyphenated last name?
Should both take a new name?
Should both keep their own name?
What will the children's surname be if there are any?

Birth Control
What kind?
Whose responsibility?

Household Duties
Who does what?

Leisure Time
Should evenings and weekends be spent together?
Who decides what to do?
Should vacations be spent together? With children? Separately?

Living Arrangements
Where will the couple live?
What kind of privacy do you need?
Shared bedroom?
Do you want to live with others?
What will you and your partner do if you want to live in different places because of jobs or for any other reasons?

Money
Will both partners work?
If so, will you pool your money?
Or will each keep own salary?
Or will the cost of living expenses be shared equally and the rest kept for yourselves?

Sexual Rights
Commitment to monogamy?
Who initiates sex?
Is either partner free not to respond?

Children
How many?
When?
Adopt?
Who will take primary responsibility for rearing the children?
Will one partner have to quit a job?

Other Relationships
Are you and your partner free to make relationships with other people?
With those of the same sex?
With those of the opposite sex?
What is to be the extent of these relationships?
Do you include each other in these relationships?

Thought Questions

1. What are some of the major developmental tasks of college students? Compare these to the major developmental tasks associated with adolescence.

2. Compare and contrast sexual behavior during the college years with that of middle adulthood. What are the differences?

3. What is Berry and Williams's model of marital satisfaction? Identify the stages.

4. What are the similarities and differences between long-term heterosexual relationships and lesbian and gay unions of the same duration?

5. What factors contribute to satisfaction and happiness in long-term relationships?

6. What changes in sexual response are associated with aging?

Test Yourself!

1. A primary developmental task of young adults is to
   a. develop friendships with peers.
   b. form a committed, intimate relationship with a partner.
   c. learn to trust others.
   d. identify one's sexual orientation.

2. Which generalization about sexual behavior among college students is most accurate?
   a. Rates of sexual activity are similar between males and females.
   b. Fewer students participate in oral sex compared to earlier generations.
   c. There is no evidence of a double standard in values for male and female behavior.
   d. The majority of students cohabit prior to committing to marriage.

3. Couples who are happily married tend to do all but which of the following?
   a. Maintain some level of individual identity
   b. Share similar interests and values
   c. Fight effectively, laying blame where it belongs
   d. Communicate honestly

4. Berry and Williams have developed a model for the phases of adult marriage. When do couples report being the most satisfied with their marriage?
   a. At the time of the birth of their first child
   b. When their children are adolescents
   c. During the honeymoon phase, at the beginning
   d. Once children move out of the house

5. The concept of "fighting fairly" includes all but which of the following?
   a. Avoiding personal attacks
   b. Taking responsibility for your behavior
   c. Being able to discuss all the things that have been bothering you
   d. Not fighting in front of others

6. Changes in female sexual response associated with aging include
   a. loss of sex drive.
   b. less clitoral response.
   c. less vaginal lubrication.
   d. loss of orgasm.

7. Changes in male sexual response associated with aging include
   a. less firm erections.
   b. loss of sex drive.
   c. increase in semen production.
   d. loss of the ability to ejaculate.

8. Marriage is a form of relationship commitment
   a. between two consenting adults.
   b. open to gay, lesbian, and heterosexual couples.
   c. shown to endure for the majority of couples.
   d. that offers financial, personal, and health benefits.

9. Long-term gay and lesbian relationships
   a. are not possible in the oppressive culture of the United States.
   b. have been proven more stable than heterosexual relationships.
   c. go through stages similar to those in a marriage, yet with economic differences.
   d. require individuals to assume traditional roles within the relationship.

10. Which statement about widowhood among women is least accurate?
    a. Women are often better able to cope with the loss than men.
    b. Women quickly remarry after the loss of a spouse.
    c. Some women feel liberated and adopt lifestyle changes, such as traveling.
    d. Traditional widows move in with their children and become involved in raising their grandchildren.

Media Menu

You can link to the following online tools by visiting
http://health.wadsworth.com/blonna1.

Face to Face Video

Heather and Cindy talk about their relationship and impending marriage.

 InfoTrac Activity

Ponnuru, R. (2003, July 28). Coming out ahead: Why gay marriage is on the way. *National Review, 55* (14).
Bradley, G. V. (2003, July 28). Stand and fight: Don't take gay marriage lying down. *National Review, 55* (14).

 Web Resources

College Sex Talk

www.CollegeSexTalk.com

A Web site operated by Dr. Sandra Caron, certified sexuality educator and professor, where students can write in questions and receive age-appropriate responses to their concerns about sexuality.

National Institutes of Health

www.nih.gov

Typing "sexuality" into the search box will link users to numerous articles examining sexuality and health.

Administration on Aging, Department of Health and Human Services

www.aoa.gov

A Web site with information on sexuality in later life, HIV/AIDS and older adults, and so forth.

National Association on HIV over 50

www.hivoverfifty.org

A site devoted to older adults infected with HIV and/or those in need of information for themselves or others.

Senior Site

www.seniorsite.com

Sexual health information for older adults.

References

Berry, R. E., & Williams, E. (1987). Assessing the relationship between quality of life and marital and income satisfaction: A path analytic approach. *Journal of Marriage and the Family, 49*, 107–116.

Block, B. (1980). *Friendship: How to give it, how to get it.* New York: Macmillan.

Blumstein, P., & Schwartz, P. (1983). *American couples.* New York: Morrow.

Cahill, S., & Slater, S. (2003). Marriage: Legal protection for families and children—A policy brief from the National Gay and Lesbian Task Force Policy Institute [Online]. Available: www.ngltf.org.

Cavanaugh, J. C. (1993). *Adult development and aging.* Belmont, CA: Wadsworth.

Cohen, S., & Syme, S. L. (1985). *Social support and health.* Orlando, FL: Academic Press.

Crawford, M., & Popp, D. (2003, February). Sexual double standards: A review and methodological critique of two decades of research. *Journal of Sex Research, 40*(1).

Doka, K. J. (1987). Silent sorrow: Grief and loss of significant others. *Death Studies, 11*(8), 455–469.

Duvall, E. M. (1977). *Family development.* Philadelphia: Lippincott.

The Elderly and HIV Conference. (2000, December). Wayne General Hospital and William Paterson University.

Ellison, C. (2000). *Women's sexualities.* California: New Harbinger.

Erikson, E. (1978). *Childhood and society* (2nd ed.). New York: Norton.

Fields, J. (2001, June 29). [Report.] *U.S. Department of Commerce News.* U.S. Census Public Information Office. Washington, DC: U.S. Government Printing Office.

Hafen, B. Q., Frandsen, K. J., Karren, K. J., & Hooker, K. R. (1992). *The health effects of attitudes, emotions, and relationships.* Provo, UT: EMS Associates.

Hales, D. (2003). *An invitation to health* (10th ed.). Belmont, CA: Wadsworth/Thomson Learning.

Hughes, R. (2003). The demographics of divorce: United States and Missouri [Online]. Available: www.missourifamilies.org.

Kart, C. (1994). *The realities of aging: An introduction to gerontology.* Boston: Allyn & Bacon.

Kurdek, L. (1989). Relationship quality of gay and lesbian cohabiting couples. *Journal of Homosexuality, 15*(3–4), 93–118.

Kurdek, L. (1993). The allocation of household labor in gay, lesbian, and heterosexual married couples. *Journal of Social Issues, 49*(3), 127–139.

Lambda Legal Defense Fund. (2003). Cases: *Lawrence and Garner v. Texas* [Online]. Available: www.cache.lambdalegal.org.

Lambert, T. A., Kahn, A. S., & Apple, K. J. (2003). Pluralistic ignorance and hooking up. *Journal of Sex Research, 40*(2), 129–133.

Laumann, E., Gagnon, J. H., Michael, R. T., & Michaels, S. (1994). *The social organization of sexuality: Sexual practices in the United States.* Chicago: University of Chicago Press.

Laumann, E. O., & Michael, R. T. (2001). *Sex, love, and health in America: Private choices and public policies.* Chicago: University of Chicago Press.

Laumann, E. O., & Youm, Y. (2001). Sexual expression in America. In E. O. Laumann & R. Michael (Eds.), *Sex, love and health in America.* Chicago: University of Chicago Press.

Lipman, A. (1986). Homosexual relationships. *Generations, 10*(4), 51–54.

Lopata, H. Z. (1973). *Widowhood in an American city.* Cambridge, MA: Schenkman.

Masters, W. H., Johnson, V. E., & Kolodny, R. C. (1992). *Human sexuality* (4th ed.). New York: HarperCollins.

McWhirter, D., & Mattison D. (1984). *The male couple.* Englewood Cliffs, NJ: Prentice Hall.

Michael, R. T., Gagnon, J. H., Laumann, E. O., & Kolata, G. (1994). *Sex in America: A definitive survey.* Boston: Little, Brown.

National Center for Education Statistics. (2000). *Percentage distribution of undergraduates by marital status: 1999–2000.* U.S. Department of Education, 1999–2000 National Postsecondary Student Aid Study (NPSAS:2000). Washington, DC: Author.

Paul, E. L., McManus, B., & Hayes, A. (2000). Hookups: Characteristics and correlates of college students' spontaneous and anonymous sexual experiences. *Journal of Sex Research, 37*(1), 76–88.

Person, E. S. (1989). *Women—Sex and sexuality.* Chicago: University of Chicago Press.

Phillis, D. E., & Stein, P. J. (1983). Sink or swing? The lifestyles of single adults. In E. R. Allegeir & N. B. McCormick (Eds.), *Changing boundaries: Gender roles and sexual behavior.* Palo Alto, CA: Mayfield.

Quam, J. K., & Whitford, G. S. (1992). Adaptation and age-related expectations of elder gay and lesbian adults. *Gerontologist, 32*(3), 367–374.

Reinisch, J. M. (1992). *The Kinsey Institute new report on sex.* New York: St. Martin's.

Thomas, J. A. (2000, October 10). Childcare and laboratory schools on campus: The national picture [Online]. National Coalition for Campus Children's Centers. Available: www.campuschildren.org.

Times will begin reporting gay couples' ceremonies. (2002, August 18). *New York Times,* National Section.

U.S. Bureau of the Census. (2002). *Median age at first marriage* [Online]. Available: www.census.gov.

Weinberg, M. S., Williams, C. J., & Pryor, D. W. (2001, April). Bisexuals at midlife: Commitment, salience, and identity. *Journal of Contemporary Ethnography, 30.*

Weishaus, S., & Field, D. (1988). A half century of marriage: Continuity or change? *Journal of Marriage and the Family, 50,* 763–774.

Zilbergeld, B. (1999). *The new male sexuality* (rev. ed.). New York: Bantam Doubleday Dell.

chapter *seven*

Human Sexual Response

Student Learning Objectives

After reading this chapter, students will be able to

- Identify the key brain structures involved in the human sexual response.

- Describe how the nervous and endocrine systems interact during sexual response.

- Explain how psychological and physiological factors interact during sexual response.

- Describe the effects of major disabilities on sexual response

- Compare and contrast a variety of sexual response theories.

- Diagram and describe the four phases of the Masters and Johnson sexual response cycle.

- Define *aphrodisiac* and evaluate the effects of aphrodisiacs on sexual response.

- Describe factors that enhance vasocongestion and sexual response.

- Describe a variety of theories of sexual response

Test your understanding of these objectives by taking the end-of-chapter quiz, available online at **http://health.wadsworth.com/blonna1.**

activity teaser: *How do you really feel about your body? Find out in the Personal Exploration Activity on page 229.*

case study 7.1

Sexual Response: John and Michelle

John and Michelle, both 23, are white.

Critical Thinking

As John and Michelle have demonstrated, sexual response can often occur despite our conscious thoughts to initiate it. How does this affect our ability to turn it off when we are aroused unintentionally?

Use your Virtual Workbook to explore your answer to this question at **http://health.wadsworth.com/blonna1.**

John is working on his computer in the apartment he shares with Michelle, his steady girlfriend of 3 years. Michelle is out with friends, having agreed to give John some quiet time to work on a paper he is writing. From his desk, he can gaze out onto the street in front of his apartment. His mind is busy trying to piece together the words that ultimately will make up his paper on Shakespeare for his English literature class. His fingers move quickly over the keyboard, his eyes riveted on the screen and his attention on his work.

As he works on the computer, he senses a car pull up, its doors swing open, and someone gets out. Without taking his eyes off the screen, John senses that this might be Michelle. He looks out the window and sees Michelle. She is wearing a short, silky, summer dress that sways with her long, athletic legs. He hears her laughter as she and her friends say their good-byes as they drive off.

Michelle enters their apartment, and, although he can't see her yet, he hears the rustling of her skirt, and a trace of Michelle's perfume wafts through the door. He hears her voice call out, "John, I'm home." The sound of her voice and the smell of her perfume cause his mind to wander and his body begins to respond. He feels his penis begin to get erect. Although he tries to fight it, his mind continues to wander, drifting from his writing to his erection, to thoughts of Michelle's warm body and past lovemaking, and back to his writing again.

Realizing that he'll never finish his writing if he allows his thoughts to keep wandering like this, John focuses his attention on his paper, and his brain begins to shut down his sexual response. After about 10 minutes, Michelle enters the room and, with a sexy smile, wanders over to John's desk and interrupts his concentration.

"Interested in taking a little break?" she asks, as she takes his glasses off his nose, wraps her arms around his shoulders, and begins to nibble on his ear. He turns, gives her a kiss, and feels his body respond to her warmth and softness.

After a couple of kisses, John decides to stop trying to fight his brain's urges and allows his body to take over. He picks up Michelle, carries her over to the bed, and they proceed to make love, both deciding that Shakespeare can wait a couple of hours.

If you were to ask the average person which part of the body is the most important for controlling sexual response, the answer most likely would be "the penis" or "the vagina." Most people equate sexual response to genital functioning. In reality, sexual response begins and ends in the brain. The brain, not the genitals, is the seat of human sexual response. Human sexual response originates with the brain's perception of desire. What makes you want to respond? What allows you to become comfortable and relax so the response will happen? In this chapter, we'll examine sexual response and try to answer these and many other questions.

Social Wellness

The quality of our social relationships plays a big part in our sexual response. Being able to relax, feel secure, and trust our partner is crucial for good sex. Another key to good sex is open communication. Getting to know your partner requires time. Intimacy builds over time as a result of shared experiences and open communication about our innermost thoughts, feelings, needs, and wants. As you can see in Case Study 7.1 with John and Michelle, an intimacy, trust, and a sense of playfulness spring from this social bond between them. Their sensuality and sexuality are easy, not forced, and are a hallmark of high-level social wellness.

Physiology of Sexual Response

Sexual response is the result of a complex interaction between psychological and physiological factors originating in the brain and spreading through various body parts and systems. We'll trace the sexual response, describing the key components and mechanisms of action that control it.

Brain

The brain has four major parts (see Figure 7.1):

1. Cerebral cortex
2. Diencephalon
3. Limbic system
4. Brain stem

The entire surface of the brain is irregular, with ridges and shallow and deep grooves, and is divided into two halves called **hemispheres.** The cerebral hemispheres form the outermost part of the brain and are divided into sections called lobes. The frontal, parietal, occipital, and temporal lobes of each hemisphere are responsible for controlling a variety of **motor, sensory,** and **associational brain functions,** which are directly involved in sexual response.

Hemispheres The two halves of the cerebrum, each controlling the functions of the opposite side of the body

Motor Relating to nerve impulses going out to muscles

Sensory Relating to nerve messages coming into the brain

Associational brain functions Connecting together individual sensory inputs

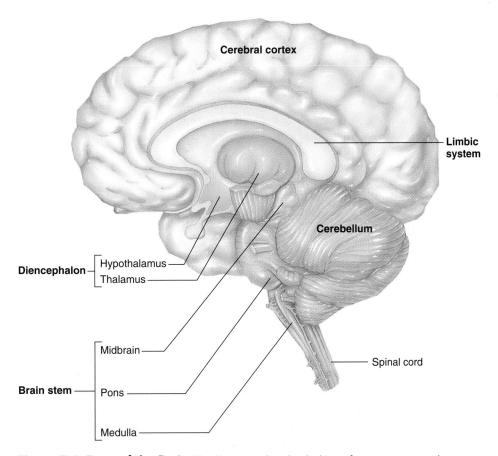

Figure 7.1 *Parts of the Brain* The brain can be divided into four main parts when studying sexuality: cerebral cortex, diencephalon, limbic system, and the brain stem.

Cerebral Cortex   The conscious awareness of sensations (sight, sound, smell, taste, and touch) is controlled by the parietal, occipital, and temporal lobes of the cerebral cortex, the thinking part of the brain. These sensations, in some combination, enter one's consciousness through the sensory areas of the cerebral cortex and are interpreted as sexual. The cortex picks up the message, and the associational areas interpret them.

Although each sensory stimulus is entered as a distinct, separate entity, they are quickly assimilated, sorted out, deciphered, and combined as a potentially sexy signal. This interplay relies on stored memories (whether real or imagined) of past experiences that influence the person's assessment of the present incoming stimuli and expectations of what is to follow.

Intellectual Wellness

Knowing how our perceptions can influence our sexual response opens the door to relearning things about our sexuality that until now might have been barriers to our sexual fulfillment. If we believe in the cognitive basis of sexual response, we can unlearn negative sexual information and learn new, healthy ways of viewing ourselves and our sexuality. Knowing about the sexual response patterns in men and women and the areas that are most responsive to stimulation can make us better lovers, regardless of whether we are straight, gay, lesbian, or bisexual. Knowing our limitations and capabilities, how to work around certain disabilities and health conditions, can help us improve our sexual response and maintain our self-respect and self-esteem. Knowing what to expect concerning sexual response can make the difference between allowing ourselves to relax and let things happen or becoming overly concerned with the process and worry that it won't happen. Knowing that our sexual desires and responses vary from day to day will help us understand the differences and enable us to relax and go with the changes. Understanding that our needs and responses won't always perfectly mirror our partner's can help us devise ways to work around these and other differences. Understanding the effects of drugs, fatigue, stress, and other substances on our sexual response empowers us and helps us moderate their effects. Knowledge also can prepare us for the future, by enabling us to anticipate the changes in sexual response associated with aging.

Thalamus The part of the brain that relays all inputs to the cerebral cortex

Hypothalamus The part of the brain that correlates activities between the nervous centers and the pituitary gland

Hormonal releasing factors Chemicals secreted by the hypothalamus that trigger the pituitary to release specific hormones

Diencephalon   The diencephalon forms the central core of the brain and contains the **thalamus** and **hypothalamus.** This area plays a crucial role in the continuation of sexual response that begins with the interpretation of an incoming stimulus as sexual.

The thalamus, a hidden region of the brain, might best be described as the relay center for all inputs to the cerebral cortex. The hypothalamus is located directly beneath the thalamus at the end of the brain stem. Despite its small size, the hypothalamus exerts a tremendous amount of control over body functioning. It works in concert with the nervous and endocrine systems, sending its messages via direct nerve transmissions and chemicals called **hormonal releasing factors.**

The nervous and endocrine systems provide the main pathways of human sexual response. The hypothalamus instantaneously sends electrical (direct nerve transmissions) and chemical (hormones) messages to switch on the body parts responsible for initiating the sexual response. The heart, responding to electrical and chemical stimulation, increases the volume of blood pumped throughout the body by raising its rate and pressure. This increased pumping of blood is necessary for supplying the extra oxygen and energy used during sexual activity.

Blood vessels supplying the genitals, brain, and skeletal muscles dilate, allowing greater blood flow to the areas involved in sexual response. The lungs re-

Jorge: Mistaken Perceptions

Jorge, 19, single, identifies as Hispanic.

Jorge is a college sophomore. He shared a story about mistaking a date's expressions of affection as an invitation to have sexual intercourse.

I'm a little embarrassed about talking about this, but I think it's exactly what we were just talking about in class. I dated a girl last semester who was really fine. I was instantly attracted to her when I saw her at the student center. I went up to her, and we hit it off, so I asked her out. We went to one of the jazz concerts on campus and hung out afterward. We walked around campus, and after a while, she kind of snuggled up against me on one of the benches by the auditorium. She smelled real good, and it felt great having my arm around her. We started to kiss and make out. Everything seemed to be going great. We were laughing and snuggling, having a great time.

It started to get late, so I suggested I walk her back to her room. Her roommates had gone home, so she invited me in, and we started making out again. I really thought she wanted to have sex. I mean, she was hot and rubbing up against me. By now I had an erection, and I started to unbutton her blouse. When I got about halfway she stopped me and said, "No." I said, "No what?" She said, "Listen, I like you a lot, but I really don't want to have sex."

I must admit, I was shocked and upset. In the past I had never gotten this far without having sex. I wasn't sure what to do. My penis was throbbing, and I really was horny. I said, "Can you take care of me?" She said "I'm really sorry. I just don't want to do this anymore. Could you please leave?"

I really didn't know if she was serious or not, so I asked her, "Are you serious?" She said she was, and I got myself straightened up and left. I was surprised, but by the time I got out of her dorm and started to walk back to my place, I had lost both my erection and my desire. I found out the next week that she had just broken up with her boyfriend that day, and I guess I came along at the wrong time. I never could bring myself to call her again.

Critical Thinking

How could you rewrite this case study to prevent this type of misunderstanding from ever happening in the first place?

Use your Virtual Workbook to explore your answer to this question at **http://health.wadsworth.com/blonna1.**

spond instantly by increasing the rate and depth of breathing. The airways expand, allowing maximum intake of air so its vital oxygen is mixed with the blood. The skeletal muscles began to contract and build tension.

Limbic System The limbic system is a complex arrangement of nerve tissue that links the emotional brain with the thinking, rational brain (cerebral cortex). In this way, the limbic system establishes a relationship between our thoughts and our feelings. Sometimes this relationship is clear-cut and appropriate; other times it is not. Sometimes our emotions get the best of us so we don't think clearly. We might interpret someone's verbal communication, body language, or behavior as conveying interest in having sex when they really are not. The cerebral cortex does have the ability to shut down sexual response through conscious control of behavior at any point.

Brain Stem The structures of the brain stem produce the autonomic functions necessary for our survival, in addition to serving as the pathway for connections between the higher and lower brain functions. A key part of the brain stem, the *reticular activating system* (RAS), is a collection of neurons running through the three regions of the brain

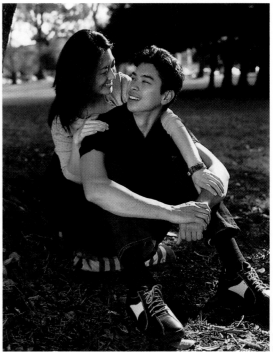

Flirting is often perceived as a sign of sexual interest.

stem. It is responsible for both arousing the brain and filtering out unnecessary information. During arousal, the RAS is responsible for magnifying and increasing our awareness of specific stimuli. It allows us to hone in or focus on details of the stimulus.

The RAS also acts as a filter. Although we don't realize it, the RAS filters out a tremendous number of stimuli, allowing us to attend to only the important information. The RAS disregards more than 90 percent of all familiar, repetitive, or weak sensory stimulation as unimportant while allowing new, unusual, or strong stimuli to penetrate. This helps us focus our attention on important stimuli.

Nervous System

The human nervous system is composed of two parts: the central nervous system and the peripheral nervous system. The **central nervous system** is made up of the brain and spinal cord. The **peripheral nervous system** consists of all other nerves and connects the spinal cord to various target organs, glands, and tissue. Figure 7.2 shows the nervous system.

The peripheral nervous system is made up of two divisions: the **somatic nervous system** and the **autonomic nervous system.** The initial information in the sexual response is passed along as electrical impulses from the brain, through the spinal cord to the peripheral nervous system, and ultimately to the specific glands, organs, and tissues involved in sexual response.

Central nervous system
The brain and spinal cord

Peripheral nervous system
All nerves coming off of the spinal cord

Somatic nervous system
The part of the peripheral nervous system under voluntary control

Autonomic nervous system
The part of the peripheral nervous system that is automatic and involuntary

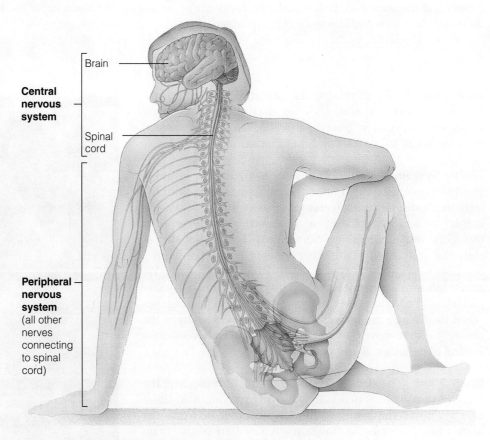

Figure 7.2 *The Nervous System* The nervous system receives and sends sexual messages electrically throughout our body.

Endocrine System

The endocrine system is responsible for the production and secretion of potent hormones that initiate and perpetuate the sexual response, in addition to a variety of other functions ranging from the stress response to growth. The endocrine system is made up of the pituitary, thyroid, parathyroid, adrenal, pancreas, thymus, and pineal glands, as well as the ovaries and the testes. These are illustrated in Figure 7.3.

The endocrine system works on the principle of feedback, with the hypothalamus acting as a thermostat that senses the level of a hormone circulating in the bloodstream. Just as the thermostat in your home senses the level of heat and turns on the heating or cooling system to regulate the temperature, the hypothalamus senses the level of circulating hormones in your bloodstream. If the level of a hormone is too low, the hypothalamus secretes specific releasing factors that travel through the bloodstream to the target endocrine gland, prompting it to begin producing hormones.

Sex Hormones The role of sex hormones in human sexual response is tremendously confusing. Part of the problem stems from categorizing "male hormones" as androgens and "female hormones" as estrogens. In fact, the primary "male hormone," testosterone, is produced in both males and females (Bancroft, 2002). In addition, the primary "female hormone," estrogen, is similarly produced in males and females. What varies is the level of each hormone and their sites of production (Bancroft, 2002).

Testosterone. Testosterone is the hormone that seems to exert the most dramatic effect on sexual response. It is the main hormone associated with sexual desire in both men and women (Bancroft, 2002). The average man produces between 6 and 8 mg of testosterone daily. Most of the male testosterone (about 95 percent) is manufactured in the testes, and the remainder is produced in the adrenal glands. The average woman produces about 0.5 milligrams of testosterone daily, manufactured in the ovaries and adrenal glands. Prior to puberty, testosterone is produced in similar quantities in boys and girls, in the adrenal glands.

Although men produce much more testosterone than women daily, women seem to have a lower threshold for testosterone sensitivity; they need less in circulation to derive the effects of this potent hormone. Regardless of the overall level of testosterone in men or women, deficiencies of this hormone result in a drop-off in sexual desire (Bancroft, 2002). Studies have shown that a drop-off in androgen levels associated with surgery, antiandrogenic drugs, and other causes can result in diminished sexual desire (Reagan, 1999). Conversely, increasing androgen levels in men and women with diminished blood levels results in heightened sexual desire (Davis, 1998).

Men are especially dependent on testosterone levels for sexual performance. When testosterone levels drop, they have difficulty obtaining and maintaining erections. Women's sexual performance does not seem to be affected as much by testosterone levels. When their levels of testosterone drop, they still are able to experience lubrication, orgasm, and other changes associated with sexual performance (Traish, Kim, Munarriz, & Goldstein, 2002).

Estrogens. Although commonly referred to as "female hormones," estrogens are also produced by men. Women manufacture estrogens in their ovaries, whereas men produce estrogen in their testes. Estrogen levels also are related to sexual response. Estrogens play a role in maintaining vaginal lubrication, thus facilitating intercourse (Traish et al., 2002).

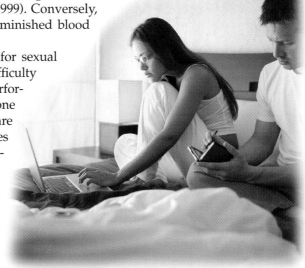

Paul Vozdic/GettyImages

Overwork can diminish one's interest in sex.

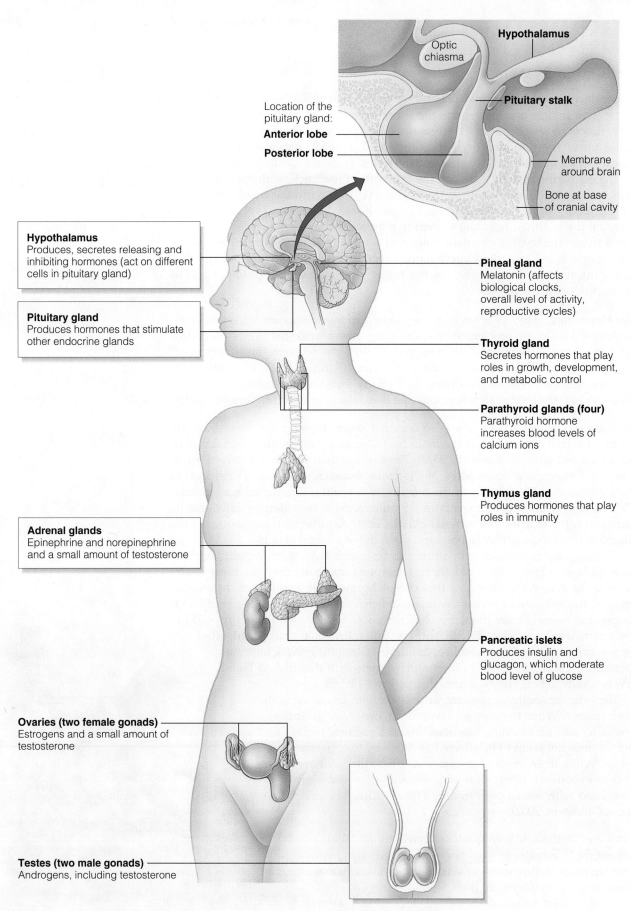

Hypothalamus
Produces, secretes releasing and inhibiting hormones (act on different cells in pituitary gland)

Pituitary gland
Produces hormones that stimulate other endocrine glands

Adrenal glands
Epinephrine and norepinephrine and a small amount of testosterone

Ovaries (two female gonads)
Estrogens and a small amount of testosterone

Testes (two male gonads)
Androgens, including testosterone

Optic chiasma

Hypothalamus

Pituitary stalk

Location of the pituitary gland:
Anterior lobe
Posterior lobe

Membrane around brain

Bone at base of cranial cavity

Pineal gland
Melatonin (affects biological clocks, overall level of activity, reproductive cycles)

Thyroid gland
Secretes hormones that play roles in growth, development, and metabolic control

Parathyroid glands (four)
Parathyroid hormone increases blood levels of calcium ions

Thymus gland
Produces hormones that play roles in immunity

Pancreatic islets
Produces insulin and glucagon, which moderate blood level of glucose

Figure 7.3 *The Endocrine System* The nervous system receives and sends sexual messages chemically throughout our body.

sex in society 7.1

Participating in Sex Research

Imagine for a moment that a team of professors from your college is going to begin a study of sexual response among college students (singles and couples) at your school and on other campuses across the country. They are recruiting volunteers to participate in the study. You are curious about this and agree to be contacted by the team to see whether you meet the study's subject protocols. They give you some preliminary reading material about the study to examine before you come in for the interview.

The material explains that the team is interested in studying the sexual response of college students to see how it has changed since the days of Masters and Johnson's research. They will be studying the sexual responses of gay and straight students under the following conditions:

Viewing erotic films alone
Viewing erotic films in a co-ed group

Solitary masturbation
Shared masturbation
Vaginal intercourse
Oral intercourse
Anal intercourse

They explain that every attempt will be made to conduct the study under the strictest standards of confidentiality. Members of the team, however, will view sexual responses through two-way mirrors and will record the responses through various instruments including video-cameras. The literature explains that this is necessary for the team to review the subjects' responses later.

Do you think you would participate in such a study? Would you participate if they paid you? How much? Do the conditions of this study create bias regarding who the subjects will be? How?

Women who have had their ovaries removed through hysterectomy and other procedures do not experience a reduction in sexual drive, although they may experience vaginal dryness and subsequent pain, which can diminish their interest and desire in sex. Women with high levels of estrogen do not experience heightened (or reduced) levels of sexual desire. Men also do not seem to be affected by too little estrogen. Excessive estrogen in men can have a "feminizing" effect that includes breast enlargement and erectile difficulties.

Progesterone. Progesterone is another major female sex hormone produced in the ovaries. It seems to play a primary role in reproduction by ensuring the viability of the endometrium. Its role in sexual desire and functioning is not understood very well. It may actually suppress the sexual interest of men and women alike (Reagan, 1999).

Models of Sexual Response

Six models of sexual response are discussed here. By far the best known is the one by William Masters and Virginia Johnson, pioneers in the study of sexual response.

Masters and Johnson Phases

In 1966, Masters and Johnson published their ground-breaking work, *Human Sexual Response*. The book was ground-breaking for several reasons. Although previous researchers (Alfred Kinsey being the most notable) had published reports concerning self-reported sexual behavior, Masters and Johnson's was the first large-scale study of sexual response. Masters (a gynecologist) and Johnson (a psychologist) were the first researchers to study sexual response in a laboratory setting. They were the first mainstream scientists to apply the scientific rigor necessary to quantify and qualify a very private act. Their work provided a graphic depiction of the actual sexual processes in action.

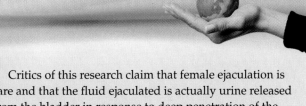

sex in society 7.2

The G-Spot

One of the more controversial topics of the past is the G-spot, named after Dr. Ernest Grafenberg. Grafenberg claimed that the G-spot is a mass of erectile tissue located on the front wall of the vagina, midway between the introitus and the cervix. He claimed that the G-spot is an erogenous zone capable of being stimulated during sex play. Once stimulated, the G-spot is purported to be capable of triggering orgasm and ejaculation. Between 10 and 40 percent of women ejaculate after sufficient stimulation of the G-spot (Ladas, Whipple, & Perry, 1982). Masters and Johnson claimed that this female ejaculate may come from the skene's glands near the bladder, which develop from the same embryonic tissue as the male prostate.

Critics of this research claim that female ejaculation is rare and that the fluid ejaculated is actually urine released from the bladder in response to deep penetration of the vagina that some intercourse positions create. Whipple and associates respond to this criticism by claiming that, although the fluid contains traces of urine, it is not urine but, rather, a new liquid released by stimulation of the G-spot.

Other critics point to researchers' inability to isolate G-spot tissue. They claim that no one has been able to identify and biopsy tissue from the part of the vagina that is dissimilar to the squamous tissue that is normally present (Ladas et al., 1982).

Masters and Johnson invented the technology and instruments necessary for studying our most intimate body parts. They devised clear, plastic, penis-shaped cameras to photograph things such as changes in vaginal lubrication. They invented electromyographic devices to measure the most intimate of all muscular contractions, those of the penis, vagina, and anus. Many of these instruments and methods also were used to treat sexual dysfunction. The Masters and Johnson Institute in St. Louis became world-renowned for the study and treatment of sexual dysfunctions.

Orgasm The stage of sexual response characterized by ejaculation in males and involuntary muscular contractions followed by relaxation in both males and females

Besides creating the technology, they operationally defined **orgasm.** An operational definition was a prerequisite for experimental research of the phenomenon. They created a language of sexuality that included words such as *orgasm*, *vasocongestion*, *myotonia*, and others that allowed professionals in the field to communicate with each other and disseminate their research findings.

Masters and Johnson were the first researchers to divide sexual response into phases that blend into one another as sexual response continues. They identified four phases:

1. Excitement
2. Plateau
3. Orgasm
4. Resolution

This sequence was the same regardless of the nature of sexual stimulation (masturbation, intercourse, and so forth) or sexual orientation (heterosexual, homosexual, bisexual) studied. The four stages are depicted in Figure 7.4 for women and Figure 7.5 for men.

Finally, Masters and Johnson discovered that the seat of women's sexual response is the clitoris, not the vagina. This broke new ground for understanding and conducting future research concerning women's sexual response. It opened the door for future research concerning issues such as the **G-spot,** differences in response patterns in women before and after a hysterectomy, and a host of other areas.

G-spot An area in the upper, rear section of the vagina named after Ernest Grafenberg, who claimed it to be an erogenous zone

Heterosexual and lesbian women (as well as their partners) have had the opportunity to apply Masters and Johnson's discoveries to enhance their sexual pleasure by better understanding their sexual functioning.

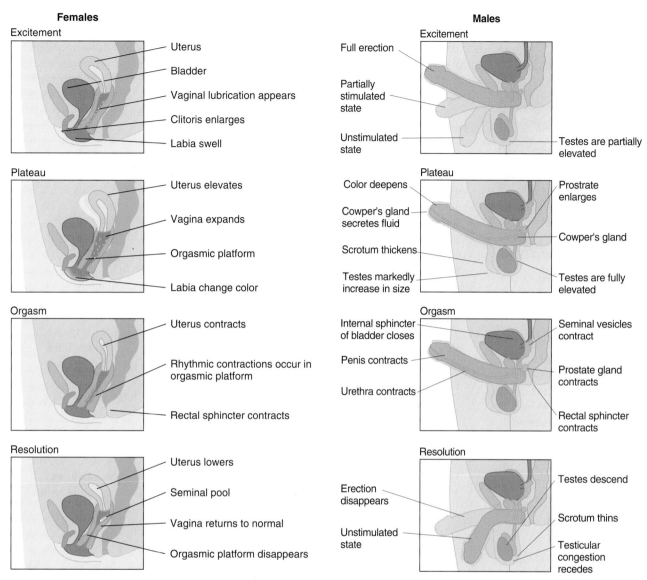

Figure 7.4 *Masters and Johnson's Sexual Response Cycle in Women* This cycle has four phases.

Figure 7.5 *Masters and Johnson's Sexual Response Cycle in Men* The cycle for men has four phases.

Excitement During the first stage of Masters and Johnson's human sexual response, excitement, sexual arousal is initiated. Excitement can be triggered by a limitless array of cognitive and sensory stimuli ranging from viewing erotic films to listening to romantic music or getting a whiff of a familiar cologne or perfume.

The excitement stage is characterized by engorgement of erectile tissue in the genitals and a buildup of muscle tension throughout the body. The brain processes sensory and motor stimuli as being sexual in nature and passes a message to the hypothalamus, which initiates the nerve and hormonal sexual response.

Many cardiovascular changes are set into motion during excitement. The heart rate increases, and blood vessels throughout the body constrict, raising blood pressure. Blood vessels in the genitals dilate, resulting in increased blood flow to the genitalia. The increased blood flow fills up the spongy tissue that

High-level cardiorespiratory fitness can enhance vasocongestion.

Vasocongestion The movement of blood flow into the genitals resulting in a variety of responses including erection in men and lubrication in women

makes up this region. Blood flow into the genitals is greater than outflow. As this tissue fills with blood, it becomes engorged, enlarging in size, deepening in color, and increasing in sensitivity. Masters and Johnson called this engorgement process **vasocongestion.** In men, the major changes associated with vasocongestion are erection of the penis and deepening of the color of the genitalia. In women, vasocongestion is responsible for labial swelling, deepening of the color of the vulva, vaginal lubrication, and increased size and sensitivity of the breasts.

Physical Wellness

Physical wellness contributes directly to healthy sexual response. When we are physically fit, our bodies respond and perform better sexually. High-level cardiorespiratory endurance can facilitate maximum blood flow and staying power. Vasocongestion hinges on efficient blood flow through the blood vessels to the genitals. Atherosclerosis, the narrowing and hardening of blood vessels, can inhibit maximum blood flow. Smoking also can speed up atherosclerosis and lead to constriction of blood flow. This affects overall health and also sexual response. Increasing the overall level of fitness (particularly, cardiorespiratory fitness and flexibility), improving the diet (minimizing fats and cholesterol), limiting use of alcohol and other illicit drugs, and maximizing body composition can increase overall physical well-being and improve sexual response.

Although being fit doesn't ensure good sex, it can enhance the physiological (body strength and endurance, increased blood flow, and the like) and psychological (higher self-esteem, positive outlook, enhanced body image) components of good sex. Conversely, having a disability or illness or being unfit doesn't necessarily preclude sexual satisfaction. People with disabilities and chronic illnesses that impact their sexual response can learn to maximize their sexual potentials and abilities, whatever they are. People who do not have the highest levels of fitness still can have good sex as they work their way toward becoming fit.

Transudation The production of vaginal lubrication because of sweating of vaginal tissue engorged with blood during vasocongestion

Myotonia Involuntary skeletal muscle contractions

Electromyographic Refers to measurement of muscle tension through electrical sensors at skin surface

Prior to Masters and Johnson's research, sex researchers believed that vaginal lubrication was caused by sweat and oil glands within the vagina. Masters and Johnson discovered, and documented through special intravaginal photography, that lubrication is a by-product of vasocongestion. Vaginal mucosal tissue becomes engorged with blood and produces a clear, slippery fluid that empties from the cells directly into the vagina. They called this process **transudation** and discovered that it was directly linked to the level of sexual excitement. Masters and Johnson found that insufficient lubrication is often the result of too little foreplay and low levels of excitement or anxiety.

The second characteristic associated with excitement is **myotonia,** the gradual heightened tension in the skeletal muscles throughout the body. Unlike the muscle tension associated with stress, myotonia is a gradual buildup that is progressive and pleasurable. Employing specially developed instruments and methods, Masters and Johnson were able to quantify the level of muscle tension in various parts of the body during sexual arousal. This was done by placing electrodes on strategic parts of the body to measure **electromyographic** activity during sexual arousal.

During excitement in men, the testes elevate, moving closer to the body. In women, the inner two-thirds of the vagina expand, and the uterus is pulled backward.

Plateau   In the second phase of Masters and Johnson's sexual response cycle, called the *plateau*, processes set into motion during the excitement phase reach their maximum levels. Vasocongestion creates peak levels of engorgement, color changes, and lubrication, and muscular tension also reaches its maximum level.

In men, the testes become fully elevated, and the prostate gland enlarges. The Cowper's gland releases clear, slippery, preejaculatory fluid (we will discuss the sperm-carrying capability of this fluid in Chapter 14). In women, the labia reach their maximum size, the vagina forms the "orgasmic platform," and the clitoris retracts under its protective hood. Both men and women experience a "sex flush," a rashlike reddish tinge to the skin of the chest and back associated with dilation of the blood vessels and increased blood flow in these areas.

Masters and Johnson found that the plateau was the most variable stage in terms of time. More experienced couples, for instance, were able to prolong the plateau if they desired, whereas younger, less sexually experienced subjects had much shorter plateau periods.

healthy sex hints 7.1
Effects of Aphrodisiacs

People are always searching for a magic potion that will enhance their sexual response and enable them to respond quicker, last longer, and become rearoused quicker. This has enabled a multimillion-dollar aphrodisiac market to flourish. Certain foods, nutrients, and other aphrodisiacs are promoted as aids to sexual response. But do they work? The answer is yes and no.

Although no true aphrodisiac (a potion that increases desire and performance) exists, if you think it's helping, it probably is, as is the case with any placebo. Because the mind and the body work together in initiating and perpetuating sexual response, it makes sense that if a person perceives that a substance will help promote sexual response, it just might.

Physiologically, however, the effects of aphrodisiacs are mixed. In general, they can be categorized by the way they work: provide energy, increase blood flow to the genitals, decrease the sensitivity of genital tissue, and increase desire in the brain.

Various "pep pills" are promoted as increasing energy levels. These are featured in fitness and "muscle" magazines and claim to enhance sexual desire by increasing overall energy levels. Though we believe that sexual desire is enhanced through high-level well-being, we think this should emanate from a healthy lifestyle, not a "pep pill."

Other aphrodisiacs, in the form of salves and creams, claim to work by enhancing vasocongestion (firmer erections, more responsiveness)—sending more blood to the genital area. In reality, vasocongestion is a result of dilation and constriction of blood vessels and changes in blood pressure, not extra surface blood in the smaller capillaries.

Still other aphrodisiacs claim to work by decreasing sensitivity, which hypothetically allows men to "last longer." These topical creams and ointments often inflame sensitive genital tissue, creating painful irritation. Using a condom to cover the head of the penis is a better way to decrease sensitivity.

Psychoactive drugs and alcohol work by altering perception. Alcohol deadens the parts of the brain that control conscious thought. This can reduce negative thoughts and feelings that might inhibit sexual response. Other drugs, such as marijuana, heighten sensations such as touch and smell. Enhancing the ability to perceive sensations can heighten enjoyment of sexual activity and promote sexual response.

Viagra, a treatment recommended for men (and under study in women) with erectile disorders associated with impaired genital blood flow, has also been touted as an aphrodisiac. Although Viagra is very effective in enhancing blood flow in people with this problem, its utility in enhancing sexual response in men and women with adequate blood flow is questionable.

The best "aphrodisiacs," in our opinion, are summarized as the following:

Become physically fit.
Develop healthy eating habits.
Reduce stress through relaxation techniques and behavior
   management.

Orgasm   The third phase of Masters and Johnson's response cycle, orgasm, is characterized by the dramatic release of tension and other physiological processes (heart rate, blood pressure, increased breathing, and so on) associated with the excitement and plateau stages. During orgasm, most of the male and female sexual structures undergo rhythmic, muscular contractions. These are responsible for the release of pent-up muscular tension in men and women and ejaculation in men.

Masters and Johnson found that women have a one-step orgasm, whereas it is a two-step process in men. The first step in men is called **ejaculatory inevitability.** During this step, men sense the release of tension and feel the inevitability of ejaculation. During the next step, **emission** contractions of the vas deferens and other structures move sperm and other ejaculatory fluids through the vas deferens and out of the urethra. Masters and Johnson found that women did not ejaculate during orgasm.

Prior to Masters and Johnson, researchers studying sexual response used much more subjective criteria for determining whether an orgasm had or had not occurred. Masters and Johnson quantified the muscular contractions, fluid expulsions (in men only), and physiological reversals associated with the release of tension as a result of orgasm.

Resolution   The last phase of the sexual response cycle is resolution, return of the body to the unaroused state. Masters and Johnson found that after orgasm, the two key physiological processes—vasocongestion and myotonia—reverse. Orgasm triggers the brain to normalize the dilation of blood vessels, heart rate, and blood pressure, allowing blood flow to return to normal and vasocongestion to reverse. With this reversal, the erection begins to shrink, lubrication ceases, and color changes disappear. In addition, the buildup of muscular tension followed by contractions stops, and muscle tissue returns to normal.

Masters and Johnson (1966) coined the term **refractory period** to describe the time required after an orgasm before a person could enter the excitement stage again. They found tremendous variability in this time between men and women, and among individual men. They found that women did not have a refractory period. Women did not need recovery time to get excited again and reach orgasm.

Vasocongestion and lubrication could remain at optimal levels if the source and intensity of stimulation and interest in maintaining activity with the partner were to continue. The significance of this finding was that it proved that women could have multiple orgasms without a refractory period. This is both a difference between men's and women's sexual response patterns and a significant finding in terms of women's ability to extend and enjoy sexual relations if they desire. For most women in Masters and Johnson's study, however, sexual stimulation ceased after their partner's orgasm. Often, this is because of preset agendas that couples have about trying to achieve orgasm simultaneously or a "me first, then you" pattern in achieving orgasm. In follow-up studies, Masters and Johnson (1976) found that most male partners did not realize that they could continue to stimulate their partners (if desired, through pubic contact or manual/oral stimulation), even if they were to lose their erection.

Unlike women, men need a certain amount of downtime before they can achieve another erection. The amount of time varies significantly. Among the variables related to the amount of time needed to obtain another erection, the most significant were age and time since last orgasm. In general, the younger the man, the shorter the refractory period. The longer the duration since the last orgasm, the shorter the refractory period. Thus, a younger man who hadn't had an orgasm in some time would become rearoused much more quickly than an older man who recently had an orgasm. Other variables, such as overall level of health, stress, and obesity, were also found to be related to the length of refractory period.

Ejaculatory inevitability The first step in male ejaculation; beginning of smooth-muscle contractions that trigger release of ejaculate

Emission The release of secretions from various organs and glands that produce male ejaculate

Refractory period The time from last orgasm to the next beginning of excitement

sex in society 7.3

Tantric Sex

For most Americans, orgasm is the whole point of sexual activities. As a culture, we're obsessed with orgasm. We keep track of orgasms like box scores for baseball: number of at-bats (sexual encounters), number of hits (orgasms), and whether they are singles (OK), doubles (slightly better orgasms), triples (really good orgasms), and home runs (really, really, great orgasms). We are not only obsessed with our own orgasms, but we also want to know about our partner's orgasms. "Was it good for you?" we ask. Our ultimate criterion is to achieve simultaneous orgasm with our partner—the ultimate: two home runs at the same time! None of these scoring measures correlates perfectly with sexual satisfaction or healthy sexuality. Frequency, intensity, and mutuality of orgasms vary in their relationship to sexual satisfaction for people.

One can even enjoy sex without orgasm. The idea of having intercourse but intentionally not having an orgasm may seem strange, but that's exactly the point of Tantric sex: an Indian sexual/spiritual practice based on *conserving orgasm*. The origins of Tantra can be traced back over 20,000 years to markings on cave walls that resemble those still in use today in Tantric training. Tantra, originally associated with fertility worship and paganism, is based on the belief that life itself is the result of sex and love.

Sacred temples decorated with the sexual positions of the Kama Sutra were built to provide places of worship for the Tantric religion in India starting in 800 A.D. Indian spiritual leaders taught their disciples about the spiritual power of sexual energy. They believed the energy that emanates from sexual arousal can be shared with one's partner and used to transcend the couple's sexual union to bring them closer to spiritual oneness with a higher power. Tantric sex is part of the spiritual form of yoga. The spiritual form of yoga is practiced to achieve a transcendent state of being (see www.tantric.com).

In the West, the practice of Tantra borrows liberally from Hinduism, Taoism, Buddhism, Native American spirituality, and Wiccan. Disciples view Tantric sex as a spiritual activity that unites partners in transcendence and also as a technique to enhance sexual intensity. Couples focus on sexual pleasuring, not the outcome of orgasm. This deemphasis on orgasm allows couples to relax and enjoy the sensations without being so goal directed. Some organizations run Tantric sex training programs and retreats.

Figures 7.6 and 7.7 show the patterns in sexual response that Masters and Johnson discovered for the men and women in their study. Figure 7.7, their classic cycle for men, shows a steady buildup in excitement followed by a moderate level of plateau. The level of stimulation in the plateau stage reaches its zenith with orgasm. This is followed by the cessation of stimulation and a rapid drop-off into resolution.

Figure 7.6 diagrams multiple orgasms in women. The pattern is similar to that in men (Figure 7.7) except that following orgasm, stimulation continues and the woman is able to achieve multiple orgasms before entering the resolution phase.

Pattern B in Figure 7.6 shows what happens when the level or type of stimulation is insufficient to trigger orgasm. Excitement builds with the stimulation, and plateau is achieved. The level or type of stimulation, however, lacks the intensity (or stops before it can build to high enough levels) to trigger orgasm, which is responsible for reversing the effects of vasocongestion. This results in a protracted resolution stage until the pelvic area and genitals return to their unaroused levels. This phenomenon in men has been called "blue balls." Although no equivalent slang term applies to women, females experience similar effects: pelvic congestion, swollen genitalia, throbbing pelvic area, and so on.

Although Masters and Johnson's findings added valuable information about the objective experience of sexual response, the analysis is physiological and is

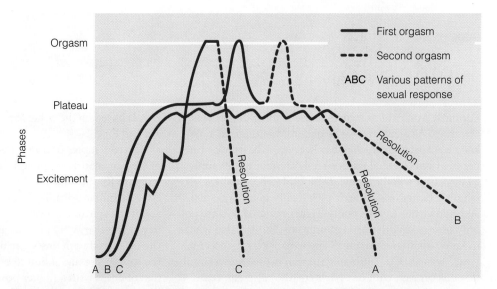

Figure 7.6 *Masters and Johnson's Sexual Response Patterns in Women* Masters and Johnson found three major sexual response patterns in women.

Source: Human Sexual Response by W. Masters and V. Johnson (New York: HarperCollins, 1966).

open to a more subjective interpretation. For instance, even though an orgasm, according to Masters and Johnson, is characterized by a certain number of muscular contractions at a certain intensity and other physiological parameters, a person could have an enjoyable sexual experience without having an official Masters and Johnson orgasm.

What operationalizing a concept such as orgasm does is to allow us to study it more rigorously. For instance, if researchers want to study the effects of alcohol on orgasm, their research will be easier and more accurate if they are able to operationally define orgasm. The same kind of rigor need not enter into our human relations.

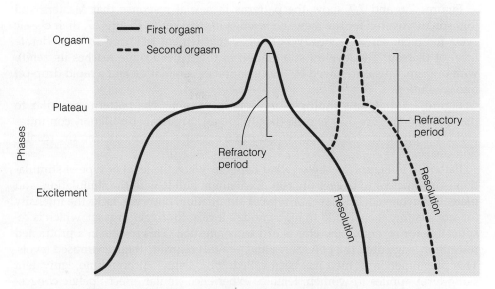

Figure 7.7 *Masters and Johnson's Sexual Response Patterns in Men* Masters and Johnson found one primary sexual response pattern in men.

Source: Human Sexual Response by W. Masters and V. Johnson (New York: HarperCollins, 1966).

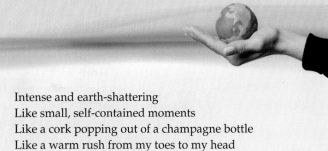

sex in society 7.4

Defining Orgasm

People have described some ways an orgasm feels like.

Like a mild explosion
Like I was soaring in the sky
Throbbing
Like an avalanche
Like pulsating bursts of energy
Like a dive into a pool
Exhilarating

Intense and earth-shattering
Like small, self-contained moments
Like a cork popping out of a champagne bottle
Like a warm rush from my toes to my head

What does an orgasm feel like to you? Can you have "good sex" without achieving orgasm?

Kaplan's Triphasic Model of Sexual Response

Helen Singer Kaplan (1974) disagreed with Masters and Johnson's four-phase sexual response cycle. She argued that the model neglects the importance of sexual desire in human sexual response. Furthermore, she agreed with others in the field who claimed that the plateau stage is really indistinguishable from excitement and that the two stages would more appropriately be merged together.

Kaplan's original model had two stages: excitement and orgasm. She modified it, however, after her work with dysfunctional individuals and couples revealed that many of them had problems with low levels of interest in sex. She then proposed a triphasic model of sexual response that included the phases of desire, excitement, and orgasm (Kaplan, 1985). She placed most of the emphasis on desire and the role of the brain in initiating sexual response.

Desire During the desire phase, some activating thought, emotion, fantasy, or sensation arises in the cortex or limbic system and triggers the activation of neural and hormonal sexual stimulation. The emphasis here is on the key role the cerebral cortex plays in initiating sexual response, and the subjective, emotional nature of arousal. As we mentioned at the beginning of this chapter, the brain is the sexiest organ in the body and plays the key role in determining whether the sexual response continues.

Excitement Kaplan accepted Masters and Johnson's findings concerning the physiology of sexual arousal. She agreed that vasocongestion is the key physiological process involved in *excitement*. She disagreed, however, with the idea of separating the plateau from excitement. She argued that the plateau is really nothing more than end-stage excitement or culmination of the excitement phase. When excitement peaks, the person reaches the plateau, or level of maximum arousal. As such, however, to clinically distinguish plateau from excitement is next to impossible, and, therefore, the two phases should be merged.

Orgasm Once again, Kaplan accepted Masters and Johnson's findings concerning the physiology of orgasm. She also described *orgasm* as the one phase that is clearly distinguishable for most people. Unlike the transition from desire to excitement, which is hard to pinpoint, the onset of orgasm is an event most people readily identify.

Criticisms of Kaplan's and Masters and Johnson's Models

Although Kaplan's model of sexual response is important because it expands Masters and Johnson's conceptualization by adding the dimension of desire to the cycle, it still left gaps in fully understanding the nature of sexual response in men and women.

Lieblum (2000), a renowned sex therapist and educator, notes how Kaplan's model doesn't always match up to women's experiences of sexual response. Lieblum describes how many women do not have spontaneous feelings of sexual desire and for those who do, it doesn't always lead to arousal. She found that most women rely on their male partners to initiate sexual activity, and they may or may not participate depending on a host of sexual and nonsexual factors such as intimacy.

Lieblum adds that for many women *and* men, arousal comes *before* desire. A man's morning erection may trigger feelings of desire and interest in initiating intercourse with a partner. The feeling of pleasurable genital sensations or touch may ignite feelings of desire in women. In other words, the order of the response is reversed from what Kaplan found.

Lastly, Lieblum (2000) found that Kaplan's and Masters and Johnson's models do not take subjective feelings of sexual satisfaction into account. A purely physiological explanation of sexual response is inadequate, according to Lieblum, because it doesn't attend to the subjective feelings of satisfaction or dissatisfaction which contribute greatly to future desire and arousal. For many women, satisfaction with sexual activity with their partner did not necessarily revolve around whether or not they had an orgasm (as it usually does with men).

Emotional Wellness

Good sexual response hinges on our emotional well-being. As Lieblum, Basson, and the other sexual response theorists in this chapter point out, our sexual response involves both physiological and psychological variables. We have to be in the right frame of mind for vasocongestion to happen. When we are nervous, angry, sad, worried, or in a number of other negative emotional states, we have trouble relaxing enough to allow our brain to trigger efficient vasocongestion. Even if we allow ourselves to become sexually excited, we may not be able to have an orgasm. The best sex is usually when we are able to let down our guard, free our mind, and relax. High-level emotional wellness allows us to do this. We are in control of our emotions; they don't control us. We feel good about ourselves and our partners, and we trust ourselves and our partners enough to relax and let the sexual response happen.

Walen and Roth's Model of Sexual Response

Walen and Roth (1987) have developed a cognitive model of human sexual response that emphasizes the importance of perception and cognitive factors in the initiation and perpetuation of sexual response. Although accepting much of Masters and Johnson's physiology of sexual arousal, they argue that a sexual stimulus is potentially erotic only until it is perceived as such. Something that is capable of turning on a person may not do so in all situations and under all circumstances. A person first must evaluate the stimulus positively. Walen and Roth's model, in short, explains that it is not just the sexual stimulus that creates the turn-on; our perception and acceptance of it are what allow our body to become sexually aroused.

Once arousal has begun, Walen and Roth accept Masters and Johnson's physiological explanation of the process of excitement. Once again, though, the role of

sex in society 7.6

Expanding Your Perception of Lovemaking and Orgasm

Sex is a goal-oriented activity for many people. It seems they view sex as a race, with both partners competing to see who crosses first with an orgasm. Even better, both partners cross at the same time and have the ultimate prize—mutual orgasms. The prize is the perfect orgasm, achieved together. The ultimate victory is the quest for perfect sex. Is this really the best sex? Is sex best viewed as a competition, a race? We like to think of sex as more of a multicourse gourmet meal. With each course the couple anticipates something special, a unique taste delight.

A before-dinner aperitif sets the mood for the evening and whets the appetite for the next course, appetizers. Appetizers delight the palate. They come in an infinite variety, each with its own special ability to please.

Next comes a soup, followed by a special salad. Each tickles the taste buds and is savored for its uniqueness. Between these courses we pause and have a refreshing sorbet to cleanse the palate. We stop and sit back, savoring the exquisite gastronomical delights we've already sampled, and we eagerly anticipate the rest of the meal to follow. We enjoy good conversation and admiring looks.

The entree comes next—not too much food, just enough to satisfy our cravings and delight our palate. We pause again to savor our meal before dessert is served. Dessert provides just a taste of sweetness to round off our meal.

Finally, we sit back, sipping our after-dinner brandy. This brings our meal to a close.

When we eat a meal such as this, who can argue that the entree is the only or most important part of the meal? Sometimes the entree isn't as special as the other parts of the meal, and we only sample it. We can view lovemaking as a feast, a multicourse meal that first involves the buildup of desire through kissing, hugging, massage, and noncoital foreplay. The lovemaking continues with a variety of techniques including oral sex, vaginal intercourse, and so on, extending the plateau as long as we desire. We pause frequently to talk, laugh, touch, have a drink, and the like. We continue into and through orgasm, and we finish by staying coupled and basking in each other's pleasure until we go limp.

If we envision sex as a feast for the senses rather than a race, perhaps we will enjoy our orgasms more when they occur and not feel as though we've missed something if we don't have them once in a while.

perception plays a part. In each of our brains is a stored bank of perceptions concerning sexual arousal. We expect and anticipate certain things to happen once we begin to get sexually aroused or engage in getting our partner aroused.

Walen and Roth propose that our perception of arousal plays into the continuation of our arousal and sexual response. Once things begin to heat up, we look for certain indicators to let us know whether everything is proceeding as planned. We ask ourselves questions ("Is my erection firm enough?" "Is my partner responding to my touch?" "Will I be able to keep this up?") to check out our expectations. If everything is proceeding as expected and planned, we can relax and our sexual response continues.

If we don't perceive arousal positively, our response can be short-circuited. Our brain can literally get in the way of our body. If negative thoughts and emotions such as fear, mistrust, or anger are part of our perception, they can short-circuit our sexual response or result in less enjoyment or lack of orgasm.

Perceptions are a problem especially when they create sexual expectations that are illogical or irrational. People who are too critical or who have too high expectations for performance can become spectators in their own sexual activity, literally sitting back and observing their (and their partner's) behavior rather than being fully involved. It's almost as if they step out of their body to critically examine what's going on. Ongoing critical evaluation can lead to unsatisfying perceptions of one's sexual response and begin to affect it adversely.

Zilbergeld and Ellison's Sexual Response Model

Zilbergeld and Ellison (1980) propose a five-phase sexual response cycle that also emphasizes the role of cognitive factors in sexual response. Like Kaplan, they separate the desire phase of sexual response from the excitement phase. They name their first phase *interest/desire* and, like Walen and Roth, stress the impact of the cognitive perception of potentially sexual stimuli. Once interest and desire are present, a person proceeds to the next phase, *arousal*, which is the initial stage of readiness for sexual activity. If aroused sufficiently, the individual proceeds to *physiological readiness*, characterized by lubrication in women and erection in men. Physiological readiness sets the stage for initiation of *sexual activity*. The next phase, *orgasm*, is similar to that of Masters and Johnson's cycle.

The last stage, *satisfaction*, is completely different from the other theories. Unlike the other stages (particularly, readiness and orgasm), satisfaction is entirely subjective. Good sex or satisfaction reflects the individual's personal level of enjoyment or fulfillment in the sexual encounter.

Spiritual Wellness

By definition, spirituality revolves around transcending ourselves and connecting with something greater than ourselves. Whether we believe our spirituality connects us with God, some higher power, or all other living things, transcendence of the self is the key to spirituality. We've often heard people describe orgasm in terms of feeling "uplifted," "out of this world," or "at one with the universe."

We believe the transcendence that orgasm offers is inherent in our sexual response and not totally reliant on our emotional connections to another. We also believe, however, that sex and orgasm with someone we love and are committed to gives a heightened level of spirituality. Sharing an intense orgasm with another person can, at times, make you feel instantly at one with the universe. If one positive human experience is capable of linking all of us together, it just might be orgasm. Humans and other animals seem to share the ability to respond sexually to one another. Sexual activity with a partner, by its nature, connects us to someone else in a unique way. A high level of spiritual wellness can help us form sexual relationships based on caring and mutual respect instead of exploitation and disrespect.

Stayton's Spiritual/Theological Model

William Stayton (2002), a Baptist minister, has an interesting spiritual/theological perspective on sexual response and pleasure. In 1965, in his early years as a minister, Stayton was asked by his church's youth group to develop an education program on sexuality. He admits to have been both excited and scared by the prospect. He was excited because he felt such information was needed and who better than the church to provide it to the congregation. He was afraid, however, because sex was very controversial, and he was not sure how his congregation would view his program.

His fears were assuaged when 60 young people, parental permission slips in hand, showed up for his first session. His program was such a success that the local school district asked him to develop a curriculum for the Glouchester, Massachusetts, board of education.

Stayton's basic premise is that it is not by coincidence that sexual response is undeniably pleasurable. The theological significance of sexual pleasure and response is that God created humans in such a way to respond to sexual pleasure. He cites Masters and Johnson's discovery of the clitoris as the center of sexual

case study 7.3

Steve and Tracy: What Good Sex Means to Us

Steve, 26, identifies as African American; Tracey, 23, is white.

Steve is a senior majoring in small business administration. He took some time off after high school and worked in construction before starting college. Tracy is an education major and a fifth-year senior, having worked her way full-time through college.

STEVE: Good sex to me is being able to relax with my partner. With Tracy, I don't have to worry about anything. I trust her.

TRACY: Yeah, that's it—trust. Before I met Steve, I went through a lot of one-night stands or real short relationships where I think the guys just wanted to get laid. I never felt I could trust any of them.

PROFESSOR: What do you mean by "trust them"?

TRACY: I guess I mean trust them about *anything*. Would they respect me and my wishes? Would they have my interests at heart or just their own? I also was worried about pregnancy and disease. Could I trust them to be disease-free, wear a condom, those sort of things? Oh, yeah, I also wanted to be able to trust that they'd respect my privacy. I didn't want them to go bragging to their friends about me or tell other people the most intimate aspects of my sex life.

STEVE: I feel the same way. I like to be able to let down my guard in order to enjoy sex. I guess you could say that, for me, it's sexy to be vulnerable with a woman. With Tracy, I can tell her about my desires, concerns, fears, and trust her to act in my best interests. I remember telling one woman I had sex with that I liked it when she played with my anus during sex but that I always worried that this might mean I was gay. I later found out she had told this to a sorority sister, and before long everyone in the house knew, as well as some members of the fraternity they were little sisters to.

PROFESSOR: How does trust affect your sexual response?

TRACY: For me, it allows me to let down my guard and relax. I trust Steve completely, and that allows my mind and body to relax. I've never been as responsive with anyone else as I am with Steve. I can get sexually aroused and have an orgasm with very little effort.

STEVE: I feel the same way. With Tracy, I feel so relaxed that things just naturally happen. I remember with other women worrying that I might not perform up to their standards, and that made it real difficult to get excited and erect. I know I can please Tracy, and even if I have an off-night, she'll understand and not use it against me.

TRACY: I hope I don't make it seem that because I'm so relaxed, there's no spark or sexual tension between Steve and me. Nothing can be farther from the truth. Even though I'm completely relaxed in bed with him, I can get aroused just thinking about sex with him. I hope this never changes.

Critical Thinking

What kinds of trust issues are important to you in your relationships with current or potential sex partners?

Use your Virtual Workbook to explore your answer to this question at **http://health.wadsworth.com/blonna1.**

response in women as evidence that God intended humans to be sexual creatures and enjoy this blessing. Why else would he make such an organ that has no other function except to provide sexual pleasure?

Stayton uses sexual research about sexual response as proof that God created humans with the ability to derive extreme pleasure from loving each other. In fact, Jesus' core teachings were about love. Stayton explains that Jesus, God's son, never, even in his teachings of self-denial, condemns sexual pleasure. Jesus' primary teachings revolved around love, not condemnation of pleasure. Stayton's "theology of sexual pleasure" is that love, spirituality, and sexuality are inextricably bound together and that God created people who are sexual in the fullest sense of the word. To be fully sexual in God's world is to be both physical and spiritual.

Love, Stayton believes, has both sexual and spiritual dimensions. Why would God create in us the ability to feel such intense sexual pleasure if it were not his intention to connect it to the pursuit of love? Doesn't "making love" have a strong spiritual component that transcends the act of sexual intercourse with the loved one? Aren't we truly at one with the universe when making love to another person?

Stayton believes that God intended sex researchers to continue his mission by guiding them to understand more about this gift he bestowed on us. Like theologians who interpret God's word through studying the Bible, sex researchers interpret God's gift of sexual pleasure by studying sexual response.

Lastly, Stayton believes that when people combine love, sex, and spirituality, God's intentions are born anew in the world. Sexual pleasure is not a hindrance to God's mission; it is part of it. He cites "creation" as something God did for humans but also as something God intended to create us to be able to derive sexual pleasure through our love for each other and to create new life.

Basson's Model

The newest sexual response model was developed by Rosemary Basson, a sex therapist, in 1999. Basson's (2000) model is both similar and different to those that preceded it and grew out of her work as a sex therapist. As we will see in Chapter 12, traditional diagnostic criteria for sexual dysfunction are based on the widely accepted sexual response phases of Masters and Johnson (arousal, and orgasm) and Kaplan's (desire) models. Basson does not believe that these models hold the key to treating women with sexual dysfunction. A new model of sexual response in women was needed that would serve as the basis for treating women's sexual dysfunction.

Basson does not take issue with the physiology of sexual response. She doesn't dispute the physiological processes involved in arousal, orgasm, and resolution. Her dispute is with the interplay of psychosocial and physiological factors during sexual arousal and the lumping of men's and women's sexual response patterns together. Basson also believes, like Walen and Roth (1987), that cognitive factors continually mediate the physiology of sexual response. Positive thoughts and feelings (trust, caring, happiness) about one's partner are necessary for intimacy to exist and sexual response to occur. Negative thoughts and feelings (anger, fear, unhappiness) can sabotage intimacy and make desire and arousal difficult, if not impossible.

Basson's model also revolves around the premise of gender-based differences in sexual response between men and women. Basson believes that emotional factors and intimacy issues are central to understanding sexual response in women. She feels that female sexual response doesn't begin with desire or arousal as it does in men; it begins with intimacy. Basson believes that for many women, the starting point for the sexual response cycle is not the desire for sex (physical sexual release) but the desire for intimacy (being close emotionally and physically with one's partner). The desire to initiate intimate contact could occur either for positive reasons or to avoid negative consequences. For instance, a woman could initiate an intimacy because she wants to hug and talk, to get close to her partner (positive reason). She might also initiate intimacy because she feels she has neglected her husband (or vice versa), and she doesn't want this to create any anger, resentment, or displeasure in her relationship with him. In either case, the primary motivation isn't a feel-

Alyssa: A Case of Fear and Mistrust

Alyssa, 20, white, identifies as lesbian.

Alyssa is a college junior. She recently broke up with Carla, her girlfriend of 2 years. She and Carla had been having sex for about 1.5 years. Alyssa has had little sexual desire and problems having an orgasm ever since she broke up with Carla about 3 months ago.

COUNSELOR: Tell me about what's been troubling you.

ALYSSA: I've been having a hard time having an orgasm lately when I have sex. I seem to be able to get excited, but something seems to keep me from being able to come.

COUNSELOR: Have you ever had this kind of problem before?

ALYSSA: No, I never had problems coming when I was going out with Carla.

COUNSELOR: When did you break up with Carla?

ALYSSA: About 3 months ago.

COUNSELOR: How many times have you had sex since then?

ALYSSA: I still masturbate about twice a week, but I've had sex only four or five times—once with a woman I met at a party and the other times with a gal from one of my classes. In each case, I didn't have sex on the first date, only after we went out a couple of times.

COUNSELOR: Do you achieve orgasm when you masturbate?

ALYSSA: Yes. Always.

COUNSELOR: Tell me about your feelings toward these two women.

ALYSSA: The first woman, Jill, is fun to be around. She's a real party gal, likes to dance, go to karaoke bars. . . . We have a good time together, but I worry about her past. I try to talk to her about her past sex life, but she kind of blows it off. It's hard to talk about this stuff. One of my girlfriends told me that she heard that Jill was bisexual and has had a lot of different sexual partners in her life. This worries me. I don't want to get AIDS.

COUNSELOR: What are you doing about this?

ALYSSA: I insisted that we practice safe sex until we got to know each other better. It basically worked. We didn't go down on each other and got off other ways, but I got the sense that she really wasn't into it. She's never said as much, but I could pick it up from her attitude. It didn't make for great sex. I kind of anticipated that it was going to be a problem, so it put a damper on things for me. I never really relaxed. I didn't come.

COUNSELOR: Tell me about the other woman.

ALYSSA: The other woman, Luz, is very nice. I know her from class last year, and she's in my psychology class this semester. She asked me out when she found out I broke up with Carla. She was very tender and understanding. She encouraged me to talk about Carla and get a lot of things out. We've had sex a few times, but I still haven't been able to come.

Luz has a real temper. I've seen her almost lose it a couple of times over silly things like getting cut off by another driver on the highway. She seems to respect me, but I worry about her going ballistic on me if I ever get on her bad side. I can't fully relax around her when we're in bed. I've heard of date rape, and I'm afraid if I ever refuse her because I'm not in the mood for sex, she might force me. Not a real good way to start a relationship, huh?

Critical Thinking

What are some of the kinds of issues you might face after the breakup of a former relationship that could impact your ability to enjoy sex in a new relationship? How does this differ if one is straight or gay?

Use your Virtual Workbook to explore your answers to these questions at **http:// health.wadsworth.com/ blonna1.**

ing of sexual tension and the desire for sexual release. It was a desire for intimacy. The woman herself may have no conscious feeling of need of sexual release (desire) to initiate an intimate connection with her partner. Once the intimate connection is made however, classic stimuli (internal and external) for sexual arousal are introduced. The woman's partner may tell her he finds her attractive, desirable, and the like (internal stimuli). They may hug, listen to music, or share a bath (external stimuli). Desire and arousal emerge from these elements of intimacy between them. In many cases, the woman makes a conscious decision to become aroused.

Another difference in Basson's theory is her belief that desire *follows* arousal and results in greater levels of arousal. Because the two are so closely related, it is often difficult to distinguish when one starts and the other ends. Basson believes that sexual response in this sense is more circular than linear. A woman doesn't move from intimacy to arousal and then to desire, and then to orgasm, and so forth. Intimacy leads to arousal, which sparks desire, which leads to greater feelings of intimacy, which leads to higher levels of arousal and therefore more desire. The cycle could end in orgasm, but it doesn't have to in order for the woman to feel satisfied and desire more intimacy. At every point in the cycle, cognitive factors (positive or negative) affect what is going on. Levels of desire, arousal, and satisfaction are always mediated by the subjective perception of cognitive factors such as trust, mistrust, fear, anger, and so on.

Another key difference is the reference to an end point of sexual response other than orgasm or resolution. Basson believes that a subjective end point relating to satisfaction is critical to understanding women's sexual response. Many women, she found, report enjoying a sexual encounter, even if it didn't end in orgasm. Men typically equate satisfaction with orgasm, but Basson found that for many women, that wasn't the case. Rather than equate "good" sexual response with achieving orgasm, Basson feels that sexual response should be evaluated on whether the person enjoyed the experience. In fact, attaining orgasm may not always be related to an enjoyable sexual encounter. Lieblum (2000) found that men and women can go through an entire sexual response cycle (including orgasm) while reporting that the encounter wasn't enjoyable. Consequently, Basson feels there should be some end point such as feelings of satisfaction, disappointment, frustration, and so on, that characterizes the cycle rather than just the presence of orgasm.

Disability and Sexual Response

Perhaps the most misunderstood aspect of persons with disabilities is their sexual response. People with disabilities are often viewed by the nondisabled as either asexual or lacking in the ability to respond sexually and in the capacity for normal and satisfying relationships (Chance, 2002).

In fact, most people with disabilities are not asexual. They have both the desire and the ability to respond sexually, seek outlets for their desire, and seek to establish satisfying sexual relationships with others. As we have learned, there are a variety of ways to define sexual response. We will examine a few different types of disabilities to illustrate how the sexual response manifests itself for persons with these conditions.

Spinal Cord Injuries

The effects of spinal cord injury on sexual response is directly related to where the injury is located. In a spinal cord injury, neural functions above the lesion tend to remain intact. Functions dictated by areas below the injury change and often cease. The lower the injury, the greater the chance the person will be able to experience some type of sexual stimulation and response.

How Do You See Yourself?

How we feel about our bodies can either enhance or inhibit sexual response and pleasure. Our society places an incredible emphasis on looks, thus often leading us to have very unrealistic expectations about how we should look. The goal of this activity is to encourage you to take a realistic look at your body and accept who you are.

Take a full sheet of paper, and cover the entire page with a drawing of your body. You do not need to be an artist, but be as realistic as possible. Make your drawing a nude one of yourself. Once you have drawn your body, put an X over the parts of your body that you think need work and a star over the parts of your body that you like or that inspire pride. Once you have finished, your entire body should be clothed in X's or stars. Take a minute and write a short analysis of what has influenced your view of your body and how this view affects the way you respond in a romantic relationship, both physically and psychologically. Conclude by making a contract with yourself to work on the parts that you are really willing to change or accept yourself as you are and like who you are. Lack of body acceptance has a very negative impact on our sexuality, so eliminate this by loving and accepting who you are.

Another variable related to how a spinal cord injury manifests itself in sexual response is when the injury occurred in the person's sexual life cycle. The older a person is when the injury occurs, the more they can draw on past sexual memories, associations, and behaviors. Being born with a spinal cord injury, having one occur during childhood, or becoming disabled in the prime of one's sexually active period all manifest themselves differently in the individual's sexual response.

Desire As we previously mentioned, there is no physical relationship between spinal cord injury and sexual desire. Alexander, Sipski, and Findley (1993) found that most men with spinal cord injuries return to sexual activities within 12 months of their injury. Although most of the subjects reported lowered sexual satisfaction postinjury, their level of sexual desire did not change significantly. A key factor influencing the subjects' sexual desire was the level of desire of their partners. The highest levels of sexual desire were correlated with high levels of partner sexual desire.

Arousal Spinal cord injury usually results in the inability of men to achieve erection through thoughts and emotions alone. "Reflex" erections occur in over 90 percent of men with spinal cord injury. These erections can be brought on through nonsexual functions such as catheter changes and having a full bladder or through direct stroking of the penis, particularly the glans and frenulum (Geiger, 1981). Although the erection is present, the man usually cannot feel it because of the absence of sensation below the spinal injury. Reflex erections are typically more difficult to maintain than tradition erections although penetration and intercourse can be achieved with the help of special rings and other devices that trap blood flow (Chance, 2002).

Sensations above the injury usually remain undisturbed. During arousal, sexual thoughts and feelings can initiate sexual excitement above the injury that manifests itself in all of the classic indicators: increased heart rate, respiration, blood pressure, and so forth.

Women with spinal cord injuries lose the ability to produce vaginal lubrication due to the lack of vasocongestion. This problem can be alleviated through the use of water-soluble vaginal lubricants.

sex in society 7.7

Redefining Orgasm

Researchers are always trying to "operationalize" the variables they study so they can minimize bias in their research. Because of this, terms such as *orgasm* have been qualified and quantified to such a degree as to include such components as the frequency and intensity of contractions of the anal sphincter muscles. This is of crucial importance when studying orgasm in the laboratory. It would be almost impossible to study the effects of an independent variable (such as alcohol use, sleep deprivation, hormone levels, and so forth) on orgasm without first operationalizing the term. In the real world, however, such precision doesn't exist and may not be necessary. Most people don't necessarily know or care about the frequency and duration of anal sphincter muscle contractions when experiencing what they would characterize as "orgasms."

This point is especially true in understanding sexual pleasure and the release of sexual tension in people with disabilities. Many disabled persons who are unable to have genitally based orgasm can experience a sense of building excitement and climax through (a) the stimulation of nongenital body parts, (b) the integration of these sensations with fantasy and memories of preinjury experiences, and (c) a sense of connection and excitement with their partners (Chance, 2002; Tepper 2001). Rather than exclude people with disabilities from the joy of sex and orgasm because they don't "measure up" to a nondisabled conceptualization of this experience, we need to embrace the diversity and richness of their experiences. By including them and inviting them to share their experiences and perceptions of sexual response and orgasm, nondisabled persons can get a better understanding of "human" sexual response.

As with men, sensations above the injury usually remain undisturbed among women with spinal cord injuries. In addition to increased heart rate, respiration, and blood pressure, women experience breast engorgement and nipple erection.

Sex flush occurs and pleasure is derived through sensations associated with stimulation of erogenous zones about the injury. Many report an intensification of pleasure associated with kissing, breast and nipple stimulation, and stimulation of the spine in the area of the injury (Chance, 2002).

Orgasm   The greatest variability in sexual response among those with spinal cord injuries is associated with orgasm. As we've discussed, orgasm traditionally is associated with ejaculation in men and a series of muscular contractions, changes in heart rate, respiration, and blood pressure in men and women. Ejaculation is a relatively rare occurrence in men with spinal cord injuries, as is contraction of the various muscles of the pelvic area.

As we've noted time and time again in this chapter, orgasm involves much more than genital contractions and the expulsion of body fluids. Orgasm is a very subjective experience involving the whole body and mind as well as one's relationship with one's partner. Many people with spinal cord injuries report a buildup of excitement and release of tension through climax despite not experiencing ejaculation or vaginal contractions.

Cerebral Palsy

Cerebral palsy is a motor function disorder caused by a permanent, nonprogressive brain defect present at birth or shortly thereafter. It manifests itself in a range of motor functions, including (a) seizures; (b) stiff, awkward movements; (c) spasmodic movements of facial muscles, hands, arms, and fingers; (d) abnormal breathing, sucking, and swallowing patterns; (e) slurred speech; and (f) hearing difficulties—to name a few of the major abnormalities (Anderson, 1994).

Although the effects of cerebral palsy present many challenges, the disorder has few direct effects on sexual response. Cerebral palsy has no direct physical affect on sexual desire in either men or women. Desire disorders associated with cerebral palsy usually originate in psychosocial issues involving the person with the disorder and his/her partner(s). Living with a person who has cerebral palsy can be a daunting challenge and place incredible nonsexual demands on partners. Additionally, engaging in sexual activity with a partner who has cerebral palsy requires special accommodations not normally present with partners who do not have the condition. These can place a strain on the relationship and tax communication skills to the limit. If these issues are not resolved, they can diminish the desire for sex in both the person with cerebral palsy as well as the partner.

Sexual arousal and excitement are also not directly affected by cerebral palsy. Vasocongestion can occur resulting in erection and vaginal lubrication. Behaviors associated with arousal ranging from holding hands, fondling, kissing, and talking are affected to some degree. Sexual behaviors can also be affected because some positions and activities may be difficult or impossible to consummate.

The ability to experience orgasm is generally not affected by cerebral palsy. The key mediating aspect regarding "traditional" genital orgasms is whether the person or his or her partner can sustain sufficient (duration and intensity) clitoral and penile stimulation to trigger orgasm. Once again, expanding the conceptualization of orgasm can help alleviate this issue. Persons with cerebral palsy and/or their partners might also find that mechanical devices such as vibrators and dildos can help moderate the duration and frequency of genital stimulation necessary to trigger orgasm (Sexual Health.com, 2003).

Environmental/Occupational Wellness

Feeling secure and being safe are essential to healthy sexuality. Our sexual response depends on a safe and comfortable environment. If we can't relax and feel safe and secure, we won't be able to relax enough to let the sexual response flow.

Have you ever been in a strange house as a guest and felt uncomfortable having sex? Think about being in a strange environment (your boyfriend's/girlfriend's fraternity/sorority house, a tent in a campground, a bed and breakfast with thin walls, your partner's parent's house) and how it feels to try to relax fully and let your sexual response flow. Even meeting potential sex partners requires a safe environment. Think about going out to a bar, club, or other public place and feeling that people there don't like you or want you around, or having to suppress your natural urges to hold hands, dance, or make out. This is what many gay and lesbian people face every day in trying to meet potential friends and lovers. This environment may also include the work site.

Your responses to the Personal Assessment, Thought Questions, and Test Yourself! quiz questions can be logged online in your Virtual Workbook at **http://health.wadsworth.com/blonna1.**

Personal Assessment

7.1 Things That Turn Me On

People become aroused in a variety of ways. Each of us has our own unique sights and sounds that get us in the mood. The purpose of this assessment is to help you take a personal inventory of your personal turn-ons and give you the opportunity to share them anonymously with your classmates.

Describe in detail the things that turn you on in the following categories:

Sights (visual images that are arousing to you):

Sounds (types of music, words, conversation that you find stimulating):

Tastes (food, drink, body fluids, or other tastes that are arousing):

Smells (perfume, cologne, body smells, other odors you find stimulating):

Touches (types, body parts, motions you find stimulating):

Thought Questions

1. How do the various regions of the brain process potentially arousing sexual stimuli and initiate sexual response?

2. How do the nervous system and the endocrine system work during sexual response?

3. What are some of the things that made Masters and Johnson pioneers in the field of sexual response?

4. What are *vasocongestion* and *myotonia*?

5. Compare and contrast the physiological changes in men and women during Masters and Johnson's sexual response cycle.

6. Compare Masters and Johnson's model of sexual response to the other models presented in this chapter.

7. Describe Basson's major criticisms of traditional theories of sexual response.

8. Evaluate the effectiveness of common "aphrodisiacs" on sexual response.

Test Yourself!

1. Sexual response begins and ends
   a. in the genitalia.
   b. in the brain.
   c. in the rectum.
   d. in the vasocongestive tissues.

2. Which best describes the role of the brain in controlling sexual response?
   a. It is central in triggering its onset but has little influence after that.
   b. It can shut down sexual response at any time.
   c. It cannot shut down sexual response without orgasm.
   d. It plays a limited role in sexual response.

3. Which statement best characterizes male and female sex hormones?
   a. They have completely opposite effects.
   b. They compliment each other.
   c. Men and women produce some of the same hormones.
   d. They act as antigens in the wrong body.

4. Testosterone is primarily associated with _____ in men and women.
   a. acne
   b. antisocial behavior
   c. sexual desire
   d. fertility

5. The role of estrogens in sexual response is mostly related to
   a. vaginal lubrication.
   b. rectal lubrication.
   c. vaginal vasocongestion.
   d. clitoral vasocongestion.

6. Which of the following is *not* a phase of the Masters and Johnson sexual response cycle?
   a. arousal
   b. plateau
   c. resolution
   d. erection

7. *Sex flush* refers to
   a. embarrassment felt over sexual desire.
   b. blood flow to the genitals during arousal.
   c. blood flow to the skin's surface during plateau.
   d. the feeling of swelling in the genitalia following arousal.

8. One of Basson's major criticisms of Masters and Johnson's sexual response cycle is
   a. men and women respond differently to sexual stimuli.
   b. men and women respond the same to sexual stimuli.
   c. most women don't respond to the same stimuli as men.
   d. most men don't respond to the same stimuli as women.

9. The main goal of Tantric sex is
   a. to meditate on orgasm.
   b. to speed up and intensify sexual response.
   c. to achieve simultaneous multiple orgasms.
   d. to deemphasize orgasm and focus on the union with your partner.

10. Walen and Roth's and Basson's models of sexual response add a cognitive component that relates to
    a. multiple orgasms.
    b. the resolution phase.
    c. arousal and sexual satisfaction.
    d. sexual abuse.

Media Menu

You can link to the following online tools by visiting
http://health.wadsworth.com/blonna1.

Animation

Female and Male Sexual Response Cycle
Female Breast Change in Sexual Response Cycle

 InfoTrac Activity

Thayton, W. R. (2002, April–May). A theology of sexual pleasure. *SIECUS Report, 39*(4), 27–32.

 Web Resources

Sinclair Intimacy Institute

www.sexualitydata.com

A database for information concerning sexual response and other areas of sexuality, written by the Sinclair Intimacy Institute staff. Provides answers to frequently asked questions through an up-to-date sexuality database with access to additional online resources.

The Church of Tantra

www.tantra.org

The home page for the Church of Tantra. It has, as its base, the belief that sexuality is a spiritual force and a pathway to direct spiritual experience. Sexuality "is the vehicle, not the destination."

The Sexual Health Network

www.sexualhealth.com

The Sexual Health Network is dedicated to providing easy access to sexuality information, education, mutual support, counseling, therapy, health care, products and other resources for people with disabilities, illness, or natural changes throughout the life cycle and those who love them or care for them.

The Masters and Johnson Institute

www.mastersandjohnson.com

Since 1957, Masters and Johnson have pioneered the field of human sexuality, in both research and treatment. In addition to relational and sex therapy, the Masters and Johnson Institute provides specialized treatment for sexual compulsivity, as well as trauma-based and dissociative disorders. Related professional training is conducted on a national basis throughout the year.

References

Alexander, C. J., Sipski, M. L., & Findley, T. W. (1993). Sexual activities, desire, and satisfaction in males pre– and post–spinal cord injuries. *Archives of Sexual Behavior, 22*(3), 217–219.

Anderson, K. N. (1994). *Mosby's medical, nursing, and allied health dictionary* (4th ed.). St. Louis: Mosby.

Bancroft, J. (2002, February). Biological factors in human sexuality. *Journal of Sex Research, 39*(1), 15–21.

Basson, R. (2000). The female sexual response: A different model. *Journal of Marital Therapy, 26*, 51–65.

Chance, R. S. (2002, Fall). To love and be loved: Sexuality and people with physical disabilities. *Journal of Psychology and Theology, 30*(3), 195–209.

Davis, S. R. (1998). The clinical use of androgens in female sexual disorders. *Journal of Sex and Marital Therapy, 24*, 153–163.

Geiger, R. C. (1981). Neurophysiology of sexual response in spinal cord injury. In D. G. Bullard & S. F. Knight (Eds.), *Sexuality and physical disability*. St. Louis: Mosby.

Kaplan, H. S. (1974). *The new sex therapy*. New York: Times Books.

Kaplan, H. S. (1985). *Comprehensive evaluation of disorders of sexual desire*. Washington, DC: American Psychiatric Press.

Ladas, A., Whipple, R., & Perry, T. (1982). *The G-spot*. New York: Holt, Rinehart, & Winston.

Lieblum, S. R. (2000, November). Redefining female sexual response. *Contemporary Obstetrics and Gynecology, 45*(11), 120–131.

Masters, W., & Johnson, V. (1966). *Human sexual response.* Boston: Little, Brown.

Masters, W., & Johnson, V. (1976). *The pleasure bond.* New York: Bantam.

Reagan, P. C. (1999, Spring). Hormonal correlates and causes of sexual desire: A review. *Canadian Journal of Human Sexuality, 8*(1), 1–29.

Sexual Health.com. (2003). Possible effects of cerebral palsy or CP on a person's sexuality [Online]. Available: www.sexualhealth.com/content/read.cfm?ID=6&theTopic=Disabilitypercent20orpercent20Illne. . . .

Stayton, W. R. (2002, April–May). A theology of sexual pleasure. *SIECUS Report, 30*(4), 27–30.

Tepper, M. (2001). Sexual healing with a disability [Online]. Available: http://www.sexualhealth.com/content/read.cfm?ID=90&theTopic=Disability percent20or percent20Ill. . . .

Traish, A. M., Kim, N. N., Munarriz, R., & Goldstein, I. (2002, October). Biochemical and physiological mechanisms of female genital sexual arousal. *Archives of Sexual Behavior, 31*(5), 393–400.

Walen, S. R., & Roth, D. (1987). A cognitive approach to sex therapy. In J. H. Geer & W. T. O'Donohue (Eds.), *Theories of human sexuality*. New York: Plenum.

Zilbergeld, B., & Ellison, C. (1980). Desire discrepancies and arousal problems in sex therapy. In S. Lieblum & L. A. Pervin, *Principles and practices of sex therapy*. New York: Guilford.

chapter *eight*

Sensuality *and* Sexual Behavior

Student Learning Objectives

After reading this chapter, students will be able to

- Compare and contrast sensuality and sexuality.
- Compare and contrast celibacy and abstinence.
- Describe a variety of nonpenetrative sexual behaviors.
- Know how to give a sensual massage.
- Evaluate the myths associated with masturbation.
- Compare and contrast a variety of positions for vaginal intercourse.
- Identify the factors associated with healthy anal sexual behavior.
- Describe a variety of oral sex behaviors.
- Explain the effects of spinal cord injury on sexual behavior.

Test your understanding of these objectives by taking the end-of-chapter quiz, available online at **http://health.wadsworth.com/blonna1.**

activity teaser: *Is your arousal boost an arousal block to your partner? Find the answer in the Personal Exploration Activity on page 246.*

case study 8.1

Delores: Sex in Pregnancy

Delores, 26, identifies as African American.

Delores is a 26-year-old nontraditional sophomore. She is married and the mother of a 6-month-old son, Greg. Delores describes her sexual experiences during her pregnancy.

Before I got pregnant, I was very concerned about the effects it would have on my sex life with my husband, Joe. We were married for 3 years and had a very satisfying sex life. I was worried about that changing. I've always liked sex, and I've kept in shape through running and lifting weights. I was concerned about gaining weight and my body changing shape. But I decided that I wouldn't limit my weight gain and make the baby suffer.

During the first trimester, my sex drive dropped a lot. I wasn't as horny as I normally was, and I had terrible morning sickness. Actually, I had morning, afternoon, and evening sickness and could hardly keep any food down. Other than that, though, nothing much changed. The frequency of sex dropped in half, but the kinds of things we did—positions—didn't change.

During the second trimester, my morning sickness disappeared, and I felt much better. I had put on some weight, but it really didn't affect our intercourse. I was concerned about bouncing around too much and things like rolling off the bed, but for the most part we didn't change our behaviors. The good news was that my sex drive returned to normal.

During the third trimester, things changed again. I had put on over 20 pounds and had a big belly. I was really concerned about deep penetration. I worried that it might hurt the baby, but my doctor reassured me that everything would be OK. I didn't have much energy, so we made love less often. We couldn't use any man- or woman-on-top positions. I've always liked the woman-on-top position with me sitting on my husband's lap, and I had to give that up, too.

I found that the only position we could use was the spoon [side-by-side] position. That allowed us to have full-body contact without putting pressure on my belly. It also allowed my husband to massage my breasts and belly. I had no desire for him to perform oral sex on me, but sometimes I liked to satisfy him that way, particularly on those days when I didn't have much energy. Overall, I think our sex life survived my pregnancy very well.

Critical Thinking

Pregnancy definitely imposes some unique challenges to our sexual desire and response. If you have never been pregnant, how do you think being pregnant will influence your sexual desire and response? If you have been pregnant before, how did it influence your sexual response and desire? Would you do anything differently regarding these issues the next time you are pregnant?

Use your Virtual Workbook to explore your answers to these questions at **http://health.wadsworth.com/blonna1.**

As Delores has shown us, one's sensuality and sexual behavior manifest themselves in many ways. In this chapter, we'll examine sensuality and how it is related to sexual behavior. We'll consider the full range of sexual behaviors, starting with celibacy.

Sensuality

As we discussed in Chapter 7, sexual response originates in our brain and senses, but what *is* sensuality? What makes a person sensual? Is it the richness and texture of her features (thick, long hair; distinct, angular nose; high cheekbones; long, exotic nails; tantalizing perfume/cologne; self-assured body language)? Is it his attitude (a deep thinker, caring/loving personality, down-to-earth simplicity)? Could it be her appreciation of life (enjoys great food, appreciates music, likes nature, enjoys physical activities)? We will answer these questions and provide hints on how to enhance and develop one's sensuality since it is the basis for all sexual response and behavior.

Although they are intimately related, sexuality and sensuality are different. **Sensuality** is the quality of being sensual, of experiencing life fully through all of the senses. **Sexuality,** you will remember, is a broad term that refers to all aspects of being sexual, encompassing a variety of biological, psychological, and cultural

Sensuality Experiencing things through all five senses

Sexuality Broad term that refers to all aspects of being sexual variables. Sensuality is a part of our sexuality. People who are very sensual have a heightened awareness of sight, sound, taste, touch, and smell. They use this increased awareness to experience life through all of these senses whenever possible. They approach each experience, every day, through this context or frame of reference. A walk in the woods or down a bustling city street is a symphony of sounds, colors, scents, tastes, and textures.

This increased sensitivity to and appreciation of all sensory stimuli carries over into their sexuality and lovemaking. The heightened awareness of all the senses enhances lovemaking. Sensual lovers delight in all aspects of their partners and their surroundings, making sex a feast for the senses. Sex isn't just a genital-driven quest for orgasm. It is a five-course gourmet meal that may include climax as the entree.

Developing Sensuality

William Burnham, a pioneering educational psychologist, believed that all humans are born as sensual creatures (Burnham, 1932). As newborns, we experience life through all of our senses. Burnham referred to this as being "fully integrated." Little separates our intellect and our senses.

A good example of this integration is how children play in the grass. Think about how toddlers play in the grass. They roll around in it, close their eyes, lie back in it, and listen to the sounds the wind makes as it blows through the high blades. They pull out handfuls of grass, throw them up in the air, and watch the blades fall to earth. They take a blade of grass and examine it carefully, rolling it around in their fingers, maybe even against their cheeks with their eyes closed. As they squeeze the grass between their fingers, they notice that oils are secreted. They smell this oil and taste it. Satiated with the grass, they move on to the next activity.

How many of us as adults take the time to get into the "grassiness" of life anymore? Have we lost our ability to revel in the "grassiness," or do we still have it but don't utilize it? We authors believe that we still have the ability to be fully integrated with the here and now of our lives but do not take advantage of it as often as we could. Along the course of our lives, most of us, for many reasons, stop experiencing life with all of our senses. We pay less and less attention to anything other than sight and sound (the primary senses we need to get through our work day). Of course we still occasionally remark about "how good something tastes" or how "nice something smells," but these observations are more often than not isolated and not part of our overall orientation to life.

What transforms the sensual child into a constrained adult? Why does this happen? Are we afraid of what others would think if they were to see us rolling in the grass at age 18 or 28 or 48 years? Or have we "been there, done that?" Are we too jaded to enjoy the simple, free, sensual delights that surround us?

We've asked our students these questions, and the results are very interesting. Often, students will just stare at us like we are crazy and then say, "Yeah, right, I can just see myself rolling around the grass like a baby, pulling up handfuls of grass." When pressed about what they would feel, they admit that such behavior would make them "feel weird" or "self-conscious." Many said, "What would other people think?" Many fear that such behavior could get them labeled by other people as "crazy" or at the very least "strange." Some even worry that a neighbor might think they are on drugs and call the police.

We asked them to think of other, less conspicuous scenarios such as sitting on the beach and playing with a handfull of sand (chosen because of the diversity of the size, colors, and textures of things found within it), watching a sunset, making bread from scratch, giving someone a shampoo, and listening to the wind blow through the trees on a brisk autumn day. In most cases the opposition to these activities was the same, but two other major issues were time and familiarity. "Who has the time?" and "Been there, done that" were often their refrains.

Often, it's not until we make the connection between their sensuality and their sexual pleasure that they begin to take the topic seriously. Losing the ability to be sensual can greatly affect our ability to experience sexual pleasure and experience eroticism through all of the senses. In many cases it can lead to dysfunction (in Chapter 12 we describe "sensate focus," a technique used by sex therapists to help dysfunctional people relearn how to be sensual). Our advice is to *make the time* now to enhance your sexuality and prevent dysfunction. By slowing down and integrating all of your senses into your daily experiences, you are setting the stage for doing the same thing in the boudoir.

healthy sex hints 8.1

Becoming a More Sensuous Person

Becoming more sensual starts with acknowledging the need to and giving yourself permission to *indulge* your senses. For some people this will involve unlearning some of the prohibitions and inhibitions you were raised with. It's OK to pamper yourself.

Sight: Enhance Visual Sensations

Most of us take our sight for granted and don't look at visual detail as something we can develop and expand. If something beautiful passes through our lives, we acknowledge it and move on. Try the following tips to develop and enhance the sights in your life.

1. Discover *flowers;* keep flowers on your desk, in your kitchen, and elsewhere in your home.
2. Immerse yourself in art (pictures, posters, photographs, drawings).
   - Paint/shoot/draw them yourself, buy art books, or cut works of art out of
   - Magazines.
   - Visit art galleries, museums, and online art sites (such as www.art.com).
   - Don't worry about what you don't know about art; focus on *what you like* and *surround yourself* with it (Marrone, 2002).
3. Take a good look at nature (sunsets, sunrises, natural beauty).
   - Star gaze.
   - Watch the sun rise and set.
   - Become an ardent cloud watcher.
   - Watch the waves crash, the tides move in and out, a local brook/stream tumble over rocks and cascade over cliffs (Eiseman, 1999).

4. Explore minienvironments.
   - Scoop a handful of sand where the water meets the shore, and spend 30 minutes examining it.
   - Take a close look at snowflakes, icicles, and frost on leaves.
   - Spend a half an hour exploring a tide pool (Eiseman, 1999).
5. Add color to your life.
   - Open your shades and let the sun shine in.
   - Drape colorful sun shades over your windows (pale orange will help trigger an endorphin release (Eiseman, 1999).

Touch: Enhance Tactile Stimulation

1. Try massage.
   - Take turns giving and receiving foot and hand massages.
   - Your feet contain over 7,000 nerve endings. Stimulating them sends pleasurable electrical impulses coursing throughout your body (Bender, 1999).
   - There are over 40,000 nerve endings in the palms waiting to be rubbed, scratched, and tickled (Kemp, 2000).
2. Knead dough.
   - Try making bread by hand and/or throwing pottery. Nothing beats these two nonsexual activities for developing an appreciation of touch.
   - Kneading dough or clay is one of life's most enjoyable tactile delights. It slows you down, stimulates the more than 40,000 nerve endings of the palms and hands, and is great practice for massage.

Types of Sexual Behavior

One way to present the many forms of sexual behavior is to place them on a continuum from celibacy to oral/anal sex. This presentation is useful in understanding safer sex options, as well as choices in fertility control.

Celibacy and Abstinence

Celibacy is defined as abstaining from sexual intercourse. Although the formal definition of celibacy refers specifically to abstaining from sexual intercourse and never marrying, many people assume that celibacy and abstinence mean total

Celibacy Abstaining from sexual intercourse

3. Give/receive shampoos.
   - There is nothing quite like having someone else wash your hair slowly and lovingly with warm water and lots of shampoo.
   - Practice on your pet. He or she will love you for it, and you will derive tactile joy from doing it.
   - Combine a long, gentle shampoo with a sensual bubble bath or shower. Take time to wash your partner with lots of soap, bubbles, and shampoo. Use a wash towel or sponge to add different textures to the experience.
4. Pet your pet.
   - Snuggling into the furry comfort of your pet's luxurious fur/hair is a sensual pleasure you both will enjoy.
   - Try to brush/comb your pet's coat at least once a week. It will slow you down and help you learn to relax and appreciate the luster of beautiful fur/hair.
5. Indulge yourself with different fabrics to wear.
   - Treat yourself to something that feels good: silk underwear; satin sheets; fleece scarves and mittens; a cashmere or angora sweater; a flannel nightshirt; leather pants, vest, or blazer. Soft, supple leather has always had a sexual appeal, as does soft, well-worn denim.
6. Be naked more.
   - Sleep naked, swim naked, run outside in the rain naked, sunbathe naked (of course, do this in places where you won't get arrested for indecency).
   - Start slowly. Sleep naked beneath clean satin, flannel, or Egyptian cotton sheets. Feel the sensations on your flesh.

Smell: Enhance Olfactory Delights

1. Use perfumes, colognes, soaps, and other scents.
   - Scientists have finally found the existence of pheromones in humans.
   - Perfumes, soaps, and other products that contain human pheromones switch on parts of the brain (hypothalamus) and increase feelings of well-being and self-confidence (Kraus, 2000; Brand, 2001).
   - Scents range from very light to heavy and from musky to fruity, to floral.
   - Goins (2001) suggests rubbing your partner's favorite scents on parts of your clothing, like your shirt collar, so he or she can smell it as you give him or her a good-bye/hello hug and kiss.
2. Light candles.
   - Use candles to set the mood (candles combine scents with color to heighten both visual and olfactory sensations).
   - Use candles in the bathroom when you take a bath.
   - Use them at night to serve as sensual night lights while you watch TV.
   - Use candles to add to the joys of a special meal.
   - Use seasonal candles to add the scents of the season to your day. For instance, pine candles have always been associated with the winter holidays (Bender, 1999).
3. Try sachet bags.
   - Use sachet bags of your favorite scent to liven your room, closet, office, or car.
   - Make your own sachet bags by using leftover pieces of cloth, cuttings from your favorite plants, pine needles, or flower petals.
4. Buy or pick flowers.
   - Flowers help develop and maintain your olfactory senses.
   - Flowers such as lilac can provide a gentle scent, while others, such as honeysuckle, can sometimes be too overpowering. Your local florist can help you identify flowers that meet your sensual demands.
5. Experience nature.
   - Walk or bicycle more. You'll be amazed at the different smells that surround you if you get out of that protective cocoon (your car).

avoidance of all forms of sexual release and the absence of sexual desire. Celibacy may or may not include masturbation and fantasy as forms of sexual release. Celibate people also have varying degrees of sexual desire. Not all celibate people lack sexual interest and desire, though; they merely choose to channel that energy and desire into different avenues of expression.

Celibacy is usually associated with a spiritual or religious sacrifice and is considered to be a lifelong commitment. Priests and nuns, for instance, declare a vow of celibacy so they may devote themselves fully to serving God and never marry. It is a conscious, willful diversion of sexual energy into nonsexual activity. Kathleen Norris (1996) uses the phrase "celibate passion" to describe how celibate monks are able to transform sexual energy into a sense of deep caring and love that she found to be unique among celibate people.

Not all people who choose celibacy, however, do so as part of a religious commitment. Actually, all of us choose to wait before we engage in intercourse. Many people choose celibacy because they are not ready to begin having intercourse, and they satisfy their sexual needs through other behaviors. We all develop at our own pace, and some of us are simply not ready as soon as others are.

We sometimes choose celibacy because we need time to recover or grieve from relationships that have ended. We need time to heal emotionally and are not interested in forming sexual relationships at the time. Others choose celibacy be-

healthy sex hints 8.1 (continued)

Taste: Sample Your World

1. Taste your partner.
   - Experience your partner with your mouth.
   - Experience all parts of his or her body.
   - Take a shower together and drink the water from his or her flesh. Lick the beaded water off your partner's nipples and body.
   - Experiment with oral sex.
   - Play with sensual eating.
   - Put together a sensual snack feast of fresh fruits, cheeses, and a bottle of wine.
   - Put it on a big platter with some crackers, and spend an hour eating it slowly in bed while you feed each other and toast your good fortune.
   - Some people like to play with things such as whipped cream or chocolate syrup in bed and lick these delights off each other (the authors have found this to create a sticky mess that can often put a damper on rather than heighten the sensual experience).
   - Try mixing tastes when you can. Moving from a tart to sweet or mild to potent taste sensation can awaken your taste buds.
   - Slow down and take smaller bites. Savor rather than devour your food, and enjoy the process of eating as well as the outcome.

Sound: Listen to the Environment

1. Make music a part of your day.
   - Music can relax you, help you forget your problems, reduce stress, recharge your batteries, and even turn you on.
   - Certain rhythms and beats mimic your body's natural tempo during sex.
   - Matching music (such as Caribbean or Latin) to the movements of your lovemaking can enhance the response (Goins, 2001).
2. Listen to nature.
   - Listen to the wind blow through the trees, the waves crash on the shore, the steam trickle through the rocks.
   - Walk in the woods; listen to the birds.
3. Become comfortable with silence.
   - Build "quiet time" into each day.
   - Allow your mind to unclutter by shutting out auditory stimuli for 20 minutes each day.
   - Listen to your partner's breathing (holding your partner or being united in intercourse and listening to his or her breathing can be both a sensual delight and a sexual turn-on).

In general, try to *slow down* and *pay attention* to the interplay of your five senses in whatever you are doing whenever you can. This will increase your awareness of how the senses work together and reinforce the importance of becoming more sensual.

case study 8.2

Susan: Choosing to Be Celibate

Susan, 31, divorced, identifies as bisexual.

I've been celibate for the past year and a half. I'm 31 years old, have a 5-year-old daughter, work full-time, and go to school full-time. Things just never worked out with my daughter's father, and ever since I've been back to school, I haven't had the energy to even think about sex. My schedule is crazy, and I don't have much free time. When I have time off, I prefer to spend it with my daughter. I don't have the time to spend on cultivating a relationship. I really want to finish school and get good enough grades to get into graduate school someday.

I don't miss intercourse. It's not that I don't like sex. Before I got married, I used to really get off on sex with both men and women. My sex life with my daughter's father was really great, and eventually I stopped having sex with anyone else but him and got pregnant. Things between us were never the same after that and since we split up, I've just been burned out on the idea of starting a new relationship. I masturbate a couple of times a week and prefer to deal with my sexual needs that way. I can see this changing someday and hope to meet a woman who can love and satisfy me and love my daughter. For now, though, I'm not looking for a relationship.

Critical Thinking

Think about your own life and periods where you have chosen voluntary celibacy. What were the circumstances surrounding your choice, and was it the right decision for you? If you have never chosen celibacy, describe a future situation where this strategy might work for you.

Use your Virtual Workbook to explore your answers to these questions at **http://health.wadsworth.com/blonna1.**

cause they do not have the time or energy to sustain a commitment (sexual or otherwise) with another person. They think they need all of their energy for school or work, especially if they are beginning a new career or starting school. They don't want to divert time and energy from these areas.

The generic definition of **abstinence** is self-restraint or self-denial. Sexual abstinence, therefore, refers to self-restraint or self-denial of sexual activities. Many people assume that abstinence means denial of all forms of sexual behavior. Actually, one can choose to abstain from unprotected intercourse but not other forms of sexual behavior.

Abstinence usually is not discussed as a lifelong spiritual or religious commitment. It is more situational; a person can abstain for a day, a week, a month, a semester, and so on. It doesn't have to be an all-or-nothing proposition. Most of us have voluntarily chosen to abstain from sexual intercourse at various times during our lives. Once abstinence is viewed as a situational choice and not a lifetime commitment, it becomes easier to accept and understand as a viable sexual option. We also believe that although abstinence is a valid option for people, it is not the only option.

Abstinence Self-restraint or self-denial, as in not engaging in sexual activity

Nonpenetrative Sexual Activity

Nonpenetrative sexual activities offer a wide variety of pleasurable behaviors that can be carried out to the point of orgasm and involve little risk of pregnancy or disease. This activity has been called "outercourse" and includes options ranging from kissing and hugging to using sex toys. To us, nonpenetrative sexual activity includes any sexual behaviors that do not involve genital-to-genital, mouth-to-genital, or insertive anal sexual contact.

Kissing is an almost universal form of sexual expression.

Thinkstock/GettyImages

Kissing

Kissing can provide intense sensual and sexual delight. The sucking, licking, rubbing, and tongue probing associated with kissing is pleasurable and carries no risk for pregnancy. Volumes have been written about kissing.

As we age, we seem to become more genitally focused and lose some of our interest in kissing. Kissing becomes an ancillary activity associated with the real objective—orgasm—rather than a satisfying activity in and of itself.

healthy sex hints 8.2

10 Good Reasons for Choosing Abstinence

Abstinence has gotten a bad rap over the years. It's almost politically incorrect to talk about abstaining from sexual intercourse (and penetrative sex, if you're gay or a lesbian). Here are 10 good reasons to choose abstinence:

1. To retain your virginity for someone special
2. To get to know your partner better (you want to become more comfortable with your partner and come to trust him or her)
3. To ascertain your partner's STD/HIV status (you'd rather wait to have intercourse but might consider safer-sex options)
4. To wait to be in the mood (you'd rather be doing something else)
5. If you're heterosexual, to avoid pregnancy if neither of you has contraception (you might consider a low-risk sexual outlet other than intercourse)

6. To find a suitable partner (sure, you've had offers, but no one turns you on)
7. To recuperate from an illness or surgery (you're not feeling very sexy or are feeling downright lousy)
8. To get a medical opinion on unusual genital symptoms (these might represent an STD)
9. To get some sleep (you're tired and need sleep, not sex)
10. To adhere to your personal moral code (regarding premarital, extramarital, and other sexual taboos that make up your personal code of ethics)

What other good reasons for abstaining from intercourse can you come up with?

sex in society 8.1

Variations on Kissing

We asked our students to talk about kissing—their likes, dislikes, the role it plays in their relationships. Here's what they had to say:

Marcia 19, single, freshman, identifies as Latina.

I love kissing. I especially like long, deep, French kissing with my boyfriend. I really enjoy deep tongue thrusting—you know, like when he tries to run his tongue all the way down my throat. What a turn-on.

Mary 18, single, freshman, identifies as Italian American.

I like gentle kissing. I like lighter pressure—soft pecks, nuzzles, gentle tongue probing. I hate it when a guy tries to ram his tongue down my throat. It's disgusting. Oh, and I hate hickeys. Why do some guys feel compelled to leave their mark on my neck? I never go out with a guy again if he tries to lay a hickey on me. How gross.

John, 20, single, junior, identifies as Asian American.

I like kissing. It's kind of like a game, tongues darting back and forth, in and out. There's almost a rhythm or method to kissing. I like to work my tongue around my girlfriend's whole mouth.

Sonja, 20, single, junior, identifies as African American.

I personally think French kissing is overrated. I prefer lip action. I like to nip and suck, just using my lips. I like it when my boyfriend nibbles on my lips and when we just use the tips of our tongues around our lips and the outer parts of our mouths. I find this kind of darting tongue action preferable to all of that deep tongue thrusting. That makes me gag.

Glen, 41, married, nontraditional senior, identifies as African American.

At this point in my life, I find that my wife and I are more gentle in our kissing. We still get into all the deep French kissing every once in a while, but most of our kissing is more affectionate than passionate. Don't get me wrong—our sex is great, and intercourse is usually pretty passionate. We just seem to kiss more as an expression of love and affection. Kissing during sex is less frequent than when we were in our 20s.

Hugging/Rubbing

Kissing is usually associated with hugging and rubbing. These activities, once commonly called *petting*, can take on new meaning if we can visualize them as viable forms of sexual expression. Hugging and rubbing, even with one's clothes on, can be intensely pleasurable and can be carried to the point of orgasm with no risk of pregnancy or disease. These activities also can serve as a prelude to other noninsertive forms of sexual activity such as masturbation and use of sex toys. A delightful way to use rubbing as a safe sexual release is to rub against your partner to the point of orgasm. Typically this is done with both partners fully clothed. You rub your penis or vulva against your partner's groin, leg, arm (or another convenient body part) to the point of orgasm.

You control the pressure, rhythm, and intensity. Although students sometimes call this "dry humping," it doesn't have to be either. You can enhance your enjoyment by doing it with your clothes off and adding oil or lotion to the equation. Try spreading lotion on your partner's breasts or chest. Take your clothes off, lie on your back, and let your partner rub your penis or vulva back and forth and up and down between her breasts or his chest until you come. Try spreading some lotion or oil on your partner's buttocks and small of his or her back. Straddle the backside and ride back and forth to the point of orgasm.

If this seems too messy, try rubbing your penis or vulva through your partner's hair and against his or her head and neck. You can use hugging and rubbing in many ways to enjoy a highly erotic sexual episode without fear of disease or pregnancy.

Massage

Nongenital massage is one of the greatest sensual delights you can share with your partner. Massage can be a stand-alone sensual activity or be part of activities culminating with orgasm. Sex therapists often prescribe nongenital massage for clients as a way to help them reestablish touching each other's bodies again. Massage allows us to explore every nook and cranny of our partner's bodies in a relaxed, sensual way.

Separating our sensuality from our sexuality is sometimes difficult when it comes to massage. The only time many of us touch others in such an intimate way is when we are being sexual. Massage is not an inherently sexual activity. It *is* sensual, though. Kneading, stroking, and manipulating another person's flesh require us to be in tune with the sensation of touch. We must be acutely aware of pressure and motion when we give a massage. Also, many of the massage oils available are scented and bring into play our sense of smell. Visually, the sight of exposed flesh has the potential for arousal.

The ability to enjoy giving and getting a massage and viewing these as sensual delights that don't have to lead to sexual activity may take time. Of course, giving a massage with the intent to arouse your partner sexually is a natural way to initiate erotic activities if that is the intention. Being able to give and receive sensual pleasure without sexual release is excellent training in becoming a compassionate lover.

Giving a massage is a natural behavior. Instinctively, we believe that if it feels good to us, it will feel good to the person we are massaging. Usually, giving a massage is easier if you use some form of lubricating oil. Some people prefer powder to reduce friction, and they like the sensation of powder. Most people, however, prefer oil. Oil should be warm or at room temperature. Cold oil on the skin can get the massage off to a bad start. The oil should sit at room temperature or be warmed in the container under hot water in the sink before starting. The oil should be poured into the hands and rubbed onto the body rather than squirted directly onto the person's skin (Good Arts, 2003).

Massage should be done with sufficient room to get completely around the person without having to lean on or jump over him or her. When straddling a person, you should not sit directly on him or her. You should be able to position yourself over the person so you can apply firm pressure during some strokes. A massage table or high bed is ideal because it allows you to stand while giving a massage. You also could kneel next to the person receiving the massage. It allows the person to lie comfortably with the face down, facilitating easy access to the neck, shoulders, and head. A professional table isn't necessary. You could place a pillow under the person's head for support and have him or her rest the head gently to the side.

Most important in giving a massage is to take your time. The other person will sense if you feel obligated to do this and are rushing through it. Giving a massage is an act of kindness and must be done slowly, lovingly, with no expectations for getting anything in return.

Several types of strokes can be used in giving a massage. All of them require maintaining contact with the partner as much as possible while moving from one body part and stroke to the next. The strokes should merge to form a sense of continuous motion with the muscles. A visual image of the muscular system may help (see Figure 8.1).

Triceps brachii

Pectoralis major

Serratus anterior

External oblique

Rectus abdominis

Adductor longus

Sartorius

Quadriceps femoris

Tibialis anterior

Biceps brachii

Deltoid

Trapezius

Latissimus dorsi

Gluteus maximus

Biceps femoris

Gastrocnemius

Figure 8.1 *Muscular System* Knowledge of the muscular system can help you when giving a massage.

Boost and Blocks to Arousal

There are so many differences in what each person finds sexually arousing and what blocks each person's arousal. Too often we don't even recognize what are our own boosts or turn-ons and our blocks or turn-offs to being aroused. Remember that arousal does not just happen as a prelude to sexual intercourse. Arousal can happen while we are walking across campus and notice a great body. The goal of this activity is to help you recognize what is sexually significant and important to you.

To identify your own personal boost and blocks to sexual arousal, keep a diary for 1 week where you list all the little things that sexually arouse you. Include not just physical but social and psychological factors that arouse you. (You can keep this in code if you don't want anyone to know what you are doing.) Notice all the little contributors such as reading an erotic passage in a novel, having someone you find attractive brush your hand, how you respond when you are being kissed, and so forth. When the week is finished, examine your list and star the ones that are the most effective in arousing you. These are the things you want to enhance in your sensual activities to increase your arousal. Next put an X by those that most effectively block your arousal, and try to eliminate these factors when possible. If you have a partner, you may want to share what you discovered about yourself and suggest he or she keep a diary for a week. Your partner can then share the findings with you. The two of you can use your list to enhance what is really important to both of you in your sensual life together.

The strokes should be rhythmic and symmetrical and will get better with practice. The whole hand should be used to master all of the strokes effectively. The fingers, palm, heel, and fist all come into play. The types of strokes are as follows (Inkeles & Austin, 1992):

1. *Kneading.* In kneading, you grasp the flesh with all four fingers of both hands and rotate your thumbs in opposite directions. Kneading works beautifully with the muscles of the arms, legs, hands, feet, back, and shoulders. You can practice kneading by making homemade bread and working on the dough.
2. *Pressing.* Pressing involves pushing against the body with the heel of the hand. For extra pressure, you can use your other hand to apply pressure against the heel of the hand involved in the pressing. Pressing can be used in long strokes or in a circular motion and is effective with thicker muscles such as those in the back.
3. *Stroking.* Stroking is done with the fingertips, either pushing away from you in circles or drawing toward you. Stroking also can employ all five fingers gently drawing flesh toward you. Stroking is good with the scalp, neck, and inner thighs and also works well as a long continuous motion along the back, torso, arms, and legs.
4. *Pulling.* Pulling is similar to stroking toward you except that it involves more pressure. Whereas stroking movements glide over the skin, pulling involves grabbing hold and gently tugging. You can pull with just your fingers, an entire hand, or both hands. Pulling is well suited for the head, hands, fingers, toes, feet, arms, and legs.
5. *Lifting.* In some cases, actually lifting a part of the body, such as the head, torso, or leg, and supporting it in your hands is relaxing. When lifting, the hands are cupped to cradle the part being elevated.
6. *Pounding.* Making a fist and gently pounding a body part can release accumulated tension. Pounding isn't for everyone or every body part. It is most effective on the back.

Anthony Saint James/GettyImages

Kneading the back is a classic massage technique.

Chrissy and Ken: Sensual Massage

Ken 23, is white; Chrissy, 22, is white.

Chrissy and Ken are single and in their senior year of college. They have been dating and having sex for 2 years and are planning to get engaged sometime before graduation in June. They have worked massage into their sexual lifestyle.

KEN: We got into massage as a way to relax and enjoy the sensual part of it. I didn't want Chrissy to think the only time she'd get a massage was when I wanted to have sex.

CHRISSY: We talk about what our needs are. If we want just a massage, we know this going into it, and that's what we do. If we're feeling sexy, we sometimes use massage to feel more sensual and get excited. We spend a lot of time massaging each other's erogenous zones.

KEN: I really get excited when Chrissy uses oil to massage my toes. I also love it when she uses long, slow strokes up my inner thighs and gently kneads the skin there.

CHRISSY: I really go wild when Ken uses small, circular strokes around my temples or kneads the base of my skull. I start to get wet when he spends a few minutes doing that.

Critical Thinking

How does your own background and upbringing affect your ability to give and receive sensual massages and derive the pleasure associated with this activity?

Use your Virtual Workbook to explore your answers to these questions at **http://health.wadsworth.com/blonna1.**

Masturbation

One of the first activities linking our sensuality to sexual behavior is **masturbation.** Masturbation usually evolves out of sensual exploration of our own body. We notice that it feels good when we unintentionally or intentionally rub (or rub up against) our genitals. In her book *Liberating Masturbation,* feminist writer, artist, and sex educator Betty Dodson (1996, p. 11) describes masturbation as "our primary sex life, our sexual base." According to Dodson, all other forms of sexual expression are a result of socialization. The expression of healthy sexual relationships between

Masturbation Individual or mutual stimulation of genitalia by hand or using other objects

healthy sex hints 8.3

Giving a Massage

You can give full-body or partial massages. Sometimes just a back massage or a foot massage will do the trick. At other times, a full-body massage, complete with scented candles, is preferred. When giving a full body massage, try these pointers:

- Start anywhere. Wherever you start, move in the direction toward the heart to facilitate venous blood flow.
- If you start with the feet, work up to the head, and finish at the hands. Or work in the reverse order.
- Or start at the abdomen, as it is the center of the body and, when stressed, is the place where blood pools.

- Cover the entire body in a systematic way. Finish a part thoroughly, then move on to the next. Don't jump around from feet to head to toes. Massage both hands/arms or feet/legs before moving to the next body part.

  After a massage, allow the person some quiet time to savor the results—and maybe even to reciprocate. Massage can be a prelude to other forms of sexual activity. In sensual massage, the focus shifts to providing more direct contact with the genitals and other erogenous zones.

individuals begins with self-exploration of sensual and sexual pleasure from the time of birth.

As described in Chapter 5, most of us learn the joy and security of cuddling, hugging, and warm, caring touch early in our lives, from contact with our parents and other caregivers. Although our earliest bonding experiences with our mother and father are not sexual in nature, they provide a sensual connection that leads to healthy sexuality.

Besides laying the foundation for developing trust and self-esteem, physical bonding with, and nurturing by, parents sets the stage for recognition and acceptance of our own body as a potential source of pleasure. Solitary sexual behavior, or masturbation, provides our first, and usually lifelong, source of sexual pleasure. Too many of us, however, associate masturbation with sinful, inappropriate behavior.

Masturbation can be a solitary sexual behavior or can be enjoyed with a partner. As a solitary behavior, masturbation may or may not be accompanied by sexual fantasy and other autoerotic activity. Couples can masturbate each other simultaneously, take turns pleasing each other, or masturbate themselves simultaneously.

Female Techniques   Masters and Johnson noted that women exhibit much greater variation in masturbatory behavior. Even when women had a similar style of stimulation, the tempo, timing, and approach to masturbation varied. The most common form of female masturbation is to stimulate the clitoris, labia, and mons by hand through stroking, pulling, or rubbing (Hite, 1976).

Most women prefer to masturbate while lying on the back. A smaller percentage chooses to sit or stand while stimulating the genitalia. Between 5 and 10 percent of women prefer to masturbate while lying on their stomach, either placing a hand between their legs to stimulate the clitoris or rubbing the vulva against a pillow or some other object (Hite, 1976). Figure 8.2 illustrates female masturbation.

Masters and Johnson reported the following patterns of masturbatory behavior in order of preference: (1) manually stimulating the vulva, (2) using a vibrator to stimulate the clitoris/vulva, (3) inserting something into the vagina, (4) rubbing up against an object, (5) pressing the thighs together, (6) using water massage, and (7) all other methods. About half of the younger women reported using sex toys (vibrators, dildos, or other devices) to

Figure 8.2 *Female Masturbation* Lying on the back and massaging the genitals with one hand is a common position for masturbation.

masturbate, choosing either to insert these or to use them to apply external vibration. A smaller percentage reports using these devices in a similar fashion to stimulate the anus during masturbation. The variety and complexity have increased markedly as more women (and their partners) express interest in these products.

Male Techniques In her study of male sexuality, Shere Hite (1981) reports the following male masturbatory techniques in order of preference: (1) stimulating the penis by hand, (2) lying down on the stomach rubbing against a bed, and (3) with water in the shower.

Few men choose to masturbate using sex toys such as vibrators, dildos, plastic sleeves, penile pumps, and inflatable dolls, although these devices are readily available. Though still relatively uncommon, proponents of these sex toys claim that they can enhance sexual pleasure, provide a change of pace from routine masturbatory practices, and add variety to safe-sex options.

Masters and Johnson found that many men masturbate by rubbing, stroking, or pumping the shaft of the penis with one hand (Masters, Johnson, & Kolodny, 1996). The tempo of movement usually builds gradually in response to the increase in arousal. Slow, deliberate touch gradually gives way to more forceful, rapid movements, often accompanied by increases in pressure and tension. A small percentage of men studied spend time stimulating the frenulum on the underside of the glans of the penis.

Uncircumcised men seem to spend more time stimulating the glans and frenulum through pulling the foreskin back and forth. Ejaculation varies more, some men preferring

Figure 8.3 *Male Masturbation*

to slow down and relax their grip and others desiring to increase pressure, squeezing out the last drops of semen. Figure 8.3 illustrates male masturbation.

Because the male penis is not lubricated, and masturbation usually involves a buildup of heat and friction, most men use some form of lubrication while masturbating. Body lotion and baby oil are two commonly used lubricants.

Health Aspects of Masturbation Early critics of masturbation posed pseudo-scientific charges that masturbation was neither "healthy" nor "normal." In fact, masturbation has no adverse health consequences. It does not cause any physical problems. It carries no risk for any physical or psychological illness. Most safe-sex educators encourage their students to masturbate to relieve sexual tension or to enjoy an orgasm whenever they want one. It is also an excellent way to learn what feels good and how their own body responds.

From a physiological perspective, a person cannot masturbate to excess. It is a self-limiting behavior; we ultimately lose our interest in it. As long as people follow basic hygienic precautions (clean hands, toys, and so on) and have adequate lubrication, they can masturbate as often as they want to. Rather than being a source of problems, masturbation is a healthy outlet for sexual desire, can reduce risk for sexually transmitted diseases in people who don't have safe sexual partners, and is an alternative to having sex with prostitutes or anonymous partners.

Intellectual and Emotional Wellness

Intellectual wellness provides the objective basis for understanding sexual behavior. It allows you to separate fact from fiction, truth from myth, science from theology. It empowers you to gain access to information and make informed choices that are free from dogma and outside pressures. Emotional wellness allows you to understand your emotions about the information without being overwhelmed by them. Perhaps nothing illustrates this interplay more than the topic of masturbation.

Centuries upon centuries of misinformation based on religious dogma, pseudo-science, and Puritanism have clouded the truth about masturbation and shrouded the topic in a veil of shame, guilt, and punishment. While the scientific "truth" about the behavior (it is a harmless outlet for sexual tension and a viable sexual behavior in itself) is well documented, the emotions it arouses often makes it difficult for people to deal with masturbation honestly and openly. People with high-level intellectual and emotional well-being about masturbation realize that it is a normal, healthy sexual behavior, and they try to work with their emotions regarding it rather than to suppress them or feel worse because of them. They talk about these issues with their partner(s) and seek help if they need it.

Patterns of Masturbatory Behavior   Masturbation is a form of autoerotic behavior. **Autoeroticism** is the dimension of the sex life defined by sexual desire or gratification, or both, experienced by a person without the direct participation of another (Lauman, Gagnon, Michael, & Michaels, 1994). Even though autoerotic activities lack a sex partner, sexual fantasies always include the imaginary presence of another person. In addition, autoerotic activity follows a specific social script appropriate to the individual, even if he or she never wishes to act out the fantasy.

Autoerotic activities differ from partnered activities because they do not require coordination with another person, can avoid many of the reality-based features of sex with a partner, and are limited only by the person's imagination. A surprising finding of Laumann et al. was the lack of imagination and repetitiveness of pornographic and fantasy themes. Table 8.1 describes women's top 10 favorite fantasy themes. These common themes permeate various autoerotic media (adult books and magazines, films, CD-ROMs, videos, telephone and computer sex) and behaviors (use of sex toys, vibrators, dildos). Table 8.2 illustrates the use of autoerotic materials by gender.

Table 8.1 Women's Top 10 Fantasies

1. Sex with current partner
2. Sex with another man
3. Sex with another woman
4. Sex in embarrassing places/situations
5. Receiving oral sex
6. Romantic sexual scenarios
7. Forced sex
8. Being found irresistable by a man
9. Working as a prostitute
10. Sex with a stranger

Source: Tracey Cox, *Hot Sex.* New York: Bantam, 1998. (Cox is a former associate editor with *Cosmopolitan* and a freelance writer.)

Table 8.2 Autoerotic Activity by Gender

	Distributions (%)	
	Men	Women
Thinking about sex		
More frequently	54	19
Less frequently		
Rarely or never	4	14
Autoerotic material		
X-rated movies or videos	23	11
Go to a club that has nude or seminude dancers	22	4
Sexually explicit books or magazines	16	4
Vibrators or dildos	2	2
Other sex toys	1	2
Sex phone numbers	1	0
Any of the above	41	16

Note: Rarely or never refers to "less than once a month" or "never"; less frequently refers to "a few times a month" to "a few times a week"; more frequently refers to "every day" or "several times a day." Fantasy is measured by the frequency with which the respondent reported thinking about sex.
Source: The Social Organization of Sexuality: Sexual Practices in the United States, by E. O. Laumann, J. H. Gagnon, R. T. Michael, and S. Michaels. © University of Chicago Press. Reprinted with permission.

Even though the content of sex fantasies is similar for men and women, the most important finding in this area by Laumann et al. is the great disparity in levels of autoerotic activity between men and women. Men are much more likely to engage in autoerotic activities and to associate masturbation with these activities. Laumann et al. attribute this to the continuing social context of masturbation among men. Masturbation is a socially acceptable concept among adolescent males and almost completely absent in the social context of adolescent females.

A final finding of Laumann et al. concerning autoerotic activity is the lack of association between autoerotic behavior and not having a primary sex partner. In fact, higher levels of autoerotic activity were associated with higher levels of partnered sexual activity. Rather than being a way to compensate for the lack of a sex partner, autoerotic activity seems to be a source of additional sexual pleasure. Laumann et al. found that individuals with higher levels of autoerotic activity were more likely than those with lower levels to engage in a broader range of sexual activities. In a sense, they have a much more elaborate set of sexual scripts. The development of sexual scripts or scenarios is influenced by a variety of sources of information, including autoerotic activities.

Autoeroticism is highly correlated with an increased incidence of techniques such as fellatio, cunnilingus, and anal intercourse (Lauman et al., 1994). Men and women who reported the highest levels of autoerotic behavior were more likely to engage in these behaviors than their peers who had lower levels of autoerotic activity.

Autoeroticism The dimension of the sex life defined by sexual desire and/or gratification experienced by a person without the direct participation of another

Social Wellness

The quality of social relationships plays a big part in sexual behavior. The foundation of social well-being is a solid relationship with your sex partner. This relationship is built on caring, trust, mutual respect, equality, and openness. Within this type of relationship, sexual communication and experimentation will flourish. It allows you and your partner to explore and understand your sexuality in a safe, caring, disease-free way.

sex in society 8.2

Masturbation: Student Reports

Although masturbation is a generally accepted form of sexual expression for our students, their feelings about it vary considerable. Some are completely accepting and open about their masturbatory behavior. Others still feel guilty masturbating and hide their behavior from their partners and friends. Here are a few reports from our students concerning masturbation:

Susan, 21, senior, is white and identifies as lesbian.

I masturbate a couple of times a month, usually when I'm stressed out. I used to feel a little guilty about it, but I've found I can deal with things a lot better if I can get rid of my tension. Usually my lover and I make love when we see each other on the weekend, but sometimes she's away on business and we miss a week. I'll usually go home and take a nice bath, relax, and make myself come. My parents were very strict when I was growing up, and masturbation was a definite no. I don't think they could imagine that I do it, and I guess that's why I still feel guilty about it.

Tom, 18, freshman, single, identifies as African American.

I would say I masturbate once or twice a week. I'm a little nervous masturbating in my room because I can't really relax, having a roommate. I'm never sure when he's going to walk in. When I go home on weekends, I enjoy it more because I can lock my door, look at my magazines, and "get off" in private. My parents have never said anything, but I think they know I do it.

Edwardo, 25, senior, engaged, identifies as Hispanic.

I masturbate about two times a week. Sometimes my fiancée and I will watch X-rated films and then masturbate each other. She'll do me, and then I do her. Other times, if either one of us isn't horny, we'll masturbate the other to orgasm. Sometimes we won't even have intercourse. We masturbate each other and finish off with oral sex. I never have had any inhibitions about masturbation. My parents always told me it was normal and OK as long as I keep it private. I don't view it as second best to intercourse, just different.

healthy sex hints 8.4

Safe Fantasy

Sexual fantasy serves several important functions. Fantasies help us expand our sexual scripts. They help us explore and expand our sexual repertoire. Sexual fantasies are a healthy sexual outlet. Coupled with masturbation, they provide a safe, exciting release of sexual tension. Sexual fantasy provides a "practice arena" to work through sexual scripts and encounters that we eventually may want to enact in real life. This safe practice carries none of the interpersonal or health risks of an actual encounter. Fantasies allow us to experience activities that turn us on but are not things we want to experience in real life. Fantasies do not necessarily represent what we really want in reality.

Sometimes, however, the lure of living out our sexual fantasies is strong. When is turning a fantasy into a reality a good idea? The following criteria may help you determine when you may appropriately cross that line:

1. The nature of the fantasy
2. The strength of the turn-on
3. The social context of the fantasy
4. The nature of your partner(s)
5. Your level of control over the specific situation
6. Whether the person is willing to lose the fantasy (sometimes living out a fantasy makes it lose its fantasy appeal)

The nature of the fantasy refers to how unusual, bizarre, or dangerous the fantasy is. The more bizarre or dangerous the fantasy, the more cautious you should be about want-

Sexual Intercourse

Many people think that being a good lover means being particularly adept at sexual intercourse. Actually, being a good lover means having certain skills (knowing how to arouse your partner, using various sexual behaviors, and so on), as well as having good psychosocial skills (knowing how to communicate, when to initiate, and the like). In this section, we will focus on a variety of intercourse positions.

Spiritual Wellness

A key component of spirituality is the sense of being connected with something beyond the self. In one sense, a person can't become more "interconnected" with another human being than through sexual intercourse. When our sexual relationships are based on respect, mutuality, and caring, our union with another person creates something that we cannot experience as individuals. In contrast, when our sexual relationships are based on exploitation, power, mistrust, fear, or other destructive intentions, we become disconnected from others, mere sexual mercenaries, out for ourselves only. Regardless of whether we are religious, we each have a moral code, a sense of right and wrong that can enhance our connectedness to others or destroy it. Those with high-level spirituality view their sexual relations with others with integrity and morality.

Vaginal Intercourse

Vaginal intercourse, also known as **coitus,** is one of the most common forms of heterosexual sexual activity, although sexual paraphernalia (strap-on or hand-held dildos and the like) allow lesbian women to penetrate their partner's vaginas if they desire. The three starting points for vaginal intercourse are face-to-face,

Coitus Vaginal intercourse

ing to turn it into a reality. If you can control for some of the other variables (items 3, 4, and 5) and safety, you might want to act it out. If you can't control these variables, you're probably better off leaving it as a fantasy.

The strength of the arousal exerts a powerful influence on whether to act out the fantasy. If a strong desire isn't there, you may not want to turn it into reality at this time. The social context of the fantasy refers to the setting in which the fantasy plays out. For example, many people are turned on by the fantasy of having sex in a public place. Public places range from semideserted beaches (where the likelihood of discovery is minimal) to the elevator at your favorite hotel (where the chance of discovery is high). Combining the risk of exposure with the consequences of being discovered (being arrested, losing your job or public stature, and the like) will help you evaluate the social context of acting out the fantasy. Some fantasies are based on giving up control. The turn-on with dominance and submission lies in being vulnerable and letting someone have control over you. Other fantasies are more

amenable to control. The greater the control, the safer is the fantasy. In general, the less control you have in the situation, the greater is your need to act out the fantasy with a trusting partner in a familiar, safe environment.

The last warning concerns losing the turn-on after you act it out. Some sexual experiences are better left as fantasies. They provide a strong turn-on that is satisfying. When you turn this into reality, however, you run the risk that the reality won't be as exciting as the fantasy. When this happens, the fantasy often loses its appeal and its ability to turn you on.

The nature of your partner(s) will help you evaluate the safety and confidentiality of acting out your fantasy. Asking your wife to tie you to the bedpost and then acting out a dominatrix scenario in the safety of your own bedroom is vastly different from going downtown to Mistress Helga's illegal place and allowing her to put manacles on you. Fantasies acted out with a well-known partner whom you can trust are much safer than those with strangers and prostitutes.

side-by-side, and rear entry. We call these starting points rather than positions because each starting point offers a limitless array of positions depending on how you place the rest of your body (arms, legs, torso, and so on).

Face-to-Face   Face-to-face positions have two variations: man on top and woman on top.

Woman on Top. The woman-on-top position, shown in Figures 8.4 (heterosexual couple) and 8.5 (lesbian couple), allows women greater control in the depth, pace, and motion of her partner's thrusting. It allows the woman on the top the greatest control in clitoral stimulation and is the easiest intercourse position for manual clitoral stimulation. Orgasm rates for heterosexual women are better for this position than any other. This position is also good for helping heterosexual male partners control premature ejaculation. The woman can get to this position in two ways: She can start with her partner on top and roll over into this position or start with her partner on his or her back and move on top. In the latter case, the partners must have enough room on the bed so they won't find themselves rolling off the bed and onto the floor.

When starting with the man on his back, the woman kneels over him with one knee on either side of his legs. Either partner can part the vaginal lips as the woman lowers herself onto the erect penis, guiding it in with a free hand.

Figure 8.4 *Woman on Top Sitting; Heterosexual Couple* This position allows for the partner on the bottom to use his hands to massage his partner's breasts and upper body.

Figure 8.5 *Woman on Top Lying; Lesbian Couple* Lying on top of one's partner while facing her allows both partners to kiss as they make love.

With the penis inside, the woman can rock or thrust her hips or move them in a circular fashion. The rocking and thrusting motions allow maximum penile penetration, whereas the circular grinding motion stimulates the clitoris more directly. Each of these three creates entirely different sensations.

Lesbians can use this position in a similar fashion with the aid of a strap-on dildo. The motions, activities, and benefits are the same as those for heterosexual couples. The partner on the bottom can be passive and allow the woman on top to control all movements or move with her, synchronizing motion with hers. The bottom partner can also initiate thrusting and grinding if the woman on top becomes tired or desires it.

In this position the woman also has more freedom to use her hands in ways similar to those of the man-on-top position. From this position she can caress and manipulate either her partner or herself. One option that the woman-on-top position offers is the ability to rotate her torso, while still being penetrated by her partner, so that her back is to her partner. In this position she can lean forward or sit back and achieve different depths of penetration and sensations. Her partner can fondle her buttocks and back while maintaining penetration.

An interesting variation of the woman-on-top position is to move from kneeling or lying on to actually sitting on her partner. By sitting on her partner, the woman-on-top position affords maximum penetration and intimacy as the couple can embrace, kiss, and talk.

Man on Top (Missionary). The man-on-top position, illustrated in Figure 8.6, is also known as the "missionary position." It is the most commonly used intercourse position in the United States. In this position, the partners stimulate each other until they are sufficiently aroused. The man then moves on top of the woman. Either partner spreads the female's vaginal lips and inserts the penis into the vagina. The man supports his weight on his elbows, hands, knees, or across his partner's entire body as his penis moves in the vagina.

The most typical penile movements involve thrusting in and out as the female either remains still or moves her hips in concert with her partner's thrusting. These motions provide direct sexual stimulation of the male's penile nerve end-

Figure 8.6 *Man on Top, Heterosexual Couple* The man-on-top position is commonly referred to as the "missionary position" and is the most common heterosexual intercourse behavior.

ings (on the shaft, glans, and corona). The woman's clitoris usually is stimulated as the clitoral hood (top of the labia minora) pulls back and forth over it or the man's pubic area rubs against it. The vagina is stimulated as the penis slides in and out. The deeper recesses of the vagina (cervical area) may or may not be stimulated depending on the depth of the strokes and the positions.

An option to thrusting in and out is a circular motion, known as *grinding*, which involves more pubis-to-pubis contact and stimulates the female's clitoris differently. This provides more direct and intense stimulation of the clitoris and the base of the man's penis and can be done even if the man has ejaculated. If he hasn't withdrawn the penis before it has become limp, he can continue stimulating his partner with the circular motion. Sometimes this can go on through his refractory period, and he can achieve another erection without removing his penis. This allows his partner to be stimulated and have additional orgasms even though he has climaxed. Many men find this type of stimulation enjoyable even though they have a limp penis and already have had an orgasm.

Variations of this starting point involve changing the position of the legs and arms. The woman on the bottom can experience a variety of different sensations and depths of penetration by wrapping her legs around the partner's ankles, legs, or waist. Or she can throw her legs over her partner's shoulders as he thrusts in and out, which affords the deepest penetration.

One of the advantages of this position is that it allows the partners to look into each other's eyes and communicate. It also allows the partners to rub and caress each other's chest and shoulders. Furthermore, it allows use of the hands to enhance stimulation by touching or rubbing the partner's genitals during intercourse.

The woman may enjoy stretching her arms over her head, arching her back. This allows her partner better access to caress the breasts and nipples. She may enjoy having the partner pin her arms back over her head. This mild form of domination/submission allows her to "lose control" in a safe way. Individuals should participate in domination/submission only with someone they trust and must understand that "no means no" if either partner wants the activity to stop.

The missionary position can also be used by lesbian women if the partner on top is using a strap-on dildo to penetrate her partner's vagina. The positioning, motions, and benefits are similar to those experienced by heterosexual couples.

Figure 8.7 *Rear Entry, Heterosexual Couple* The rear entry intercourse position is commonly referred to as "doggie style."

Rear Entry The rear entry starting point (Figure 8.7) is also known as "doggie style" because it is the way in which dogs and most other animals have intercourse. In rear entry positions, the partner enters the woman's vagina from behind. This usually is accomplished with the woman kneeling on her hands and knees and the man kneeling behind her, either between or straddling her legs. Either partner parts the vaginal lips and guides the penis in.

This position creates deep vaginal penetration but little direct clitoral stimulation. For this reason, either the man or the woman stimulates the clitoris manually. This position also offers stimulation of the anus and perineum through pressure and friction from the man's pubis rubbing or grinding against it. Once engaged, the woman can lower her head and raise her hips higher to achieve maximum penetration.

The rear entry position can also be used by lesbian women with the aid of a strap-on dildo for vaginal penetration. The positioning, motions, and benefits are similar.

Two other rear entry position variations are (1) the couple can lie down with the man on top of the woman, or (2) they can lie on their sides. The latter is commonly known as the "spoon" position. One disadvantage of this position is that the partners do not face each other, which makes communication and kissing more difficult.

Side-to-Side The side-to-side vaginal intercourse can involve face-to-face positioning (Figures 8.8 and 8.9) or rear entry positioning. Because neither partner is bearing the full weight of the other, the side-to-side position is ideal for leisurely lovemaking or the rest period between more vigorous sessions. The easiest way to get into the side-to-side position is by rolling into it from the man-on-top or woman-on-top or the rear entry position.

Figure 8.8 *Side-by-Side, Heterosexual Couple* The side-by-side facing and rear entry intercourse positions are very comfortable and are often used to relieve pressure on the partner.

Figure 8.9 *Side-by-Side, Pregnant Heterosexual Couple*

Figure 8.10 *Rear Entry Anal Intercourse, Gay Couple* The rear entry position is commonly used by gay couples.

Besides being a comfortable position for leisurely lovemaking, the side-to-side variation has many advantages. It also is good for obese people, as it minimizes weight-bearing. The rear entry variation (Figure 8.9) is good for pregnant women whose developing fetus and protruding abdomen make the man-on-top position impossible. The side-to-side position also facilitates good communication and kissing while leaving the hands free for hugging and forms of manual stimulation.

Anal Intercourse

In anal intercourse, a man inserts his penis into his partner's rectum. Heterosexual and homosexual couples both practice anal intercourse. Like vaginal intercourse, anal intercourse can take place from the three starting points: side-to-side, rear entry, or face-to-face. The advantages and disadvantages associated with these starting points for vaginal intercourse are similar to those for anal intercourse. Rear entry is the most commonly used starting point for anal intercourse, although anal penetration can be accomplished through all of the positions previously described (Figure 8.10).

Oral Sex

Oral sex, also known as oral-genital sex, mouth-genital sex, giving head, and going down, is the stimulation of the partner's genitals with the lips, mouth, tongue, and face. The three main types of oral sex are fellatio (mouth-to-penis contact), cunnilingus (mouth-to-vulva contact), and anilingus (mouth-to-anus contact). All three are common forms of sexual expression for straight, gay, lesbian, and bisexual people.

Fellatio Oral stimulation of the penis

Fellatio   Also known as a "blow job," **fellatio** involves licking and sucking a man's penis. The term is derived from the Latin word *fellare*, which means "to suck." During fellatio, the partner begins by licking and sucking the flaccid penis while holding it. As the penis begins to grow, a man usually enjoys having his penis move in and out of his partner's mouth. The man can accomplish this by gently thrusting his hips, driving the penis in and out of his partner's mouth. The partner can do this by moving his or her head up and down, moving the penis deeper into the mouth and then letting it slide back again.

The sliding motion is accompanied by sucking, which can vary in intensity depending on the man's preference. The tongue is used to lick, flick, or swirl around the penis as it moves in the mouth. Using these tongue motions to stimulate the

healthy sex hints 8.5

Reducing Health Risks Associated with Anal Intercourse

Although the anus is richly endowed with nerve endings and has erogenous potential, it differs from other body parts and requires a few special considerations. One major difference between the tissue of the anus and rectum and that of the vagina concerns the blood vessels that supply the area. The blood vessels of the anus and rectum are very close to the surface. Any minor tearing or scraping of this tissue will result in bleeding and exposing these blood vessels to germs that could enter the bloodstream in this way.

Another major difference involves lubrication. Unlike the vagina, anal and rectal tissue does not produce natural lubrication as a product of vasocongestion. Therefore, care must be taken to adequately lubricate the anal opening and rectum with some other product. Saliva or a commercial water-based sterile lubricant is advisable. Saliva is not as slippery as most commercial products, such as K-Y Jelly, but it is free and can be used at any time. Because petroleum-based products can erode the latex in condoms, these products, such as Vaseline, should not be used in conjunction with a condom.

Lubricants should be spread liberally on the penis and the anus. Gently inserting a lubricated finger into the rectum will lubricate this area and relax the sphincter that keep the anus closed. (Make sure your fingernails are trimmed!)

The lubricated penis is inserted gently and begins controlled thrusting to work the penis deeper into the rectum. Once the penis is inserted comfortably into the rectum, the couple can decide on the nature and intensity of pelvic thrusting. From this rear entry starting point, couples can try most of the positions described in the section on vaginal intercourse.

Sex involving the anus and rectum also carries an increased risk for transmitting a range of infections ranging from hepatitis B to HIV. Organisms that are transmitted through contact with fecal matter or blood are easily transmitted through insertive or receptive anal intercourse or anilingus.

To reduce the likelihood of disease transmission and increase sexual response associated with anal stimulation:

1. Do not engage in anilingus or anal intercourse with an anonymous (don't know at all) or a casual (don't know that well) partner.
2. Before engaging in anal activities, be sure your sex partner is HIV-negative and free of other STDs. This means getting to know your potential partner better and sometimes being tested.
3. With disease-free partners, shower normally with soap and water before having sex to provide adequate hygiene.
4. Always use a water-based lubricant when anal penetration is involved.
5. Do not insert foreign objects (other than specially designed dildos, vibrators, and the like) into the rectum. Be careful not to let things you insert slip past the anal sphincter muscle. The object can get "lost" in the rectum and may require surgical removal.
6. If your partner's STD/HIV status is unknown, use a condom for anal intercourse.

glans and the coronal ridge (particularly the underside where the shaft meets the glans) provides maximum stimulation for the man.

These movements, if continued, usually provide enough stimulation to trigger orgasm. Many men find that a combination of oral and manual stimulation is necessary to provide enough stimulation for orgasm. The partner can grasp the penis at its base or along the shaft and pump it while simultaneously stimulating it with the mouth and tongue. Grasping the penis in one hand while licking and sucking it can also give the partner a sense of control over the depth and intensity of the man's thrusting.

When the penis is thrust into the throat, it typically initiates a gag reflex, which can be minimized by using your hand to control the depth of the partner's thrusting. To minimize this, the partner can relax the throat muscles and control the depth of thrusting by holding the penis.

Couples need to discuss their feelings about ejaculation. As discussed in Chapter 3, the male ejaculate is typically about 1 teaspoon of fluid when he comes. The ejaculate is milky-white in color, has a slippery texture resembling egg whites, and leaves a salty aftertaste. Most men enjoy the sensation of ejaculating into the partner's mouth. This also can be enjoyable to the partner. If the partner finds swallowing ejaculate distasteful, an alternative is fellatio to the point of orgasm, then to withdraw the penis and ejaculate outside the partner's mouth, or to switch to some other form of sexual behavior prior to the point of orgasm.

Environmental Wellness

In this chapter, we openly discuss sexual behaviors from a scientific/health perspective. We discuss the pros and cons of such things as oral and anal intercourse, heterosexual, homosexual, and bisexual variations on these behaviors, and how to engage in them with minimal health risks. We realize, however, that people don't engage in these behaviors in a vacuum. There are still places in the United States where century-old statutes regarding *sodomy* (a term that can be broadly interpreted to include such things as oral sex between consenting marital partners) laws are still enforced. You need to know what laws are still on the books regarding sexual behavior in your city, town, county, and state. This is vital information that can help you make informed choices about your sexual behavior and lifestyle.

Cunnilingus The oral stimulation of a woman's vulva through licking, sucking, and nibbling or rubbing with the face is called **cunnilingus.** It is a common sexual practice of straight, lesbian, and bisexual men and women. Although cunnilingus (from the Latin words *cunnus* [vulva] and *lingere* [to lick]) by definition refers to oral stimulation of the vulva, often the perineum and outer parts of the vagina are also stimulated during this act.

Cunnilingus typically begins as the partner kisses and licks the partner's inner thighs, abdomen, and mons area. The partner then gently parts the labia majora and uses the tongue to lick, flick, or swirl around the vaginal lips, clitoris, and introitus. Pressure can be applied by pressing the tongue against the vulva with greater force. Circular motions are often used to stimulate the vulva in a somewhat different fashion. Care must be taken not to apply too much pressure directly to the clitoris, as it is the part of the female sexual anatomy that is most richly endowed with nerve endings.

The mouth can be used to gently suck on the vaginal lips and clitoris. Gently sucking one or more lips into one's mouth can provide intense pleasure. The clitoris also can be sucked on gently. Some women find it arousing to have their

Cunnilingus Oral stimulation of the vulva

partner gently nibble the vaginal lips and clitoris. The tongue also can be used to penetrate the vagina with thrusting motions.

The face (chin, cheeks, and forehead) can become involved in cunnilingus while the mouth and lips are busy providing stimulation. A partner can intentionally use the face to provide additional stimulation through direct pressure or circular motion. For instance, the bridge of the nose can provide clitoral stimulation while licking or sucking on the labia.

As with fellatio, cunnilingus can be performed with or without manual stimulation. Many women derive pleasure from having their partner insert a well-lubricated finger into their vagina or anus while performing cunnilingus. Saliva or vaginal lubrication can be used to make the fingers slippery. The partner also can stimulate the woman's clitoris with manual stimulation while licking or sucking on another part of the vulva.

Anilingus Oral stimulation of the anus

Anilingus   Although it isn't as common as fellatio or cunnilingus, **anilingus,** also known as *rimming,* is another form of oral sex practiced by people of all forms of sexual orientation. During anilingus, a person kisses, licks, or sucks the partner's anus. The motions and activities of anilingus are similar to both cunnilingus and fellatio.

Performing anilingus affords a good opportunity to stimulate the perineum, an area richly endowed with nerve endings. Some men and women enjoy having their partners insert their tongues into their anus during anilingus. Others prefer that their partner insert a well-lubricated finger into the rectum. When performing anilingus on a woman, care must be taken to avoid spreading *Escherichia coli* bacteria into the vagina. The tongue or fingers never should be inserted directly from the anus to the vagina without first being washed.

Another concern is the spread of hepatitis and other STD organisms through anilingus. We do not recommend performing anilingus with a casual sex partner or someone whose STD status is unknown, as this could result in ingesting disease-causing organisms. (This topic is discussed in greater detail in Chapter 15.)

Figure 8.11 *Mutual Oral Sex, Heterosexual* Mutual oral sex is often referred to as *sixty-nine* because of the shape couples form when engaged in it.

Figure 8.12 *Mutual Oral Sex, Lesbian Couple*

Mutual Oral Sex   The term used to describe simultaneous cunnilingus and fellatio is *sixty-nine*. This usually is accomplished in the side-to-side starting point, with each partner's head at the other's genitals (see Figures 8.11 and 8.12). From this position, both partners have easy access to their partner's genitals. From the side-to-side starting point, it is easy to roll into the man or woman on either the top or bottom positions. By being on the top or the bottom, a person can control for deeper penetration of the tongue when performing cunnilingus, or the penis during fellatio. Mutual oral sex is enjoyed by heterosexual, gay, and lesbian couples.

Sexuality and Disability

Physical disabilities can manifest themselves across a broad spectrum of afflictions. People who are physically or developmentally challenged can maximize their sexual potential by being creative despite their limitations. They experience sensual and sexual pleasures the same way people without disabilities do. Although they may have some restrictions concerning what they can and cannot do, they still can enjoy robust sexual activity and satisfying relationships.

Disabilities, Body Image, and Self-Esteem

For some people with physical disabilities, the main obstacles to sexual activity are social—finding and attracting partners and overcoming self-imposed or societal attitudinal barriers to sex. For these people, sexual behavior is affected very little by the actual physical disability. Their disability affects their body image and their perception of themselves as desirable. Their disability doesn't create a physical barrier to engaging in specific sexual acts or behaviors. Rather, it is their perception of the disability that creates the barrier.

Ostomy is the perfect example of this and will be covered in greater detail in Chapter 11. A *colostomy* can be described as a resectioning of the colon to a stoma that empties the contents of the colon into a bag attached to the abdominal wall. This procedure does not normally affect sexual response, and it doesn't impede engaging in a variety of sexual behaviors ranging from oral sex to different forms of intercourse. However, learning to manage these and other sexual activities while wearing a colostomy bag (or temporarily removing it) depends on the willingness of the person with the disability to accept the colostomy and work around it (Chance, 2002).

Physical Wellness

Physical well-being implies the absence of sexually transmitted diseases, which can severely curtail sexual activity and pleasure. It also includes daily hygiene and health behaviors, both of which play a role in enjoying sexual behavior. High-level physical fitness can enhance sexuality, and nowhere is this more evident than in relation to sexual behavior. High-level physical wellness enhances everything related to sexual behavior. It influences our ability to perform sexually. Although the goal is not to become a sexual acrobat, a high level of fitness will increase our strength, flexibility, and endurance—all elements that can enhance sexual ability and creativity. People with physical disabilities or illnesses may not be able to achieve the same levels of fitness as those who are not disabled or ill. However, they can strive to get the most out of their abilities and maximize their individual fitness level to achieve their sexual potential despite their limitations.

Disabilities and Physical Barriers

For others, the disability directly affects sexual behavior. Arthritis and low-back injury/pain can be used to illustrate this. A woman with arthritis in her hands, for instance, might find masturbation difficult and have to adjust, perhaps enlisting the aid of a vibrator, dildo, or the willing help of a partner. The pain in her hands and fingers, her limited range of motion, lack of strength, and physical deformity (depending on the severity of her arthritis and her ability to control it with a therapeutic regimen) all affect her ability to stimulate herself sufficiently through masturbation.

A man with a lower-back disc-related injury can experience chronic pain which makes certain sexual behaviors impossible. For instance, positions that require him to support his partner's weight (partner-on-top vaginal intercourse, partner sitting on top while seated on a chair, and so forth) would be difficult, if not impossible, to accomplish. He might have to substitute side-by-side, rear entry vaginal intercourse, or mutual oral sex, behaviors that don't require him to support the full weight of his partner.

Neurological Disabilities

Some disabilities such as spinal cord injuries (covered in detail in Chapter 7) and Parkinson's disease will actually affect the transmission of nerve messages that trigger sexual response. Men with spinal cord injuries and Parkinson's disease rarely achieve erections except through reflexive neural activity, and they lose their ability to ejaculate. This makes vaginal intercourse difficult, if not impossible, for them. However, these men might find that although they can no longer get erections, they can still enjoy cunnilingus and other forms of nonpenetrative sexual pleasuring (Yang, 2000; Alexander, Sipski, & Findley, 1993). Chance (2002) reports that some men with spinal cord injuries pride themselves in their abilities to satisfy their partners orally.

case study 8.4

Charlotte: Spinal Cord Injury

Charlotte, 30, single, identifies as African American.

As a young woman, Charlotte was a promising athlete. She was a multifaceted track star who at 20, while on spring break, got into a serious automobile accident that put her into a coma for 4 days and left her paralyzed from the waist down.

I was very bitter for several months following the accident. I didn't want to talk to anyone and was angry all of the time. I broke off my engagement and retreated into a world of antidepressant drugs and disability checks. I hated rehabilitation and didn't work hard at all. I couldn't accept myself without my legs. They had been the source of my greatest accomplishments and my best feature.

After about 6 months, we had a guest lecturer at the rehabilitation center. A social worker spoke to us about redefining our selves, including our sexual selves. I hadn't even begun to think about redefining myself let alone redefining my sexuality. She made me realize how much I missed my partner and the intimacy and sex we had. I really used to love oral sex (giving and receiving) and how my partner kissed and caressed my breasts when we made love. I really began to wonder whether I could really recapture that again with another man.

I slowly came around and began to take my rehabilitation seriously. I also started paying attention to myself as a whole person, capable of satisfying myself and someday my partner. I started taking night classes again and eventually went back to college full-time where I met my present husband. He was a graduate student in the counseling department, and it took me a long time to believe that he really loved me and wasn't just looking to "help" some poor cripple out.

I'm glad I gave him a chance because he is the best thing that ever happened to me. He helped me rediscover the intimacy, passion, and sex in my life. Sure, there are things I can't do sexually any more, and I can't have vaginal orgasms like I used to, but that is becoming less and less important in my life.

We've adopted a little girl, and I am thoroughly enjoying motherhood and hoping I can still teach her a thing or two about running high hurdles.

Critical Thinking

When you strip away all of the emotions and take into account the energy needed to work through a situation like Charlotte's, it makes you think about how you would react if you were in her shoes. How do you think you would react if it were you instead of Charlotte who had gone through this ordeal? Is there really ever a good reason to react the way she did initially?

Use your Virtual Workbook to explore your answers to these questions at **http://health.wadsworth.com/blonna1.**

Chronic Lifestyle Diseases

Chronic illnesses such as cardiovascular disease, obesity, and diabetes can affect sexual behavior. These and other chronic diseases, besides influencing body image and sexual desire, impact strength, endurance, and coordination. People with these conditions can find themselves unable to sustain sexual activity for sufficient duration to achieve orgasm. They might also find certain sexual positions unattainable because of excess body weight.

Redefining Sex

The major challenge for people with disabilities is redefining sexual activity and the goal of sexual behavior. Most people in American culture define sexual activity as genital intercourse and orgasm the goal of sexual behavior. For certain people with physical disabilities, however, that activity and goal are unattainable (Chance, 2002). It is essential, then, that people with physical disabilities set their own activities and goals for sex and not evaluate their happiness in terms of societal expectations. We have seen that activities such as massage, masturbation, and oral sex, with or without orgasm, can be as satisfying as penile-vaginal intercourse.

In some cases, people with physical disabilities develop new levels of sensitivity and sensuality. Research has shown that people with spinal cord injury can develop new erogenous zones and are more than able to become aroused when stimulated (Chance, 2002).

Persons with developmental disabilities usually do not face the same limitations as those with physical disabilities. Rather, their greatest challenge is protecting themselves from unintended pregnancy, disease, and abuse. Care must be taken not to lump all developmentally disabled people together because their abilities vary across a broad spectrum. Many are able to make informed decisions about their sexuality and risk reduction.

In this book, we cannot describe all of the potential variations in lovemaking associated with a full range of physical disabilities. We suggest that people with disabilities use the information in this chapter as a starting point to experiment with different forms of sexual behavior. They may find that accessories such as chairs or stools can be helpful when trying various positions. Communication with the partner is of primary importance, to ensure that the erotic and safety needs of both are being met.

Your responses to the Personal Assessment, Thought Questions, and Test Yourself! quiz questions can be logged online in your Virtual Workbook at **http://health.wadsworth.com/blonna1.**

Personal Assessment

8.1 Online Sensuality Test

Take an online sensuality assessment developed by Discoveryhealth.com. The test is one of many contained on its Web site (see Web Resources). Go to **http://discoveryhealth.queendom.com/sensuality_abridged_access.html.**

8.2 Favorite Sexual Behaviors

People satisfy their sexual needs in a variety of ways. We each engage in unique activities and behaviors to satisfy our sexual desire. The purpose of this activity is to illustrate how different positions satisfy different sexual needs. This will enable you to take a personal inventory of your personal turn-ons and have the opportunity to exchange them anonymously with your classmates.

1. Which autoerotic sexual activity do you find most enjoyable, and why? (If you do not engage in autoerotic activity, simply state this.)
2. Which partnered sexual activity do you find most satisfying? Why? (You could also include masturbation in this category.)
3. Describe your favorite sexual position within this category (for instance, if you enjoy vaginal intercourse most, which starting point and position do you find most enjoyable?).
4. Describe your favorite sexual fantasy. (If you do not fantasize, simply state this.)

Thought Questions

1. What is sensuality? What does "sensual lover" mean?
2. What is Burnham's concept of integration? What contributes to adults losing this capacity?
3. What are some guidelines for giving a massage?
4. What is the difference between celibacy and abstinence? When are each appropriate?
5. What are five nonpenetrative forms of sexual activity?
6. What are the pros and cons of the man-on-top and woman-on-top intercourse positions?
7. What are the advantages of the side-by-side and rear entry intercourse positions?
8. Describe how a person with disabilities might "redefine" sexual behavior and the goal of sexual activity.

Test Yourself!

1. Burnham's concept of "integration" refers to
   a. interracial sex.
   b. a merging of the senses and the intellect.
   c. acting childlike in response to sexual stimuli.
   d. integrating childish things into sensuality.
2. Which of the following best characterizes the relationship between sensuality and sexuality?
   a. They are the same.
   b. Sexuality is an important part of sensuality.
   c. They are completely different.
   d. Sensuality is an important part of sexuality.

3. The major distinction between abstinence and celibacy is
   a. celibacy is something that only involves the clergy.
   b. celibacy is very rare while abstinence is much more common.
   c. abstinence is usually viewed as a situational choice, not a lifetime commitment.
   d. abstinence makes the heart grow fonder.

4. Which of the following is generally *not* considered outercourse?
   a. mutual masturbation
   b. sensual massage
   c. coitus
   d. use of sex toys

5. Most health experts would agree that masturbation
   a. is an acceptable sexual outlet for children and teens only.
   b. can be carried out to excess and needs to be controlled.
   c. is not acceptable adult sexual activity.
   d. is an acceptable sexual outlet for people of any age.

6. Lauman et al. found that adults who masturbated on a regular basis
   a. had higher levels of sex with their partners.
   b. had lower levels of sex with their partners.
   c. did not have steady partners.
   d. preferred solitary sex to partnered sex.

7. Which of the following statements best characterizes how sexual health experts perceive anal sexual intercourse?

   a. It is a source of STDs and should be avoided.
   b. It can be a pleasurable sexual activity if care and extra lubrication are used.
   c. It is similar to vaginal intercourse because of the naturally occurring lubrication.
   d. It is a homosexual activity.

8. Which response best characterizes sexual intercourse during pregnancy?
   a. Should be avoided
   b. Should be avoided after the first trimester
   c. Can be facilitated through side-by-side or rear entry intercourse positions
   d. Is best accomplished using the man-on-top position

9. Which answer best describes people with physical disabilities such as multiple sclerosis and Parkinson's disease?
   a. Are almost always unable to engage in sexual intercourse
   b. Are uninterested in sexual intercourse
   c. Can't make the necessary adjustments to enjoy sexual intercourse
   d. Can enjoy sexual intercourse if they are able to make the necessary adjustments

10. Which answer best describes people with developmental disabilities such as Down's syndrome?
    a. Are too immature to have sexual intercourse
    b. Do not respond sexually the way "normal" people do
    c. Have the same desires as people without such disabilities
    d. Can't be trusted to have sex and not get pregnant

Media Menu

You can link to the following online tools by visiting
http://health.wadsworth.com/blonna1.

 InfoTrac Activity

Felleux, Z. (1998, October). A great week of sex. *Men's Health*, 13(8), 96–99.

 Web Resources

Good Vibrations

www.goodvibes.com

This is the definitive site for all of your sexual aids. The site offers an online catalog for sexual toys, book, films, and related materials and information from the sensual to the erotic.

Discovery Health

http://health.discovery.com/tools/assessments.html

This is the Discovery Channel's health Web site. It contains a variety of assessments related to health.

Intimacy Institute Sexuality

www.bettersex.com/gateway.asp

This is the home page of the Sinclair Intimacy Institute. It provides products and information on sexual response and a host of other topics.

The Pantone Color Institute

http://cn.pantone.com/colorinstitute/colorj.html

This one of the institute's color pages that provides a quick game regarding color and its effects on us. Click on the icon and play the game, or go to the institute's home page: www.pantone.com/aboutus/aboutus.asp?idArticle=49.

The Celibate FAQ

www.glandscape.com/celibate.html

A personal Web page with frequently asked questions and answers on celibacy. The site gives reasons for celibacy, advantages, and disadvantages, plus booklists and other resources. Questions raised include, What kind of people are celibate? What are the advantages/disadvantages of celibacy?

National Abstinence Clearinghouse (NAC)

www.abstinence.net

An alliance of nationally known educators formed to promote the practice of abstinence. The NAC provides a resource center and training for educators and parents. Many links are provided for related topics in the area of abstinence.

The Kama Sutra

www.bibliomania.com/nonfiction/vatsyayana/kamasutra

The Kama Sutra, by Vatsyayana (1883), online and translated by Sir Richard Burton. The timeless Indian sex manual that merges yoga, spirituality, and sex.

Tracey Cox.com

www.traceycox.com

This is the home page for Tracey Cox, writer of *Hot Sex* and other self-help sex books.

References

Alexander, C. J., Sipski, M. L., & Findley, T. W. (1993). Sexual activities, desire, and satisfaction in males pre- and post spinal cord injury. *Archives of Sexual Behavior, 22*(3), 217–229.

Bender, M. (1999). The secret to living a sensuous life. *Cosmopolitan, 227,* 236–242.

Brand, H. (2001). Sexual chemistry (the use of pheromones). *Soap, Perfumery & Cosmetics, 74*(9), 19.

Burnham, W. H. (1932). *The wholesome personality.* New York: Appleton Century.

Chance, R. S. (2002). To love and to be loved: Sexuality and people with disabilities. *Journal of Psychology and Theology, 30*(3), 195–209.

Dodson, B. (1996). *Sex for one: The joy of selfloving.* New York: Crown.

Eiseman, L. (1999). *Colors for your every mood.* New York: Capitol.

Goins, L. (2001). 5 secrets for making sex supersensual. *Cosmopolitan, 230*(4), 156–160.

Good Arts. (2003). *Sensual massage* [Online]. Available: www.goodarts.com.

Hite, S. (1976). *The Hite report: A nationwide study of female sexuality.* New York: Dell.

Hite, S. (1981). *The Hite report on male sexuality.* New York: Knopf.

Inkeles, G., & Austin, K. K. (1992). *The new sensual massage.* Bayside, CA: Arcata Arts.

Kemp, K. (2000). How to touch a naked man. *Cosmopolitan, 228*(4), 194–206.

Kraus, D. K. (2000, October 27). Realm of the senses. *San Francisco Business Times,* pp. 29–33.

Laumann, E. O., Gagnon, J. H., Michael, R. T., & Michaels, S. (1994). *The social organization of human sexuality: Sexual practices in the United States.* Chicago: University of Chicago Press.

Marrone, S. (2002). Indulge your sensual side: Eat a mango, sniff some cinnamon, and other fun, fast ideas for putting more pleasure into your life. *Redbook, 198*(5), 84–86.

Masters, W. H., Johnson, V., & Kolodny, R. (1996). *Human sexuality.* New York: HarperCollins.

Norris, K. (1996, September–October). Celibate passion. *Utne Reader,* 51–53.

Yang, C. C. (2000). Female sexual function in neurologic disease. *Journal of Sex Research, 37*(3), 205–208.

chapter *nine*

Atypical Sexual Behavior

Student Learning Objectives

After reading this chapter, students will be able to

- Distinguish between normal, atypical, and paraphiliac sexual behavior.
- Describe the four typical measures used to assess normalcy.
- Assess their own attitudes, values, and beliefs about what is normal.
- Describe the key characteristics of a variety of paraphilias.
- Evaluate the paraphiliac risks associated with the Internet.
- Evaluate the health risks associated with body piercing.
- Differentiate transvestic fetishism and transsexualism (gender identity disorder).
- Describe the origins of atypical sexual behavior and paraphilias.
- Evaluate various ways of treating atypical sexual behaviors and paraphilias.

*Test your understanding of these objectives by taking the end-of-chapter quiz, available online at **http://wadsworth.com/blonna1**.*

activity teaser: *Discover your true feeling about different sexual behaviors in the Personal Exploration Activity on page 285.*

case study 9.1

Greg: Exhibitionism or Mooning?

Gregg, 20, single, is white.

Critical Thinking

Many people experiment with a host of sexual behaviors such as "mooning." What distinguishes Greg's mooning from someone else's prank?

Use your Virtual Workbook to explore your answers to this question at **http://health.wadsworth.com/blonna1.**

Greg was the first client assigned to Dr. Blonna during the supervised clinical training component of the master's degree in counseling. Greg was on probation as a first-time sex offender convicted of exhibitionism. As a condition of parole, Greg had to seek counseling for a proscribed period of time. In Dr. Blonna's words:

I'll never forget Greg. I was a 25-year-old man, not too much older than Greg. I was still working through issues related to my own sexuality and found Greg quite a challenge. He was referred to counseling because he had been arrested for exposing himself to a young woman.

It was hard for me to understand the significance of exhibitionism. I had been raised as a typical man of the 1950s and 1960s and viewed exhibitionism with amusement more than a clinician's understanding of it as a paraphilia. Indeed, I was only a few years removed from engaging in mooning and streaking as fraternity pranks. In time, my work with Greg crystallized the significance of his behavior and the furtive nature of exhibitionism.

Greg was a reluctant client at first. He did not want to be in counseling, and the first couple of sessions were almost totally devoid of any conversation. Gradually we began to establish a relationship, and Greg started to talk about his exhibitionism. It became quite evident after that point that Greg's behavior was vastly different from mooning and other juvenile sexual behavior that, although offensive, has an entirely different motivation. Mooning, streaking, and other prank public displays of nudity are not intended to serve as sexual come-ons. Greg's behavior had an entirely different purpose.

Greg was immature—both socially and sexually retarded. He was painfully shy, could not communicate with women effectively, and had limited dating experience. His sexual experience was limited to autoerotic activities and a handful of sexual liaisons with prostitutes. He lacked self-esteem and self-confidence and had a hard time maintaining eye contact. He also admitted, while in counseling, that he was a voyeur and had masturbated several times while watching a few women in his neighborhood get undressed. He had a couple of peeping vantage points that allowed him to peer into the windows of apartment buildings in his neighborhood.

After seeing Greg for several sessions, it was obvious that exposing himself was his way of coming on to women sexually. He really believed that women, upon seeing his nakedness (and throbbing erection) would literally throw themselves at his feet and perform oral sex on him or ask him back to their place to have intercourse. He believed that his "manhood" would speak for itself and make traditional forms of establishing a sexual relationship unnecessary. In reality, Greg lacked the conversational and other social skills necessary to meet women and establish a sexual relationship.

As we can see with the illustration of Greg, sometimes there is a fine line between what is considered "normal" sexual behavior and what isn't. Normative behavior can be classified as sociological, biological, psychological, and statistical. Sexual behavior that is *sociologically* normal falls within the laws, mores, and customs of a society. Most of this behavior is culturally defined and passed from one generation to the next as a result of socialization. *Biologically* normal behavior is characterized as healthy and natural and helps perpetuate the species in positive ways. *Psychologically* normal sexual behavior is sexual activity that does not result in emotional distress or in neurotic or psychotic functioning. Finally, behavior that is considered *statistically* normal is sexual behavior in which the majority of people engage.

Given these four categories of "normality," defining abnormal sexual behavior might seem easy. Anything falling outside the parameters established by these four categories would be considered "abnormal."

The words *normal* and *abnormal* are commonly used labels because they characterize sexual behavior in easy-to-understand, stereotypical patterns. Furthermore, dichotomizing normal and abnormal makes it easier to stigmatize and discriminate against people who are not in the norm. A more commonly accepted term to describe behaviors that the majority of the population does not practice is *atypical* sexual behavior. Atypical sexual behavior is described as behavior that is not statistically typical. The term *atypical* does not carry the same pejorative tone as *abnormal*.

Paraphilias

Paraphilias are atypical or unusual sexual behaviors that become the focal point for an obsessive preoccupation or need. The paraphilia is almost always the central focus of the person's sexual repertoire, and arousal and orgasm are difficult, if not impossible, in the absence of the paraphilia.

Paraphilia An unusual or atypical sexual behavior that becomes the focal point for an obsessive preoccupation or need

Paraphilias generally revolve around three common themes: (a) nonhuman objects, (b) suffering or humiliation involving oneself or one's own partner, and (c) children or other nonconsenting persons. In addition, to qualify as a paraphilia, a behavior has to occur over a period of at least 6 months and cause clinically significant distress or impairment in social, occupational, or other important areas of functioning (American Psychiatric Association [APA], 2000).

The fourth edition, text revision, of the *Diagnostic and Statistical Manual of Mental Disorders* (DSM-IV) lists eight categories of paraphilias and one catchall category. The eight officially recognized categories are as follows:

exhibitionism
voyeurism
fetishism
frotteurism
pedophilia
sexual masochism
sexual sadism
transvestic fetishism (APA, 2000)

The catchall category "not otherwise specified" includes the following paraphilias, which are less common and don't meet the criteria to be included in any of the other eight categories:

telephone scatologia (obscene phone calls)
necrophilia (sex with a corpse)
partialism (focus on certain parts of the body)
zoophilia (sex with animals)
coprophilia (contact with feces)
klismaphilia (enemas)
urophilia (undue attention to urine) (APA, 2000)

A person often exhibits more than one paraphiliac behavior (APA, 2000). Also, someone who exhibits true paraphiliac behavior and someone who casually experiments with atypical behavior are different. True paraphilia creates almost obsessive recurring, intense sexually arousing fantasies, urges, and behavior, and it is the main focal point for sexual arousal.

In addition, the person recognizes that the paraphilia causes significant enough emotional, social, occupational, or other distress to interfere with daily functioning. Someone who casually experiments with episodic paraphiliac behavior (such as occasionally liking his lover to tie him to the bedpost) and does not suffer negative emotional or other consequences is considered a person who simply enjoys occasional atypical sexual behavior.

Exhibitionism

The paraphiliac focus of **exhibitionism** involves deriving sexual arousal by exposing one's genitals to unsuspecting strangers. The overwhelming majority of people with this paraphilia are men between 18 and 40 years of age. Sometimes the person masturbates while exposing himself or fantasizing exposing himself (APA, 2000). Often the sexual gratification is derived from the sheer shock value of the act and the reaction from the victim. The greater the reaction, the more the person has proven his masculinity.

Men who reveal exhibitionism tend to be shy, passive, and sexually inhibited. Exhibitionism is generally perceived to be unrelated to rape or sexual assault. In some instances, the man with this paraphilia believes that his victim will be sexually aroused by his nakedness and that it will provoke a sexual encounter with her.

Exhibitionism is often confused with "mooning" (baring one's buttocks to unsuspecting passersby). Generally, those who moon do not derive sexual gratification from the act, and it usually is a prank typically associated with adolescents. In a sense, exhibitionism is culturally disparate. Male and female exotic dancers get paid to expose themselves. Nude or partially nude dancing and other forms of exotic entertaining are designed to be sexually arousing and are legal, yet streaking, which is not sexual, is illegal.

Voyeurism

The paraphiliac focus of **voyeurism** is exactly the opposite of exhibitionism. The voyeur derives sexual excitement and pleasure from observing unsuspecting people (usually strangers) who are naked, disrobing, getting dressed, or in the act of having sex. The pleasure is derived from the act of "peeping" and is not intended to lead to an encounter with the unsuspecting stranger. Sexual release usually occurs through masturbation either while peeping or later with the voyeuristic memory of the encounter. The person may fantasize having sex with the stranger (APA, 2000).

Voyeuristic behavior can be depicted along a continuum. At the extreme is the person who can achieve sexual release only by observing others having sex. At the other end of the continuum is the person who watches others to augment sexual pleasure with a partner. This person might get turned on by watching exotic entertainers to fuel a sexual episode with a partner.

Fetishism

The paraphiliac focus of **fetishism** is deriving sexual arousal and gratification from nonliving objects. The overwhelming majority of people with fetishes consists of men who derive sexual pleasure from items of women's clothing such as underwear, bras, stockings, shoes, and boots. Typically, the man with paraphiliac fetishism masturbates while holding, stroking, smelling, or licking the object. To a lesser extent, the person may ask his partner (or pay a prostitute) to wear the item of clothing while they engage in sex or he masturbates (APA, 2000).

A person with a true paraphiliac fetish usually strongly prefers and needs the object to experience sexual desire. Often, a person with a fetish is unable to obtain or sustain an erection without the object being present. Fetishes often are linked to significant childhood experiences and are in place by adolescence (APA, 2000).

Frotteurism

The paraphiliac focus of **frotteurism** is deriving sexual arousal and pleasure from rubbing one's genitals against an unsuspecting, nonconsenting person. The male rubs his genitals against his victim's buttocks and thighs while simultaneously fondling her breasts or genitalia, or both. This typically occurs in crowded public places such as busy sidewalks, subways, buses, and other public places where the perpetrator can make a quick escape and avoid arrest (APA, 2000).

Environmental/Occupational Wellness

The overwhelming majority of paraphiliacs are harmless, and as long as their behavior is private and with consenting adults, it does not represent a threat to society. In other instances it does. Legislation was passed in New Jersey and a host of other states to protect children from sex offenders in their communities. The New Jersey legislation, "Megan's Law," was enacted in response to the brutal murder of a young girl, Megan Kanka, by a neighbor who was a known sex offender. Essentially, the new law requires that neighbors be notified that a convicted sex offender has moved into their neighborhood. The hope is that such notification will enable parents and other neighbors to protect their children by keeping them away from the sex offender. In 1994, 12 new laws were enacted in California specifically targeting sex offenders. Provisions of these laws include, among others, a state-maintained toll-free phone number that alerts people to registered sex offenders living in their area, stiffer penalties for first-time offenders convicted of child molestation or rape, and the barring of unsupervised visits of sex offenders to their children.

The workplace can present many challenges to persons with atypical behavior. Transsexuals, and those with certain paraphilias such as fetishism, face daily stress (and often outright discrimination) as they struggle to earn a living and cultivate a career while living with atypical sexual desires and behavior.

Pedophilia

The legal aspects of **pedophilia** are discussed in detail in Chapter 16. The paraphiliac focus of pedophilia is fantasizing about engaging in sexual activity with a prepubescent child. Those sexually attracted to girls, in general, prefer 8- to 10-year-olds. Those attracted to boys favor slightly older children. The two subtypes of pedophilia are (a) exclusive (individuals who are sexually attracted to children only) and (b) nonexclusive (individuals who are sexually attracted to both adults and children) (APA, 2000).

Pedophilia Engaging in sexual activity with or fantasizing about prepubescent children

Individuals with pedophilia show a wide range of sexual activity with their victims. Not all pedophiles are child molesters. According to the law, a pedophile is an individual who fantasizes about sexual contact with children, whereas a child molester actually commits that act in some form (Davis, McShane, & Williams, 1995).

Most pedophiles masturbate while watching their victims undress, fondle themselves, or engage in sexual activities with another child or an adult. These activities can be live (paying children to perform in person or observing live sex shows broadcast over the Internet) or available through print (magazines, newspapers, and the like) and other electronic media (including movies, videotapes, and CD-ROMs).

Child molesters engage in a variety of sexual activities with their victims. This may consist of rubbing or fondling the child. Other child molesters penetrate the child's mouth, vagina, or rectum with their fingers, penis, or a foreign object. Some people with pedophilia obtain these sexual favors by gaining their victims' trust, affection, or loyalty. Others use physical force and psychological pressure and terror to obtain sex and control their victims.

The Internet and Pedophilia

The Internet and the World Wide Web have become a major source of concern for law enforcement officials around the world trying to stem the tide of child pornography and pedophilia-related abductions and murders that originated in chat and other services available on the Web. The cases of Marc Dutrox of Belgium and Ronald Riva of California are just two of many that have brought attention to the problem of pedophilia and its many manifestations on the Internet.

Dutrox was convicted of kidnapping and murdering young girls in Belgium. The suspected head of a Europe-wide pedophile sex ring, Dutrox used the Internet to meet and lure his victims.

Riva, an unemployed truck driver, former prison officer, and father of four, was discovered when the mother of one of his victims (a 10-year-old girl) pressed charges of child abuse against him. The girl claimed that Riva had abused her when she stayed overnight at a slumber party for one of his daughters.

The case broke wide open when detectives discovered that Riva's house contained equipment (similar to that used in videoconferencing) that was set up to broadcast live "photo shoots" on the Internet. Police also discovered computer files containing child pornography and links to another man, Melton Lee Myers, who had similar equipment.

The investigation ultimately linked the two to a worldwide pedophile ring with members based in the United States, Finland, Australia, and Canada. The group was abusing children as young as 5 years old and broadcasting pictures and live child-sex shows on the Internet (Cusack, 1996).

The Web and Internet have made it almost impossible to control kiddie porn, and the number of federal "cyber-cops" (federal agents who scour the Internet for such material) has increased from a handful to more than 100 operating in the United States alone (Kaplan, 1997). Besides having a voracious appetite for pornography, which has contributed literally tens of thousands of child sex visual images to the Internet, pedophiles and child molesters have taken advantage of sophisticated broadcasting techniques to stay ahead of the law. Child pornographers often "morph" the head of one child onto the body of another, making identification of the child and proof of sexual abuse almost impossible. The naked images of adults in child pornography are limited almost exclusively to shots from the torso down.

Additional obstacles to tracking pedophiles, child molesters, and child pornographers include the sheer volume and worldwide scope of their activities. Keeping abreast of new sites, linking perpetrators, and identifying victims is indeed difficult. Often, just as investigators are making progress, a site closes down and relocates with a new Web address or country of origin.

One potential inroad being explored is forcing service providers to sever relationships with sites that have been known to contain child porn. A key component of the Communications Decency Act, which the U.S. Supreme Court struck down as unconstitutional in 1997, was the provision to hold providers (such as America Online) liable if their customers could gain access to obscene and indecent material. At present, a global effort is under way to come up with a way to control access of child pornography via the Internet.

Numerous state and federal laws have made the possession of any sexual image of kids under age 18 illegal. Nonetheless, the underground market for all forms of child pornography and prostitution is thriving (Kaplan, 1997). Pedophiles have victimized their own children, stepchildren, foster children, or relatives' children. Less often victims are children adopted through foreign services, bought through underground slave trade, or exchanged with other pedophiles. People with pedophilia have been known to use extraordinary means to obtain child pornography or actual live victims. In recent years, several pedophiles have made headlines by arranging encounters with children while posing as adolescents in Internet chat rooms.

Pedophilia usually is chronic and is more difficult to treat than other paraphilias. The recidivism rate for men attracted to boys is more than twice that of men attracted to girls (Davis et al., 1995).

Sexual Masochism

The paraphiliac focus of **sexual masochism** is deriving arousal and pleasure through being beaten, bound, humiliated (physically or mentally), or made to suffer in some other fashion (APA, 2000). Although fantasizing about being the victim of masochistic acts is common, true paraphilia involves engaging in the behaviors.

Many different masochistic acts typically are sought with a partner. These include being bound (physical restraint involving being tied, strapped, taped, chained, or handcuffed), spanked, bitten, paddled, whipped, beaten, shocked with an electrical current, cut, or pierced/pinned (infibulation). Another common masochistic desire is to be humiliated by being urinated or defecated on, to be forced to crawl and bark like a dog, and to be verbally abused. **Infantilism** involves being treated like an infant and forced to wear a diaper.

The last category of masochistic paraphilia involves **hypoxyphilia** (also known as *autoerotic asphyxia*), or oxygen deprivation, by noose or wire (ligature), chest compression, plastic bag, mask, or chemical (such as amyl nitrate, a powerful vasodilator that reduces the flow of oxygen to the brain). This behavior is particularly dangerous because mishaps in applying these procedures for sexual arousal could result in death. Little is known about this behavior since information about individual cases is usually derived from postmortem physical and psychological evaluations of the victim. Investigation is made even more difficult by the victim's family attempting to cover up the sexual nature of the death (Friedrich & Gerber, 1994). It does not seem that hypoxyphilia is attempted suicide (Hickman, 2002). Rather, in most cases it is accidental, a result of ritualized autoeroticism where oxygen deprivation is part of the sexual attraction and risk taking. Most people who engage in autoerotic asphyxia are males with a history of sexual abuse, physical abuse, choking behavior (sometimes associated with asthma), exposure to traumatic family experiences, and other risk taking (Friedrich & Gerber, 1994).

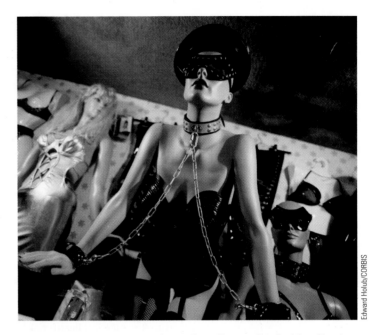

Many sex shops cater to sexual paraphernalia associated with sadism and masochism.

Sexual masochism Deriving sexual pleasure from being humiliated or forced to suffer pain

Infantilism Deriving sexual pleasure from being treated like an infant

Hypoxyphilia Deriving sexual pleasure from activities that involve oxygen deprivation

Piercing has become so popular that many states have adopted guidelines for ensuring the health and safety of the practice.

Sometimes, individuals with sexual masochism engage in masochistic acts by themselves. They self-inflict pain and humiliation through pinning, binding, shocking, or engaging in hypoxyphilia. Men with sexual masochism often concurrently have fetishism, transvestic fetishism, or sexual masochism (APA, 2000). The practice of body piercing has its etiology in sexual masochism. Piercing erogenous body parts such as the labia, nipples, and scrotum by paraphiliacs represents self-mutilation associated with masochism and the desire to humiliate and injure oneself. Most body piercers, however, have the procedures done for personal adornment, a reflection of style (Association of Professional Piercers [APP], 2002).

Physical Wellness

The continuum of atypical sexual behavior, as we've discussed, ranges from the relatively benign (occasional use of a fetish object) to the very dangerous (sadomasochistic beatings and torture). As we've mentioned throughout this text, healthy sexuality promotes physical well-being and behaviors that enhance health. Engaging in many of the atypical sexual behaviors can put your physical health in jeopardy. It is crucial to follow all of the warnings associated with these behaviors. There are ways to reduce the physical health risks associated with atypical sexual behavior.

healthy sex hints 9.1
Reducing the Health Risks Associated with Body Piercing

Body piercing, like other forms of adornment such as tattooing, branding, and ear piercing, carries some risk. The risks vary and are related to the body part being pierced, the piercing equipment, sterilization procedures used (or lack thereof), and the skill of the provider. The following hints can help reduce the risks associated with body piercing:

1. Think long and hard about your motivation for getting your body pierced. Make sure you understand the risks associated with the procedure.
2. Talk with people who have had piercing done. Ask what kind of experiences they had.
3. Before getting pierced, ask your physician about vaccination for hepatitis B, a blood-borne infection passed through contaminated needles.
4. Do not pierce yourself or let an inexperienced person (such as your best friend, who pierced her own ears) pierce you.
5. Go to a reputable piercing parlor that has been in business for some time. Ask for references from former customers.
6. Make sure the piercing parlor you choose uses an autoclave (a tabletop sterilizing device that uses heat and pressure to kill germs) to sterilize equipment. Ask to

see the certificate verifying that the autoclave has been recently inspected. If only boiling water is used to clean equipment, head for the door.
7. If a tattoo artist uses individually sealed, sterile needles, ask him or her to open these in front of you. Request the same for the containers of ink being used for your tattoo.
8. Talk to your physician to learn about special considerations concerning the body part being pierced. Particularly risky parts (because of increased likelihood of infection or permanent damage) are the eyelids, the tongue, the nipples, the clitoris, and the frenulum of the penis.
9. Don't have piercing done if you are pregnant or nursing.
10. Follow after-care instructions to the letter. If you suspect infection, consult a doctor immediately.
11. Wear only jewelry that is 14K gold, niobium, or surgical-grade stainless steel. These contain fewer alloys and are less likely to cause allergic reactions.

Source: Association of Professional Piercers (2002), *Procedure manual* (Chamblee, GA: Author).

Sexual Sadism

The paraphiliac focus of **sexual sadism** involves deriving sexual arousal and pleasure by inflicting physical or psychological pain and suffering on another person. The person may engage in sadistic activities with either a willing victim (usually someone with sexual masochism) or a nonconsenting victim (APA, 2000). Sexual sadism incorporates a range of acts, including all of those discussed previously under the topic of sexual masochism. In extreme cases, people with sexual sadism seek sexual arousal through extreme brutality, torture, mutilation, and murder. Typically, they engage in such behavior with nonconsenting victims and have had the condition for several years. The fantasies of sexual sadism usually are present in childhood, and the behavior begins in early adulthood and becomes chronic.

Sexual sadism Deriving sexual pleasure from inflicting pain or humiliation

Emotional Wellness

The difference between someone who engages in atypical sexual behavior and the true paraphiliac is in the emotional distress and social dysfunction the latter experiences. An individual or couple can engage in almost all of the atypical behaviors of paraphiliacs without this representing a paraphiliac sexual condition. A person can be emotionally healthy and still enjoy an occasional walk on the wild side. Actually, some people engage in atypical sexual activities to add a spark to their sex lives. When the behavior becomes an obsession, however, and carries with it emotional distress and social dysfunction, it becomes a paraphiliac sexual disorder.

Transvestic Fetishism

Transvestic fetishism differs from other forms of fetishism in that the fetishist derives sexual arousal by cross-dressing (dressing up as a female or wearing an article of female clothing). The transvestic fetishist typically masturbates to orgasm while dressed in that clothing.

Transvestic fetishism Deriving sexual pleasure from wearing women's clothing

The disorder is known only in males. It runs the full spectrum of behavior from routinely wearing a single item of female clothing (such as silk panties) under the male clothing to spending thousands of dollars on customized gowns and makeup and participating in the transvestic subculture (APA, 2000).

Men with transvestic fetishism do not have gender identity disorder (think they are really females), and most are heterosexual in sexual orientation. When not cross-dressed, men with transvestic fetishism look like the average man. Men who do not have transvestic fetishism but occasionally like to put on articles of female clothing often do so with the willing participation of their female partners.

Gender Identity Disorder

Gender identity disorder (GID) is also known as **transsexualism.** Gender identity disorder is characterized by four criteria:

- a strong and persistent cross-gender identification;
- persistent discomfort with his or her sex or a sense of inappropriateness in the gender role of that sex;
- the absence of any genetic or physical abnormality (intersex condition such as androgen insensitivity);
- significant accompanying clinical psychological distress and impairment in social, occupational, or other functioning.

Transsexualism (a gender identity disorder) A strong and persistent cross-gender identification

From James to Jenny

Jenny, 46, is white.

Critical Thinking

Should the medical profession be engaged in helping people change their biological gender? Why?

Use your Virtual Workbook to explore your answers to these questions at **http://health.wadsworth.com/blonna1.**

James Finney Boylan was living an idyllic life. He was a successful novelist and a professor of creative writing at Colby College in Maine. He was a loving husband with two sons. There was just one thing wrong. Since childhood, James felt he was living the wrong life. James had a secret: He was a woman trapped in a man's body.

In her book, *She's Not There: A Life in Two Genders,* Jennifer Finney Boylan chronicles her journey to womanhood. In 1998, James accepted the reality of his situation and began the process of transition, including psychotherapy, hormone treatments, electrolysis, and voice coaching. She underwent gender reassignment surgery in 2002.

Boylan began his transformation by telling his wife "Grace" about the psychological torment he was enduring because of his gender identity issues. In one particularly poignant moment, Boylan apologizes to his wife for all that she is enduring as they are watching the first *Lord of the Rings* movie: In the words of Bilbo, "I am sorry. Sorry you have come in for this burden, sorry about everything."

Boylan's children seem to take the metamorphosis in stride, even inventing a name to call her that makes sense: "Maddy," a combination of *Mommy* and *Daddy*.

Boylan takes a leave of absence from his duties at Colby, announcing to his colleagues via a letter that when he returns he will be Jennifer Finney Boylan. Boylan's close friend and colleague at Colby, Pulitzer Prize–winning novelist Richard Russo, initially cannot accept his friend's decision and evokes him to "be a man." Eventually, however, Russo comes to support his friend's decision and even accompanies Boylan and Grace to Wisconsin for the surgery.

Now Boylan notices that as a female her moods are more wide-ranging; she often feels more vulnerable and cries easily. She also deals with body image issues, being more conscientious about ordering a salad rather than the slab of ribs James would have requested. She also says that she is now attracted to men.

Today Jenny and Grace are in a new kind of relationship. Not husband and wife, or lesbian partners, but something different. They are still legally married and are committed to being partners in parenting. They are not currently seeking relationships with other people. At the end of this particular personal journey, Jenny Boylan is finally enjoying the life that she always felt was meant to be.

A strong and persistent cross-gender identification has several markers for children. The following constitute evidence for a strong and persistent cross-gender identification:

- a repeated stated desire to be, or insistence that he or she is, the other sex;
- in boys, a preference for dressing in female attire or simulating girls' clothing; in girls, wearing only stereotypical boys' clothing;
- a strong and persistent preference for cross-gender sex roles in make-believe play or fantasy;
- desire and participation in the stereotypical games and pastimes of the other sex;
- a strong preference for playmates of the other sex.

In adolescents and adults, the criteria for a strong and persistent cross-gender identification are met by the following symptoms:

- stated desire to be the other sex,
- frequent passing as the other sex,
- desire to live or be treated as the other sex, and
- conviction that he or she has the typical feelings and reactions as the other sex.

sex in society 9.2
The Underground World

In the 1970s Lou Reed, an avant garde artist and the lead singer for the Velvet Underground, sang about taking a walk on the wild side. The wild side in this case was the underground world of transsexuals—a world replete with its own bars, clubs, magazines, and clothing outlets.

Today you still can experience this underground world on certain streets in every major city in the United States, from New Orleans to New York City to San Francisco, and find a world filled with all of the transpeople—transsexuals, transvestites, and the transgendered. You'll find boutiques catering to transsexuals that carry everything in "women's" clothing from panties to feather boas in sizes designed to fit the average truck driver. You'll also find shoe stores that cater to spiked heels in sizes 10, 11, and 12 in every width. At night these districts come alive as club-goers of all sexual persuasions flock to see their favorite female impersonators, although some of the actors and actresses already have gone through sex reassignment surgery and can hardly be called impersonators.

The World Wide Web has opened the globe to the transcommunity. You now can view entire catalogs of merchandise on your computer and shop from the privacy of your own home. There are social organizations, self-help groups, political action committees, legal aid societies, chat rooms, list serves, travel clubs (they find the best places for transpeople to vacation), auto clubs, discount purchasing cooperatives—and the list goes on and on. The amazing thing is that most of these people, places, and services operate outside the realization of mainstream society.

Supporting the second criterion is discomfort and inappropriateness with one's gender role. Boys strongly and persistently assert that their penis and testes are disgusting and wish they would disappear. They also have a strong aversion to typical rough-and-tumble play and stereotypical boys' toys, games, and activities. Girls have a strong and persistent resistance to sitting while urinating and assert that they do not want to grow breasts or menstruate. They also have an aversion to feminine clothing (APA, 2000).

Adults with gender identity disorder are preoccupied with ridding themselves of their primary and secondary physical sexual characteristics through hormone therapy and surgery. Transsexuals feel, and have always felt, that they were literally born the wrong sex, as if nature had made some mistake with their genitals.

Leavitt and Berger (1990) identify two forms of transsexualism: primary and secondary. *Primary* transsexuals are individuals who feel strong cross-gender identification from their earliest recollections of their childhood. Often, these individuals have clear cross-gender identification by age 3. *Secondary* transsexuals begin to develop strong cross-gender identification in adulthood. Because secondary transsexuals have gone through infancy, childhood, adolescence, and early adulthood with same-gender identification, shifting to their new cross-gender identification is more difficult.

There is much controversy surrounding the classification of GID, especially among secondary transsexuals. Transgender activists and those who serve transgendered clients claim that the "significant enough emotional, social, occupational, or other distress" that "interferes with their daily functioning" (quotes indicate DSM-IV criteria necessary for diagnosis) experienced by most transgendered men and women is not due to their gender identification but by societal reaction to it (Carroll, Gilroy, & Ryan, 2002; Klein, 2002; Isay, 1997). Citing this and other controversies

Jennifer Finney Boylan recently wrote about her journey from male to female in the book She's Not There: A Life in Two Genders.

sex in society 9.3

Jan Morris: A Conundrum

Jan Morris started out in life as John Morris, later to be knighted and become Sir John Morris. John Morris—man, husband, father, athlete, soldier, explorer, writer, world traveler, climber of Mount Everest—was the epitome of every man's fantasy. He had power, prestige, wealth, and fame. Beautiful women wanted to be around him. He held the world in his hands.

John Morris had everything he wanted except for one thing: he really wanted to be a woman. He'd gladly have given it all up (and did) to become the woman he always

wanted to be. In the book *Conundrum,* one of the first of its genre, Jan Morris explains the crux of what being a transsexual means—feeling as though nature made a mistake. Morris recalls early recollections of feeling literally trapped within the wrong body. Her whole life, up to the point of having sex reassignment surgery, consisted of trying to do things to convince herself that maybe she actually did belong in that body. Ultimately she realized that she didn't, and she had the surgery necessary to become a female.

surrounding the diagnostic category, Isay (1997) appealed to the American Psychiatric Association for the removal of the classification gender identity disorder. In a rebuttal to Isay (1997), Friedman (1998) acknowledges the problems associated with misdiagnoses of some transgendered persons (especially adult, homosexual men) but supports the continuation of the inclusion of the classification in the DSM-IV. Friedman notes that children with GID have much more psychopathology compared to other children. Elimination of the GID classification, Friedman claims, would cause these children to fall through the cracks and not receive the psychiatric care they need.

The Origin and Treatment of Atypical Sexual Behavior

Many different theories abound about the causes and treatment of atypical sexual behavior and paraphilias. Implied in "atypical" is the need to fix something that is wrong. Therefore, we reemphasize the difference between individuals who occasionally engage in behaviors that are atypical and cause no harm to another person and individuals who have paraphilias that cause themselves and others pain and suffering. The difference lies in the psychological distress and impairment in social, occupational, and other functioning between the two types of behavior.

Ethical Considerations

Society has an ethical and moral obligation to protect paraphiliacs and their victims from harm, even if they do not realize they are at risk. A sexual masochist, for instance, should be protected from the violence and suffering that may coexist with that paraphilia.

The need for treatment is less clear with problems such as gender identity disorder. Is this really a psychological disorder? Is the condition really a problem that requires treatment, or should their desire to be the other sex be respected? Many question the essential duality of maleness and femaleness. As mentioned in Chapter 4, gender is best viewed as a continuum rather than an absolute value (100 percent male versus 100 percent female).

The ethics of sexual reassignment surgery (surgically removing the genitals and reconstructing the genitalia of the desired, opposite sex) has been the subject of much debate. Should people who have GID be allowed to have sex reassignment surgery? Would it make more sense to try to help these people learn to accept both the fact that they have the genitalia of one gender and the identity of another? Why do we have to fit them into only one neat niche? These and other questions related to the diagnosis and treatment of atypical and paraphiliac sexual behavior are still being debated and may never be fully resolved.

Spiritual Wellness

When discussing spiritual wellness, we must take care to separate people who engage in occasional atypical sexual behavior from paraphiliacs. Spirituality, as we've mentioned throughout the book, emphasizes the interconnectedness of people and treating all people with respect and dignity. Paraphilias such as sadism, masochism, and pedophilia are based on seeking gratification by inflicting pain, humiliation, or dominance over another. Hurting others represents an absence of spirituality.

Etiology

Many explanations have been set forth for the causes of atypical sexual behavior and paraphilias. Three of the more commonly accepted views revolve around a psychoanalytic appraisal, a behaviorist explanation, and an eclectic etiology.

Psychoanalytic Appraisal   A classic psychoanalytic explanation for atypical or paraphiliac sexual behavior is the fixation of libidinal energy at a specific point in development. An individual becomes "stuck" and, with advancing age, constantly regresses to that point in psychosexual development. The immature level of sexual development is a result of not having been allowed the full expression and passage of libidinal energy at the age-appropriate stage.

Sexual masochists' need to be humiliated by having their partner urinate or defecate on them, for instance, is attributed to unresolved issues at the anal stage. Perhaps this person was rushed through toilet training or belittled for soiling his underpants. Whatever the specific issue, the unresolved transition through this period results in the fixation of sexuality at this stage of development.

Behaviorism   The behaviorist focuses on some facet of learning and argues that atypical sexual behavior and paraphilia stem from some associative learning experience. Perhaps it was extremely harsh parental punishment for some minor sexual act such as observing Mom in the shower or being caught masturbating. Or it may be pairing an act (observing a woman undressing, for instance) with a pleasurable sexual experience (such as masturbation) that is positively reinforcing. This type of behavior is likely to be repeated.

Eclectic Perspective   John Money (Money & Lamacz, 1989) offers an eclectic explanation to atypical sexual behavior and paraphilia. He has developed a biosocial theory of sexual and gender development (see Chapter 4) based on what he called "lovemaps" ("templates" in the brain for patterns of eroticism and love). These templates, according to Money, are developed between 5 and 8 years of age as a result of biological and psychosocial forces.

During this period of development, Money believes children begin to link sex, love, and lust. The child usually develops a normal, healthy connection between romantic love and lust (sexual desire). Each of us has a unique lovemap based on

case study 9.3

The Marv Albert Case

Marv, 66, married, is white.

Critical Thinking

Because most paraphilias are deeply ingrained and difficult to extinguish, what do you think the goal of treatment should be? Why?

Use your Virtual Workbook to explore your answers to these questions at **http:// health.wadsworth.com/ blonna1.**

The sporting world was shocked when Marv Albert, a longtime radio and television sportscaster, was arraigned in Virginia on charges of forced sodomy and a variety of other lesser charges. Albert's more than 30-year career as the play-by-play announcer for NBC and other networks made him a celebrity, and his trademark "Yes-s-s-s!" following key baskets during New York Knicks broadcasts was known across the United States.

Albert's accuser, a longtime lover, charged him with biting her in several places on the back and forcing her to perform fellatio on him. She claimed that Albert's behavior was in response to his disappointment in the woman's unwillingness to bring a third partner in a ménage à trois, another man, to a rendezvous at a local hotel. The woman further asserted that she had a long history of such trysts with Albert, even several years ago while he was still married. She also claimed that Albert had a penchant for cross-dressing, watching X-rated videos, and biting during sex.

Albert countered by claiming that the woman liked "rough sex," and the biting was part of their sexual repertoire. He confirmed their long-term relationship but claimed that he never had forced her to do anything. Her accusations, Albert asserted, were in response to his informing her that he would be getting engaged and married and would be ending their relationship.

During the investigation, a second woman, a hotel manager from Washington, DC, surfaced, claiming that Albert had tried to force her to have sex with him also. She claimed that Albert had placed a call for room service, and when she arrived, Albert met her at the door wearing only women's panties and a garter belt. He had an obvious erection and tried to force her to have sex with him. She said she fought him off and left the room.

The case ended with Albert's and the woman's attorneys working out a plea bargain in which the sportscaster agreed to a lesser charge of assault (a misdemeanor) in exchange for dropping the forced sodomy charge (a felony). Albert eventually received a suspended 12-month sentence with a promise to expunge his record of all charges if he would seek counseling and honor all of the conditions of his probation.

The case sent shock waves throughout the United States, touching off a flurry of talk-show programs concerning rough sex, biting, cross-dressing, and other paraphiliac behavior. Included in the debate was a discussion of whether someone like Albert could ever be "rehabilitated." Experts testified claiming that the goal of Albert's treatment would be to teach him how to control his urges to engage in such behavior in public with strangers or nonmarital partners. Albert is now back on the airwaves.

a combination of biology (genetic inheritance, gonadal and hormonal influences) and psychosocial learning (parental and other models of love and affection). Healthy lovemaps are imprinted in our brain and create our idealized lover, love affair, and erotic imagery.

Atypical sexual behavior and paraphilia, according to Money, are a result of a distorted or "vandalized" lovemap that does not make a healthy connection between romantic love and lust. Love and lust are imprinted as disparate entities. Because the two are not linked, sexual desire (lust) is not attached to normal romantic involvements but, rather, becomes attached to the inanimate objects, humiliating behavior, and the like, that evolve into paraphilias. Sexual desire is something apart from intimacy and affection. Lovemaps can become distorted for a variety of reasons including incest, physical abuse, extremely harsh parental punishments for normal sexual activity in childhood, repressive parental attitudes, and lack of displays of affection between parents.

Is It Really So Bad?

It is really easy to react negatively when we hear of some "different" sexual behavior and to immediately label it as harmful. However, even though we may never want to engage in any paraphiliac sexual behavior, many of the behaviors cause no real harm to the person or others. The goal of this activity is to try to identify those behaviors that are truly harmful from those that, however odd they seem, are really rather harmless.

Take a sheet of paper and label three columns—one "harmless," one "harmful," and one "both harmful and harmless." As you continue to read about the different behaviors, try to keep an open mind and forget the judgments you have already formed about these behaviors. After reading about each behavior, list it in the column where it seems to fit the best. Notice what factors cause you to give each the label you assign. Based on what label you give each behavior, do you think there should be criminal penalties for the behavior? Keep in mind that many of these behaviors carry severe criminal penalties or at least very negative social attitudes. Is it possible that our society is overreacting because the behaviors do not fit what most consider to be normal? Should our laws and attitudes be changed for those you listed in the harmless category?

Treatment

Most paraphiliacs enter treatment as a result of being arrested for their behavior. They do not seek treatment on their own or enter willingly. Paraphilias are extremely difficult to treat, and "cure rates" are low. Regardless of which view one holds regarding the etiology of paraphilias, most experts agree that atypical and paraphiliac behavior originates early in life, manifests itself in fantasy and desire, and evolves into full-blown behavior and lifestyle by young adulthood. As such, the person has a long history of behavior that has been reinforced over time through pleasure (masturbation or other sources of orgasm). The prognosis for eliminating such behavior is not good.

Biomedical and Surgical Treatment   One way to treat people with paraphilia is to attempt to lower their level of sexual desire through chemical (drugs) and surgical (castration) procedures. Drug therapy consists of administering drugs that either inhibit the production of testosterone or block its effects on the brain. As we discussed in Chapters 2 and 3, testosterone is the main androgen linked to sexual desire in men and women. Drugs such as cyproterone acetate (CPA) and medrohxyprogesterone (MPA-Depo-Provera) interfere with the effects of progesterone. They have been shown to have limited effectiveness in treating pedophiles, rapists, and other male sex offenders (Wincze, Bansal, & Malamud, 1986; Cooper, 1986). Until the 1980s, castration was used to reduce the sexual desire of sex offenders. The surgical removal of the testicles eliminates the production of most testosterone but does not prevent sexual excitement and erection.

Although decreasing testosterone levels lower sexual desire, it does not eliminate desire entirely. Also, no evidence is available to show that reducing testosterone levels, and thus sexual desire, has any permanent effect on the focus of sexual behavior. Testosterone is linked with sexual desire, not sexual orientation or the focus of sexual activity. Drug therapy seems to work by lessening the compulsion to engage in paraphiliac behavior (Walen & Roth, 1987). It doesn't eliminate the desire but, in conjunction with other approaches invoking the patient's support system, helps control the desire enough to allow intervention.

Treatment for transsexualism (gender identity disorder) often involves surgically reconstructing the patient's genitalia. The overwhelming majority of transsexual surgical reassignments involve male-to-female transitions. In male-to-female transsexual reassignment surgery, a new clitoris, vulva, and vagina are constructed from penile and scrotal tissue. Internal structures remain the same. In female-to-male surgery, a penis and scrotum are constructed from vulval and vaginal tissue. In this case, artificial testes (with implants) are constructed, and removable penile implant rods can be inserted into the structure to achieve an erection.

Transsexual reassignment surgery is part of a four-part treatment process that also involves psychotherapy, hormone therapy, and living as the other gender. The goal of psychotherapy is to help the client readjust in his/her new role. The client begins taking hormones of the new gender to either "feminize" (in male-to-female reassignment) or "masculinize" (in female-to-male reassignment) the client's body. Lastly, before surgery is performed, clients must live as the new gender (complete with cross-dressing) for a year to learn what it is like to function as a member of society in one's new gender (Meyerowitz, 2002; Money & Wiedcking, 1980).

Behavior Modification   Behavior modification is used to desensitize paraphiliacs to their paraphilias and sensitize them to new, aversive stimuli. **Aversion therapy** is a behavior modification technique that pairs an aversive stimulus (such as electric shock) with the behavior that is targeted for change. Covert sensitization is a type of aversion therapy sometimes used with paraphiliacs. In **covert sensitization,** an aversive fantasy (not behavior) is paired with the paraphiliac fantasy in an attempt to extinguish it. For example, a voyeur is asked to visualize a past fantasy that accompanied one of the voyeuristic episodes. As the person visualizes the pleasing fantasy (say, peeping on an unsuspecting woman), the therapist introduces an aversive fantasy image (such as vomiting uncontrollably). By pairing the new aversive image (the vomiting) with the previously arousing image (peeping at the victim), the therapist links the negative image to the paraphilia.

Aversion therapy A behavior modification technique that pairs an aversive stimulus with the behavior targeted for change

Covert sensitization A type of behavior modification in which an aversive fantasy is paired with the paraphiliac fantasy in an attempt to extinguish it

Intellectual Wellness

High-level intellectual functioning can help a person know when an atypical behavior pattern represents a true paraphilia. Knowledge can help people understand that they have a problem and how to seek help in dealing with it. Paraphilias, however, tend to have such a strong hold over people that knowledge alone usually isn't enough to motivate them to seek help. Even so, knowledge can play a part in helping them learn how to live with their obsession and channel it into more acceptable forms of expression.

Skills Training   The focus of skills training is to enhance interpersonal skills. Paraphiliacs often rely on the paraphilia because of their inability to engage in satisfying interpersonal sexual relationships. Often they lack the self-esteem, confidence, and behavioral skills to meet potential sex partners and cultivate sexually satisfying relationships.

In skills training, they learn a variety of behaviors ranging from communicating (how to initiate conversations, meet new people, and the like) to coping with stress. As individuals become more proficient with these skills, they can learn to rely less and less on their paraphilia for sexual arousal (Zilbergeld, 1992).

Social Wellness

People who engage in atypical sexual activity (particularly partnered activities) can be socially healthy. They may engage in atypical activities to add spice to their sex lives. Most people with full-blown paraphilias, however, are not doing well socially. Their paraphilia often originated from disordered social functioning and learning. The paraphilia takes the place of functional adult social and sexual relationships. Many paraphiliacs experience sexual release through solitary masturbation in the presence of their paraphiliac object of desire.

Thought Questions

1. What are some of the many facets of "normal" sexual behavior?

2. What does "atypical" sexual behavior mean?

3. When does atypical sexual behavior become a paraphilia?

4. How do a person's morality and ethics influence atypical sexual behavior?

5. How have the media treated some of the more common paraphilias such as voyeurism and exhibitionism?

6. What is the difference between a true transsexual and someone with transvestic fetishism?

7. What are the origins of paraphilias?

8. What are three treatment approaches for paraphilias?

9. Describe the controversy associated with sexual reassignment surgery.

Test Yourself!

1. Which of the following is *not* considered a category of normative sexual behavior discussed in this chapter?
   a. Biological norm
   b. Anthropological norm
   c. Statistical norm
   d. Sociological norm

2. *Abnormal behavior* is generally considered
   a. an outdated term, replaced by *atypical behavior*.
   b. an outdated term, replaced by *nonnormative behavior*.
   c. an acceptable term synonymous with *atypical behavior*.
   d. an acceptable term still widely used by most experts in the field of human sexuality.

3. Atypical sexual behavior becomes paraphiliac when
   a. it is the major recurring theme in the person's sexual fantasies.
   b. it is obsessive and interferes with a normal sex life.
   c. it becomes repetitive and obsessive.
   d. it causes obsessive preoccupation or need and interference with daily functioning.

4. Occasionally tying your lover to the bedpost to simulate loss of control during sex is an example of
   a. a fetish related to rope.
   b. an atypical sexual behavior.
   c. a paraphilia.
   d. an abnormal sexual behavior.

5. Which behavior is often mistaken for mooning or other forms of consensual public sexual activity with a partner?
   a. voyeurism
   b. frottage
   c. urophilia
   d. exhibitionism

6. A sexual sadist is someone who derives sexual arousal and pleasure from
   a. inflicting pain and/or humiliation on sexual partners.
   b. experiencing pain and/or humiliation at the hands of sexual partners.
   c. "snuffing" a partner with no direct sexual involvement.
   d. torturing a partner with no direct sexual involvement.

7. A sexual masochist is someone who derives sexual arousal and pleasure from
   a. inflicting pain and/or humiliation on sexual partners.
   b. experiencing pain and/or humiliation at the hands of sexual partners.
   c. "snuffing" a partner with no direct sexual involvement.
   d. torturing a partner with no direct sexual involvement.

8. The best answer to describe the major differences between transsexuals and transvestites is
   a. transsexuals derive sexual arousal and pleasure from cross-dressing.
   b. transvestites derive no sexual arousal and pleasure from cross-dressing.
   c. transvestites feel they are members of the opposite gender and are "trapped" in the wrong body.
   d. transsexuals feel they are members of the opposite gender and are "trapped" in the wrong body.

9. John Money's "lovemaps" theory of atypical sexual behavior and paraphilia says that paraphilias develop as a result of
   a. neurolinguistic programming that distorts lovemaps.
   b. unhealthy lovemaps that link love and lust.
   c. unhealthy lovemaps that imprint love and lust as distinct entities.
   d. people who vandalize other people's lovemaps.

10. The prognosis for treatment of people with paraphilias is
    a. excellent over time using conventional behavioral modification.
    b. fair using short-term aversion therapies such as electric shock.
    c. not good regardless of the treatment modality.
    d. pretty good if the patient is highly motivated.

Media Menu

You can link to the following online tools by visiting
http://health.wadsworth.com/blonna1.

Face to Face Videos

Heather, a pre-op transgendered person talks about her journey and upcoming surgery.

Jason and Jeanette and Rex and Kia discuss safe sex and the S&M lifestyle.

Film

Gender Identity Disorder

InfoTrac Activity

Kinnon, J. B. (2000, April). Pierced to death. *Ebony, 55*(6), 142–146.

Web Resources

The American Psychiatric Association (APA)

www.psych.org/index.cfm

A medical specialty society recognized worldwide. Its 37,000 U.S. and international member physicians work together to ensure humane care and effective treatment for all persons with mental disorder, including mental retardation and substance-related disorders. The APA is the voice and conscience of modern psychiatry and envisions a society that has available, accessible quality psychiatric diagnosis and treatment.

Above & Beyond

www.abgender.com

This outrageous site is a smorgasbord of resources (everything from shopping to emotional support) devoted to the transgender community.

Transgendered Suite

www.tgni.com

A major site for transgender information, support, and services. It provides everything from general information to a transgender dating service.

The Association of Professional Piercers (APP)

www.safepiercing.org

An international nonprofit association dedicated to the dissemination of vital health and safety information related to body piercing to piercers, health care providers, and the general public. The group believes that it is the obligation of all professionals in the field to assume responsibility for their continued education. The organization dedicates itself to enabling this responsibility to be met.

The New Zealand Edge; John Money Page

www.nzedge.com/heroes/money.html

The New Zealand Edge is a nonpolitical organization dedicated to fostering understanding of the country and its contributions to the world. This linked page is their page devoted to John Money.

References

American Psychiatric Association. (2000). *The diagnostic and statistical manual of mental disorders* (4th ed., text revision). Washington, DC: Author.

Association of Professional Piercers. (2002). *Procedure manual.* Chamblee, GA: Author.

Carroll, L., Gilroy, P. J., & Ryan, J. (2002, Spring). Counseling transgendered, transsexual, and gender-variant clients (practice and theory). *Journal of Counseling and Development, 80*(2), 131–140.

Cooper, A. J. (1986). Progesterone in the treatment of male sex offenders: A review. *Canadian Journal of Psychiatry, 31,* 73–79.

Cusack, J. (1996). The murky world of Internet porn: The "Orchid Club" shakes up the law. *World Press Review, 43*(11), 8–10.

Davis, L., McShane, M. D., & Williams, F. P. (1995). Controlling computer access to pornography: Special conditions for sex offenders. *Federal Probation, 59*(2), 43–48.

Friedman, R. C. (1998, January 19). Gender identity. *Psychiatric News: Viewpoints* [Online]. Available: www.payxh.org/pnews/98–01019/gender.html.

Friedrich, W. N., & Gerber, P. N. (1994, September). Autoerotic asphyxia: The development of a paraphilia. *Journal of the American Academy of Child and Adolescent Psychiatry, 33*(7), 970–975.

Hickman, W. (2002, August 8). A real swinger—Part IV (autoerotic asphyxiation cases). *Mondau Business Briefings.*

Isay, R. A. (1997, November 21). Remove gender identity disorder from DSM. *Psychiatric News: Viewpoints* [Online]. Available: www.psych.org/pnews/97/-11-21/isay.html.

Kaplan, D. E. (1997). New cybercop tricks to fight child porn: Police struggle against an online onslaught. *U S. News & World Report, 122*(20), 29.

Klein, J. A. (2002, December). A sex of one's own. *The Nation* [book review, *How Sex Changed: A History of Transsexuality in the United States*], 274(19), 33–39.

Leavitt, F., & Berger, J. C. (1990). Clinical patterns among male transsexual candidates with erotic interest in males. *Archives of Sexual Behavior, 19*(5), 491–505.

Meyerowitz, J. (2002). *How sex changed: A history of transsexuality in the United States.* Boston: Harvard University Press.

Money, J., & Lamacz, M. (1989). *Vandalized lovemaps.* New York: Prometheus.

Money, J., & Wiedcking, C. (1980). Gender identity/role: Normal differentiation and its transpositions. In B. B. Wolman & J. Money (Eds.), *Handbook of human sexuality.* Englewood Cliffs, NJ: Prentice Hall.

Walen, S., & Roth, D. (1987). A cognitive approach. In J. H. Geer & W. T. O'Donohue (Eds.), *Theories of human sexuality.* New York: Plenum.

Wincze, J., Bansal, S., & Malamud, M. (1986). Effects of medroxprogesterone acetate on subjective arousal, arousal to erotic stimulation, and nocturnal penile tumescence in male sex offenders. *Archives of Sexual Behavior, 15*, 293–306.

Zilbergeld, B. (1992). *Male sexuality: A guide to sexual fulfillment.* Boston: Little, Brown.

chapter *ten*

Intimate Relationships

Student Learning Objectives

After reading this chapter, students will be able to

- Describe the key elements of healthy relationships.
- Identify issues related to meeting potential partners.
- Describe ways to meet partners safely online.
- Define intimacy and trace its development in relationships.
- Define love and describe how it develops in relationships.
- Compare a variety of theories regarding love.
- Evaluate a variety of barriers to intimacy.
- Describe various techniques used to overcome barriers to intimacy.
- Identify characteristics of unhealthy relationships.
- Become aware of markers for abusive relationships.
- Examine a variety of ways to end unhappy relationships.

*Test your understanding of these objectives by taking the end-of-chapter quiz, available online at **http://health.wadsworth.com/blonna1.***

activity teaser: *The couple that laughs together, stays together. See the Personal Exploration Activity on page 307.*

case study 10.1

"Fitting In and Finding My Niche"

Lily, 20, identifies as biracial.

For some reason, the questions about "What are you?" at times are more frequent here at college than they were in high school. I notice people looking at my eyes, more than my skin tone, and wondering. My dad is white; my mom is Thai. So, am I "Asian American"? "Thai American"? When I got here, there were two clubs for Asian students; one was Chinese American, and that didn't fit. The other was Asian American, yet at the meetings most of the students were of Indian descent. I didn't really feel like I fit there, either.

I find myself hanging with the African American students most. White students see me as different, and while my black friends know my background, they don't seem to care. I have a black boyfriend right now, and his friends accept me. My parents don't know about him, though. I don't think they'd approve. Funny . . . they're a mixed-race couple, yet some groups are more comfortable for them than others.

I've joined a sorority and have friends there. My boyfriend and I are in a good place, so I'm just taking one day at time. He hasn't tried Thai food with me yet, but I'm working on it!

Critical Thinking

Do students on your campus socialize across racial lines? How important are issues of race for you when choosing friends? Romantic partners?

Use your Virtual Workbook to explore your answers to these questions at **http://health.wadsworth.com/blonna1.**

Intimacy Connectedness to another person characterized by mutual caring, openness, self-disclosure, honesty, attentiveness, sharing, commitment, trust, empathy, and tenderness

Our quality of life depends to a large extent on the types of relationships we develop. Relationships define our connectedness to others and provide opportunities for **intimacy.** Intimate relationships are characterized by honesty, caring, sharing, trust, commitment, empathy, and tenderness. Forming healthy relationships with others is a skill a person develops and practices. For relationships to be intimate, we have to be ourselves and let others be who they are. Good relationships derive from good role models and require giving thought to the outcome of our actions. As Lily explained in the case study, her social comfort was connected to her race to some degree. For others, connections may be stronger along gender lines or sexual orientation.

As we age, we form social relationships with others on many levels—family, friends, working colleagues, neighbors, and partners. Although this chapter focuses primarily on partner relationships, we have to realize that becoming sexually intimate with someone does not necessarily mean that we automatically have an emotionally intimate relationship.

We learn patterns of relating to others from our families, friends, and past experiences. Some people are extroverted and outgoing, and they enjoy having many different types of relationships. Developing relationships is easy for them. Other people are introverted and enjoy doing many things alone. They develop fewer relationships in their lives and may have difficulty forming new relationships. Regardless, human contact is essential for health and wellness.

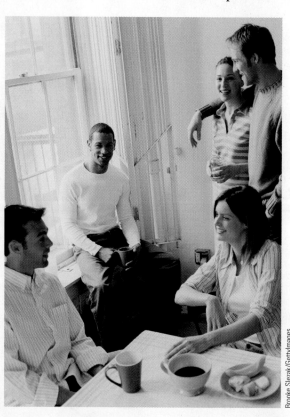

Brooke Slezak/GettyImages

College provides opportunities to meet a wide variety of people.

Intellectual and Social Wellness

College affords many opportunities to meet and learn from different types of people. Many of us grow up in communities where those around us are of similar race, religion, and social class. Institutions of higher learning commit themselves to meeting the needs of diverse students and enabling the exchange of a variety of perspectives. Challenging opinions, listening to the views of others, and learning about difference all contribute to greater intellectual well-being.

Dating and being in relationships provide opportunities to broaden one's social network, to meet new people and make new connections. Being with others and forming intimate relationships is critical to social well-being. We all need people we can count on, who are our friends, and who see us through the good times and bad. Sharing activities with others is part of social health. Lifelong friendships may develop in college, and for some college also becomes the source for one's lifelong romantic partner as well.

Establishing Relationships

The dynamics of forming close, intimate relationships with friends are different from the dynamics of developing intimate relationships with sexual partners. A look at the shelves of a bookstore quickly reveals rows of books offering advice on how to find a partner, keep a partner, satisfy a partner, and be satisfied with a partner. But you won't find rows and rows of books on how to make and keep friends. The same holds true for music. The lyrics of country, rock, and blues passionately describe the ups and downs of emotions related to love relationships. The intensity of feelings related to platonic friendships just doesn't compare.

Friends share activities, thoughts, and feelings. They help each other out. When a life experience tests a friendship, we often hear the comment "That really let me know who my true friends are!" With friends, we are relaxed and able to "be ourselves." Now switch the scenario to a boyfriend, girlfriend, or partner. A healthy romantic relationship, one that is founded on intimacy, requires the same expectations, yet we may find ourselves not being authentic with our thoughts and feelings, second-guessing the other person, and sometimes tolerating behaviors we would never accept from our friends. The erotic piece of the puzzle is what changes the interaction. We often become self-conscious in ways we hadn't anticipated, and we might lose our identity in pursuit of the relationship. Healthy relationships are based on being able to clearly identify who we are, what we want, how we want to be treated, how we want to live, and recognizing that we deserve to want what we want.

Meeting People

The first step toward developing an intimate relationship is connecting with a potential partner. People can meet in many ways, not all equally comfortable or familiar. College is sometimes viewed as an ideal place to meet someone and form an intimate relationship, yet some students graduate without experiencing a serious dating relationship. Unlike years past, when many college women in particular had been told that they had 4 years to earn their "Mrs. degree," students today are likely to feel less pressure to be married upon graduation. Even when students do not have marriage as a goal, though, they have the desire to form intimate relationships.

Much of the research that examines partner and mate selection has been conducted on samples of college students using laboratory experiments and questionnaires; such research has limitations and may not explain how the population at large develops couple relationships (Wiederman, 2001b). For example, young adults who don't go to college may choose partners in different ways and from different social situations than those who attend college. Important partner characteristics and strategies for meeting people may change as one ages—young, typical, college students may have important criteria that do not match those who are divorced, have children, and may be in their 30s or 40s. Furthermore, the process of attraction and partner selection often includes socializing with someone on multiple occasions and evaluating how that "chosen person" reacts to expressed interest. Being part of a college community may afford opportunities to see a partner regularly, yet exposure to and participation in the types of situations that test relationships over time may be limited. Overall, it is important to distinguish between what may be reported as a "preference" for a partner and what goes on in actual social experiences.

Before looking at issues of where and how to meet a prospective partner, people have to be ready for a relationship. Are they open to a relationship? Are they comfortable with themselves? If they were hurt in a previous relationship, they may not have let go of the "old baggage." Too often people approach a new relationship with defensiveness, negative past associations that become expectations with a new partner, and patterns of relating that prevent new relationships from developing.

Feeling comfortable when meeting people and forming relationships is a social skill and, as such, is behavior that is modeled, taught, and practiced. People have to feel comfortable enough with themselves to believe they are worth getting to know—fundamental to self-esteem. People who consider themselves "shy" may find social settings very intimidating. They may not be able to identify the behaviors and words needed to make social contact with others.

Shyness

Zimbardo's (1977) classic work on shyness provides a framework for understanding what is a nearly universal experience of being shy at some point in one's life. More than 80 percent reported feeling shy at some time, 25 percent described themselves as chronically shy, and 4 percent described themselves as being shy all the time, in all situations, with virtually all people. The ability to overcome shyness is essential to forming relationships.

Shyness is revealed in a number of ways. People who are shy may experience or demonstrate one or more of the following characteristics:

Speaking softly
Not making eye contact
Being reticent/reluctant to relate to others
Blushing
Experiencing "butterflies" in the stomach
Feeling embarrassed
Feeling self-conscious

Although everyone has those experiences and feelings at times, shyness becomes a problem when the level and frequency of those experiences impede the development of relationships. Shy individuals might be operating from a negative script in which they deem themselves unacceptable and unworthy, and they typically lack the social skills of knowing how to initiate conversation and make connections. Zimbardo found that overcoming shyness is possible if individuals are willing to work on making changes in the way they think about themselves and others and in how they behave.

Shyness can become painful enough that professional intervention may be warranted. Individuals may choose to avoid social situations, cancel out at the last minute, avoid pleasurable activities, and/or choose to spend the majority of time at the computer rather than in face-to-face interactions. Additionally, chronic low moods, use of alcohol and drugs to manage social situations, or excessive time spent on academic work and professional activity to the exclusion of socializing can be symptoms of painful shyness (Henderson, Zimbardo, & Rodino, 2001).

Another impediment to forming intimate relationships is the fear of being rejected. Some people enter social situations with an expectation that they will be rejected. They become anxious about being rejected, expect to be rejected, and overreact to what may be ambiguous behavior in others (Downey & Feldman, 1996). Again, having a frame of mind that allows one to approach others in a positive way, without worrying about rejection, is more likely to lead to better interactions and a possible relationship.

Group Socializing

Reports from some colleges and universities reveal that students do not date in traditional ways; they prefer to socialize in groups rather than pair off (Gabriel, 1997). Traveling with a small circle of five or six friends, they go to movies, parties, and dinner, feeling safe within their group. This is an excellent way to discover what types of people you enjoy being with and what you are looking for in a partner.

In a study of 9,100 undergraduates from campuses across the United States (Gabriel, 1997), students reported a preference for casual sex rather than deeply committed emotional relationships. Increasingly, sexual liaisons result from partying, drinking, going to someone's room, and then having little contact with that person later. The term *hooking up* defines that experience for all its ambiguity. Two people can kiss and fondle extensively, sleep together fully clothed, or have sexual intercourse. Developing a long-term relationship is another matter. Some students explain their reticence for developing committed relationships by their lack of witnessing successful relationships among their parents and other adults they know.

Where and How to Meet People

As our lifestyles become busier, "meeting that special someone" can become a project in and of itself. Individuals may purposely go to a social event in the hopes of finding a prospective partner. Friends may purposely invite a range of people to a party—some single, some coupled—hoping that additional pairing occurs. Although it may not be productive to set purposeful goals to meet someone, and it can be frustrating when a social event doesn't introduce a new potential partner, individuals have to put themselves in social situations where potential social opportunities exist. An essential strategy for meeting people involves widening the scope of one's activities.

College offers a comfortable social environment in which to form relationships. Academic classes, clubs, parties, sorority and fraternity functions, rallies, student newspapers and yearbooks, and the like, involve students in activities while simultaneously providing environments to meet others.

If similarities in race, culture, or religion are important, campus organizations whose members align themselves with the relevant similarities may be places to meet. Because of issues of "coming out" and the added burden of attempting to determine someone's sexual orientation, lesbian, gay, and bisexual students may want to meet through organizations in which sexual orientation is the foundation for the group.

sex in society 10.1

Finding That Special Someone on the Internet

The strategies available for meeting a potential partner have become more complicated than in decades past. Although college still provides a very social environment, the expectations of the "real" world after graduation may increasingly lead to organized searches for a partner through dating services and the Internet. Some people are in search of a long-term partner, while others focus on finding partners for sexual behavior without commitment. Parties, personal introductions, the bar scene, and other venues may still lead to romance, yet for the very busy, the Internet may become a tool for organizing one's own social life. With work expectations, commutation, and other demands on one's time, the possibilities afforded by a system that is available 24 hours a day, every day, become very attractive.

Some of the popular sites are Yahoo!Personals, Match.com, eHarmony.com, web.tickle.com, Salon.com, Springstreetnetworks.com, and Friendster.com. Individuals can create personal profiles, rewrite them over time, read and reread profiles of potential partners, take personal assessments that identify interests and better matches, and so forth. Some sites require a membership fee; others are free. Millions of Americans reportedly visit online dating services, with over $200 million being spent on dating fees in the first half of 2003 (Egan, 2003, p. 66).

While the increased availability of personals in newspapers and magazines provides one mechanism for meeting, the Internet increases the amount of information that can be transmitted. Many sites allow members to place their photographs online. Readers can react to a photograph and decide whether someone seems attractive. Pictures can be deceptive, however, and real face-to-face meetings potentially disappointing. Someone could easily be older, heavier, or shorter than what was conveyed in a photograph; even if those qualities are of minimal importance, there is still the issue of sexual chemistry and whether a potential romantic relationship will develop. On the positive side, by the time a couple decides to meet for the first time, they may have already established good lines of communication.

Overall, healthy relationships form with people, not computers. The technology may change some of the dynamics of meeting and communicating, but in the long run being with someone who is right for you is the goal.

As a result of the Anita Hill versus Clarence Thomas hearings related to sexual harassment, the culture has started to redefine and pay attention to settings where developing romantic attachments is deemed inappropriate and, at the minimum, adds complications, obvious and subtle. Consequently, although dating someone in your class can become awkward if the relationship doesn't work out, dating someone with whom you work can be more complicated, as work situations often involve competition and power. Sexual harassment laws and policies usually define the prohibitions associated with work-based relationships, with policies against romantic and sexual involvement most directed at power imbalances. Specifically, prohibitions and sanctions focus on relationships that could develop with a professor or supervisor; such individuals have the power of determining grades, promotions, graduate school recommendations, hiring, transfers, salaries, or firings.

Outside the school environment, you may find that dating becomes more of a project than you had anticipated. Work hours, busy schedules, and a desire to avoid the bar scene have led to technological interventions for dating. Personal advertisements, which used to be a feature in select newspapers and magazines, now have worked their way into mainstream newspapers (see Figure 10.1), cable television, and the Internet. Sophisticated video dating services, in which registered members can review tapes of people they might want to meet, have flourished in some areas. Hefty membership fees and promises made by some dating services, however, have sometimes resulted in dissatisfied consumers suing for fraud.

Finding a partner via the Internet allows people of all backgrounds to do some initial screening from the privacy of their own homes. Sex in Society 10.1 highlights some of the issues related to finding a partner online. As humorously depicted in Figure 10.2, caution when meeting someone for the first time is advisable. Healthy Sex Hints 10.1 outlines guidelines for safe online relationships.

Females Seeking Males

Call 1-000-000-0000
$2.39 per minute
You must be 18 years of age or older to use this service.

Prince Charming
Educated professional SWM 40, 6', 180 lbs. Likes movies & nature. Seeking SWF, 20–40. Ad #000

Try Bi
Disease-free W couple, 30, seeks bi-GWM, 30+. Ad #XXX

Casual Only
SWM 34, 5'11", lives in XXXX County, seeks a well-built, clean-shaven, SM, 21–45, who likes to have fun, for discreet relationship. Ad #0000

Hardworking
Personable, humorous SWM, 37, 5'11", self-employed, seeks sensitive slender SWF, under 32, to share a serious, loving relationship with. Ad #XXXX

Figure 10.1 *A Sample of Personal Ads* Personal ads usually are coded for age, race, and sex of the desired partner.

healthy sex hints 10.1

Guidelines for Safer Online Relationships

Meeting people online can be fun and exciting. Unfortunately, it can also be very dangerous, as evidenced by news reports of predators and children. Recommendations for teens may differ from those for college students and older adults, yet some basic guidelines prevail:

Do not use your real name in your e-mail address or disclose it, or disclose your address or telephone number to someone you have only met online.

Do not give details about yourself, such as the state in which you live or other information that would make it easy for someone to find you.

If after chatting with someone you decide to meet them in person, here are additional guidelines to follow:

Ask the person to give you information that will help you determine whether he or she is "for real," such as any employers, name of his or her school, or other references. Ask the person to send a picture so that you will recognize him or her. Remember, too, that any information provided can be easily faked.

Meet in a public place like a mall or restaurant.

Bring a cell phone with you so that you can call for help if needed.

Consider taking a friend with you when you meet, and have the friend stay throughout the entire first meeting. It would also be a good idea to have a friend call you

on the cell phone during the meeting to make sure that everything is OK. Be sure your friends know where you are so that they can send help if you need it.

Never go to this person's car or anywhere else alone and out of view of others.

Tell a friend or other trusted adult where you are going and who you are meeting. Tell that person you will call when you get home. (Have that friend be prepared to call your parents and the police if you do not call by the specified time.)

If you plan to meet this person a second time, suggest that the second meeting take place at your home. If you live with your parents, make sure the visit takes place while at least one parent is there so that your mom or dad can meet him or her. If you live with friends in an apartment or dormitory, again, make sure a friend meets him or her.

Any person who cares about you and is interested in a real relationship with you will be more than willing to make you feel safe and secure about the relationship, and they will not mind the precautions that you are suggesting. Anyone who refuses to meet in public, or who refuses to meet your parents or friends, is not someone you can trust, no matter how wonderful they might seem.

Source: Prepared by E. Casparian, New Jersey Network for Family Life Education, New Brunswick, NJ, 2003.

Figure 10.2 *Close to Home*

Choosing a Partner

When asked to describe what makes someone attractive to them, students have responded with a combination of physical attributes and personality characteristics. Some responses are specific, and others are more general. A sampling from the authors' files includes the following:

I like a guy who is not overly muscular, has a hairy chest, and nice buns.
I like big breasts, a round butt, and long hair.
He must be clean, have good teeth, and not smoke.
The smile is important to me. And eyes—I can tell a lot from the eyes.
I like to bike and mountain-climb. I need a partner who likes the outdoors and has a sense of adventure.
She has to have some brains, not be too skinny, and like sports.
I always like blondes—blond hair, blue eyes.
My partners have always been dark—dark skin, dark eyes, and dark hair.
He has to be nice, have a good sense of humor, and enjoy family.
I like women fully shaved.

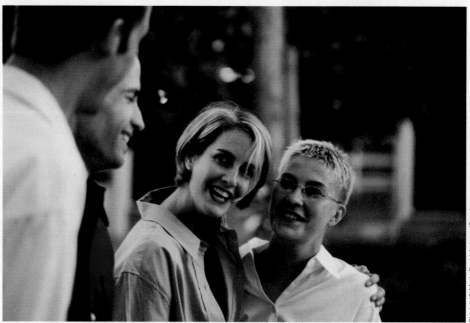

Attraction is based on a variety of physical and personality attributes.

I'm very involved with my church and want to wait to have sex until I'm married. I find it hard sometimes to meet people at school who share my views. Anyone I'd get involved with has to be religious.

I like them all. My partners have all been different. Looks don't matter that much to me. It's what's inside their head that counts.

Adjectives such as *nice* and *good* point to the subjectivity of attraction. Some of us have qualities that do not allow someone a chance. Some males refuse to get interested in females who are taller than they are, and some females refuse to get involved with males who are shorter. Gay men who work out with weights and value large muscles might ignore men who don't exercise regularly. And lesbians who present themselves with a natural, no-makeup face might reject a woman who uses cosmetics.

Research on partner choice and attraction leads to certain generalizations. Most people are drawn to partners from similar backgrounds and form relationships with people who are close in age, race, ethnicity, and social status. Table 10.1 presents findings from the National Health and Social Life Survey (NHSLS) conducted by the National Opinion Research Center (NORC), in which race, education, age, and religious background were found to be similar in a significant number of couples (Michael, Gagnon, Laumann, & Kolata, 1994).

The authors reported that about 90 percent of couples were of the same race. Having similar educational backgrounds was also the predominant pattern as individuals chose sexual partners. Men who had less than a high school education seldom had a partner who had gone to college, and men with a college degree almost never reported having sex with women who had much less or much more education than they did (Michael et al., 1994) Similarly, 81 percent of the women who did not finish high school chose men with a high school degree or less, and women who had graduate degrees reported never choosing partners who had not finished high school. Religion and age comparisons also yielded choices based on similarity. The authors of the NHSLS study concluded that couples with more marked differences in background tend to be the exception rather than the rule. Most people choose partners and marry someone who is the same race, same educational background, same religion, and within 5 years of their age.

Our society tends to be structured in segregated ways. Consequently, where you live, work, and with whom you socialize have an influence on your choice of partner (Michael, et al., 1994).

healthy sex hints 10.2

Tips for Assessing the Health of a Relationship

- Are you comfortable with yourself—know who you are, what you want, what you believe in? This is a critical first step toward being able to relate to others.
- When you're with this person, do you feel good about yourself? Are you complimented? Praised? Do you feel you receive a lot of support?
- Is your relationship based on shared interests? Are your personal values close enough in perspective to allow for becoming close? Do you have a sense of mutual respect?

- Can you tolerate differences? If you two are different, are those differences critical? For example, can your relationship surpass differences in age, race, sexual orientation, money, and political outlook?
- Can you maintain a sense of individuality within the relationship?

Table 10.1 Partnerships in Which the Two Partners Are Similar in Social Characteristics

Type of Similarity	Type of Partnership (%)			
	Marriage	Cohabitation	Long-term Noncohabiting	Short-term Noncohabiting
Racial/ethnic	93	88	89	91
Age	78	75	76	83
Educational	82	87	83	87
Religious	72	53	56	60

Notes: Observations are partnerships, including all sexually active partnerships in the past 12 months. Excluded are marriages or cohabitations that began more than 10 years before the interview date. Respondents with more than one sex partner in the past 12 months are represented more than once (up to a maximum of nine partnerships may be included for any one respondent). Short-term noncohabiting partnerships are those lasting less than 1 month and where no more than 10 sexual episodes occurred. Long-term noncohabiting partnerships include those lasting more than 1 month and/or involving more than 10 sexual episodes.

Age similarity is defined as no more than 5 years between partners' ages. *Educational similarity* is defined as a difference of no more than one educational category where the categories include less than high school, high school graduate, some college or vocational training, 4-year college, and graduate degree. Race/ethnicity categories include white, black, Hispanic, and Asian. Religions include none, mainline Protestant, conservative Protestant, and Catholic.

Source: Sex in America, by Robert T. Michael et al. Copyright © by CSG Enterprises, Inc., Edward O. Laumann, Robert T. Michael, and Gina Kolata. By permission of Little, Brown, and Company.

Problems of definition exist in overvaluing the NHSLS findings. The topic of race alone is so complicated that critics of traditional demography recommend dispensing with that social classification altogether. Anthropologists have documented hundreds of races, so to describe groups using a few traditional categories—white, black, Hispanic, Asian—is of limited value. For example, discussion of race has been part of many articles on pro golfer Tiger Woods; though some consider him "black," his background is so diverse that "multiracial" seems to be a more accurate description.

Attraction

Researchers have long concluded that people prefer romantic partners who are physically attractive and that there is some cultural consistency in what is deemed attractive (Berscheid & Walster, 1974; Dion & Dion, 1987; Hatfield & Sprecher, 1986). An image of the ideal female and male physique emerges from the media and advertising, and though it may be hard to attain in reality, the standard is set in many people's minds. How we each think we measure up to cultural ideals also may influence our sexual self-esteem. Are we acceptable? Are we attractive? We have found in our classes that just as students can identify what they find attractive in others, they can identify aspects of themselves they deem attractive, as well as characteristics they do not like. Individuals will become sexually healthier when they can accept themselves or make constructive changes that allow them to interact in a healthier way.

Research on attraction has indicated different values between the sexes. Males place more emphasis on physical attributes than females do. Females value interpersonal warmth, personality, and earning potential over appearance (Bailey, Gaulin, Agyei, & Gladue, 1994; Nevid, 1984; Sprecher, Sullivan, & Hatfield, 1994; Wiederman & Allgeier, 1992). Regardless, looks alone do not define attractiveness, nor can looks sustain a relationship. Most of us have admired someone for their looks only to discover that this person had a voice that detracted from their appearance or thoughts and values that we found objectionable, making that person unappealing after all. Over time, looks diminish in importance, as we develop loving feelings toward our partners and accept them "warts and all."

Social psychologist Donn Byrne (1971) developed a theory of attraction focusing on rewards and punishments. He postulated that we tend to like people who reward us by making us feel good about ourselves and tend to dislike people who punish us and are nasty. Researchers have also documented that people tend to be attracted to those who share similar attitudes on issues (Smith, Becker, Byrne, & Przybyla, 1993). Relationships can develop and function well when we get along with our partners. Although this point sounds like common sense, too many people invest time and energy in relationships that are not working, with people who do not treat them well, and where they do not feel good about themselves.

Environmental/Occupational Wellness

People today seem to spend more and more hours at work. Many students juggle classes and jobs. Consequently, the people one meets and spends a lot of time with can be classmates, coworkers, teachers, and employers. What continues to be a thorny question is whether people should become romantically involved with those at work. Prohibitions about workers becoming involved romantically may be included in sexual harassment policies. Colleges and universities also have such policies, dictating the acceptable parameters of romantic relationships. At work, romantic involvements may be permitted as long as the two involved are not in the same division or unit. At the university level, professors are not to get involved with those they grade and mentor. In reality, the prohibitions do not always prevail.

For LGBT (lesbian, gay, bisexual, transgendered) individuals, romantic relationships become more complicated. If one is "out" at work and school, secrecy and fear of reprisals can be minimal. Job discrimination based on gender and sexuality is outlawed in many states, yet harassment still occurs both overtly and subtly.

Our overall health is enhanced when we can share and be open about the positive love relationships we have.

Sexual Chemistry

Many times friends and family offer to "fix up" a person with someone they're "sure you'll like." A man may be told, "She's attractive, very nice, interested in a lot of different things." Or a woman may be told, "I have just the man for you! He's smart, handsome, talented, and has a great sense of humor." So, with such glowing testaments, they agree to a blind date. They go out. They have an OK time but can't see anything romantic developing. They don't disagree about their date's attributes; he or she is objectively attractive, has a nice personality, and so on, but just doesn't excite the other person. The explanation to the matchmaker is "Well, there was just no chemistry—no spark." Despite a host of attractive traits, chemistry may be lacking.

People respond to the smell of others, and bad breath may turn us off. Certain colognes, perfumes, and aftershaves are designed to turn us on. On an unconscious level, we may be responding to **pheromones,** which are sex-attractant chemicals, more familiar in lower animal forms. For example, a female dog "in heat" puts out an odor that male dogs can pick up from some distance. Even

Pheromones Body chemicals that attract potential sexual partners though human attraction is not grounded so heavily in reproductive issues, odors may have a larger role than previously thought (Kohl & Francouer, 1995).

Studies have begun to look at the impact of chemicals in male sweat and female vaginal secretions, examining their role in increasing attraction between a male and a female; their role in same-sex couples has yet to be assessed. The intense feelings associated with the early phases of a relationship, when we feel excited and caught up with the newness of the relationship, may have a chemical connection to higher levels of phenylethylamine (PEA) and possibly dopamine and norepinephrine, stimulants the body produces. As a consequence, we literally can be on a "romantic high" that can be explained through chemistry (Botting & Botting, 1996).

The general assumption about attraction is that one's sexual orientation will direct you toward the person of the appropriate sex. Lesbians will be with lesbians, gay men with other men, heterosexual men with women, and heterosexual women with men. Those identifying as bisexual become free to be attracted to both men and women.

In practice, however, such categories can be both misleading and complicated. The *New York Times* in October 2001 devoted its whole Sunday magazine section to exploring changes in love and relationships in the 21st century. The themes that were addressed brought to the public awareness topics not previously addressed in such a medium. To illustrate the complexities associated with the fluidity of sexual identity, personal health, and greater openness, the stories of various couplings were shared in detail. Individuals identified as lesbian reported falling in love with men, much to the chagrin of activist friends. A bisexual man, married to a woman, was open about his sexual affairs with other men (D'Erasmo, 2001). Another case described in detail was that of a lesbian who partnered with another woman, who later transitioned to a man. The lesbian struggled with her identity—in love with and now living with a man with whom she is having a family, albeit by donor insemination. The man has compromised his transitioning by having a double mastectomy, taking testosterone, but forgoing the genital modification known as phalloplasty. The mere cost of genital surgery, estimated to be in the realm of $50,000, was part of his decision as well (Corbett, 2001).

Compatibility

In the long run, what makes a relationship work is how compatible the two individuals are. A healthy relationship allows two people to be who they truly are, with no attempt to change their partners. The values and lifestyles of the two, therefore, must mesh closely.

Popular books abound, offering advice on finding the right partner and making the relationship work. Although the advice is plentiful, those providing it may base their guidance not on solid information but rather on their own perspectives. Clinical psychologists, for example, may develop advice after working with a variety of clients on their problems. Likewise, identifying patterns of behavior drawn by surveying college students has limitations.

Nonetheless, some of the "popular" authors can provide helpful, down-to-earth, practical advice. One author whose approach works well from a wellness model is Barbara DeAngelis (1992), author of *Are You the One for Me? Knowing Who's Right and Avoiding Who's Wrong.* DeAngelis advises her readers to develop a compatibility checklist along 10 dimensions, identifying qualities that are important to them in each category. When two people are in an actual relationship, assessing compatibility takes time, as some things are learned early in a relationship and others over a period of months, if not longer.

sex in society 10.2

Compatibility List

According to author Barbara DeAngelis (1992), "Your Compatibility List can help you understand what is and what isn't working between you and your mate, and make it easier to decide whether it's time to separate. If you're looking for a new relationship, your Compatibility List acts like a shopping list, directing you toward partners who are right for you and helping you avoid partners you don't need and who will be a waste of time." Here is her list:

Directions: Use the following 10 categories to identify qualities you possess and those you want in a partner. Being as specific as possible will make the list more useful. When comparing results, you need to keep in mind how flexible you can be, how frequently you need traits to be exhibited, and which aspects of a relationship may work even if you two don't match.

1. *Physical style:* appearance, eating habits, personal fitness habits, personal hygiene
   Example: I exercise regularly. I would want a partner who likes to work out and exercise.
2. *Emotional style:* attitudes toward romance and affection, expression of emotions, approach to relationships
   Example: I'm very affectionate and need a lot of support. I would want a partner who would be affectionate and care about my interests.
3. *Social style:* personality traits, ways of interacting with others
   Example: I'm very outgoing and love to have family and friends around. I would not want a partner who only wanted to be with me and stay at home.
4. *Intellectual style:* educational background, attitude toward learning, world affairs
   Example: I'm a college graduate and read the newspaper daily. I also love books, both fiction and nonfiction. I would want a partner who is aware of what is going on in the world and also loves to read. My partner would have to at least have an associate's degree, although I would prefer someone who has finished a 4-year college program.
5. *Sexual style:* attitudes, skill, ability to enjoy sex
   Example: I love to try new things and be adventurous. I would want a partner who enjoys sex and is creative.
6. *Communication style:* patterns of communication, attitude toward talking, other forms of expression
   Example: I know that I tend to scream when I'm angry.

My family is a bunch of screamers. While I may need to work on that behavior, I'd need someone who would understand that the screaming is more style than substance and wouldn't let the volume get to him [her].

7. *Professional/financial style:* relationship with money, attitudes toward success, work, and organizational habits
   Example: I work hard and budget my money carefully, never owing more than a couple hundred dollars on a credit card. I couldn't be with someone who gambles and is always in debt.
8. *Personal growth style:* attitudes toward self-improvement, ability to be introspective and change, willingness to work on a relationship
   Example: I tend to think a lot about what I value and how I came to be who I am. If a relationship is important to me, I would do anything—even seek professional help if necessary—to make it work. I wouldn't want a partner who couldn't look at how we were getting along and work on the relationship.
9. *Spiritual style:* attitudes toward a higher power, spiritual practices, philosophy of life, moral views
   Example: I'm very involved with my church, working with youth groups and helping at local shelters. My partner wouldn't have to be exactly the same faith but would have to respect my beliefs and have a sense of his or her own.
10. *Interests and hobbies*
    Example: I love to travel, and I do my best to take at least one exciting vacation to some place new each year. I would want a partner who also likes to travel, or at least would be willing to travel.

After reviewing your list, think about how open you are to changing any of your answers. If you are without a partner, thinking about your interests becomes valuable in assessing how well you two match. As you get to know someone, finding dissimilar answers and styles in too many areas highlights a lack of compatibility. Most important, not all areas are equally important.

Source: From *Are You the One for Me?* by Barbara DeAngelis Ph.D. Used by permission of Dell Publishing, a division of Random House, Inc.

Maintaining Healthy Relationships

In plain language, a healthy relationship is one that is good for you. Finding a compatible partner is part of the process, yet the number of relationships that break up and marriages that end in divorce indicate that initial assessments can change or be wrong in the first place.

Relationships that are good for you make you happy most of the time. They are fun, serve as sources of strength and support, and provide connections that improve the quality of your life. You can be who you are and be appreciated for your uniqueness. If you are unhappy, depressed, sad, and feeling that you are hiding your true self, those feelings should serve as a barometer to the health of the relationship. As with Jessica, in Case Study 10.2 (see page 310), it is not easy to recognize what is really going on between two people. Putting your needs and self aside to "keep a relationship going" is not good, as it fosters imbalance of power and interest in the relationship. Other people often can identify relationships as unhealthy when those in the relationship cannot.

Physical and Emotional Wellness

Relationships enhance physical and emotional wellness in a variety of ways. Being in love energizes a person and may actually boost the immune system. Because the partners want to please each other, they may take better care of themselves. Emotional health is aided by involvement with others. As young children, most of us learn to trust and form loving relationships. As we get older, we have the opportunity to develop our own partner relationships. Having someone with whom to share thoughts and feelings, who will love us for who we are, who can give constructive feedback and support—all contribute to emotional well-being.

Having intimate relationships usually means that someone is physically there for us, sharing daily experiences and also caring for us. Traditional marriage vows speak to "in sickness and in health"; couples in commitment ceremonies also vow to be there for each other in the good times and bad. A partner can help the other be healthier as well as manage illnesses that come along.

Plenty of evidence also indicates that unhealthy relationships can have a negative impact on physical and emotional well-being. Being stressed about a relationship, depressed about a partner, being the recipient of anger, and so forth, affect not only mood but our physical bodies as well. Individuals may find that they have difficulty eating, sleeping, and concentrating, and in order to find solutions to relationship problems, they need to seek out professional help, in the form of both counseling and medication.

Jealousy

Feelings of jealousy, particularly if out of control and increasingly intense, can spell the end of a relationship. The news too often announces murders committed by a jealous lover, current or from the past. Jealousy can result from a number of factors: low self-esteem, fear of loss, bruised pride, insecurity, and, in some cases, a sense of "lost property" (Hatfield & Rapson, 1996). Individuals may react with feelings of jealousy in response to behaviors they find threatening. For example, a woman may get upset at seeing her boyfriend be kissed by a female friend. Another woman may not care about gestures of affection but not be able to handle a current boyfriend even having a cup of coffee with a woman he used to date.

Let's Have Some Fun Together

An important element of a healthy relationship is laughing and having playful, fun times together. Some experts believe that when a couple stops laughing together, this signals trouble in the relationship. It takes creativity and work to make sure you do interesting activities that strengthen a relationship. The purpose of this activity is to develop a creative list of interesting things to do with a date or your partner so you can keep the joy in your relationship.

Your goal is to make a list of 30 activities that you would enjoy doing with a date or partner. They should not be expensive and should be easily accessible—you should not have to travel great distances to do these. First, list as many as you can think of that you would enjoy. Once you have exhausted your own ideas, start interviewing your friends and acquaintances to see what they can add to your list. Only add those that you would really like to do. When you have interviewed as many people as possible, share your list with your partner and put a check by those activities your partner would also enjoy doing. Decide which ones you want to do first and try to add one new activity each week. If you are not in a relationship at the present time, try these with your dates or with your friends. You should experience more laughter and enjoyment in your times together.

Men and women have been found to respond to feelings of jealousy in different ways. Jealous women are more likely to focus on the emotional involvement of their partner with another person, whereas men may focus on the sexual activity of their partner with another person. Researchers continue to find gender differences in how distressing infidelity becomes to the relationship, with women identifying emotional infidelity as the most distressing and men choosing sexual infidelity (Cann, Mangum, & Wells, 2001; Buss, Larse, Westen, & Semmelroth, 1992). Men are more likely to respond with rage and violence, and women are more likely to blame themselves and display more possessive behavior (Hatfield & Rapson, 1996).

When asked in a classroom setting, college students have voiced the opinion that some amount of jealousy is good for a relationship and shows love for the partner. In actuality, the foundation for jealous feelings is not based on love, nor are these feelings likely to be healthy for a relationship. The survival of a relationship can be connected to how each partner handles infidelity. Students are more inclined to refer to someone "cheating on them." When asked in a human sexuality class, "How many of you living on campus know of individuals who are sexually involved here yet have a boyfriend/girlfriend back home?" The response is embarrassed laughter with comments of "Oh, lots of people 'cheat.' This is college." At the same time, if the partner at home discovers the infidelity, the relationship may or may not survive. And, of course, discovering that your partner has had sex with someone else because of a newly diagnosed STD can certainly intensify reactions.

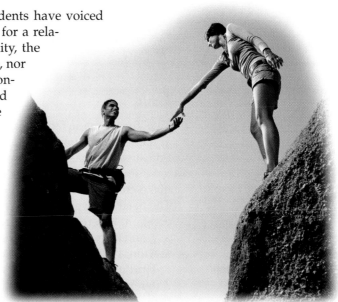

Shared interests are important to a relationship.

Ian Logan/GettyImages

307

Critical Thinking

When couples get into a cycle of an on-again/off-again relationship, what can help them figure out whether to stay together?

Use your Virtual Workbook to explore your answer to this question at **http://health.wadsworth.com/blonna1.**

case study 10.2

Jessica: "Finding My True Love"

Jessica, 31, is white.

Jessica, now engaged to be married, shares the journey of finding the right partner:

I used to be a real romantic. There was one true love "out there somewhere" for me. I am much more grounded in the realities of relationships today than I used to be, but there is still nothing to match those intense feelings of love for someone.

My first true love was Tim. We met at a party senior year of high school and dated each other exclusively from that moment on, spending Christmas with each other's families, going out alone or with friends every weekend, and sharing a very romantic senior prom. Graduation was both joyous and sad, as we had to face the prospect of separation, with each of us going away to different colleges.

We talked about our feelings for each other and decided we wouldn't date anybody else at our respective schools. We called frequently, saw each other on vacations, and spent the summer together. I still get knots in my stomach thinking about the summer after junior year. One week Tim said he loved me. The next he wasn't sure. We would fight. I would cry. He would apologize. We'd be fine for a while, and then the cycle would start up again. My parents tried not to interfere, but they could see how miserable I was. At the end of August, we decided to break up and date other people.

Tim and I became one of those on-again/off-again couples. I always loved him and hoped we'd get married. He was never sure. After college he accepted a job in California and asked me to live with him. I followed him west, attended graduate school, and was sure that our being together would solidify the relationship. We had our ups and downs, but I kept thinking that things would work out. He was transferred to Chicago, and after I graduated, I followed him there. We lived together for a year, and then Tim broke off the relationship. I had really been miserable with him for a long time, taking a lot of emotional abuse and neglect. I had few friends, low self-esteem, and most of the affection I received was from our dog.

That was a few years ago. The memories are very strong, yet finally the anger has subsided. I was angry at Tim. And angry with myself. As the saying goes, I "couldn't see the forest for the trees." I invested a lot of time with one person and lost myself too much in the process.

I am now with Mark. We, too, have had our ups and downs, a temporary hiatus from being a couple, but now we're engaged. I am honest about my feelings, I am independent yet want to be part of a couple, we each have our own and shared group of friends, and we truly want the same lifestyle.

Am I still a romantic? In some ways, yes. But I've also learned that good relationships don't "just happen." Both people work at it.

Love

Tina Turner made famous a song with the lyrics "What's love got to do with it?" The emotion of love is tied closely to our emotions and expectations from relationships and has been a topic for songwriters and researchers. Studies on love have attempted to classify the emotion, develop theory, examine love styles, make cross-cultural comparisons, and recognize the complexity of the emotion. The need to love a partner is important for individuals, regardless of sexual orientation. Whereas U.S. culture so often has focused on heterosexual love, lesbian, gay, and bisexual adults also share the need to develop loving relationships (Aron & Aron, 1991; Peplau & Cochran, 1988).

Finding a comfortable definition of love is not easy. Some advise of the need to differentiate "love" and "lust." Others talk about being able to tell the difference between "love" and "infatuation." Hatfield and Rapson (1996) distinguish between passionate love and companionate love. **Passionate love** has an intense quality, in which the individual can feel lovesick, head-over-heels in love, and to-

Passionate love Feelings characterized by intense longing for another, infatuation, ecstasy when reciprocated, and emptiness when not shared by the other tally infatuated. There is an obsessive focus, intense longing, and, if reciprocated, a sense of fulfillment and ecstasy.

In contrast, **companionate love** is what we ideally experience as relationships endure. It is characterized by feelings of deep attachment, commitment, and intimacy. Companionate love encompasses feelings of affection and tenderness we feel for those with whom our lives are deeply connected.

Companionate love
Feelings that include deep attachment, commitment, and intimacy

Theories of Love   Robert Sternberg (1986) has developed a theoretical model for examining love. Shown in Figure 10.3, love is conceptualized as a triangle with three faces: passion, intimacy, and commitment. Each person within a love relationship brings his or her triangle to that relationship, albeit with varying dimensions. When two people are well matched, they tend to find satisfaction within their relationship.

Sternberg identifies six different kinds of love that evolve in response to the varying dimensions:

Liking—Intimacy only, such as may be found between friends
Infatuation—Passion only, with high physical and emotional attraction
Romantic love—A combination of intimacy and passion, similar to liking with the addition of physical attraction
Companionate love—A combination of intimacy and commitment; may have had romantic components, but the key element is the emotional bond between the two people.
Fatuous love—A combination of passion and commitment, which may lead to two people quickly living together but over time realizing that they lack a deep, emotional intimacy
Consummate love—Ideal love, combining passion, intimacy, and commitment. Though we may strive to achieve this, it is hard to sustain over time.

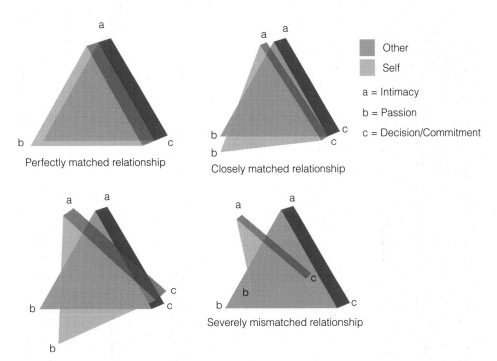

Figure 10.3 *Sternberg's Triangular Theory of Love*
Source: Sternberg, R. (1986) A triangular theory of love. *Psychological Review, 93,* 119–35.
Sternberg R. (1988) Triangular love. In R. Sternberg and M. Barnes (eds.) *The Psychology of Love.* New Haven, CT: Yale Univ. Press.

Another typology for examining styles of love is credited to John Lee (Lee, 1974). Recognizing that some styles can be combined, Lee describes six styles of love:

Eros—Focuses on physical beauty and has a strong sensual component
Mania—Characterized by a lot of roller-coaster emotions, with anxiety and ecstasy at the extremes
Ludus—Love for fun and play—nothing too serious
Storge—Marked by much affection, gradually deepening into love
Agape—Type of love that is undemanding, patient, and does not expect reciprocation
Pragma—Practical love; lovers carefully assess compatibility in background, values, and interest to find a good match.

Anthropologists provide us with data from other cultures, indicating that love and strong feelings of attraction may almost be universal emotions. Helen Fisher (1993), a popular anthropologist and author, posits that the human animal may have evolved with feelings of attraction that are somewhat time limited. Romantic love tends to wane after a 4-year period, which she claims matches the amount of time it takes to rear a child beyond infancy. Divorce statistics, as well as her study of 62 cultures around the world, lend support to her theory that couples stay together for a period of time and then may get interested in forming new partnerships.

Researchers have found differences in love styles based on gender (Hendrick, Foote, & Slapion-Foote, 1984). In a survey of an extremely diverse group of college students, females tended to be more manic, storgic, and pragmatic than males, who seemed more ludic and erotic. Women were found to be more conservative in their views toward love and relationships, incorporating concerns over finding a mate who would be a good provider and partner. Males, on the other hand, tended to respond early on to beauty and the playful aspects of relationships, and they were less concerned with commitment.

From Theory to Practice   Most of us want to find a partner with whom we can make a relationship work. Not all relationships function in exactly the same way, yet some characteristics predict a greater likelihood of "success." The style of love may change as people age. The style of love may improve with experience. The style of love may interfere with one's getting into and sustaining the kind of relationship desired. Recognizing your values, style, and how well you "match" to your partner, therefore, becomes valuable as you seek out love and a partner.

Research and therapeutic practice have yielded insights into the variety of relationships couples create and sustain. Lonnie Barbach (2001) writes about the use of power in relationships, with each partner needing to carve out areas of control. Individuals can use "forceful power" in which needs and wants are stated, asked for, and in some cases demanded. In contrast, individuals can also use "withholding power," in which love and nurturance are withheld. For intimate relationships to be successful, neither form of power is desirable. Individuals can use their power around how money is spent, with whom the couple or each individual in the couple socializes, and even around sexual contact. Meeting one person's needs can be viewed as purposely disregarding the other's needs, and a power struggle ensues with misunderstandings, anger, and resentment. The power relationship between the couple impacts their love and commitment. Those who can successfully negotiate differing needs develop healthier and happier relationships (Barbach, 2001).

Pepper Schwartz (2001) has identified many myths about successful relationships that warrant being questioned. A few examples are "You can't be in love with two people at the same time," "Little annoying habits are unimportant in long-term relationships," and "You should always be 100 percent honest with your partner." Because human relationships are complex, she takes issues with commonly held guidelines governing behavior.

Loving more than one person can happen as we commit to a partner yet hold loving feelings for a past partner; deciding to act on those feelings is different from having them. When couples date, they may not mind that one person is neat while the other messy; living in a home with two very different styles of where to place clothes, papers, and other items or different attitudes toward personal hygiene may prove more challenging than they had when dating. Finally, although most people feel that honesty in a relationship is fundamental to building trust and intimacy, Schwartz argues that there are times when information may need to be kept secret for the health of the relationship. Individuals are entitled to some areas of privacy, and partners may really only want to know information that they can deal with. Schwartz does caution that there are times, however, when keeping secrets can be destructive to the relationship. For example, if one person had unsafe sex outside the relationship, putting their partner's health in jeopardy, getting medical attention and discussing the situation are imperative. If real feedback is needed about behaviors such as drinking, the intimate partner is in an ideal situation to provide it. And for those for whom honesty is viewed as the key component of the relationship, keeping secrets from a partner is fundamentally incompatible with maintaining an intimate relationship.

Sexual Activity Within Relationships

We examined adult choices about sexual behaviors in greater detail in Chapter 6. In the context of relationships, individuals decide on preferences for particular behaviors, frequency of activity, and whether their behavior will occur exclusively with one partner. Research on the timing of sexual activity has often been framed with a heterosexual and marital bias. Hence, students can find reports on **premarital sex,** coitus occurring before marriage, and **extramarital sex,** coitus occurring outside of marriage. The demographics in the United States, however, indicate that there are currently more unmarried adults than at other times in history, with an estimated three-quarters of unmarried men and two-thirds of unmarried women engaging in some form of partnered sex over the course of a year (Waite & Joyner, 2001). Consequently, making marriage as the central core from which other situations vary can be problematic.

Because of such realities, terms that are more generic and focus on the primary relationship become preferred. The term **monogamy** by strict definition refers to the practice of having one spouse at a time, but more commonly it refers to having one sexual partner. Despite much of the research on sexual behavior outside the primary relationship using the term *extramarital,* the terms **dyadic,** referring to the couple, and **extradyadic,** referring to sexual activity with someone other than the primary partner, are preferred and considered to be less biased (Wiederman, 2001a).

In drawing conclusions from research, definitions become important. What is "sex"? What makes someone a "partner"? And how do individuals categorize their sexual activity within their relationships? For example, a young couple can regularly engage in mutual oral sex yet report that they have "not engaged in premarital sex." Because gay and lesbian couples have been unable to marry, engaging in "premarital sex" is not even possible.

Christopher and Sprecher (2000) reviewed years of research focused on sexuality within relationships. As couples were together longer, whether married or in long-term gay and lesbian relationships, there was a decline in the frequency with which they engaged in lovemaking. Researchers also found that sexual satisfaction is associated with relationship satisfaction, regardless of the sexual orientation of the couple. Cohabiting couples and those dating had slightly lower lev-

Premarital sex Usually refers to coitus, sexual intercourse, before marriage

Extramarital sex Usually refers to coitus, sexual intercourse, outside marriage

Monogamy Commonly used to refer to having one sexual partner, whether married to that person or not

Dyadic sex Referring to the sexual behavior of a couple, the two people in a relationship

Extradyadic sex Referring to sexual behavior outside the primary relationship. This term replaces *extramarital sex,* which is confined to heterosexual marriages.

els of sexual satisfaction when compared with married couples. Factors such as race, religion, and social status were not related to the frequency of sexual activity or sexual satisfaction.

Waite and Joyner (2001), in analyzing data from the National Health and Social Life Survey, propose that couples bring different expectations about sex to their relationships depending on whether they are married, cohabiting, or dating. For married individuals, there is a long-term contract with each being able to learn what pleases the other; satisfying a spouse enhances the emotional component of the relationship. Cohabiters have a lower level of commitment to each other and may not feel as compelled to develop partner-specific skills. Single individuals may be dating more than one person, aware that a long-term relationship may or may not be possible, yet the connection may be sexual regardless. Overall, viewing a relationship to be long-term, being emotionally invested in it, and being sexually exclusive were hypothesized to increase emotional satisfaction and physical pleasure from sex. As with other research, commitment becomes an important variable for both men and women when examining their emotional satisfaction with the relationship. The researchers found that physical pleasure and emotional satisfaction were higher when the sex was used to express love for the partner.

Never-married, young adults can and do decide to remain virgins. Primarily, researchers have identified that young adults may not feel that enough love is present in the relationship, they express a fear of sexually transmitted diseases and unwanted pregnancies, their belief system supports virginity, and/or personal feelings of insecurity and inadequacy interfere with experiencing coitus (Christopher & Sprecher, 2000). What is critical is that decisions to be sexually active involve mutual consent and comfort. For some, a solid, committed relationship is key.

Because there are strong social sanctions against extradyadic sex, it can be difficult to assess its prevalence. Asking whether a person has been "unfaithful" or "has cheated on his or her partner" may affect research findings. When students in our human sexuality classes have been asked, "How many of you know couples who claim to be monogamous yet date more than one person? For example, have a girlfriend/boyfriend at home, but go out up here at school?" the majority of hands go up. At times students have added, "Oh, everyone cheats," or "We're too young to be that committed." Once marriage is thrown in, however, there seems to be less willingness to approve of multiple partners.

healthy sex hints 10.3
Guidelines for Healthy Relationships

Both people in a relationship have the right to

Ask for what they want.
Be accepted for who they are.
Be treated with respect.
Express their thoughts and feelings.
Not be forced to do anything.
Feel safe when alone with each other.
Give and receive expressions of affection.
Make some mistakes and be forgiven.
Say no and not feel guilty.
Have fun.

No one in the relationship has the right to

Tell the other person where and when he or she can go out.
Act like a boss and order the other person around.
Degrade and humiliate the other person, in either public or private.
Isolate the other from friends and family.
Pressure the other to give up interests and goals.
Read the partner's personal materials without permission, search private property, or follow the other around.
Physically intimidate and harm the other person.

Researchers have attempted to determine rates of extradyadic sexual activity, yet there are problems with definitions and the meanings of the behavior to the participants (Wiederman, 2001a). Clearly, our students based their responses on observations and impressions of their peer group. Formal researchers have looked at married and cohabiting couples, and although those who cohabit have higher rates of extradyadic sex than married couples, and the rates for married couples in contemporary studies are relatively low, there are still significant numbers of people who have had sex with someone other than their spouse at least once. The variables found to be associated with more permissive extramarital attitudes are high education, low religiosity, premarital sexual permissiveness, and being male (Christopher & Sprecher, 2000).

Abusive Relationships

Patterns of physical and mental abuse are obvious markers of an unhealthy relationship. Both forms of abuse may develop slowly but tend to increase as the relationship becomes more involved. Being put down, insulted, blamed for a partner's problems ("It's your fault. . . ."), pushed, shoved, or beaten are all forms of abuse.

Abuse often begins in the dating relationship, with intimate partner violence recognized as a significant public health problem. Rates of dating violence among high school and college students is reported to be between 9 and 41 percent, depending on definitions of abuse and methods of sampling (Freedner, Freed, Yang, & Austin, 2002). Lesbian, gay, bisexual, and transgendered youth when abused have the added threat of being "outed" to others who may not know of their sexual orientation. In a study of adolescents Freedner et al. found that sexual orientation in general did not make a difference as to whether dating violence occurred. However, bisexual males were more than five times more likely and bisexual females more than four times more likely to be threatened with "outing" compared to their gay and lesbian peers. Lesbians had greater odds of being scared for their safety compared to heterosexual females (Freedner et al., 2002). Cruz (2002) argues that for gay men, incidences of abuse may not even be accurately remembered, as violence is part of gendered socialization—that is, men get angry, and that anger is often expressed in violent ways.

Typically, the abuser has been abused him- or herself and has learned inappropriate ways of dealing with feelings of anger and frustration. Some abusers have violent personalities, and others have no respect for their partner's right to think and behave independently. Some of the warning signs that a person may be violent include the following:

Loss of temper on a daily basis
Frequent physical fighting
Significant vandalism or property damage
Increase in the use of drugs or alcohol
Increase in risk-taking behavior
Detailed plans to commit acts of violence
Announcing threats or plans for hurting others
Enjoying hurting animals
Carrying a weapon

Further warning signals include gang membership, threatening others regularly, trouble controlling feelings of anger, feeling constantly disrespected, and failing to acknowledge the feelings or rights of others (American Psychological Association, 2003).

Regardless, without the abusive person's getting professional help and being willing to change, the abuse will continue and the "relationship" will be between an abuser and a victim, rather than two adults in a healthy relationship. Shelters exist across the United States for victims of domestic violence, with women over-whelmingly being those at greatest risk. Although those outside a violent relationship may wonder why a victim "doesn't just leave," professionals in the field know that financial dependency, children, and fear make such flight difficult. Statistics support the fact that when a woman chooses to leave, she is at the most vulnerable point for becoming a victim of violence and possibly murder (Francese, 2001).

At the same time, those who recognize their violent tendencies can work to learn to control violent urges and develop healthier ways to relate to those they claim to care about. Breathing exercises can help the individual learn to relax when angered. Talking to oneself with such ideas as "I'm not going to let him/her get to me" and "Calm down" can be useful. It is critical that violent individuals learn what sets them off and develop appropriate ways to diffuse their angry reactions (American Psychological Association, 2003).

Sexual Orientation and Relationships

Love and relationships among gay, lesbian, and bisexual adults have been subject to many myths. Perhaps one of the biggest problems lies in the secrecy involved. To be open about the relationship poses barriers that heterosexual couples seldom face. This translates into day-to-day losses such as relating stories of weekend fun with coworkers on Monday and the larger risk of losing one's job if coworkers find out about the gay or lesbian orientation. As José explains in Case Study 10.3, there can be a heavy emotional price to pay for having to keep a love relationship secret from friends and family.

Research comparing heterosexual couples and gay and lesbian couples has revealed some differences, although the similarities, such as valuing communication, sharing experiences, and laughing together, far outweigh the differences identified. The differences in values one brings to a love relationship are tied more closely to gender than sexual orientation (Peplau, 1981; Metz, Rosser, & Strapko, 1994). Similarly, gender was a more significant variable when examining differences in styles of conflict resolution. Overall, lesbians were found to make greater efforts to resolve conflicts and do so with less physical and verbal aggression compared to gay and heterosexual couples (Metz et al., 1994).

Perhaps because gay and lesbian marriages aren't sanctioned, or perhaps in response to the realization that gender role stereotyping is problematic when both partners are of the same sex, same-sex relationships tend to reject the traditional marriage model. (Increasingly, though, heterosexuals aren't following that model, either.) Compared to heterosexual couples, gay and lesbian relationships are more egalitarian, sharing household responsibilities and finances (Peplau, 1981).

Another reported difference has been greater openness to sexual relationships outside the primary one, although that pattern is more prevalent among gay men than lesbian women. The ability to separate sex and love theoretically diminishes feelings of jealousy. It could be easily argued, however, that couples who have an emotional investment in each other do not welcome outside involvements, regardless of sexual orientation.

Breaking Up and Ending Relationships

Just as relationships can be formed in healthy ways, they can be ended in ways that are not destructive. When feelings are mutual, both parties realize that the relationship is not working, and the breakup may not be as difficult. The experience of having a partner break up with you without your awareness of any problems, however, is quite another matter. Ending a relationship in any case is emotionally difficult and painful for most of us.

case study 10.3

José and Marco

José, 26, identifies as Latino American.

I'm the only son in my family and until recently was the middle child. My older sister was married, and my younger one is single. When my older sister died, my younger sister Selena and I felt increased pressure from our parents to provide grandchildren. My mother, in particular, is very religious and goes to church every day. She prays for her family, and her faith helped her deal with my sister's death. Now she prays to be blessed with a grandchild. Only one of us is going to be able answer those prayers—and Selena doesn't even have a boyfriend.

I get angry at my situation sometimes and realize that things might be easier if I would come out to my parents. On the other hand, my mother is very religious, and the church hasn't been all that welcoming. My father never gets into deep conversations, and I fear his disappointment. They've met Marco but just think he's one of my good friends. Since they live in Texas and I'm in San Francisco, it's easier to maintain the lie. Marco and I have caller ID on the phone, so we usually can tell who's calling before answering. The "right" person answers the phone.

My parents think I live alone and just have had little success dating women. I took a female friend to my senior prom, but other than her, I've never introduced my family to a girlfriend. They seem to be comfortable accepting my stories, although my mother tells me I should "settle down" and make a family.

When my sister died, it was hard to go home and not have Marco with me. And it continues to be hard to visit family without my partner. Straight people don't have to play these games. I'm getting sick of the secrets and know that I cut myself off from family because I expect them not to like me if they knew. I may be wrong, but I'm just not ready to take the risk.

Critical Thinking

If José were with a woman rather than a man, what are some of the specific ways his story might be different?

Use your Virtual Workbook to explore your answer to this question at **http://health.wadsworth.com/blonna1.**

Romantic relationships end for a myriad of reasons. For college students, the reasons may include being too busy with academics and sports or music commitments, transferring schools and being apart, finding someone new who excites you and with whom you want to get involved, getting pressure from family because a partner is of an "unacceptable background," and other reasons. Sometimes a health crisis tests a relationship, and where one partner expected support, none was forthcoming. Whatever the reason, for at least one of the partners, the relationship wasn't working.

healthy sex hints 10.4

Unhealthy Behaviors After Ending a Relationship

Though some behaviors can be expected following a breakup, others become increasingly problematic if they persist. If the breakup is disrupting your life, get some help from a counselor or therapist. These symptoms indicate a problem:

Sleeping too much or too little
Using drugs and alcohol excessively
Inability to eat
Inability to concentrate on work

Inability to study
Wanting to drop classes
Wanting to drop out of school
Driving recklessly
Making harassing phone calls to the ex-partner
Following the ex-partner around
Harassing an ex-partner's new boyfriend or girlfriend
Being violent toward the old partner or his or her property
Wanting to commit murder or suicide

As examined earlier in Chapter 6, divorce rates in the United States remain high. Although it may seem ironic that couples entering their second, third, or even fourth marriages do so with great fanfare and formal vows, remarriage after divorce is not uncommon. Somehow "in sickness and health, 'til death do us part" doesn't have the same validity it did decades ago. Nonetheless, ending a long-term relationship can be accompanied by depression, illness, and cycles of grief that mimic those associated with a loved one's death. In point of fact, some "ends" to relationship have included murder and murder/suicide.

For college students dealing with the end of a relationship, it may be important to seek help from campus counseling centers. Whereas some students seem able to accept the end of the relationship, and move on, others find it extremely difficult to continue with their studies. College students may also need to seek counseling when their parents divorce and/or remarry. Some parents wait until their children are out of the house before initiating separation and divorce. Universities recognize the need to provide psychological health services to students. Academic success can certainly be compromised by the energy diverted from studying to healing "a broken heart" or managing the array of emotions connected to seeing loved ones end their relationship.

Spiritual Wellness

Feelings of love and connectedness go hand in hand with spiritual wellness. To be able to be yourself and be loved for who you are contributes to our spiritual needs. The intensity of love feelings becomes apparent when we experience loss. "Loss of a loved one" is rated the highest mean measuring personal stress, and the emptiness we feel highlights how much the loved one contributed to our lives.

Depending on why a relationship ended (such as mutual change in interests, divorce, death, and the like), our emotional responses can vary. Nonetheless, it is a time to reflect on ourselves, who and what are important in our lives, and how we plan to move on. Our spiritual health is enhanced when we develop and maintain intimate relationships with family and friends as well as partners.

Personal Assessment

10.1 How Jealous Are You?

One feeling that often causes conflict between two people is jealousy, perhaps because men and women often experience and express jealousy in different ways. If partners are unable to communicate openly about an issue, a conflict may result. The following exercise is designed to help bring to light your experiences with jealousy so you may better understand yourself and your partner. If you currently do not have a partner, simply respond to the questions in terms of your last relationship or a hoped-for future one.

Directions:

Read each statement carefully, then respond yes or no in the blank following the statement.

1. You have found at times that you actually like feeling jealous. _____
2. Your spells of jealousy seem to follow a pattern, one after another. _____
3. Sometimes you get so jealous you lose your appetite or overeat. _____
4. When you hear about, or think about, your partner's former lovers, you are jealous. _____
5. You avoid close relationships with people other than your partner because such situations may cause your partner to be jealous. _____
6. You are very jealous of your partner's friends, yet you tell people you are not the jealous type. _____
7. You are apt to display fits of jealousy with no apparent cause. _____
8. You are often jealous of your partner's friends even when you know your partner has no romantic feelings toward them. _____
9. At social gatherings you are aware of every move your partner makes. _____
10. Jealousy has led you to spy on your partner. _____
11. You want to know where your partner is at all times. _____
12. It would definitely be a crisis if you were to discover that your partner had one sexual encounter with another person. _____
13. The feeling of loneliness is common to you. _____
14. You have thought of taking revenge on a person you felt was a rival. _____
15. You feel that jealousy is proof of your love for your partner. _____
16. You are jealous of your partner's hobbies. _____

Scoring:

If you have responded yes to more than five of these statements, you are allowing jealousy to control your life. To continue in this way is to leave yourself open to considerable pain and anguish. When jealousy arises, talk about it and reaffirm your commitment to your partner. You need to listen to each other.

Reactions:

Use the space provided to respond to the following questions.

1. Which statements, to which you responded yes, are of most concern to you? After discussing them with a friend or partner, explain what you plan to do differently.

2. Do you feel you are trying to control this person who is important to you? Why or why not?

Source: Your Sexuality: A Self Assessment (2nd ed.), by R. Valois and S. Kammermann, New York: McGraw-Hill, 1992, pp. 111–112. Reprinted with permission.

Thought Questions

1. What is intimacy? How can a person be intimate but not have sex with a partner or have sex with someone but not be intimate?

2. What are three barriers to intimacy? Does gender role impact on our ability to form intimate relationships? If so, how?

3. Explain Sternberg's model of love.

4. Give an example of a love mismatch, according to Sternberg.

5. How does romantic love differ from consummate love?

6. What are three characteristics of happy couples?

7. What are three common problems that lead to breakups and divorce?

Test Yourself!

1. Intimacy is characterized by all but which of the following qualities?
   a. Honesty
   b. Controlled emotions
   c. Openness
   d. Trust

2. Intimate friendships and intimate romantic relationships
   a. both enhance our social health.
   b. both have an erotic component.
   c. essentially induce the same emotional responses in the participants.
   d. differ substantially in their expectations of openness.

3. Which of the following statements about shyness is true?
   a. It is common for most people to feel shy at some point or other.
   b. People who are shy have low self-esteem and need professional help.
   c. Most people who are shy feel that way in all situations.
   d. Some levels of shyness help foster intimate relationships.

4. Laws and public policies have been put into place to prevent dating
   a. between two students in the same class.
   b. between supervisors and employees at work.
   c. between athletes on the same team.
   d. between two adults more than 5 years apart in age.

5. Marla met Chuck in a chat room, and they then began an online relationship. After a month, they decided that they wanted to meet face-to-face. They should follow all but which of the following pieces of advice?
   a. Let a friend know where they've gone and when they will return.
   b. Find a quiet place to be alone so that they can get to know each other.
   c. Take a cell phone.
   d. Have their own means of transportation.

6. Research on partner choice indicates that most people choose someone
   a. of a higher socioeconomic class so that there is more money to live on.
   b. regardless of the person's background, as long as there is compatibility.
   c. within a 10-year age differential, older or younger.
   d. of the same race and religion.

7. Research on attraction has revealed
   a. lesbians are only attracted to other lesbians.
   b. most men prefer large-breasted women.
   c. variations in what and who is perceived as attractive.
   d. similarities in what gay and straight men find attractive.

8. Being compatible with a partner means
   a. you share all the same values.
   b. you find each other physically attractive.
   c. you share similar values, interests, and goals.
   d. you have the same level of education.

9. John and Karen have been dating for 1 year. Prior to John, Karen dated Carlos and has remained friends with him. John is jealous. According to research, what best explains John's feelings of jealousy?
   a. Carlos is very attractive.
   b. John also likes Carlos.
   c. Karen had been sexually involved with Carlos.
   d. Karen had been in love with Carlos.

10. Theories of love are useful to couples in that they
    a. recognize different styles of love and attachment.
    b. guide couples on how to love each other.
    c. provide a framework for understanding couple behavior.
    d. teach the individual how to become a loving partner.

Media Menu

You can link to the following online tools by visiting
http://health.wadsworth.com/blonna1.

Face to Face Video

Our panel discusses intimacy within their different partnerships.

Animation

Sternberg's Triangular Theory of Love

 InfoTrac Activity

Boo, K. (2003, August 18). The marriage cure. *New Yorker, 79*(23), 105.

 Web Resources

Go Ask Alice

www.goaskalice.columbia.edu

This site is sponsored by the Columbia University Health Service yet will answer questions mailed from anywhere.

Students will find the answers to questions about love and relationships, conflicting feelings, and other topics.

Planned Parenthood

www.teenwire.com

Sponsored by Planned Parenthood, teens and young adults can write in for information about all aspects of sexuality, including concerns about relationships.

Resource Directory for Internet Dating Sites

www.internetdating.net

The site leads the user to a variety of options from regional and international sites to religious and singles' travel sites. Each category provides a list of links.

American Association of Sex Educators, Counselors, and Therapists

www.aasect.org

Professional certifying organization that provides links to professional help nationwide.

References

American Psychological Association. (2003). *Warning signs: Fight for your rights: Take a stand against violence.* Pamphlet. Washington, DC: Author.

Aron, A., & Aron, E. (1991). Love and sexuality. In K. McKinney & S. Sprecher (Eds.), *Sexuality in close relationships.* Hillsdale, NJ: Erlbaum.

Bailey, J., Gaulin, S., Agyei, Y., & Gladue, B. (1994). Effects of gender and sexual orientation on evolutionary relevant aspects of human mating psychology. *Journal of Personality and Social Psychology, 66,* 1091–1093.

Barbach, L. (2001). *For each other: Sharing sexual intimacy.* New York: Penguin.

Berscheid, E., & Walster, W. (1974). Physical attractiveness. In L. Berkowitz (Ed.), *Advances in experimental social psychology* (Vol. 7). New York: Academic Press.

Botting, D., & Botting, K. (1996). *Sex appeal.* New York: St. Martin's.

Buss, D. M., Larse, R. J., Westen, D., & Semmelroth, J. (1992). Sex differences in jealousy: Evolution, physiology, and psychology. *Psychological Science, 3,* 251–255.

Byrne, D. (1971). *The attraction paradigm.* New York: Academic Press.

Cann, A., Mangum, J., & Wells, M. (2001, August). Distress in response to relationship infidelity: The roles of gender and attitudes about relationships. *Journal of Sex Research, 38*(3), 185–190.

Christopher, F. S., & Sprecher, S. (2000, November). Sexuality in marriage, dating, and other relationships: A decade review. *Journal of Marriage and the Family, 62,* 999–1017.

Corbett, S. (2001, October 14). When Debbie met Christina, who then became Chris. *New York Times Magazine,* Section 6, pp. 84–87.

Cruz, J. M. (2002, October 4). *Domestic violence: Is it an LGBT issue?* Paper presented at the Second Annual Lesbian, Gay, Bisexual, Transgender and Allies Student Leadership Conference, William Paterson University of New Jersey.

DeAngelis, B. (1992). *Are you the one for me? Knowing who's right and avoiding who's wrong.* New York: Dell.

D'Erasmo, S. (2001, October 14). Polymorphous normal. *New York Times Magazine,* Section 6, pp. 104–107.

Dion, K. L., & Dion, K. K. (1987). Belief in a just world and physical attractiveness stereotyping. *Journal of Personality and Social Psychology, 52,* 775–780.

Downey, G., & Feldman, S. I. (1996). Implications of rejection sensitivity for intimate relationships. *Journal of Personality and Social Psychology, 70*(6), 1327–1343.

Egan, J. (2003, November 23). Love in the time of no time. *New York Times Magazine,* p. 66.

Fisher, H. (1993). *Anatomy of love: The national history of monogamy, adultery, and divorce.* London: Simon & Schuster.

Francese, T. (2001, November). The battered woman's experience and theories of violence. Class presentation by the Passaic County Office of Women, William Paterson University.

Freedner, N., Freed, L., Yang, Y., & Austin, S. (2002, December). Dating violence among gay, lesbian, and bisexual adolescents: Results from a community survey. *Journal of Adolescent Health,* 469–474.

Gabriel, T. (1997, January 5). Pack dating: For a good time, call a crowd. *New York Times,* Education Supplement, pp. 22–23, 38.

Hatfield, E. (1996). *Love, sex, and intimacy: Their psychology, biology, and history.* New York: HarperCollins.

Hatfield, E., & Rapson, R. L. (1996). *Love and sex: Cross cultural perspectives.* Boston: Allyn & Bacon.

Hatfield, E., & Sprecher, S. (1986). *Mirror, mirror. . . . The importance of looks in everyday life.* Albany: State University of New York Press.

Henderson, L., Zimbardo, P., & Rodino, E. (2001). Painful shyness in children and adults [Online]. American Psychological Association. Available: http://helping.apa.org.

Hendrick, S., Foote, F. J., & Slapion-Foote, J. (1984). Do men and women love differently? *Journal of Social and Personal Relationships, 1,* 177–180, 184, 193–195.

Kohl, J. V., & Francouer, R. T. (1995). *The scent of eros: Mysteries of odor in human sexuality.* New York: Continuum.

Lee, J. (1988). Love styles. In R. Sternberg & M. Barnes (Eds.), *The psychology of love.* New Haven, CT: Yale University Press.

Metz, M. E., Rosser, B. R., & Strapko, N. (1994, November). Differences in conflict-resolution styles among heterosexual, gay, and lesbian couples. *Journal of Sex Research, 31*(4), 293.

Michael, R. T., Gagnon, J. H., Laumann, E. O., & Kolata, G. (1994). *Sex in America.* New York: Little, Brown.

Nevid, J. (1984). Sex differences in factors of romantic attraction. *Sex Roles, 11,* 401–411.

New York Times. (2001, October 14). Love in the 21st century: An issue exploring how the American couple has changed. *New York Times Magazine* [whole issue].

Peplau, L., & Cochran, S. (1988). Value orientations in the intimate relationships of gay men. In J. DeCecco (Ed.), *Gay relationships.* New York: Haworth.

Peplau, L. A. (1981, March). What homosexuals want in relationships. *Psychology Today,* 28–34, 37–38.

Schwartz, P. (2001). *Everything you know about love and sex is wrong: 25 relationship myths redefined to achieve happiness and fulfillment in your intimate life.* New York: Perigee.

Smith, E., Becker, M., Byrne, D., & Przybyla, D. (1993). Sexual attitudes of males and females as predictors of interpersonal attraction and marital compatibility. *Journal of Applied Social Psychology, 23*(13), 1011–1034.

Sprecher, S., Sullivan, Q., & Hatfield, E. (1994). Mate selection preferences: Gender differences examined in a national sample. *Journal of Personality and Social Psychology, 66,* 1074–1080.

Sternberg, R. (1986). A triangular theory of love. *Psychological Review, 93,* 119–135.

Waite, L. J., & Joyner, K. (2001). Emotional and physical satisfaction with sex in married, cohabiting, and dating sexual unions: *Do men and women differ?* In E. O. Laumann & R. Michael (Eds.), *Sex, love and health in America.* Chicago: University of Chicago Press.

Wiederman, M. W. (2001a). Infidelity: What proportion of people had extradyadic sex? In *Understanding sexuality research.* Belmont, CA: Wadsworth/Thomson Learning.

Wiederman, M. W. (2001b). Mate selection: What determines peoples' choice of particular partners? In *Understanding sexuality research.* Belmont, CA: Wadsworth/Thomson Learning.

Wiederman, M., & Allgeier, E. (1992). Gender differences in mate selection criteria: Sociobiological or socioeconomic explanations? *Ethnology and Sociobiology, 13,* 115–124.

Zimbardo, P. G. (1977). *Shyness.* Reading, MA: Addison-Wesley.

chapter *eleven*

Sexual Communication

Student Learning Objectives

After reading this chapter, students will be able to

- Compare a variety of communication models.

- Describe some of the key elements that make sexual communication different and difficult.

- Assess the importance of communication in sexual relationships.

- Describe a variety of verbal sexual communication techniques.

- Describe a variety of nonverbal sexual communication techniques.

- Compare and contrast verbal and nonverbal sexual communication techniques.

- Describe some barriers to effective sexual communication.

- Describe how disabilities impact sexual communication.

Test your understanding of these objectives by taking the end-of-chapter quiz, available online at http://health.wadsworth.com/blonna1.

activity teaser: *Are you comfortable with the language of sex? Find out with the Personal Exploration Activity on page 334.*

Sirahana

Sirahana, 22, single, identifies as Iranian American.

Critical Thinking

How have your cultural beliefs and traditions influenced your relationships with current or former partners?

Use your Virtual Workbook to explore your answer to this question at **http://health.wadsworth.com/blonna1.**

Sirahana was a senior with a major in finance, enrolled in the human sexuality class to fulfill her free elective requirement and to learn more about herself. Normally an "A" student, Sirahana was having trouble with a couple of assignments that required her to write brief reactions about the influence of culture and religion on her sexuality.

She came to see Dr. Blonna about this matter and explained that the assignments forced her to examine things about her life and culture that were painful to her. She had been able to avoid these subjects because she had lived away from home for the past 4 years and was able to hide them from her parents. In a couple of months, however, school would be ending, and her parents expected her to move in with her Iranian family.

Sirahana would have to make some tough choices. She had a steady boyfriend, Sean, who was Irish Catholic. She had never told her parents about Sean because their relationship started out as a casual, lighthearted romance that neither thought would last. Little by little, it blossomed as their attraction for each other grew. She practically lived at his off-campus apartment and wanted to move in full-time once school ended in the summer. They had talked seriously about marriage and eventually children, neither one wanting to let their religious beliefs stand in the way of their love.

Sirahana explained that she was feeling a tremendous amount of guilt over her desire to live apart from her family with Sean. Her parents, culture, and religion all expected her to follow tradition by living at home and ultimately marrying someone of her own faith. It was such a strong expectation that she felt utterly paralyzed at the thought of talking to her parents about it. She also knew that she loved Sean and wanted to start a new life with him. She didn't want to move back home.

She liked the freedom of her current life and felt less and less drawn by the covenants and traditions of her religion and culture. She also loved and respected her parents and deeply appreciated all they had done to put her through school and rear her. She wanted to talk to them, explain exactly what she was feeling, and help them understand, but she didn't know how or where to begin.

Communication

Communication The process by which information is exchanged between individuals through a common system of symbols, signs, and behaviors

Communication is defined as the process by which information is exchanged between individuals through a common system of symbols, signs, or behaviors. It involves all the modes of behavior that an individual uses to affect another person. It encompasses spoken and written words as well as nonverbal messages such as gestures, facial expressions, bodily messages or signals, and artistic symbols (Watzlawick, Beaven, & Jackson, 1967).

Communicating, as Sirahana has shown us in Case Study 11.1, involves a whole range of issues from emotional comfort and security, to cultural considerations, and finally to discrete behavioral skills. Communicating about sexuality-related issues is even more complex and often more difficult because of this. Communication is the foundation of healthy sexuality. It is essential to obtaining sexual information for oneself as well as communicating information to others. Sexual communication poses unique challenges because of the difficulty of communicating in general, plus the personal nature of sexuality. Communicating effectively requires skill, patience, and commitment as well as an understanding and mastery of sexual information. Honest and accurate sexual communication is essential in developing and maintaining good relationships and fostering healthy sexuality.

Metacommunication

Communication also includes the interpersonal relationship between communicators. When we are in the presence of others, it is impossible not to communicate. Activity and inactivity, speech and silence—all communicate messages. Communication occurs at two levels: the *content* level (what is actually being said) and the *relationship* level (what is going on between the communicants). This second relationship level is referred to as **metacommunication,** or communication about communication. **Pragmatics** refers to the relationship between communicators, and relationships are of two types—symmetrical and complementary. **Symmetrical relationships** are based on equality. Each communicator treats the other in a like fashion, minimizing differences and conflict. Symmetrical relationships are comfortable and facilitate communication. When we are involved in symmetrical relationships, we are relaxed, our conversation is not forced, and we perceive periods of silence as comfortable and not awkward (Watzlawick et al., 1967).

Complementary relationships are based on differences. Communicators maximize their differences, causing inequality and disharmony. Complementary relationships crackle with the tension in the air. Communication is forced, and periods of silence seem interminable. Complementary relationships often result in stress (Watzlawick et al., 1967).

Metacommunication
Communication about
communication

Pragmatics The relationship
between communicators

Symmetrical relationships
Relationships based on
equality

Complementary
relationships Relationships
based on differences

Social Wellness

All interpersonal communication has a social basis. It is not just about putting thoughts and feelings into words. It also is about the relationship between you and the person with whom you are communicating. As we have seen, metacommunication proposes a framework for communicating based on symmetrical (equal) and complementary (confrontational) relationships. Symmetrical relationships foster good communication, whereas complementary ones discourage effective dialogue.

Transactional Analysis

Eric Berne's (1960) **transactional analysis** (TA) model examines relationships that are either symmetrical or complementary. Berne proposed that all of us have three sources of behavior, or ego states: child, adult, and parent. Each ego state manifests itself in a different communication style. Figure 11.1 illustrates the three ego states of TA.

1. *The child.* The child manifests itself through childish use of verbal and nonverbal communication. The child uses coyness, naiveté, charm and seduction, boisterousness, giggling, and whining and is spontaneous, irresponsible, and manipulative. Our childish ego state is playful and free of restraint.
2. *The adult.* The adult is rational and objective, uses logic and analysis, and exhibits sound decision making based on accurate perception and analysis. The adult is fair, responsible, sociable.
3. *The parent.* The parent incorporates feelings and behaviors learned from authority figures. The parent communicates the conscience of the person through words, actions, postures, behaviors, expectations, and the use of guilt or reward. The parent can be nurturing (protects, cuddles, and cares for) or critical (corrects and condemns).

Figure 11.1 *Berne's Three Ego States*
Berne identified three ego states: the parent, the adult, and the child.

Source: Transactional Analysis in Psychotherapy, by Eric Berne (New York: Grove Press, 1960).

Figure 11.2
Transactional Mismatch
Miscommunication occurs when people talk to each other using different ego state levels.

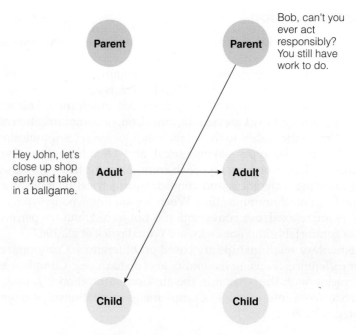

One adult addresses another adult. The second adult receives the message in an adult ego state and responds as if to a child ego state.

Transactional analysis (TA)
Eric Berne's communication model based on three ego states—parent, adult, and child

According to Berne, when we communicate, our message is sent from one of our three ego states and is received by a specific ego state of another. Ideally, the ego state from which we send messages matches that of the person to whom we are talking. Thus, if we are speaking from our adult state to another person, that person should be receiving our message in his or her adult state. If this is not the case, a mismatch occurs. A mismatch is similar to the complementary message in

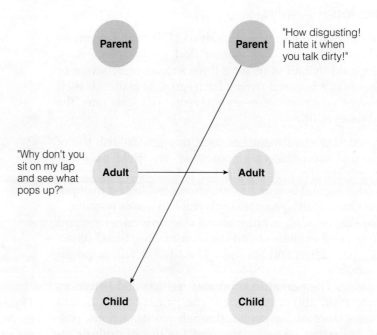

Figure 11.3 *Sexual Transactional Mismatches*
Sexual transactional mismatches occur when lovers communicate about sex using different ego state levels.

One person initiates from his adult state, using humor to signal his sexual interest. His partner responds sternly from her critical parent state, treating him like a child.

Susan: An Awkward Communication Circumstance

Susan, 37, single, and lesbian, is white.

Susan, a professor, is attending an out-of-town conference with some friends. She is sitting at the bar in her hotel, waiting for friends to come down and go out to dinner with her. She is nursing a drink, trying to relax.

A man seated two stools to her right tries to draw Susan into a conversation he is having with a group of his friends about the sexual differences between men and women. Susan doesn't know any of these people. She finds them not only a little drunk but also pretentious, shallow, and untrustworthy. She immediately feels uncomfortable. Susan feigns interest in what they are talking about, nodding her head while looking over their shoulders to try to spot her friends. She politely adds a comment here and there but can't relax around them as they carry on about a variety of issues she doesn't care about and trade barbs with each other. She also feels uncomfortable talking about this subject with a group of strangers who don't realize she is gay. These are characteristics of a complementary relationship.

Eventually Susan's friends arrive, and she quickly excuses herself and joins them. She is able to let down her guard, be herself, and enjoy the rest of the evening in symmetrical conversation among peers she respects and feels comfortable around.

Critical Thinking

We are often forced to endure social situations like the one Susan encountered that made her feel uneasy. How would you have responded to the man at the bar if you were Susan?

Use your Virtual Workbook to explore your answer to this question at **http://health.wadsworth.com/blonna1.**

Watzlawick et al.'s (1967) metacommunication model. Mismatches between messages sent from one state and received by another can be a source of stress and sexual miscommunication.

Figure 11.2 illustrates a mismatch that occurs when we are talking to a peer and we use our parent ego state instead of our adult state. Our friend, receiving in an adult ego state, expects us to send an adult message. Instead, we send a parent message assuming we are sending to an assumed child ego state, which creates a mismatch and is a source of stress.

Figure 11.3 illustrates another mismatch between two lovers. One is in a playful mood and communicates a sexy message from his adult state. His lover, in an adult state, receives the message, is confused, and sends back a parent message. The critical nature of the message and the condemning tone send a stressful message that resonates within the partner's child state. Mismatches like this can cool the fires of desire if they are not cleared up.

Forms of Communication

The basic forms of communication are one-way and two-way.

One-Way Communication

One-way communication is an information-giving process that does not involve or rely on feedback. Speeches, lectures, movies, TV programs, concerts, and radio broadcasts are examples of one-way communication. One-way communication is a direct and powerful way to transmit information about sexuality. Much of what we learn about sexuality in our culture is disseminated through one-way communication.

Print and broadcast media use sexual themes in their programming and to sell their products. Movies, TV programs, and music videos weave visual sexual images into their plots. Song lyrics provide auditory sexual information. We absorb most of what we learn about the cultural context of sexuality through this passive transfer of sexual information through mass media. Mass media convey messages about how our culture views sex. Mass media communicate sexual information to entertain or sell products, not to inform and educate us. Although the impact of this exposure is powerful and conveys messages about sex, the portrayal is often shallow and inaccurate and doesn't offer the opportunity for a dialogue. It also doesn't afford the opportunity to personalize the information and explore how it relates to us as individuals.

Two-Way Communication

Two-way communication goes beyond information-giving by including **feedback.** Feedback ensures a dialogue, the key component of two-way communication. It gives us the opportunity to share information, ask questions, seek clarification, and explore ideas and feelings that go beyond those initially presented. **Dialogue** represents a true exchange of information. This is why two-way communication is essential for communicating about sexuality. Two-way communication increases the likelihood that each person will express his or her needs and wants and will understand each other clearly. One way to explain two-way communication is through a circular model of communication.

A Circular Model of Communication Effective communication is a circular process that involves sending and receiving coded messages, as illustrated in Figure 11.4. A sender, wishing to communicate, puts the idea and feeling of the message into a form that can be transmitted. This process of formulating a message, choosing appropriate words, symbols, tone, and expressions to represent it is called **encoding.** The receiver perceives and translates the message using his or her personal storehouse of knowledge and experience in a process called **decoding.**

Encoding and decoding take place within the context of the communicator's interpersonal and physical relationship. What is being said involves not only the

Feedback A verbal or nonverbal response sent from a person receiving a message to the person sending that message

Dialogue An exchange of information in communication

Encoding Selecting the signs, symbols, emotions, and words to transmit a message

Decoding The use of knowledge, memory, language, context, and personal history and experience to interpret a message

Figure 11.4
A Circular Model of Communication
A circular model of communication assumes that senders and receivers provide feedback to each other.

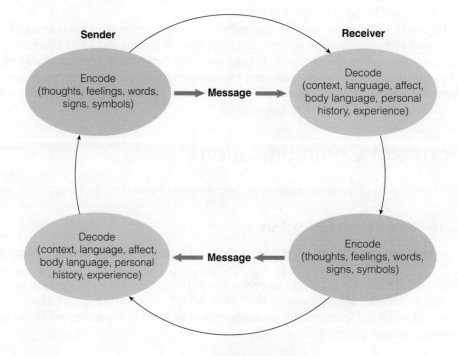

actual message but also the physical environment of the communication as well as the relationship of the sender and receiver. A sender might alter the message depending on whether the environment is friendly or unfriendly, familiar or unfamiliar, safe or unsafe, formal or informal (Sawyer & Behnke, 2002).

In addition, a sender might send a different message in the same environment depending on the nature of the relationship with the receiver. The message might be affected by whether the sender and receiver are friends or enemies, strangers or known to each other, peers or of unequal status (Sawyer & Behnke, 2002). Communication involves sending and receiving both verbal and nonverbal messages. Each type of message is capable of transmitting information and is part of the encoding and decoding process.

Verbal Communication

Verbal communication is two-dimensional in that it involves transmitting both thoughts and feelings through words. The *cognitive* domain is concerned with communicating our thoughts about things. The *affective* domain involves putting our feelings into words. Many people find communicating cognitive information easier than expressing feelings.

Specificity Specificity is crucial in effective verbal communication. The more specific the message, the more likely it is to be transmitted clearly. Vocabulary plays a big part in the specificity of our verbal communication. Having a large working vocabulary allows us to specify exactly what we want to say.

Sexual Vocabulary One of the things that makes sexual communication difficult is the lack of a common sexual vocabulary. U.S. culture has no uniform set of agreed-on words, phrases, and sexual language level. Often we are unsure of the proper terminology for sexual topics such as anatomy and physiology and sexual behaviors. Insecurity about sexual terminology, coupled with emotional discomfort, makes talking about sex difficult.

Language Level The level of language we use also plays a part in effective verbal communication. The four levels of language are childhood, street, everyday discourse, and scientific language (Mandel, 1980).

1. *Childhood language* is simple, cute, and fun and often is used to disguise embarrassment. Lovers have their own brand of childhood language. They may use it to describe their sexual anatomy and physiology, sexual desire, or need for pleasure. Pet names and phrases are part of this language. Lovers often use childhood language to refer to their genitalia or sexual desire. People also use childhood language when they make mistakes and seek forgiveness. "Ooops, sowwy about that," we might say in mock childhood tones.

2. *Street language* is tough, expressive, and emotional. Street language can be disarming and often is used to level the playing field when communicators do not share equal power or prestige. Tough talk can bestow power and superiority. Street language also serves to create bonds between members of subcultures by sharing a language that members of mainstream society do not understand. Rap music incorporates the power and raw sensuality of street language into a unique art form.

3. *Common discourse* is the language level of mainstream society. It is the generally accepted form of language with which most of us communicate. Most people use its words, expressions, and speech patterns in communicating information that is neither intimate nor scientific. It is the language taught in schools and used in most communications.

sex in society 11.1

He Said/She Said

Do men and women communicate differently? Research about this subject over the past 20 years has yielded mixed results. Men and women are socialized differently, and many researchers believe this difference emerges in the way we communicate. Women are socialized to show their feelings, whereas men have been taught to keep their feelings hidden (Michaud & Warner, 1997). Men have been taught to keep their fears and doubts disguised, because showing these is considered a sign of weakness. Men are socialized to believe that admitting weakness is unmanly (Tannen, 1990).

These beliefs can affect the way we communicate with our partners. Wives send clearer and more emotional messages than their husbands do (Noller & Fitzpatrick, 1991). Wives tend to frame their message in an emotional context, whereas husbands deemphasize affect and focus instead on issues and facts. Husbands send more neutral, less expressive messages that are harder to interpret (Tannen, 1990).

Michaud and Warner (1997) found that men and women communicate differently when dealing with problems. When dealing with "troubles talk," these researchers found that women were much more likely to offer sympathy than men were. Men were much more likely to tell a joke. Women were much more likely to be supportive, whereas

men were more likely to avoid the trouble. Lastly, Tannen (1990) found that women were much more likely to listen as a way to offer support, whereas men were much more likely to try to "solve" the problem by offering advice.

McGinty, Knox, and Zusman (2003) found that female college students were more likely to engage in nonverbal feedback and were more proficient at using it than their male counterparts. Female college students in the study were also more proficient at decoding nonverbal feedback than the males who participated. McGinty et al. (2003) also found that males and females differ in how they communicate according to the nature of the relationship. There were significant differences in the communication patterns of students in "involved" versus "casual" relationships. The former group was significantly more concerned about nonverbal communication than the latter. The involved students also demonstrated greater skill in communicating nonverbally with their partners than the casual daters did (McGinty et al., 2003). Involved daters were also "less confused" about their communications than the casual daters were and reported "working harder" on communicating (both verbally and nonverbally) clearly (McGinty et al., 2003).

---

4. *Scientific/professional language* is the discourse of the work world and professional community. It is the language that professional peers use as they communicate about the subtleties of their chosen professions. Like street language, it usually is understood only by those who share its culture. Computer programmers, doctors, and other professions have unique vocabularies, complete with acronyms only they understand.

When we communicate with our partners, we must use the level of language with which they are most comfortable. Miscommunication can occur when the language levels of two communicators are not the same. A language level in common is a good starting point for effective sexual communication.

Nonverbal Communication

Body language Sending intentional or unintentional messages through body postures and movements

How we say things is just as important as *what* we actually say. **Body language** describes the nonverbal messages we send through posture, gestures, movement, and physical appearance, including adornment. Our body language intentionally or unintentionally sends messages to receivers (Andersen 1999).

Lovers use nonverbal communication to express feelings, ask for things, and reinforce pleasurable activities. A moan, a hug, a seductive look—these can speak a thousand words. Placing a partner's hand in the correct spot or squeezing it when you are being touched as you want can accomplish as much as explaining these things through words.

Body Language

Positive, or open, body language is demonstrated by a relaxed posture, steady eye contact, nods of the head, and an occasional smile or happy expression. These are cues that you are an approachable sender or a receptive receiver (McGinty et al., 2003).

Negative, or closed, body language has visible signs of tension such as clenched fists or tight jaw muscles, a closed posture (arms folded, body shifted sideways, and the like), and facial expressions ranging from anger to disbelief. Negative body language can indicate either apathy or disturbance about something.

Physical Appearance

Physical appearance can convey a variety of messages. A messy, sloppy, or ungroomed appearance may send encoded messages ranging from positive ("I'm comfortable enough in your presence to relax") to negative ("I don't care enough about you or myself to pay attention to my appearance"). Clothing and adornment might intentionally or unintentionally be erotic and seductive. This can affect both the encoding and the decoding process, as the sender might be trying to convey one message ("I'm trying to look my best"), while the receiver may perceive another ("This person is trying to manipulate or come on to me sexually").

Silence

Silence is a form of nonverbal communication that can be either a source of stress or a sign of comfort. Silence also can be used to hurt and control people. Silence is a stressor when wordless pauses are perceived as signs of a breakdown in communication. Conversely, silence communicates comfort and acceptance between friends and lovers who understand that a loving bond is present despite a lack of conversation. Silence is a necessary part of effective communication that is often overlooked. We need time to listen, digest, and understand messages. Silence allows us time to reflect as we formulate our thoughts and words.

Touch

A firm handshake, a reassuring touch on the arm, a gentle squeeze of the buttocks, the placing of a partner's hand on the genitals or breast—all convey messages without speaking a single word (McBurney, 2002). Appropriately used, touch adds another dimension of communication that sometimes reaches deeper than mere words.

Often we find it easier to communicate our sexual desires through touch than words. For instance, a man might take his partner's hand and place it on his penis and squeeze it rather than ask, "Please squeeze my penis this hard." A woman might draw her partner's head upon her breast rather than ask, "Please suck on my nipples." A person might moan or groan rather than say, "I like it when you suck on my penis like that," or "It feels good when you rub my clitoris like that."

When used inappropriately, however, the effects of touch can be devastating. A pat on the head can be a sign of endearment to a child but can embarrass or infuriate another adult. A squeeze on your friend's shoulder can show him you understand his problems and care about him. The same squeeze on your secretary's

True intimacy doesn't require constant talking. Holding hands and walking silently can communicate love, trust, and a variety of other emotions.

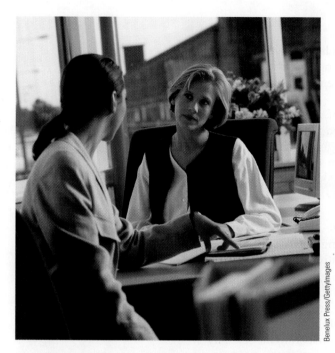

Benelux Press/Getty/Images

Professionals use desk and chair placements as a way to establish comfortable space requirements.

shoulder, however, can convey an entirely different meaning. A pat on a teammate's buttocks can show appreciation of a great play or an extreme effort. The same pat on a coworker's buttocks can be perceived as sexual harassment.

Space

The space between sender and receiver also affects communication. Four space zones common to communication in North America are as follows (Hall, 1973):

Intimate space (less than 18 inches)—space reserved for communication between intimate partners
Personal space (18 inches to 4 feet)—space appropriate for close relationships that may involve touching
Social-consultive space (4 to 12 feet) space for non-touching, less intimate relationships that may involve louder verbal communication
Public space (more than 12 feet)—space used for formal gatherings such as addressing a large group.

Stress and sexual tension can arise when we violate these commonly accepted space parameters. For example, we find ourselves backing up to reclaim our violated space when a non-intimate person gets within the boundaries of our intimate space. Sometimes we place objects as barriers between us and other people to define our space and set allowable communication zones. Culture plays an important part in determining what is acceptable and unacceptable concerning space.

Intellectual Wellness

Intellectual wellness can facilitate communication. Effective communication, whether of a generic or sexual nature, involves three sets of skills: initiating, listening, and responding. Because these are skills, they can be developed and improved, regardless of one's current level of functioning.

Initiating Skills

Initiating sexual communication is different for new and for established relationships. Initiating skills are critical in meeting new people. Initiating skills also are important for discovering what our partners desire, as well as for communicating our own wants and needs, likes and dislikes. Partners in established relationships have a history of intimacy and trust that foster communication. The context of their communication differs greatly from that of two people who are attracted to each other but have not established an intimate relationship yet.

Despite the nature or length of the relationship, however, research shows that men and women often misread emotional cues and misinterpret nonverbal messages (Senecal, Murard, & Hess, 2003). This makes it particularly important to take responsibility for any perceived miscommunication and initiate a dialogue with one's partner to clear this up.

Nonverbal Initiating Skills

Initiating communication starts with nonverbal messages. Think about how you act when you meet for the first time someone to whom you are attracted. You make eye contact and hold it a little longer than you would if you were not interested in meeting the person. Eye contact leads to a smile, a brush of the hair, followed by another look that signals approachability.

Take the case of John and Susan. They are in the same biology lecture class of 150 students. For a couple of weeks they have noticed each other and seem mutually attracted. Today Susan decides she wants to meet John. She intentionally sits closer to him—about four seats down in the same row. She smiles at him as she takes her seat. She sees that he notices her and returns her smile. Buoyed by this, she glances over again, tossing back a long shock of hair while reestablishing eye contact—this time for a moment longer. She decides to approach John after class and initiate a conversation with him. If John hadn't noticed Susan, returned her glance, or maintained eye contact, she might have received a different message and decided not to pursue meeting him any further.

Nonverbal communication between lovers in a long-term relationship is similar—but different because of their shared intimacy, comfort level, and experience together. Nonverbal messages are still important, though, to signal approachability and desire to communicate. They still need to establish eye contact, set the appropriate distance, and adopt a relaxed and approachable posture. Lovers can soften or strengthen their intentions with techniques such as a flirtatious look, lingering eye contact, a smile, or a serious look

Initiating nonverbal communication also can involve props for both new and established lovers. Peering over the top of a book you are reading or the drink you are nursing provides a small security blanket. The feigned dropped handkerchief is the quintessential prop that heroines in classic movies used to gain the attention of their heroes.

Leaving on the table a magazine opened to a story about sex is one way to send a message that you are interested in discussing the subject. Putting a sex manual on your coffee table or bedstand is a way to send messages of interest and approachability to your partner. Renting an erotic or romantic video is a way to introduce the topic of sex without saying a word.

Verbal Initiating Skills

Whether a person is trying to meet someone for the first time or to talk to a partner of 15 years about a sexual topic, he or she has to initiate the communication. Waiting and hoping that your partner or someone in whom you are interested will initiate is a sure way to end the communication before it begins.

Take the case of Susan and John again. Clearly, from his nonverbal messages, John is at least approachable. Susan now is responsible for initiating. Deciding what to say in first-time encounters can be excruciating. A simple rule of thumb is to be honest. Susan could simply say, "Hi, I'm Susan. I'm a little embarrassed, but I've noticed you for the past couple of weeks, and I'd like to meet you." It's now up to John either to reinforce his nonverbal display interest or to pass it up. Susan also could draw from their shared experience of the biology lecture. She might initiate by saying something like, "Hi, I'm Susan. I'm having trouble understanding something the professor just said. Can we talk?"

Four common initiating techniques that can be used in both first-time and longtime relationships are open-ended questions, paraphrasing, declarative statements, and simple yes/no questions.

sex in society 11.2

Cultural Considerations in Communication

Communicating effectively requires awareness of, and sensitivity to, various cultural influences related to verbal and nonverbal communication. The following are a few examples of common cultural consideration to keep in mind.

Verbal Communication

Cultural groups and subcultures do not necessarily share a common language. Although English is the first language spoken by most Americans, and common discourse is the level most frequently used to communicate, this is not the case for many individuals and groups. For many Americans, English is a second language, and common discourse (including slang) is often misunderstood. For these Americans, certain subjects, words, and gestures may be misunderstood or taboo.

For Americans traveling abroad for pleasure or business, this consideration is even more important. Sharing personal information, using hand gestures, squeezing an arm, and giving a peck on the cheek are all examples of communication behaviors that are common to everyday discourse among Americans. These would be consider major gaffes when used by Americans traveling in such places as China and Japan (Dou & Clark, 1999).

Perception of time and the relationship of the past, the present, and the future also vary by culture. The predominant culture in the United States is time-urgent and future oriented. Being aware of the present and doing something now to plan for the future (such as exercising now to prevent heart disease in the future) are commonly accepted. In daily life, people are oriented to specific times of the day and strict schedules. Some other cultures are much less interested in time and are not as oriented to specific schedules. For example, many Native American homes do not even have clocks, as people of some tribes are more concerned about the present and live one day at a time (Ivey, D'Andrea, Ivey, & Simek-Morgan, 2002).

Nonverbal Communication

A variety of nonverbal factors also vary from culture to culture. Cultures differ in their norms for territoriality and personal space. In general, people of Arabic, Southern European, and African origins sit or stand relatively close to each other when talking. People of Asian, Northern European, and North American countries are more comfortable being farther apart when they are talking (Ivey et al., 2002).

Body language varies significantly according to culture. The dominant U.S. culture places a high value on direct eye contact when speaking. In contrast, Native Americans consider continuous direct eye contact to be insulting and disrespectful. Rules about eye contact also vary by gender in certain cultures. In Islamic cultures, women are taught to avert the eyes, whereas eye contact is OK for men. The meaning and acceptability of a myriad of other nonverbal behaviors, such as pointing fingers, shaking hands, and other forms of touch, vary by culture (Ivey et al., 2002).

The following general suggestions can be helpful in verbal and nonverbal communication with people from cultures different from one's own:

- *Slow down.* People for whom English is a second language sometimes have a hard time keeping up with and understanding English when it is spoken too rapidly.
- *Minimize nonverbal distractions.* Be conservative rather than flamboyant in your use of gestures, personal space, and other nonverbal communication.
- *Look for feedback.* People who don't understand, can't keep up, or are uncomfortable with something you do or say often give nonverbal or verbal cues. These can be as overt as asking for clarification or as subtle as a turned head or lack of eye contact. Seek clarification of these cues.
- *Avoid talking louder.* Sometimes, when we are not sure we are being understood, we raise our voice, assuming that the person can't hear us. Talking too loudly, however, can be perceived as threatening or condescending and is rarely helpful.
- *Show respect.* Being humble and respectful of cultural differences conveys the message that you care and want to understand and improve communication.
- *Use an interpreter.* If necessary, get someone to translate your message into the person's primary language.
- *Seek information.* Take advantage of opportunities to learn more about cultural differences in communication (read, travel, go to workshops, and so forth).

Spiritual Wellness

Sometimes our moral and ethical standards affect our emotions and impact negatively on our ability to communicate. We each have our own personal moral code with a unique set of values and ethics that develop over a lifetime. Taboos against behaviors ranging from masturbation to oral sex are often deep-seated and rooted in religious training. This can make it very difficult to initiate discussions and pose conflicts in communicating about some of these behaviors.

Open-Ended Questions Open-ended questions are excellent for initiating a dialogue because they cannot be answered with a simple yes/no response. Imagine that you want to explore how your partner likes to be touched. You initiate using an open-ended question such as, "Tell me more about how you like to be touched," or "What else can I do to make you feel good?" Open-ended questions require information from the other person. Your partner can't respond with a simple yes/no answer. Open-ended questions will get your partner talking and draw out additional detail and emotion.

> **Open-ended questions** Sentences that require information from the other person

Paraphrasing Paraphrasing means interpreting the meaning of a message and restating it in one's own words. Paraphrasing is another way to initiate a conversation and obtain additional information by getting a person to talk. Imagine that you want to follow up on something your partner said about sex last night. You could initiate a conversation by paraphrasing your partner's comments from the previous evening. For instance, in discussing last night's conversation about sexual technique, you might say, "I was thinking about what you said last night. What I heard you say was that you like it when I squeeze your scrotum firmly," or, "So, what you were saying last night is that you really enjoy it when I bite gently on your nipples," or, "I sense from last night that you don't like it when I put my tongue in your ear." Paraphrasing requires interpretation, or reading between the lines. Your partner usually will let you know if you are on target or off base in your interpretation of the initial message.

> **Paraphrasing** Restating a message in one's own words

healthy sex hints 11.1

Open-Ended Questions to Keep a Sexual Dialogue Flowing

Close-ended questions provoke simple answers. Most closed-ended questions tend to be answered with one- or two-word replies. Open-ended questions (often referred to as *open-ended statements*) require the person to elaborate. They usually cannot be answered with a simple response.

Close-Ended

"Did you do like this/that?"
"Do you still love me?"
"Can you remember the last time we made love?"

Open-Ended

"Tell me more about. . . ."
"How do you feel about. . . .?"
"Describe that more fully."
"What are your thoughts about. . . .?"
"Explain that more completely."
"What made you decide to do that?"

My Personal Sexual Dictionary

Sexual communication is made even more difficult by the lack of a comfortable vocabulary that does not offend anyone. Most of us have heard an amazing number of different words for the various sexual anatomy and sexual acts. To make our own sexual communication easier, we may find it helpful to identify which words we are comfortable using and hearing used. In this activity, you will create your own personal list of sexual terms that you like and enjoy using.

For the following sexual terms, list all the words you feel comfortable using and enjoy hearing. These can be words you have made up, words from your childhood, slang, words you as a couple have made up, or technical terms. The terms for making your list are *vagina, penis, intercourse, masturbation, breast,* and *testicles.* When you have listed all your favorites, ask your partner to do the same and then compare your list. If one of you has listed a word that the other finds offensive, discuss what about the word offends. Decide as a couple what words you want to eliminate and what words you want to use together. You may find this activity makes asking for what you want and need sexually a little easier when you have a comfortable communication tool. If you are not in a relationship now, do this exercise with a friend. You may find you are quite different in your likes and dislikes.

Declarative statement A verbal initiating technique that does not require a response to a message

Simple Declarative Statements Sometimes simple **declarative statements** about a sexual topic can initiate a dialogue. These are not as direct as the previous two techniques because they do not specifically require a response. They can be useful, however, especially to test the waters to see how someone feels or what he or she thinks about some sexual topic. Imagine you just read some sexually provocative story in a magazine and are interested in discussing it with your partner. You could simply state this as a declarative sentence: "I just read a fascinating story in this magazine about what men desire most in sexual relationships." By tossing out this simple declarative statement, you could assess whether your partner wants to pursue the discussion and gauge his or her feelings about it. You might follow up with an open-ended statement or let it pass if your partner shows no interest.

Yes/no questions A verbal initiating technique involving a question that requires only a yes or no response

Yes/No Questions The weakest way to initiate a dialogue—and the way most of us start conversations—is to ask direct **yes/no questions.** These are questions that can be answered by a simple yes or no. They don't require explanation or embellishment in the way that open-ended statements and paraphrasing do. Although they are useful for verifying facts ("Do you like it when I touch you like this?" "Does this feel good?"), when they are overused, they can shut down a dialogue.

Listening Skills

Passive listening One-way listening; provides no feedback

There are two types of listening: passive and active. In **passive listening** the listener merely soaks in what the initiator of the message is sending. Passive listening is what we do when watching television, a movie, the radio, and so on. It is one-way communication. Although passive listening can be an effective way to receive sexual information, it is not the most effective form of listening to another person when trying to establish or maintain a dialogue.

Active listening Listening with understanding and providing feedback

Active listening is much better than passive listening for dealing with interpersonal communication because, by definition, it requires feedback. Active listeners show that they are listening by providing both nonverbal and verbal feedback. For this reason, active listening is demanding. It takes a lot of energy and concentration, and the listener can easily get distracted and lose interest.

Letting the sender know that the receiver is listening actively can be accomplished through a variety of nonverbal cues. First, the listener adopts a relaxed pose and maintains eye contact. Additional techniques include nodding the head and smiling. Simple verbal cues such as "uh huh," combined with eye contact and head nodding, are enough to let the speaker know the receiver is listening.

Responding Skills

The message receiver reacts to the initiator's message and encodes some type of feedback using verbal or nonverbal communication. If the message was understood and no further clarification is necessary, the receiver can make a simple declarative statement, acknowledging the message with agreement, disagreement, or new information. If the receiver disagrees, or has problems, he or she can use **"I" language** to express opinions. An example is "I hear what you're saying, and I understand your point, but I disagree with that position. I see it differently."

Often, responding skills go beyond merely providing feedback and are used to get additional information needed to understand an issue or to solve a problem. Keeping the conversation going or requesting more information relies on being able to draw more information out of the initiator. Open-ended statements, paraphrasing, and simple yes/no questions, discussed earlier in the chapter, can be used to respond as well as initiate. An additional responding technique that can be powerful is mirroring.

"I" language Taking responsibility for feelings by saying "I feel . . ." versus "You make me feel . . ."

Open-Ended Statements

The open-ended statement is an excellent responding technique because it provides feedback and also keeps the dialogue going. A response such as, "I hear what you're saying—tell me more about how you feel about masturbation," lets the sender know you are with him or her and want additional information.

Paraphrasing

Paraphrasing lets senders know you are listening but goes one step further by giving them an idea of how you interpret their message. For instance, a response such as "What I heard you say is that you can accept masturbation as a form of sexual release in general but personally don't feel good about it" lets the sender know you are listening and also provides the opportunity for the sender to know what you think he or she said. The sender usually will let you know if your interpretation is accurate or if you missed the point.

Mirroring

A powerful technique for providing feedback and keeping a person talking is **mirroring**—restating the person's exact words while mimicking the body posturing. This is done intentionally for impact. Mirroring is useful when someone says something that has strong emotional connotations. The message was so powerful that you do not want to risk weakening or misinterpreting it. Let's say a friend tells you she was so angry at the lewd comments a stranger made to her as she walked by him that she felt she could kill him. You would mirror it by saying, "You were so angry you felt you could kill him!" This usually prompts the person to continue and go into the greater detail you desire.

Mirroring Restating the message exactly, including body language

Yes/No Questions

The weakest type of response in a dialogue—and the way most of us seek additional information about something—is to ask direct yes/no questions. Although these are useful for verifying facts ("Do you like it when I touch you like this?" "Does this feel good?"), they are easy to overuse, can make people feel defensive, and can shut down a dialogue.

Once the receiver encodes a response, the communication process shifts back to the sender. We have now come full circle from sender encoding, receiver decoding, receiver encoding, and providing feedback that now becomes information to be decoded by the sender. And the cycle begins all over again.

Barriers to Sexual Communication

Impediments to communicating sexually include failure to initiate, picking an inappropriate time or place, not being specific enough, lack of active listening and assertiveness, saying no when we mean yes, and failing to make requests.

Failing to Initiate

One of the biggest barriers to effective sexual communication is failing to initiate. Whether you want to meet someone or discuss a problem with something your long-term lover says or does, you are responsible for bringing it to the person's attention. Failing to initiate is the initiator's problem, not the receiver's.

The best time to address issues and problems is when they occur. Taking time to clear things up, before they are allowed to progress, can prevent problems from escalating. Often, however, situational constraints prevent this. Other people may be around, you're in the middle of something else, or you don't have enough time right then. In these cases, you should tell the other person you need some time alone with him or her to discuss something important. The two of you should be in a neutral territory where you feel safe and emotionally strong, with enough time so neither of you feels rushed. In the case of meeting someone new, initiators should wait until they can speak to the person alone, away from friends.

When using "I" language, communicators take responsibility for their feelings. This is especially important when discussing sexual concerns. For example, let's say your boyfriend has made fun of your outfit in front of three other mutual friends. Rather than blame your boyfriend by saying, "You really made me feel bad," you could say, "I felt bad when you criticized my outfit in front of our friends." Rather than blame your friend for what you are feeling, you own your feelings and state them in "I" language.

The situation and feelings about what happened should be stated in clear, simple terms. General statements like "I hate it when you treat me like a sex object" or "I hate it when you do things like that" should be avoided. Good communicators specify exactly what the other person did that they dislike. It's better to say things like "I don't like you to talk about my sexual behavior or level of desire in front of your friends," or "I really feel like a fool when you talk about my sexual needs in front of my friends." Specifying exactly *what* you dislike (talking about sexual needs) and the context (in front of your friends) clarifies the situation and leaves no room for misunderstanding.

Using "I" language when trying to meet others shows the other person that you are being responsible for your feelings and you really care: "Hi, I'm Rich. I find myself agreeing with a lot of your viewpoints about things. I really liked what you said in political science class today. Can we talk about it over a cup of coffee in the Student Center?"

Physical Wellness

Good communication takes time and energy. Often we are too tired, too stressed, and too busy to communicate effectively. Sometimes when our energy level is low, we simply don't have the energy to think clearly and communicate well. Spending our energy on talking and active listening seems beyond our ability during times of low energy. Stress also robs us of energy, puts us on edge, and contributes to our being overly defensive. It's hard to communicate effectively when we are on edge. We don't listen effectively and have empathy when we are stressed out.

Inappropriate Time and Place

Choosing the appropriate time and place to initiate a discussion about sexuality is important. To be able to relax, each person needs to feel safe and secure. This is important for establishing new relationships as well as strengthening existing ones.

In new relationships, talking in public in less intimate settings is sometimes better. A booth in a restaurant, a bench in the park, under a tree on campus all afford privacy yet are public enough to ensure safety and security until you get to know each other better.

When dealing with problems or concerns in an established relationship, time should be sufficient to discuss the issues completely. Privacy and undisturbed time are ensured by shutting off the TV, putting the answering machine on the phone, closing the door to your room, and giving each other undivided attention. Some people prefer the privacy of their bedrooms when talking about sex. As one student explained, "I like to talk about sex in the bedroom—not when we're making love, but at other times. I like to close the door, prop up a few pillows, unplug the phone, and talk. Sometimes we'll have a glass of wine, relax, and let our feelings flow."

Other people prefer discussing sex outdoors. A student described it this way: "I like to get outdoors to talk to my wife about sex. We go for a long walk somewhere in the mountains or in a local park along the canal. There's something open but private about strolling slowly, hand in hand, and discussing our feelings. It works for us."

Environmental/Occupational Wellness

Some of the barriers to effective communication are environmental in nature. Privacy, safety, and a nonthreatening, nondistracting environment are essential for effective sexual communication. Most people find that talking about intimate personal issues in public places is somewhat threatening. A walk in the woods or along the beach or in a park sometimes can create a facilitative setting and mood for communicating about sexual matters.

The workplace can be a particularly challenging place to communicate. Men and women of different cultures and ages all come together around a common work theme. The potential for miscommunication is great, so extra care must be taken to communicate effectively and to take responsibility for miscommunication.

Lack of Specificity

Being critical of a partner's behavior at times is normal in any long-term relationship. Being critical of someone's *behavior*, however, is different from being critical of the person. A sure-fire way to sabotage an attempt to discuss sexual concerns is to criticize the partner rather than the behavior. It is important to criticize the behavior, not the person. People have to understand that the other still loves them but does not like a certain behavior. The partner probably is unaware of how the behavior affects the other. The more precision in describing exactly what a person did or said, the better is the chance of clearing up the problem without hurting the person's feelings. "I really feel hurt when you reject my sexual advances" is a lot easier to deal with than "You're a jerk for rejecting me."

Sexual messages are difficult to interpret clearly, even under the best of circumstances. People in long-term relationships are no exception. Mixed messages—contradictory messages—usually are a result of nonverbal cues not matching verbal messages or people saying something they don't really mean. For instance, if a partner asks, "Do you like it when I do this?" and the response is, "Yeah, sure," while the body is tight and the facial expression is pained, the message is mixed.

We send mixed messages for various reasons. In some cases, we are unsure where we stand or how we feel. The message is mixed because feelings are mixed. Sometimes we send mixed messages because we are unable or unwilling to be assertive and say no or tell the other person how we really feel. In the worst case, we send mixed messages because we play games and deliberately want to keep people off balance and unsure of our position. This approach may be linked to unhealthy sex role stereotyping based on positioning for power and control in relationships.

The bottom line in mixed messages is that they impair the communication process, making it difficult to understand the true meaning of what is going on. Healthy sexuality revolves around effective communication, based on personal knowledge and the desire to communicate honestly.

Failing to Listen Actively

Many sexual communication problems, too, revolve around failure to listen actively. Instead of giving undivided attention and providing feedback, we get caught in a variety of bad listening habits that impair our ability to listen actively.

healthy sex hints 11.2

How to Be a Better Listener

1. *Keep yourself in good mental and physical shape.* We listen better when we are mentally and physically alert.
2. *Keep eye contact with the speaker whenever possible.* This will assure the speaker that what he or she is saying is being heard.
3. *Listen actively rather than passively.* In other words, exert energy and use body language to reflect what the speaker is saying. Nod in agreement, smile or laugh at the speaker's humor, and the like.
4. *Avoid distracting mannerisms.* Things such as hair twirling, fingernail inspecting, and similar behaviors convey boredom or disinterest.

5. *Ask questions* when you don't understand something the speaker is saying. Repeat what the speaker has said, in different words, to convey understanding.
6. *Resist the temptation to let your mind wander.* It's easy to do considering that a person can think much faster than he or she can speak.

The best listeners make the speaker feel like he or she is the only person in the world at that moment. By following these tips, you can join the ranks of good listeners.

Lack of Assertiveness

Assertiveness is a positive attribute, based on mutual respect and democracy in relationships. Assertiveness means understanding one's own wants and needs and pursuing these without infringing on others' ability to do the same. **Aggressiveness,** on the other hand, means pursuing one's needs and wants without regard to how this affects the rights of the others. Often, aggressive people get their needs met at the expense of others. Nonassertive people fail to pursue their needs and wants while allowing others to meet theirs. They fail to stick up for their rights and allow others to take advantage of them, often denying what is going on (Smith, 1993).

Assertiveness is important to effective communication. Many people are not assertive because they confuse assertiveness with aggressiveness. In an attempt to control what they perceive as aggressiveness, they act nonassertively and fail to meet their needs while allowing hostility and frustration to build up inside themselves, weakening their communication and relationships.

Assertiveness Pursuing one's own needs and wants without infringing on others

Aggressiveness Pursuing one's own wants and needs without regard for the rights of others

Saying Yes When We Mean No

When people are nonassertive, they say yes to others' demands when they really want to say no. They spend an inordinate amount of time pleasing others without being reciprocated. They forsake their sexual needs and wants while granting the partner's desires. Although sharing and sacrificing are important to relationships, they become a problem when this behavior is always one-way and not reciprocated.

When people are nonassertive, they are filled with resentment and hostility toward their partner as a result. It's a vicious cycle. Originally, in an attempt to avoid conflict, discomfort, or hurting the partner's feelings, they say yes when they really mean no. This response temporarily relieves them from feeling guilty. Unfortunately, however, when they do this, they get trapped into doing things they really don't want to do. When this result happens, they begin to feel miserable because they've lost control of their lives and lost their self-respect. Not only do they feel stressed because of this situation, but it also affects their sexual response. Desire and arousal are difficult when a person feels stressed and angry.

healthy sex hints 11.3

Assertiveness Bill of Rights

The following "Assertiveness Bill of Rights" may help strengthen your resolve to speak up for yourself:

You have the right to judge your own behavior, thoughts, emotions and to take responsibility for their initiation and consequences upon yourself.

You have the right to offer no reason or excuses for justifying your behavior.

You have the right to judge if you are responsible for finding solutions for other people's problems.

You have the right to change your mind.

You have the right to make mistakes and be responsible for them.

You have the right to say, "I don't know."

You have the right to be independent of the goodwill of others before coping with them.

You have the right to be illogical in making decisions.

You have the right to say, "I don't understand."

You have the right to say, "I don't care."

Source: Terrap Treatment Centers, Menlo Park, CA, 1999.

The only way to stop the cycle is to begin to say no. This brings us full circle to the same situation as the initial one: having to say no. If people are assertive to begin with, they can avoid the aggravation and stress.

Failing to Make Requests

Assertiveness is directly related to requesting things you desire and saying no to things you don't want to do. People have many reasons for not making explicit sexual requests. As we've already discussed, language poses a unique barrier. Feeling comfortable with sexual language is important, and finding a comfortable language level helps. If sex has been a taboo topic of conversation while growing up, it may be difficult to talk about openly. People enter their first relationship without having had the benefit of knowing that talking about sex is OK. Shaking this taboo is sometimes difficult. You can become more comfortable by proceeding slowly, acknowledging your fears and discomfort, and allowing yourself to take chances and grow out of your old ways of thinking and feeling.

Another barrier is not taking responsibility for one's wants, needs, and feelings. First, the individual has to find out who he or she is as a sexual person. Then the person has to accept this. The third step is to share it with the partner. The partner can't know who the other is, what he or she needs, and how to please that person without the other person's taking responsibility to communicate this.

Our sexuality is continually growing and evolving. A married student expressed it this way in class:

> *My wife is always saying that she shouldn't have to explain what she wants sexually. We've been together for 10 years, and I should know how to please her and what her needs are. I*

healthy sex hints 11.4
Saying No

Saying no isn't always easy, but it is essential if you are to be assertive and reduce your stress. You have the right to say no. The following are clear guidelines:

1. *Face the other person from a normal distance.* If you are too far away, you may appear timid. If you crowd the person, you border on aggressiveness.
2. *Look the person directly in the eyes.* Averting eye contact is a sure giveaway that you'll cave in.
3. *Keep your head up and your body relaxed.* Don't be a shrinking violet.
4. *Speak clearly and firmly, at a volume that can be heard clearly.*
5. *Just say no.* You don't have to clarify why.
6. *Be prepared to repeat it.* Sometimes people are persistent. Be prepared to say it again.
7. *Stick to your guns.* Don't give in. It gets easier with practice.

If you feel a need to explain why you are declining, here are a few tips for setting the stage:

1. Thank the person for the offer: "Gee, thanks, but *no*. I really can't [don't want to] . . ."
2. Express appreciation: "I really appreciate the offer, but *no*. I'm not interested/too busy/don't want any . . ."
3. Affirm your friendship: "I enjoy your company, and I'd like to do something together, but *no*."
4. Reject the offer, not the person: "Please don't take this personally. I like you, but *no*, I don't . . ."

have a hard time with this. My own needs change from day to day and from sexual encounter to sexual encounter. One day I may want her to take the lead and initiate sex and be dominant while I lie back and let her take me. The next time we make love, I might want to initiate. I know she's the same way, but I can't tell in advance without her communicating her desires to me.

We need to take responsibility for what we're feeling and make requests accordingly, using "I" language.

Gender and Cultural Considerations

Often, lack of assertiveness is based in religious, cultural, or gender role expectations and transcends lack of skill or desire to assert oneself. Some cultures require subjugating one's personal desires to those of the dominant partner in the relationship. In many cultures, the male partner is the dominant member of the couple. Women are expected to put their needs behind those of their partner and behave in ways expected of them. Respecting the wishes of the partner and the culture is taught to be more important than one's own needs. The conflict between these traditional ways of behaving and U.S. cultural values focusing on the individual and self-actualization is a source of stress and sexual dissatisfaction for many women.

Models of Communication

Two models relevant to sexual communication are the DESC model and rational emotive behavior therapy.

The DESC Model

A useful model that combines assertiveness and effective verbal communication is the DESC model (Bower, 1976; Greenberg, 2003). It is a powerful tool that helps a person make requests, deliver criticism more effectively, and become more precise in assertiveness.

The DESC model has four parts:

D—describe: Paint a verbal picture of the situation or the other person's behavior that is a source of stress. Be as precise as possible: "Honey, when you use language like 'I'm feeling horny—let's fuck,'. . . ."

E—express: Express your feelings about the incident using "I" language: "I feel seedy and cheap" or "I feel very uncomfortable."

S—specify: Be specific in identifying alternative ways that you would prefer the person to speak or behave: "I'd like you to soften your language and say, 'I'm feeling sexy—let's make love.'"

C—consequences: Identify the consequences that will follow if the person does (pro) or doesn't (con) comply with your wishes: "In the future, if you do soften your language, I'll be much more likely to get in the mood and want to make love with you (pro)." "If you don't, and you continue to use such crude language, I can't guarantee that I won't be turned off and not feel sexy."

When using this model, precision is important in describing the other person's offending behavior or actions. Again, the offensive behavior, not the person, should be the object of criticism. And the person should take responsibility for his or her feelings and use "I" language when describing them. Rather than blaming the partner and saying, "You make me feel cheap and seedy," the person should be clear and take responsibility by stating, "I feel cheap and seedy when you use those coarse words."

Emotional Wellness

Emotional wellness affects the ability to communicate clearly. Communicating effectively is difficult even under the best of circumstances. Communicating about sexuality poses unique challenges because of the sensitive nature of the topic. Even though people may want to communicate more effectively, emotions sometimes get in the way. They might feel embarrassed talking about their most intimate desires, thoughts, and feelings. They also might feel guilty about some of these things. These emotions often make it difficult to think clearly and logically. A first step in sexual communication is to identify how we are feeling and to take responsibility for owning these feelings. Once we assume ownership for our feelings, we can use "I" language to communicate them to our intimate partner.

Rational Emotive Behavior Therapy (REBT) and Irrational Thinking

Sometimes we fail to communicate clearly because our sexual thinking is irrational or illogical. Our sexual perspective, or belief system—as Albert Ellis (1993), the father of rational emotive behavior therapy (REBT), calls it—is disordered. Ellis believes that our *perception* of our partners and specific sexual situations (not the actual person or situation) gives them meaning and determines whether they become a source of dissatisfaction and miscommunication.

For instance, Khalid and Teri have been lovers for a year and have been happy with their sexual lifestyle. They make love about once a week and engage in a variety of sexual behaviors they find enjoyable. Last night, after they came home from the movies, Khalid wanted to make love and Teri didn't. She was tired and wanted to get to bed early. Feeling rejected, Khalid began to have doubts about their sexual relationship, wondering, "What's wrong with her? Teri should be in the mood when I am. What's wrong with our relationship?" In reality, nothing is wrong with their relationship. They are happy, enjoy each other's company, and have a satisfying sex life together. The only problem is Khalid's perception of this specific situation.

In their clinical work with neurotic patients, Albert Ellis and Robert Harper (1998) identified a group of 10 commonly held irrational or illogical beliefs about life. These beliefs form the basis of a belief system that gives one a distorted perspective for assessing potentially stressful situations. Using and understanding Ellis and Harper's theory can be simplified by grouping the 10 illogical/irrational beliefs into four categories (Walen, DiGuisseppi, & Wessler, 1980).

Awfulizing statements: These exaggerate the negative aspects/impact of a situation.
Shoulds/musts/oughts: These are beliefs that put illogical demands on oneself and others.
Evaluation-of-worth statements: These imply that some people or things are worthless or a complete waste of time.
Need statements: These are beliefs that set unrealistic, unattainable requirements for happiness.

We often blow things out of proportion, set unrealistic demands for our behavior and that of our partners, misinterpret sexual comments, or have irrational fears about discussing our wants, needs, desires, or problems with our partners. These illogical/irrational beliefs result in undesirable emotional, intellectual, physical, social, and behavioral consequences. Ellis and Harper (1998) use an ABC model to describe this interaction. In this model, the presence of an activating event, A, triggers a series of irrational/illogical beliefs, B, about A. These illogical beliefs about A (not the activating event itself) are the cause of a variety of negative consequences, C. We'll illustrate the model again using Khalid and Teri:

A—activating event:
> Khalid wanted to make love with his girlfriend Teri when they came home from the movies, but she didn't. She said she wasn't in the mood and wanted to get to bed early.

B—irrational/illogical beliefs:
> "My girlfriend should always be in the mood."
> "My girlfriend should always be in the mood when I am."
> "Partners should always be sexually available."
> "People who are in love should always please their partners sexually."
> "She must not love me anymore."
> "She must be having an affair with someone else."
> "I'm not good enough for her."

C—Consequences
> Physical—muscle tension, upset stomach, tension headache
> Emotional—anger, depression
> Mental—irrational thoughts
> Social—retreating into isolation, breaking off all physical touching
> Behavioral—starting to drink to excess

REBT uses logical thinking and positive self-talk as an aid to reducing sexual problems. Ellis and Harper's (1998) ABCDE technique attempts to help us understand our illogical beliefs and self-talk and learn to substitute more rational thoughts in their place. The ABCDE technique builds upon Ellis's ABC model of **illogical thinking** by adding D (dispute) and E (evaluate). D involves disputing each illogical B and substituting a more logical belief in its place. When all of the illogical beliefs have been disputed, the effectiveness of the dispute in defusing the consequences is evaluated.

> **Illogical thinking** Thought based on inaccurate or irrational perception of information

The ABCDE technique would work like this:

A—Khalid's girlfriend Teri rejecting his offer to make love
B—Khalid's irrational beliefs about A
> "My girlfriend should always be in the mood."
> "My girlfriend should always be in the mood when I am."
> "Partners should always be sexually available."
> "People who are in love should always please their partners sexually."
> "She must not love me anymore."
> "She must be having an affair with someone else."
> "I'm not good enough for her."

C—Consequences of B
> Physical—muscle tension, upset stomach, tension headache
> Emotional—anger, depression
> Mental—irrational thoughts
> Social—retreating into isolation, breaking off all physical touching
> Behavioral—starting to drink to excess

Ellis and Harper's 10 Illogical Beliefs

Often we are sexually dissatisfied because of illogical or irrational beliefs and expectations we have about sex and our relationships. Ellis and Harper found that when these beliefs form a belief system that is predominately irrational, we are more prone to stress and sexual dissatisfaction. Throughout the course of their clinical work, Ellis and Harper noticed recurring themes or patterns. They distilled these beliefs into 10 that form the basis of an irrational belief system or way of viewing the world. This way of viewing the world could relate to any subject. When it forms the basis of our sexual belief system, it can create sexual problems and make it difficult to communicate effectively. The beliefs are the following:

1. You must have love or approval from all the people you find significant.
2. You must thoroughly prove adequate, competent, or achieving.
3. When people act obnoxiously or unfairly, you should blame and damn them and see them as bad, wicked, or rotten individuals.
4. You have to view things as awful, terrible, horrible, and catastrophic when you get seriously frustrated, treated unfairly, or rejected.
5. Emotional misery comes from external pressures, and you have little ability to control or change your feelings.
6. If something seems dangerous or fearsome, you must preoccupy yourself with it and make yourself anxious about it.
7. You can more easily avoid facing many life difficulties and self-responsibilities than undertake more rewarding forms of self-discipline.
8. Your past remains all-important, and, because something once strongly influenced your life, it has to keep determining your feelings and behavior today.
9. People and things should turn out better than they do, and you must view it as awful and horrible if you do not find good solutions to life's grim realities.
10. You can achieve maximum human happiness by inertia and inaction or by passively and uncommittedly enjoying yourself.

Source: Guide to Rational Living, by A. Ellis and R. Harper (Hollywood, CA: Wilshire Book Company, 1998). Reprinted with permission.

D—Dispute

Khalid decides to tackle this problem by analyzing each of these illogical beliefs and substitute more rational thoughts in their place.

1. "It's irrational for me to think that Teri should always be in the mood."
2. "It's impossible for us both to always be in sync with our sexual desire."
3. "Each partner has the right to say no when he or she is not in the mood to make love."
4. "People can be in love but on any given day not feel sexually responsive."
5. "Teri's not wanting to have sex doesn't necessarily mean she doesn't love me."
6. "Her not wanting to have sex with me doesn't necessarily mean she's doing it with someone else."
7. "I'm great for Teri. This has nothing to do with that."

E—Evaluate

As a result of working through the dispute and coming up with a more rational belief system concerning what happened, Khalid experiences the following changes: Physically, his muscles begin to relax and he can get to sleep again. His tension headache subsides. Emotionally, Khalid feels like a tremendous weight has been lifted from his shoulders. He feels he is thinking clearly again. Khalid stops drinking and asks Teri whether she wants to snuggle and fall asleep while he reads his book.

Communicating About Disabilities

As we have discussed, communicating sexual needs and wants is often difficult for many people because of their upbringing, the uniqueness of the subject, and the lack of a uniform language of sex. Communicating about special sexual considerations due to disabilities presents a unique challenge for the person with disabilities and his or her partner. Not only does the person have to work through personal issues surrounding sexuality in general, but he or she also has the added challenge of describing how the disability impacts sexual needs and wants (Bullard & Knight, 1981).

As we've seen, disabilities can affect sexual anatomy and physiology, sexual response, and sexual behavior. Describing these effects and the special considerations they bring to the sexual encounter can be a daunting experience for the most proficient communicator. We'll use colostomy as the disability to illustrate these challenges.

Ostomy

Ostomy is a general term used to describe an artificially created opening in the body. The prefix associated with the ostomy denotes the organ where the opening is. A *colostomy* is an opening of the colon, for example, and an *ileostomy* is an opening to the ileum (Alterescu, 1981). The actual connection of the opening to the abdominal wall is referred to as the *stoma*.

Many people are squeamish about the association of an ostomy to organs associated with human waste (urine and feces), and they have a hard time discussing the impact of the ostomy on their sexuality. A colostomy, for instance, redirects the movement of feces from the rectum and anus to the colostomy bag, which is attached to the stoma through a ring and sealed bag secured to the abdominal wall with adhesive material. The bag fills up with waste on a schedule that coincides with the person's bowel movement behavior. The consistency of the fecal material and the frequency of accumulation will vary according to the person's diet, exercise behavior, and overall health. Assuming the person with the colostomy returns to a normal lifestyle following surgery, eventually the person can expect a bowel pattern similar to what he or she experienced prior to the surgery. A person with a colostomy can learn how to clean, change, sanitize, and maintain the colostomy bag to ensure a return to a normal life and control of bowel functioning with normal hygiene.

In reality, having a colostomy does not necessarily impact sexual response and behavior. The physiological changes that occur during arousal and orgasm are, in most cases, unchanged by the procedure. A person who has undergone a colostomy may experience nerve damage, pain, and the development of scar tissue. These can impact sexual arousal and the enjoyment of sexual activities (Alterescu, 1981). These complications can occur with any surgery, however, and are not exclusive to colostomy. A person with a colostomy can also have temporary mechanical problems associated with securing the ostomy bag to the abdominal wall and securing a leak-free attachment between the ring and the collection bag.

In most cases, sexual problems associated with colostomy are due to psychosocial factors related to the patient's self-perception, depression, and relationship concerns or problems. Desire and the frequency of sexual activity can be affected if the person with the colostomy perceives it negatively and as something that interferes with sexuality in a negative way. Alterescu (1981) has compiled the following list of questions that many colostomy patients have:

Will my partner(s) still consider me desirable and attractive?
Will I still be capable of maintaining social usefulness as a worker and mother/
father?

Will I (male patient) be capable of achieving/maintaining an erection and ejaculating?

Will I be able to make adjustments in clothing?

Will I experience pain during intercourse?

Will my pouch interfere with my sexual activities?

How will I explain the existence of my pouch to my new partner?

Will my ostomy keep me from being the person I want to be?

Questions like these must be answered honestly and completely by the person with a colostomy and his or her partner in order to have a satisfying sex life. The communication skills discussed in this chapter will help people with a colostomy or other disabilities understand these concerns, transmit them to their partner(s), and keep the dialogue open regarding these issues so they don't lead to deeper response and relationship problems.

Foremost, this chapter has demonstrated how the responsibility for sexual communication lies with the individual. People with a colostomy or any other disability must discuss the nature of their disabilities with their intimate partners and helping professionals if necessary. They must seek to learn all they can about how their disability impacts their sexuality and take responsibility for transmitting this information to their intimate partners.

Your responses to the Personal Assessment, Thought Questions, and Test Yourself! quiz questions can be logged online in your Virtual Workbook at **http://health.wadsworth.com/blonna1.**

Personal Assessment

11.1 Sexual Communication Satisfaction Questionnaire

This questionnaire assesses your satisfaction with your sexual communication with your partner. Use the following scale to indicate how strongly you agree or disagree with each statement:

1 = Strongly agree   4 = Disagree

2 = Agree   5 = Strongly disagree

3 = Neither agree nor disagree

1. I tell my partner when I am especially sexually satisfied.
2. I am satisfied with my partner's ability to communicate his/her sexual desires to me.
3. I do not let my partner know things that I find pleasing during sex.
4. I am very satisfied with the quality of our sexual interactions.
5. I do not hesitate to let my partner know when I want to have sex with him/her.
6. I do not tell my partner whether or not I am sexually satisfied.
7. I am dissatisfied over the degree to which my partner and I discuss our sexual relationship.
8. I am not afraid to show my partner what kind of sexual behavior I find satisfying.
9. I would not hesitate to show my partner what is a sexual turn-on to me.
10. My partner does not show me when he/she is sexually satisfied.
11. I show my partner what pleases me during sex.
12. I am displeased with the manner in which my partner and I communicate with each other during sex.
13. My partner does not show me things he/she finds pleasing during sex.
14. I show my partner when I am sexually satisfied.
15. My partner does not let me know whether sex has been satisfying or not.
16. I do not show my partner when I am sexually satisfied.
17. I am satisfied concerning my ability to communicate about sexual matters with my partner.
18. My partner shows me by the way he/she touches me if he/she is satisfied.
19. I am dissatisfied with my partner's ability to communicate his/her sexual desire to me.
20. I have no way of knowing when my partner is sexually satisfied.
21. I am not satisfied in the majority of our sexual interactions.
22. I am pleased with the manner in which my partner and I communicate with each other after sex.

Source: "Sexual Communication, Communication Satisfaction, and Solidarity in the Developmental Stages of Intimate Relationships," by Lawrence R. Wheeless, Virginia Eman Wheeless, and Raymond Baus (1984), *Western Journal of Speech Communication, 48* (3), 224. Copyright © 1984 by Western Speech Communication Association. Reprinted by permission.

Thought Questions

1. What makes communicating about sex different from communicating about other subjects?

2. Define metacommunication. What are the parts of a metacommunication model?

3. What four sets of skills are involved in two-way communication?

4. What is "I" language? Give examples of using "I" language.

5. How do we communicate about sexuality nonverbally? Is nonverbal sexual communication accurate?

6. What is the best thing to do if miscommunication becomes apparent? Whose responsibility is it? Why?

7. Give examples of four open-ended sexual statements.

8. What is the impact of language level on sexual communication?

9. What are three barriers to effective listening?

10. What are two barriers to correcting miscommunication?

11. What should you do if you reach a communication impasse?

12. Describe the effects of a disability such as colostomy on sexual communication.

Test Yourself!

1. Which statement best characterizes communicating about sex?
   a. It is easier than communicating about other topics because everyone likes sex.
   b. It is harder than communicating about other topics because of the subject and the personal nature of the material.
   c. It is easier because of the personal nature of the subject matter.
   d. It is harder because the subject is personal and immaterial.

2. Metacommunication focuses on
   a. the actual content being discussed.
   b. the content and the relationship between the communicators.
   c. the content and the metaphysical nature of human sexuality.
   d. the relationship between the communicators.

3. The key to successful communications using Berne's transactional analysis model is
   a. communicating on the same ego state as your partner.
   b. communicating on a different ego state than your partner.
   c. trying to keep your ego state out of objective communication with your partner.
   d. keeping your ego out of communications.

4. Which of the following represents a true exchange of information between two people?
   a. Selflessness
   b. Monologue
   c. Dialogue
   d. Information giving

5. Which statement best describes how men and women communicate?
   a. Research shows that men tend to focus more on wanting to solve problems, whereas women want to share emotions.
   b. Research shows that men and women are very similar in their communication patterns.
   c. Research shows that women tend to focus more on wanting to solve problems, whereas men want to share emotions.
   d. Research shows that women and men focus equally on problem solving and sharing emotions.

6. Nonverbal forms of sexual communication
   a. generally are not very useful in communicating sexual content.
   b. are often just as effective in communicating sexual needs and wants as verbal forms.
   c. should be avoided until you get to know a person better.
   d. have no place in effective sexual communication.

7. What is the relationship between language level and sexual miscommunication?
   a. Miscommunication can occur when the language levels of the two communicators differs.
   b. Miscommunication occurs because people from different countries have different words to describe things.
   c. It is easiest to avoid miscommunication by using scientific/professional language, which is the most precise language level.
   d. Miscommunication is less likely to occur if both partners use a lower language level.

8. "I" language refers to
   a. maintaining eye contact when you are communicating.
   b. being very assertive about your sexual needs and desires.
   c. taking personal responsibility for feelings.
   d. putting blame for problems on others where it belongs.

9. Using open-ended statements is effective when you want your partner to
   a. expand on how he or she feels about an issue.
   b. get a simple yes or no answer to a simple question.
   c. leave things kind of open to debate.
   d. put off closure on the subject.

10. DESC is a communication model that is useful for
    a. using verbal aggressiveness to resolve communication problems.
    b. using verbal assertiveness to resolve communication problems.
    c. describing communication problems that are descriptive in nature.
    d. expressing deep-seated sexual problems to your partner.

Media Menu

You can link to the following online tools by visiting
http://health.wadsworth.com/blonna1.

 InfoTrac Activity

Van Gorp, K. (2001, Fall). You're not hearing me! Communication problems within a couple. *Marriage Partnership,* *18*(3), 18.

 Web Resources

General Communication Skills

http://discoveryhealth.queendom.com/access_communication_skills.html

This site presents a test that evaluates your general level of communication skills and offers detailed, personalized tips.

Communication in Sexual Behavior

www.couns.msu.edu/self-help/suggest.htm

Michigan State University Counseling Center site with a wide range of topics to improve communications: asserting your interpersonal rights, improving communication skills, maintaining a relationship, communicating in sexual behavior, establishing sex guidelines, saying no without feeling guilty, criticizing others, blaming, and avoiding the self-defeating "should."

Manhattan College Counseling Center

www.mancol.edu/stntlife/relcom.html

Suggestions for improving communication skills in relationships. These hands-on exercises provide sentence completion methods in which students complete statements with their partner.

RealWorld University

www.rwuniversity.com/articles.cfm?cid=28

RealWorld University's (RWU) mission is to help students succeed in college and in life by helping them identify and pursue their purpose, strengthen their character, overcome life's obstacles, and maximize their potential. RWU addresses some of the toughest challenges facing college students today by sharing proven strategies, solutions, and advice from some of the country's leading educators, authors, speakers, and college graduates.

DiscoveryHealth.Com's Love and Relationships Page

http://health.discovery.com/centers/loverelationships/loverelationships.html

This is the love and relationships page of DiscoveryHealth.Com. It offers a variety of assessments and links to other pages devoted to this subject.

References

Alterescu, V. (1981). Sexual functioning following creation of an abdominal stoma. In D. G. Bullard & S. E. Knight (Eds.), *Sexuality and physical disability*. St. Louis: Mosby.

Andersen, P. A. (1999). *Nonverbal communication: Form and function*. Mountain View, CA: Mayfield.

Berne, E. (1960). *Transactional analysis in psychotherapy*. New York: Grove.

Bower, S. A., & Bower, G. H. (1976). *Asserting yourself: A practical guide for positive change*. Reading, MA: Addison-Wesley.

Bullard, D. G., & Knight, S. E. (Eds.). (1981). *Sexuality and physical disability*. St. Louis: Mosby.

Dou, W. L., & Clark, W. (1999, Summer–Fall). Appreciating the diversity in multicultural communication styles. *Business Forum, 24*(3–4), 54–62.

Ellis, A. (1993). Reflections on rational emotive therapy. *Journal of Consulting and Clinical Psychology, 61*(2), 199–201.

Ellis, A., & Harper, R. (1998). *A new guide to rational living*. North Hollywood, CA: Wilshire.

Greenberg, J. S. (2003). *Comprehensive stress management* (8th ed.). Boston: McGraw-Hill.

Hall, E. (1973). *The silent language*. Menlo Park, CA: Cummings.

Ivey, A. E., D'Andrea, M. D., Ivey, M. B., & Simek-Morgan, L. (2002). *Theories of counseling and psychotherapy: A multicultural perspective* (5th ed.). Boston: Allyn & Bacon.

Michaud, S. L., & Warner, R. M. (1997, October). Gender differences in self-reported troubles talk. *Sex Roles: A Journal of Research, 37*(7–8), 527–541.

Mandel, B. (1980, Summer). Communication: A four part process. *Hotliner, 1*(4), 6.

McBurney, L. (2002, Spring). Touch me—not there! How to be sensual without necessarily being sexual. *Marriage Partnership, 19*(1), 26–29.

McGinty, K., Knox, D., & Zusman, M. E. (2003, March). Nonverbal and verbal communication in "involved" and "casual" relationships among college students. *College Student Journal, 37*(1), 68–72.

Noller, P., & Fitzpatrick, M. A. (1991). Marital communication. In A. Booth (Ed.), *Contemporary families: Looking backward, looking forward*. Minneapolis: Council on Family Relations.

Sawyer, C. R., & Behnke, R. R. (2002, Fall). Behavioral inhibition and the communication of public speaking state anxiety. *Western Journal of Communication, 66*(4), 12–23.

Senecal, S., Murard, N., & Hess, U. (2003, January). Do you know what I feel? Partners' predictions and judgements of each other's emotional reactions to emotion-eliciting situations. *Sex Roles: A Journal of Research*, 21–38.

Smith, J. C. (1993). *Creative stress management*. Englewood Cliffs, NJ: Prentice Hall.

Tannen, D. (1990). *You just don't know: Women and men in conversation*. New York: Morrow.

Walen, S., DiGuisseppi, R., & Wessler, R. (1980). *A practitioner's guide to RET*. New York: Oxford University Press.

Watzlawick, P., Beaven, J. H., & Jackson, D. D. (1967). *Pragmatics of human communication*. New York: Norton.

chapter *twelve*

Sexual Dysfunction, Sex Therapy, *and* Sexual Enhancement

Student Learning Objectives

After reading this chapter, students will be able to

- Describe the relationship between sexual dysfunctions and the phases of the sexual response cycle.

- Describe the key components of sexual desire disorders.

- Describe the key components of sexual arousal disorders.

- Describe the main elements of orgasmic disorders.

- Describe the main elements of sexual pain disorders.

- Describe the psychological causes of sexual dysfunctions.

- Evaluate recent criticisms of the current conceptualizations of sexual disorders based on the classic sexual response cycle.

- Describe the medical and pharmacological causes of sexual dysfunctions.

- Differentiate prior learning and immediate causes of sexual dysfunctions.

- Evaluate the effects of legal and illicit psychoactive substances on sexual dysfunction.

Test your understanding of these objectives by taking the end-of-chapter quiz, available online at **http://health.wadsworth.com/blonna1.**

activity teaser: *How can you improve your sexual response? Find out with the Personal Exploration Activity on page 381.*

case study 12.1

Orgasmic Disorders: Christine

Christine, 25, single, is white.

Christine is a college senior. She has been having sex with her boyfriend, Nick, for about 3 months and has not been able to have an orgasm yet. She met with Dr. Blonna.

I'm not sure whether I have a problem, but I've been having sex with my boyfriend, Nick, since the end of the spring semester—about 3 months—and haven't had an orgasm yet.

He's a real nice guy, and I think I love him. I've been dating lots of guys since my boyfriend Tom and I broke up 3 years ago, and Nick is very special. I met him at the college gym, and we were instantly attracted to each other. He is in great shape, is very outgoing, a former athlete, and has a great sense of humor. In a way, he's a great big kid, always joking.

We started having sex from the first date and all spring made love about three to five times a week, but I never had an orgasm with him. Even though I don't come, sex with him is a lot of laughs. The only problem is that he kind of rushes through it and doesn't last very long. I haven't said anything because I kind of hoped he would get better with time.

During the summer, things cooled off because he had a summer house with a bunch of fraternity brothers and was at the shore every weekend (Friday to Sunday night) from Memorial Day to mid-September. I went down a few times but was really turned off because everyone did nothing but get drunk, act out, and sleep the days away.

Since September, we've picked up where we left off last spring, but I still can't come with him. When I masturbate by myself, I have satisfying orgasms, but not with Nick. I'm afraid that if I tell him, he'll get upset and maybe our relationship will suffer. The problem is that I like him a lot and would like the relationship to grow, but the sex is a real problem. I'm not sure what to do about the relationship.

Critical Thinking

What evidence is there to support the idea that Christine's dysfunction may be more related to her relationship with Nick than anything having to do with herself?

Use your Virtual Workbook to explore your answer to this question at **http://health.wadsworth.com/blonna1.**

Sexual dysfunction A disturbance or disorder in desire, excitement, orgasm, or resolution of the sexual response cycle

Sexual dysfunctions, as Christine illustrates, are complex phenomena, involving our bodies, minds, past history, relationships, and a host of other factors. According to the *Diagnostic and Statistical Manual,* **sexual dysfunction** is a disturbance or disorder in desire, excitement, orgasm, or resolution of the sexual response cycle (American Psychiatric Association [APA], 2000). As we discussed in detail in Chapter 7, the interaction of all five senses plays a key role in the sexual response: becoming sexually aroused, maintaining interest, having an orgasm, and feeling satisfied.

Sensory arousal combines with emotional arousal (limbic system) and conscious thought (cerebral cortex) as our sensing, feeling, thinking brain triggers and directs the organs, glands, and tissues that regulate our sexual response. Although something as common as developing and maintaining an erection seems like a fairly primitive response, in reality it is a complex result of many reactions within a complicated interdependent system. As such, sexual response isn't always an all-or-nothing phenomenon. Levels of performance and satisfaction vary. Everyone experiences some level of dysfunction throughout the course of life. Sometimes it is produced by illness, stress, fatigue, or a variety of other causes. Dysfunction is not just a heterosexual issue, either. Gay, lesbian, and bisexual people also experience sexual dysfunction.

Our perception, gender role, and beliefs about aging all factor into determining whether a sexual problem is or is not a dysfunction. As we'll describe, one of the mediating factors in determining dysfunction is whether the "problem" causes emotional distress or relationship difficulties. One's perception of the issue plays a big part in determining whether it is even a problem. If a person or partner does not perceive a sexual "problem" (premature ejaculation, for instance) as troubling, is it a dysfunction or even a problem?

Gender role also factors into the mix. For years women were taught that they were not supposed to initiate sex. Does a woman who wants sex but won't ask for it from her partner because she thinks this isn't the "proper" thing to do have a sexual dysfunction? What about our expectations of sex as we age? If we expect a decline in sexual performance and response because we view this as a normal part of aging, do these changes constitute a dysfunction? We'll address these and many other questions in this chapter.

Basson et al. (2000) carry the issue of gender-based differences a step further. They argue that emotional factors and intimacy issues are the central issues in understanding sexual response and subsequent dysfunction in women. Women, according to these researchers, are much more likely than men to have intimacy issues as the basis of low sexual desire and sexual arousal disorders. In fact, as we will examine in more detail later in this chapter, Basson et al. found that many women who have low sexual desire have no problem becoming aroused physiologically (evidence of lubrication and so forth) and achieving orgasm.

If you recall from Chapter 7, sexual functioning combines physical, intellectual, emotional, social, spiritual, and environmental well-being. We need a minimum level of physical health to ensure that all of the component body parts and systems are able to perform the myriad tasks necessary for sexual response to occur. The health of our social relationships impacts on our ability to trust our partner, relax, and let the sexual response happen. Our emotional health contributes to our self-esteem, feeling good about ourselves, and feeling comfortable with our partner. Our intellectual health contributes to being able to understand and improve our sexual technique and to make informed choices about fertility control and protecting ourselves against STDs. Our spirituality helps us connect with our inner sexuality and others in a deeper way. And a healthy environment allows us to feel safe and comfortable in our sexual space. Stevenson (2002), in an eloquent editorial, describes the interplay of the mind–body continuum in sexual response and dysfunction. He explains how the body does not exist independent of the mind and how sexual dysfunctions can never be diagnosed independently without an examination of the whole person.

Therefore, although we will use the classic diagnostic and etiologic criteria for sexual dysfunctions for practical purposes (since they are the most widely accepted), they must always be examined within the context of the whole person, not merely as just physical or psychological problems.

Physical/Medical Causes of Sexual Dysfunction

Research findings over the past decade concerning the causes of sexual dysfunctions have created a dramatic change in our understanding of these conditions and approach to their treatment. In the past, sexual dysfunctions (particularly **erectile dysfunction,** formerly known as *impotence*) had been thought to be caused primarily by psychological factors. Most experts in the field now believe the exact opposite, especially regarding erectile disorder. Sexual dysfunction can be caused by a host of physical causes, ranging from disease and injury to the side effects of legal and illegal drugs (Richardson, 1991; Buvat, Buvat-Herbaut, Lemaire, Marcolin, & Quittelier, 1990; Kita, 1997; Leland, 1997; Horvitz, 1997).

Recent studies show that understanding sexual dysfunction may not be such a simple either-or phenomenon. It may well be that dysfunction in men is primarily related to blood flow and physical causes (therefore very amenable to pharmacological fixes such as Viagra), whereas problems in women are more related to psychosocial issues such as intimacy (*Drug Week,* 2001). The differences may be so

Erectile dysfunction A disturbance or disorder related to obtaining an erection

Aerobic exercise can reduce the risk for developing certain sexual dysfunctions.

great that prominent researchers in the field are calling for a reexamination of the nature of sexual response in women to shed light on how to treat sexual dysfunctions. This may ultimately change the very way dysfunctions are diagnosed and treated in men and women (Lieblum, 2000).

Cardiovascular Disease

In a study of approximately 1,300 men in the Massachusetts Male Aging Study, nearly half of the subjects (all were between 40 and 70 years of age) had experienced erectile difficulties in the previous 6 months (Heapes, 1994). Furthermore, men being treated for heart disease and high blood pressure were up to four times more likely to be completely impotent than men without these conditions. These findings implicate vascular problems (blood flow) as the major culprit in erectile problems. All forms of cardiovascular disease rob the blood and body of adequate oxygen through circulation.

Behaviors that increase the risk for cardiovascular disease also can increase the likelihood of incurring erectile disorders. Smokers have been found to be four times more likely than nonsmokers to have severe erectile dysfunction (Heapes, 1994).

Physical Wellness

High-level physical wellness can enhance sexual performance and satisfaction and lessen the risk for dysfunction. Physical wellness plays a crucial role in the desire and excitement phases of sexual response. Physical wellness is also linked to vasocongestion, as blood flow leading to engorgement of genital tissue and lubrication are affected adversely by obesity, arteriosclerosis, and other physical health problems. Being fit (especially attaining high levels of cardiovascular fitness) and maintaining recommended body composition promote efficient vasocongestion.

Other Diseases

Other physical causes of sexual dysfunction range from structural defects or changes (congenital abnormality of the penis or vagina, scar tissue, fibroids, tumors), to sexually transmitted disease, endocrine disorders, neurological problems, and spinal cord injury, to deficiency diseases (insufficient hormonal production, malnutrition, vitamin deficiency), to allergic reactions (say, to spermicide). These and other medical causes can affect any or all of the phases of the sexual response cycle, resulting in a wide variety of sexual dysfunctions. Table 12.1 describes a variety of chronic diseases and disabilities and their effects on sexual functioning.

Injuries and Surgery

Certain injuries also can cause erectile disorder and other forms of sexual dysfunction. An estimated 600,000 or more cases of erectile dysfunction are attributed to accidents and injuries to the underside of the penis (Kita, 1997). Athletic

Table 12.1 Effects of Select Medical Physical Conditions on Sexual Response

Condition	Effects of Sexual Response
Cardiovascular disease	*Men and women:* sexual arousal disorder; loss of sexual desire
Spinal cord injuries	Vary according to severity and location *Men:* often lose ability to have typical erections (may have "reflex" erections); often lose ability to ejaculate *Women:* decreased vaginal lubrication; lose genital and orgasmic sensations
Complications from surgery (hysterectomy, cesarean section, tubal ligation, episiotomy	*Women:* damage to nerves and blood vessels involved in vasocongestion; sexual arousal disorder; orgasmic disorder
Multiple sclerosis and other neurogenic diseases	*Men:* loss of erections and ejaculation *Women:* orgasmic disorder
Diabetes	*Men:* male erectile disorder; small percentage suffers from retrograde ejaculation and less intense ejaculation *Women:* varies—some experience less lubrication and sexual arousal disorder; female orgasmic disorder
Cancer	
Breast	Vary based on treatment and psychological reactions
Cervix	Minimal if treated early (bleeding; discharge)
Uterus	Vary according to amount of scarring; hysterectomy is sometimes related to sexual desire disorder in women who feel a diminished sense of femininity
Prostate	Can cause sexual arousal disorder and orgasmic disorder
Testicles	Infertility; no physiological changes but psychological stress is related to sexual desire disorder in some men who feel a diminished masculinity
Anorexia	Sexual desire disorders; sexual arousal disorders
Bulimia	Sexual desire disorder

Sources: Masters, Johnson, and Kolodny (1996); O'Donohue and Geer (1993); Lowinson, Ruis, Millman, and Langrod (1992); Kita (2001).

injuries resulting from being kicked or struck in the groin can damage the area. Extensive bicycle riding (100-mile rides) can damage the blood vessels on the underside of the penis. Falls that crush the penis against an object (such as a railing or fence) can damage the blood vessels that supply blood to the penis.

Female-centered sex therapists suggest that such injuries to women can also damage nerves and blood vessels in the pelvic region associated with sexual response in women. "Straddle" injury trauma associated with accidents such as falls from gymnastic balance beams and narrow bicycle seats can affect blood flow and nerve transmissions in women also (Kita, 2001).

Sexual dysfunction can also be traced to nerve and blood vessel damage associated with surgery. Common surgical procedures such as episiotomy, cesarean section, hysterectomy, and tubal ligations are often related to subsequent sexual dysfunctions. Cosmetic surgery involving the pelvic area (genital, cosmetic surgery, vaginal tightening, and labial reconstruction) is also associated with some forms of female sexual dysfunction (Kita, 2001).

Substance-Induced Sexual Dysfunction

Substance-induced sexual dysfunction can affect any stage of the sexual response cycle. The essential feature of this condition is the link between a clinically diagnosed sexual dysfunction and a specific substance, legal or illegal. The three diagnostic criteria of this condition are as follows:

1. The sexual dysfunction causes marked distress or interpersonal difficulty.
2. Depending on the substance involved, the condition may involve impaired desire, arousal, or orgasm or sexual pain and is fully explained by the direct effects of the substance.
3. The dysfunction is not better accounted for by a dysfunction that is not substance induced. A diagnosis of substance-induced sexual dysfunction represents a recurrent or persistent condition and should not be confused with the effects of episodic substance intoxication.

healthy sex hints 12.1

Enhancing Male Potency by Increasing Wellness

Greg Gutfield (1994) summarized findings from studies documenting the effects of a healthy lifestyle on sexual potency. These findings show that many of the roadblocks to good sex can be removed through simple lifestyle changes aimed at improving overall health status.

Three of the major culprits in sexual potency—heart disease, diabetes, and high blood pressure—often can be prevented by regular exercise and a healthy diet. Both of these also aid tremendously in weight management and controlling obesity, a major risk factor for all three conditions. The common denominator is *vascular health*. Impaired blood flow leads to poor sexual response. Increasing exercise and eating a healthy diet (low-fat, high-carbohydrate, moderate protein) enhances blood flow and vascular health.

Stress is another factor that can undermine sexual potency. Chronic stress can lower testosterone, the key hormone related to sexual desire. Less testosterone means less sexual desire. Stress also can make us angry. Men who respond to stressors by losing control and getting angry were much more likely to suffer from erectile disorder then men who were not angry. Of the men who scored highest on measures of anger, 35 percent reported moderate erectile disorder and 20 percent complete erectile disorder. Stress management and relaxation will help moderate testosterone levels, reduce anger, and help restore potency.

Smoking increases the likelihood of erectile dysfunction and is a major risk factor in cardiovascular disease (Heapes, 1994). Smokers are four times as likely as non-smokers to develop complete erectile disorder. The negative effects of smoking can be reversed by quitting.

Use it or lose it. "The more erections you have, the more you're likely to have" (Gutfield, 1994). Having at least three erections per week can reduce the risk for erectile disorder. Erections improve blood flow to the penis. Frequent erections help promote circulation and bring oxygen-rich blood to the area.

To improve your erectile function, make these three simple lifestyle changes:

1. Exercise regularly.
2. Eat a balanced diet.
3. Stop smoking.

Both **psychotropic** (mind-altering) **drugs** and **somatotropic** (body-altering) **drugs** may have side effects that can produce sexual dysfunction. In some cases, the use of drugs to influence sexual response is intentional (for example, using alcohol to decrease sexual inhibitions). In other cases, the effects of drug use on sexual response are unintentional or unexpected (for instance, the contributing effects of prescription antihypertensive medications on male erectile disorders) (Parrish, 1997).

Psychotropic drugs Substances that are mind altering

Somatotropic drugs Substances that are body altering

Prescription Drug Interactions

The effects of prescribed and over-the-counter drugs are many and varied. They range from decreased vaginal lubrication associated with antihistamines (over-the-counter use by allergy sufferers) to erectile dysfunction associated with certain forms of antihypertensive medication. The commonly prescribed antidepressant drug Prozac (fluoxetine) has been shown to cause erectile disorder and **anorgasmia** in small numbers of male and female users, respectively (Rosen, 1991). Table 12.2 outlines common medical drugs and their associated sexual dysfunctions.

Anorgasmia An inability to achieve orgasm

Anyone who takes these drugs should have a thorough understanding of their potential sexual side effects. A potential complication associated with taking medications is the effect of combining two or more medications. The effects can range from a simple additive effect (the effect of one medication added to the effect of the other) to a **synergistic effect** (the effects of two or more drugs creating

Synergistic effect An enhanced, unpredictable drug effect caused by combining two or more substances

Table 12.2 The Effects of Select Medical Drugs on Sexual Response

Drug	Medical Use	Effect on Sexual Response
Hormones Estrogen and Progesterone	Replacement therapy in menopause; birth control; prostate cancer prescription	May decrease sexual desire in women; sexual arousal disorder in men
Steroids Diannabol and others	Treatment for hypogonad disorder (deficiency in gonadal function); promote growth; treatment for aplastic anemia	*Men:* atrophy of testicles; cessation of sperm production; growth of breasts; sexual desire disorder *Women:* masculination of clitoris; excessive facial and body hair
Hypertensive medications Diamox Catapres Inderal Tanormin	Control high blood pressure	Loss of sexual desire; sexual arousal disorders; orgasmic disorders
Gastrointestinal drugs Tagament Librax	Treat gastrointestinal distress and similar problems	Decreased sexual desire; sexual arousal disorders
Antihistamines	Control allergic reactions, stop runny nose, itchy eyes	Inhibit lubrication; painful intercourse
Psychiatric medications (major tranquilizers)	Control psychotic episodes	Decreased sexual desire; sexual arousal disorders; orgasmic disorders

Sources: Witters, Venturell, and Hanson (1992); Jones and Jones (1977); Masters et al. (1996); O'Donohue and Geer (1993); Lowinson et al. (1992).

a third, enhanced, and often unpredictable effect), which can be associated with sexual dysfunction. This possibility can be especially troubling for people with chronic diseases who must take more than one medication regularly. They must guard against mixing over-the-counter medications with alcohol or illegal substances, as well as medically prescribed drugs.

Psychotropic Drugs

Mind-altering drugs, both legal and illegal, have the potential to affect sexual response. The complexity of our vascular, neurological, and endocrine interactions during sexual response makes us particularly susceptible to the effects of psychoactive substances. The sexually related side effects of psychoactive drugs are variable. As with all psychoactive drugs, the user's psychological well-being and environment can affect the outcome of the drug experience. A placebo effect can occur if a user has certain expectations for the drug.

Depressants   Tranquilizers, barbiturates, and alcohol are all central nervous system (CNS) depressants. They reduce, depress, or slow down brain and nervous system functioning. Although they are all classified as depressants, their intended use and effects are different. Barbiturates and alcohol have a more diffuse, less targeted effect on the nervous system. Benzodiazepines (the most frequently prescribed tranquilizers) selectively target neural receptors. In addition, tranquilizers and barbiturates are prescribed as medical drugs for treating psychological

healthy sex hints 12.2
Dealing with Side Effects of Drugs

Drugs have many different effects. The *intended effect* is the desired outcome of taking the product. The intended effect of hypertension medication, for instance, is to lower blood pressure.

Side effects are secondary outcomes that result from taking the medication. Some side effects are beneficial, such as regulation of the menstrual cycle when taking oral contraceptives. The drug is intended to prevent the release of an ovum, and, as a side effect, it regulates the menstrual cycle. Many side effects, however, are not beneficial for sexual response. A side effect of some hypertension medication, for instance, is a reduction in sexual desire.

All drug manufacturers are required by law to provide information about side effects concerning their products. Pharmacists also are required to discuss side effects with consumers.

Ultimately, you have the responsibility for making sense of it all. Here are some tips for understanding possible adverse side effects of prescriptions:

1. Make sure you know what disease or condition you have been diagnosed as having *before* you leave your health care provider.

2. Be sure you know the name of your medication and its intended effects.
3. Understand exactly how to take it (dosage schedule, contraindications, and so forth).
4. Ask your health care provider, "What possible effects will taking this medication have on my sexual response?"
5. If the medication carries any potentially negative sexual side effects, ask, "What other medication can I take that will treat my disease [or condition] without affecting my sexual response?"
6. When you pick up your prescription, read the package insert. Ask the pharmacist to clear up any questions you have about the medication.

If you experience any negative side effects that detract from the quality of your life, go back to your health care provider.

disorders. Their social use is illegal. Alcohol is a legal, nonmedical drug whose primary use is social.

Tranquilizers originally were divided into two categories: minor (primarily used to treat anxiety and insomnia) and major (antipsychotic drugs used to treat severe mental illness such as schizophrenia). Benzodiazepines (Valium-like drugs) are the most frequently prescribed CNS depressants. The pharmacologic effects of benzodiazepines are so different from those of the antipsychotic drugs that the terms *minor* and *major tranquilizers* are rarely used today.

The primary medical use of Valium-like drugs is to reduce anxiety and treat neuroses. They work by depressing limbic functioning and thereby altering mood. Because these drugs can reduce anxiety and improve mood, they sometimes are used by people in an attempt to enhance sexual desire.

Barbiturates have a less specific, more diffuse sedative/hypnotic effect on depressing nervous system functioning. Barbiturates are used primarily as sedatives, to treat insomnia. Barbiturates are rarely used to treat anxiety these days, having been replaced by safer drugs (such as the benzodiazepines). In low doses, barbiturates can induce a lazy, sleepy state. Because of this, barbiturates sometimes are used incorrectly and illegally to enhance sexual response by inducing a relaxed, less inhibited state of mind. In high, toxic doses, barbiturates can induce coma.

The alcohol people drink is more precisely termed ethyl alcohol, also known as ethanol. **Ethyl alcohol** is available either in its pure form, grain alcohol, or more commonly as the active ingredient in a wide variety of alcoholic beverages. Alcohol is a strong central nervous system depressant.

Ethyl alcohol A grain alcohol that is a central nervous system depressant

---

healthy sex hints 12.3
Mixing Alcohol and Medicines

Sometimes alcohol increases the effects and the risks of a medicine to potentially dangerous levels. About 100 prescription medicines can produce unwanted effects when mixed with alcohol. A few examples are presented here:

Analgesic Pain Medication
Salicylates (aspirin)
Ibuprofen (Advil, Motrin)
Effects: Stomach and intestinal bleeding; bleeding ulcers

Antidiabetic Agents
Chlorpropamide (Diabinese)
Tolbutamide (Orinase) Insulin
Effects: Altered control of blood sugar, most often hypoglycemia

Barbiturates
Secobarbitol (Seconal)
Phenobarbital (Barbita)
Pentobarbital (Nembutal)
Effects: Greater sedative effect; drowsiness; confusion

Benzodiazepines
Alprazolam (Xanax)
Diazepam (Valium)
Triazolam (Halcion)
Effects: Greater sedative effect; impaired motor coordination (such as driving ability)

Monamine Oxidase (MAO) Inhibitors
Isocarboxazid (Marplan)
Phenelzine (Nardil)
Tranylcypromine (Parnate)
Effects: Certain alcoholic beverages contain tyramine, which can cause severe high blood pressure; may be fatal.

Make sure you understand the risks associated with mixing alcohol with your prescription medications. If you have any doubts, ask your physician or pharmacist.

Source: Adapted from "Alcohol and Medications: Ask Before You Mix," publication #B-20, National Council on Patient Information and Education, 666 Eleventh St. N.W., Suite 810, Washington, DC 20001. Reprinted with permission.

Unlike the other categories of depressants (tranquilizers and barbiturates), alcohol is not a prescription medical drug with specific intended effects. Alcohol creates a sedative/hypnotic effect similar to that of barbiturates. Alcohol decreases the inhibitory centers of the brain and is used primarily for its ability to reduce inhibitions. Therefore, people often use alcohol to enhance sexual desire. In larger doses, alcohol has effects similar to those of other depressant drugs.

When a person consumes an alcoholic beverage, about 20 percent of the alcohol enters the bloodstream immediately through the stomach lining. The remainder enters the body when the stomach's contents enter the intestines. Because the brain has a large blood supply, it absorbs a lot of alcohol. The measurement of alcohol content of blood in circulation is termed **blood alcohol concentration (BAC).** Physical and psychological effects on the body at different blood alcohol levels are shown in Table 12.3.

Small elevations in BAC are characterized by a "mellow" state, in which the body is relaxed and the person is less inhibited than usual. At this stage, sexual desire—and sexual performance—may be enhanced. With increased alcohol intake, though, the person's judgment rapidly becomes impaired, which impacts sexual decisions. Because alcohol is classified as a depressant, the initial high may be followed by a low. Some drinkers become suicidal.

Physiological responses (including sexual performance) are compromised with increasing BACs. The person may have trouble walking a straight line and maintaining balance, and the speech may become slurred. Sometimes the person

Blood alcohol concentration (BAC)
A measurement of percentage of alcohol in blood; also termed *blood alcohol level* (BAL)

Table 12.3 Effects of Various Blood Alcohol Concentrations

BAC (%)	Effects
0.01	Mild, if any; slight changes in feeling, mood elevation
0.03	Feelings of relaxation and exhilaration; slight impairment of mental function
0.08	Diminished inhibitions; difficulty performing motor skills; impaired judgment; impaired visual and hearing acuity
0.10	Typically, little or no judgment and poor coordination
0.12	Difficulty performing gross-motor skills; impaired vision; definite impairment of mental function
0.15	Major impairment of physical and mental functions; erratic and irresponsible behavior; distorted judgment; feeling of euphoria; difficulty responding to stimuli
0.20	Confusion; decreased inhibitions; inability to move without assistance; inability to maintain upright position; may fall asleep
0.30	Severe mental confusion; difficulty in comprehension and perception; difficulty responding to stimuli; extreme distortion of sensibility; produces sleep in most people
0.40	Nearly complete anesthesia; severely depressed reflexes; possible unconsciousness or coma
0.50	Unconsciousness or deep coma; possibly death
0.60	Total depression of nerves that control heart and breathing centers; death

vomits. At higher levels, the drinker may pass out. Chronic drinkers often have a problem with erectile dysfunction. Alcohol intoxication can even result in death. Because of the many variables—gender, weight, food consumption, simultaneous use with other medications, and so forth—the actual effects vary from person to person and cannot be predicted.

The legal drinking age is 21 in all states. Also, because of the high accident rates involving drinking and driving, laws are becoming more restrictive. A person is considered legally intoxicated at BAC levels between 0.08 and 0.10 percent, depending on the state. Sexual assault, rape, domestic violence, and crime in general are also associated with overuse of alcohol. *Moderation* is the operative word.

Stimulant Drugs Stimulants work by increasing or speeding up nervous system functioning. Three major physiological effects of stimulants are higher energy and alertness, heightened cognitive functioning, and less appetite. The major legal stimulant

Although alcohol in limited amounts can reduce inhibitions, excess consumption can make sexual arousal difficult.

drugs are **amphetamines,** which come in a wide variety of brands. The major illegal stimulants are designer amphetamines (chemically synthesized variants of legal products) and cocaine (in powder and crack forms). Amphetamines are available by prescription for three intended medical purposes: treatment of narcolepsy (inadvertent falling asleep), attention deficit hyperactivity disorder (ADHD), and weight reduction.

People often use stimulants illegally in an effort to enhance sexual response. Cocaine and intravenous injection of amphetamines have been reported to create an intense burst of energy that users have described as "orgasmic." Users also report that amphetamines can help prolong sexual activity. The use of stimulants seems to interfere with the brain's ability to trigger orgasm. Although these drugs might enhance the excitement and plateau stages, some users are unable to achieve orgasm under any circumstances (Goldberg, 1997).

Hallucinogens Hallucinogens are a class of drugs that distort the perception of reality by altering the perception of all sensory inputs—sights, sounds, tastes, touches, and smells. Hallucinogens work by interfering with the normal function of sensory processing systems within the brain. Routine interpretation of sensory input is altered, causing hallucinations.

Some people use hallucinogens to improve their sexual response by enhancing the perception of touch and other sensations. Users also report a sense of time distortion; sexual activities seem to last longer.

Three of the best-known hallucinogens are lysergic acid diethylamide (LSD), methylenedioxymethamphetamine (MDMA), and phencyclidine (PCP). Hallucinogens are illegal except as part of certain American Indian tribal ceremonies.

Marijuana For many years, marijuana, or cannabis, was classified as a mild hallucinogen. Most drug authorities now place marijuana and its variants (hashish and hash oil) in its own category because of the varied effects. The effects of marijuana result in part from the varying amounts of the active ingredient, tetrahydrocannabinol (THC). High levels of THC can produce a mild hallucinogenic effect, which leads to changes in perception of sensory stimuli. Users report a heightened sensitivity to visual and auditory stimuli and an increased craving for certain kinds of foods.

Amphetamines A central nervous system stimulant that is administered by ingestion, injection, snorting, or inhalation

Hallucinogens A class of drugs that distort the perception of reality by altering the perception of all sensory inputs

The effects of marijuana on sexual response are variable. Many users report increased sexual pleasure because of enhanced sensations, as well as a distortion of space and time. This creates a "time warp" in which the sexual act seems to hang suspended.

Other users, in contrast, report that the same mildly hallucinogenic state creates a kind of paranoia that cancels out these same effects. The loss of control brought on by the distortion of perception of time and space is frightening and can diminish sexual pleasure and disorders in sexual response. Long-term marijuana use has been shown to lower testosterone (the sex hormone most related to sexual desire) and sperm levels.

Marijuana use is illegal except in two instances: (a) as an adjunct to glaucoma treatment (to relieve pressure within the eye) and (b) as a way to reduce nausea symptoms associated with chemotherapy for cancer. In both instances, strict legal regulations control its use.

Narcotics Narcotic drugs are pain killers. They work by diminishing the transmission of pain throughout the nerve pathway. The common opium-derivative narcotics are opium, heroin, and codeine. A common myth concerning heroin addicts is that they are sexually aggressive. To the contrary, one of the side effects of heroin addiction is a diminished interest in sex.

Table 12.4 The Effects of Select Psychoactive Substances on Sexual Response

Drug	Chronic Use or Effects of Small Doses	High Dosage
Depressants		
Benzodiazepines		
Valium	Diminished anxiety and improved	Loss of interest in sex
Librium	social and sexual functioning	
Tranxene		
Barbiturates		
Amytal	Cerebral disinhibition; increased	Loss of desire; sexual
Nembutal	relaxation	arousal disorders; loss of
Luminal		motor control
Seconal		
Tuinal		
Alcohol	Cerebral disinhibition; increased relaxation	After time, loss of desire; sexual arousal disorders; loss of motor control
Stimulants		
Amphetamines	Increased energy and interest in	After time, loss of desire
Cocaine	sex; ability to prolong sexual activities; "rush" similar to orgasm	and interest; loss of control; orgasmic disorders
Hallucinogens		
Marijuana	Heightened awareness and	Decrease in testosterone;
LSD	sensations; time distortion (sex	loss of desire
MDMA	seems to last longer)	
Narcotics		
Opium	Feelings of warmth; reduction in	Loss of desire; sexual
Heroin	aggression; sleepy/mellow state	arousal disorders; orgasmic
Morphine		disorders
Methadone		
Codeine		

Cautions

Any illegal drug carries the potential for toxicity, overdose, and serious physical danger because illegal substances are not regulated or controlled. Therefore, a person has no idea where or how the substance was produced, and there is no way to quantify the amount of the active ingredient in the drug or the presence of any additives. Marijuana, for instance, has varying amounts of THC and can be cured or mixed with a variety of other substances. Heroin and cocaine can be "cut" (diluting the original volume and pure form by adding ingredients to increase the volume) with anything ranging from talcum powder to rat poison.

Penalties for using illegal drugs are variable and far outweigh any perceived benefits associated with enhanced sexual response. Sexual response can be greatly diminished by spending the rest of one's life in prison.

All of the four categories of drugs (depressants, stimulants, hallucinogens [including marijuana], and narcotics) have the potential to cause sexual dysfunction. Table 12.4 summarizes the effects of psychoactive drugs on sexual response.

Psychological Causes of Sexual Dysfunction

The two basic psychological causes of sexual dysfunction are (a) prior learning and (b) immediate causes. **Prior learning** refers to factors related to childhood development. *Immediate causes* are factors that have their origins later than childhood learning.

Prior learning Factors relating to childhood development

Prior Learning

Most theorists agree that childhood learning shapes many of our fundamental attitudes, values, and beliefs about sexuality. Humans are capable of experiencing sexual and sensual pleasure from birth to death. Infants of both sexes seem to derive great pleasure from touching and rubbing their genitals against bedding and clothing. They also seem to thrive when physical bonding, breastfeeding, and other forms of intimate physical touch are established early in infancy (Montague, 1977). When this seemingly innate sexual potential is thwarted through overt or covert child-rearing practices, the seeds of subsequent sexual problems in adulthood are planted.

The messages we receive during childhood—particularly those from our parents and other primary caregivers—contribute heavily to healthy or unhealthy psychosexual development. Sex therapists widely report the relationship between severe antisex parenting and the development of sexual dysfunction in later life. Children who are reared in environments where nudity, masturbation, and childhood inquiry and discussion of sexuality are severely punished are more likely to develop sexual problems than their peers who are reared in more tolerant environments.

In one study, adults with the former type of childhood histories were less interested in sex, derived less pleasure from sexual relations, had more inhibitions about sexual expression, and had higher levels of shame, guilt, anxiety, and disgust than those with less rigid backgrounds (Purcell, 1985). The "sex-as-sin" message and subsequent sexual problems came from a strict or orthodox religious orientation; the more rigidly orthodox, the greater the extent of dysfunction.

Another researcher warned about associating sexual dysfunction with religious orthodoxy. Hyde (1994) notes the lack of suitable research designs and methodology associated with sex therapists' reports concerning the etiology of sexual dysfunction. Without suitable control groups, it is impossible to discern whether orthodoxy or some other factor is the problem.

Lilian's Thoughts About Her Parents' Sexuality

Critical Thinking

Many students can't visualize their parents having sex. What are some of the reasons for this?

Use your Virtual Workbook to explore your answer to this question at **http://health.wadsworth.com/blonna1.**

Lilian, 19, single, lesbian, identifies as African American.

Lilian is a freshman. She shared these feelings about her parents as sexual beings.

I never viewed my parents as sexual creatures. They never talked about sex once in my presence. My mom briefly explained menstruation to me and what to expect when I get my period, but when I interrupted and told her we had already gone over that stuff in school, she abruptly stopped and seemed relieved.

My brothers told me that my mom and dad never talked to them about sex, either. My parents are not very warm people. They never hug and kiss in public and very rarely express themselves physically.

I guess they love each other, because they seem to care about each other and respect one another's needs. It's just that they don't seem interested in sex at all. I'd never ask either of them about a sexual issue. My lover's mom kind of fills that role for me. She thinks its kind of sad that I can't talk to my own mom about it.

To tell you the truth, I can't even imagine my parents ever having sex. I guess they had to have it three times to conceive my brothers and me, but I can't even visualize it. It doesn't gross me out or anything. I just can't seem to create the picture. Funny, isn't it?

Even covert practices can sabotage the development of healthy sexuality. Parents who are uneasy about sexuality may choose to deal with this subject by ignoring it. Saying nothing still sends a strong message to children about sexuality. Omitting such an integral part of life from all discussion leaves a void that children clearly perceive. They learn early that something must be wrong, shameful, or dirty about sex if it doesn't ever come up as a topic of conversation. Students often report anecdotally in class their feelings that their parents must have made love only once (for their conception) or as many times as they have siblings, because they never discussed sexuality, their desire for each other, or other sexual themes when the children were around.

Other messages about sexuality relate to gender role expectations. Males and females in U.S. culture often are reared with different sets of sexual standards and expectations. Rather than viewing sexual needs and expression as a human universal, they are reared with the belief that men and women have differing needs and wants that are gender-specific. Society also has different rules and codes of conduct concerning how to satisfy these needs. Men are expected to be more assertive in pursuing their sexual needs. Women are expected to be more demure, to rely on men to pursue them and satisfy them.

These gender role expectations can create anxiety, shame, guilt, and fear—all attributes that detract from sexual pleasure. As early as 1970, Masters and Johnson noted that rigid sex roles and a double standard concerning sexual expression were often at the root of much of their clients' sexual dysfunction.

Fifteen years later, another study found that nontraditional, less rigid gender roles were related positively to increased enjoyment with sex, greater levels of experimentation with sexual positions, oral sex, initiation of sexual encounters, and assertion of one's sexual needs and wants (Kobilinsky & Palmeter, 1985).

Male sexual dysfunction is often related to performance anxiety stemming from rigid male gender role socialization. (Zilbergeld, 1992). Many men grow up with an idealized picture of male sexuality that positions men as all-knowing, ever-ready, and being responsible for initiating sexual encounters and pleasing their partners. This view puts tremendous pressure on men to live up to those expectations.

Immediate Causes

Immediate causes of sexual dysfunction are identified as (a) failure to engage in effective sexual behavior because of either ignorance or unconscious avoidance; (b) anxiety related to performance, fear of failure, or perceived inability to please a partner; (c) perceptual and intellectual defenses against erotic feelings; (d) failure to communicate effectively with one's partner; and (e) stress and fatigue.

Ignorance/Avoidance Failure to engage in effective sexual behavior often arises from simple ignorance. Sexual dysfunctions related to the arousal and orgasm phase often are related to lack of knowledge concerning effective techniques for achieving optimal levels of stimulation. Ignorance is often compounded by shame and guilt related to sexual experimentation, assertiveness, and admission of what is arousing. Some people unconsciously avoid exploration of the sensual and erotic and fail to take advantage of opportunities to explore sexual satisfaction.

Achieving sexual pleasure is a skill that can improve with better technique. If one perceives sexual activity as something that is learned rather than innate and allows oneself to pursue self-improvement, many sexual problems and dysfunctions can be remedied. All five phases of sexual response can be enhanced by improving technique. People can learn how to increase desire, enhance arousal, maximize plateau, increase the likelihood of orgasm (and multiple orgasms), and enjoy resolution and the refractory period.

Good communication can enhance technique, especially when practicing with a partner and discovering what works with him or her. But, as one man said, "The way I got to become such a good lover was that I practiced a lot by myself when I was at home." Through introspection, guided readings, practice activities, and a variety of other techniques, technique and performance can be enhanced.

Social Wellness

Sex with another person is a unique social experience that cannot be separated from the emotions the two people bring to the encounter. High-level social wellness revolves around healthy relationships. And healthy relationships are based on trust, respect, commitment, love, and affection. Good sex flows out of this safe and protected context.

When trust, respect, and affection are displaced by mistrust, disrespect, and fear, relationship problems ensue. Communication, which is central to good sex, often breaks down when couples are having relationship problems. When sexual needs and desires are not communicated clearly, sexual response suffers.

Performance Anxiety Sexual anxiety resulting from fear of failure, the demand for performance, or an excessive need to please one's partner can literally short-circuit sexual response. Any type of anxiety interferes with the ability to relax and allow vasocongestion and other sexual processes to occur. Anxiety can interfere with the level of sexual desire and ability to get aroused and to create sufficient stimulation to trigger orgasm. Anxiety interferes with the ability to become fully involved in the moment, allowing one to be immersed in the sexual episode.

Anxiety related to a current sexual encounter is often rooted in past sexual episodes. Failure to become sufficiently aroused and maintain an erection in the past often leads to anxiety related to the present ability to perform satisfactorily. Being asked to perform sexually on demand can create resentment and anxiety related to current functioning. In a sense, anxiety fosters the anticipation of failure.

Performance anxiety Fear, worry, or panic associated with one's perceived sexual behavior

Anxiety is perhaps the greatest psychological factor associated with erectile disorder. Although **performance anxiety** is often characterized as a "male problem" because men usually are viewed as responsible for their partner's orgasm, women also suffer from this malady. The person worries over every facet of the sexual encounter: "Am I attractive enough . . . sexy enough?" "Is my penis big enough?" "Are my breasts large enough?" "Is my underwear sexy?" "Will I be able to get [sustain] an erection?" "Will my technique work?" "What if he [she] asks me to do something I'm not comfortable with or know how to do?" "Will we come together?"

These and countless other thoughts and concerns set up an expectation-anxiety-performance-feedback loop that initiates and perpetuates sexual problems. The expectation of failure or poor performance produces anxiety ranging from mild worry to panic. Anxiety creates physiological and psychological roadblocks that impair good performance, resulting in the kind of poor performance the person feared to begin with. In a sense, it creates a self-fulfilling prophecy. The fears are answered by "I told you so," confirming the failure. This outcome seals one's fate by making it twice as hard to correct the problem and improve performance.

Spectatoring Becoming an outside observer of one's own sexual encounter while it is occurring

Defenses   Anxiety also contributes to the perceptual and intellectual defense against erotic feelings called **spectatoring.** Spectatoring occurs when the person becomes an outside observer of his or her own sexual encounter. In a sense, the sexual encounter is reduced to an intellectual activity in which the participant steps away and critically analyzes his or her own behavior.

Whether driven by narcissistic preoccupation with self, voyeurism, or performance anxiety, spectatoring turns the participant into an observer of his or her own sexual encounter. In a sense, the spectator examines the performance of self or partner rather than becoming fully involved in the sensations and experiences. The result is a lack of enjoyment in the experience, as well as dysfunction with any phase in the response cycle.

Communication Problems   We sometimes have trouble communicating our sexual desires, needs, and wants because of feelings of shame, guilt, or fear. Maybe we have learned that sex and sexual needs are a taboo subject.

Furthermore, we may be uncomfortable with the language of sexuality. Our culture does not have a common sexual language. This makes it difficult to understand, articulate, and communicate about sexuality with our partners. Consequently, we suppress our needs and problems, anger and resentment build, and eventually this repression short-circuits the delicate balance among the neurological, vascular, and endocrine factors necessary in the sexual response.

Stress and Fatigue   Finally, stress and fatigue can precipitate sexual dysfunction. When associated with other aspects of life such as work, child-rearing demands, money problems, and poor health, stress and fatigue can rob a person of vital energy and a zest for living. Stress and fatigue can affect all phases of the sexual response cycle.

When men are stressed, their testosterone levels drop. Testosterone, you may recall, is the hormone most related to the level of sexual desire.

Visual Image Source Limited/Index Stock Imagery

Open communication is essential for dealing with sexual problems.

sex in society 12.1

Cultural Considerations in Sexual Dysfunction

As we have seen, sexual dysfunction, like sexual response, is a very complex phenomenon. Basson et al. (2000) have shown that the origin of sexual desire is different for men and women. Desire disorders in women may really be related more to problems associated with intimacy than with desire.

Just as gender affects desire, response, and dysfunction, so does culture. We have seen what a big role communication plays in sexual dysfunction. The American therapeutic model emphasizes open communication between marital partners. Both partners hold equal status in the therapeutic relationship. Each are expected to take an active role and to be responsible for their therapy. How does sexual desire and dysfunction play out in cultures where this is *not* the norm?

Media coverage of Middle Eastern countries such as Iraq, Iran, and Afghanistan, where a radical version of Islam is practiced, paints an entirely different view of spousal relationships and communication between spouses. Women are clearly subservient in the marriage. They do not have equal status, power, or responsibility in the marriage. Women are routinely tortured and put to death for committing even the smallest transgression against their spouses.

In such a climate, is something like *sexual satisfaction* or *dysfunction* even in the vocabulary? Is the right to experience sexual pleasure (for the sake of pleasure itself) even a part of sexual relations between partners?

For years, organizations such as the National Organization for Women (NOW) have lobbied international organizations from the United Nations to Amnesty International to stop barbaric practices such as clitoridectomy (see Chapter 2) and various forms of torture commonly used against women in Iran, Iraq, and Afghanistan. Until women in these cultures have even the most basic human rights, healthy sexual rights will have to be put on hold.

When these men participated in stress management activities, their testosterone levels and levels of sexual desire returned to normal (Singer-Kaplan, 1974). Common sense tells us that when we are tired and stressed, the last thing we seem to be interested in is sex. For the sexual response to begin and orgasm to occur, people need to relax and let the body take over. This reaction often is not possible if a person is feeling overwhelmed or just needs a good night's sleep.

Occupational Wellness

Work-related stress is often associated with low sexual desire. Other job-related issues ranging from rotating shifts to excessive travel and long-standing separation (such as in military assignments) are also implicated in sexual dysfunction. As we have seen, injury and illness are also associated with sexual dysfunction. Some jobs and work sites are more risky than others and can indeed be hazardous to one's health.

Types of Sexual Dysfunctions

The APA (2000) classifies sexual dysfunctions as the lifelong type, acquired type, generalized type, and situational type. *Lifelong* disorders have been present since the onset of sexual functioning. *Acquired* disorders have developed after a period of normal functioning. *Generalized* dysfunctions are not limited to specific types of stimulation, situations, or partners. *Situational* dysfunctions are limited to certain types of stimulation, situations, or partners.

The APA classification of sexual dysfunctions is based on traditional models of sexual response and a four-phase conceptualization of human sexual response: desire, excitement, orgasm, and resolution.

The *desire phase* originates with fantasizing and thinking about engaging in sexual activities. Sexual dysfunctions that relate to this phase are called *sexual desire disorders*.

The *excitement phase* is characterized by the buildup of sexual excitement and tension, manifested through vasocongestion. Penile tumescence and erection are physical evidence of desire in men. In women, vaginal lubrication and expansion and swelling of the vulva indicate arousal. Sexual dysfunctions related to this stage are called *sexual arousal disorders*.

In the *orgasm phase,* built-up sexual tension is released, followed immediately by psychological feelings of satisfaction and satiation. Sexual dysfunctions related to this phase are referred to as *orgasmic disorders*.

The *resolution phase* is characterized by a physiological return to the predesire stage. *Sexual pain disorders* may be present during intercourse or in the resolution phase.

As we mentioned in Chapter 7, Lieblum (2000) proposes a need to redefine sexual response in women based on the emerging work of Basson. Basson et al. (2000) question the presence and ordering of the traditional phases of sexual response and suggests a new model of sexual response. If such a new model of sexual response (particularly one that is more consistent with women's response patterns) becomes widely accepted, it should spur the development of a new paradigm for treating sexual dysfunctions in both men and women.

Dysfunction Versus Disinterest

When discussing sexual dysfunctions, we must recognize the normal continuum of sexual interest and desire in all people. Some people are much more interested in sexual activity than others. The level of interest, desire, and fantasy are variable and are not the only criteria for a diagnosis of sexual dysfunction. To qualify for a diagnosis of either hypoactive sexual desire disorder or sexual aversion disorder, the condition must (a) be persistent and recurrent, (b) cause marked distress or interpersonal difficulty, and (c) not be the result of another medical or physical condition. Little interest in sexual activity, low desire, and no fantasizing aren't necessarily dysfunctional unless they are accompanied by the three diagnostic criteria. Individuals with low levels of sexual desire still can be happy, productive, and sustain satisfying long-term relationships as long as their partners have similar sexual traits.

Hypoactive sexual desire disorder should not be confused with voluntary celibacy or abstinence. Some people perceive celibacy as a sexual dysfunction because they believe it is "abnormal" and abstinence is "unnatural." Celibacy is not a sexual dysfunction. Not all celibate people lack sexual interest and desire. Most of us choose to be celibate and abstain from sexual activity at times in our lives, for a variety of reasons.

Sexual Desire Disorders

Sexual desire disorders include hypoactive sexual desire disorder and sexual aversion disorder.

Hypoactive Sexual Desire Disorder   **Hypoactive sexual desire disorder** is a dysfunction characterized by very low levels (or complete absence) of sexual desire. Individuals with this condition do not initiate sexual activity and may en-

Hypoactive sexual desire disorder A dysfunction characterized by very low or complete absence of sexual desire

Hypoactive Sexual Disorder: The Case of Rhonda

Rhonda, 45, married, is white.

Rhonda is a part-time evening student. She has been married for 20 years and has three children, ages 19, 17, and 14. A homemaker for the past two decades, Rhonda has returned to school to earn a second degree in computer science (she already has a bachelor's degree in English). Rhonda met with one of the authors for counseling.

I'm not even sure why I came to see you. I've never discussed this with anyone before. We were discussing hypoactive sexual disorder in class today, and I think I have it. I've been married to Ed over 20 years. We met in college in the seventies, fell in love, and were married in 1976. Our sex life was great for the first 10 years of our marriage. Even with the pregnancies, the kids, staying home, and all, sex was always a strong part of our relationship. It all changed about 10 years ago. Ed and I had been drifting apart a little. His career had taken off, and I was home with the kids. He felt we didn't have as much in common any more, and I was getting boring. It's hard when you're raising three kids almost by yourself. Ed is on the road almost 40 percent of the time, traveling all over the world for his job. One day he's in Japan, the next in Indianapolis. Meanwhile, I'm schlepping one kid off to soccer, another to band practice, and the third to the mall to work.

Anyway, we began to pull back from each other sexually. Sex became such a hassle. Half of the time Ed claimed he was too tired or busy with work. Other times he'd pop in, fresh from some exciting business trip to Europe or somewhere exotic, and expect me to be Miss Bubbly, drop everything, and jump in the sack with him. I really resented that and just withdrew.

Our sex life slipped from two or three times a week, when he was home, to two or three times a month. There were even some months when we didn't have sex at all.

It seems as though for the past 2 years I don't even care if we don't have sex at all. I'm not even sure if I miss it, but I know something is terribly wrong. I guess I thought these kinds of feelings were inevitable after being together for 20 years.

Critical Thinking

Are Rhonda's feelings about sex "inevitable" after 20 years, or are there ways to keep sexual desire and activity levels continuous after such a long time together?

Use your Virtual Workbook to explore your answer to this question at **http://health.wadsworth.com/blonna1.**

---

gage in sexual relations only begrudgingly at the insistence of their partner. They have little or no motivation to seek sexual stimulation and are increasingly undisturbed by this lack of opportunity.

Three APA (2000) criteria are necessary to diagnose hypoactive sexual desire disorder: (a) persistent or recurrent deficiency or absence of sexual fantasy or desire for sexual activity; (b) marked psychological or interpersonal distress attributable to the disorder; and (c) no other psychological disorder (such as major depression or posttraumatic stress disorder), medical condition, or direct physiological effects of a drug or medication.

The onset of hypoactive sexual desire disorder can be as early as puberty but usually begins in adulthood, after a period of adequate sexual interest. This dysfunction often is associated with chronic stress, interpersonal difficulties, and problems related to intimacy and commitment.

Although loss of sexual desire can be chronic or episodic, depending on the underlying relationship and psychological problems, hypoactive sexual desire disorder is a chronic condition. Temporary loss of sexual desire is a common by-product of recovery from depressive disorders.

Sexual Aversion Disorder Sexual aversion disorder is characterized by disgust and active avoidance of any genital sexual contact with a sexual partner. People who have sexual aversion disorder report anxiety, fear, disgust, or revulsion when

Sexual aversion disorder A disorder characterized by disgust and active avoidance of any genital sexual contact

case study 12.4

Sexual Aversion Disorder: The Case of Josh

Josh, 25, single, is African American; Suzanne, 30, is divorced and white.

Josh, a senior, is an excellent student and works for a large investment firm. He is finishing his degree in finance. He grew up in a strict, conservative family and remembers being severely punished for masturbating when he was a child. He came to the office of one of the authors to seek guidance concerning a sexual problem he had. Josh began by saying, "I feel really strange talking to you about this, but you seem very understanding and I need to talk to someone."

After receiving some reassurances and permission, he began his story.

I met this wonderful woman, Suzanne, at work this semester. She is 30 years old, divorced with no kids, and is one of the stock traders for the company. She is gorgeous, funny, and bright. We hit it off immediately. I'm not a virgin, and I've been engaged in the past, but I'm hardly what you'd call sexually experienced. I like sex and all that, but I'm kind of conservative and not into any kinky stuff. Intercourse is okay, but oral sex repulses me. I start to get nauseous just thinking about it.

Anyway, Suzanne and I began dating, and from the start she was very passionate. She wanted to have sex on our first date, but I held off, told her I was tired and needed to get up early the next day. I wasn't ready for her and needed time to get to know her. I was surprised she wanted to see me again, but she did, and we talked about my need to get to know her better before we began to have sex. She said she really liked me and it was OK—we wouldn't rush into a sexual relationship.

After about a month, we finally had sex. We went back to her place after dinner and a movie, and she had a glass of wine. We started to kiss and undress, and everything was great until she started to kiss me on the chest and stomach. I felt her head begin to go lower, and as she reached my penis, I began to stiffen up and push her away. I guess she thought I was teasing, because she persisted and even laughed. When I began to lose my erection, she knew something was wrong and stopped. I was so embarrassed I didn't know what to say.

She told me it was OK, that we'd try to work it out, but I just couldn't perform that night. I told her we'd have intercourse the next time, but I just couldn't enjoy oral sex. I really like her and want to make this relationship work. My fiancée broke our engagement because of this same issue 3 years ago, and I don't want to lose Suzanne.

confronted with a sexual opportunity with a partner. The aversion may be to a specific aspect of sexual contact (such as genital secretions or vaginal penetration) or to all sexual stimuli, including kissing and touching (APA, 2000).

People with this disorder may have extreme psychological distress, panic attacks, and physical symptoms such as dizziness, nausea, and breathing difficulties. These symptoms often are accompanied by impaired relationship functioning and unusual "covert" strategies to avoid sexual contact (immersion in work, going to sleep early, neglecting personal appearance, abusing substances, and so forth).

Sexual Arousal Disorders

Sexual arousal disorders differ from sexual desire disorders in that the latter are related to lack of desire and the former to the inability to achieve sufficient levels of arousal. The arousal phase of sexual response depends on vasocongestion, which affects erection in men and vaginal lubrication and expansion and swelling of the external genitalia in women. Vasocongestion involves a complex interplay between psychological variables (desire, trust, affection) and physiological variables (unrestricted blood vessels, a healthy endocrine system). Similarly, the causes of sexual dysfunction related to vasocongestion can be psychological, physiological, or both.

Female Sexual Arousal Disorder   The major characteristic of this female dysfunction is the persistent or recurrent inability to attain or maintain sufficient vaginal lubrication and swelling to complete the sexual activity. Vasocongestion is impaired, and the vagina and external genitalia do not become fully engorged with blood. As a result, penetration is restricted, which may result in painful intercourse, avoidance of sexual relations, and a disturbance of the relationship. Female sexual arousal disorder is often accompanied by a sexual desire disorder and female orgasmic disorder.

The three APA diagnostic criteria for female sexual arousal disorder are (a) persistent or recurrent inability to attain or maintain an adequate lubrication/swelling response; (b) marked psychological distress; and (c) not caused by another psychological condition (such as major depression), the effects of a medication or drug, or a general medical condition.

Women who have sexual arousal disorder simply do not become sufficiently aroused to have or enjoy sexual relations. Sexual arousal disorder often is accompanied by sexual desire disorders and female orgasmic disorder.

Male Erectile Disorder   Often called *impotence*, male erectile disorder is the persistent or recurring inability to attain or maintain an adequate erection for the completion of sexual activity. This disorder has different patterns. Some men with the disorder are unable to attain an erection at all. Others are able to get an erection but lose it upon penetration. A third group of males are able to attain an erection and complete penetration but lose their erection during thrusting. Some men with this condition report having morning erections or being able to attain erection during masturbation. Others are unable to attain an erection through masturbation. Approximately 5 percent of men at age 40 are unable to get erections. This number climbs to 15 percent at age 70 (Parrish, 1997).

The three APA diagnostic criteria for male erectile disorder are (a) marked distress or interpersonal difficulty, (b) no other coexisting psychological condition, and (c) no direct physiological effects of a substance or preexisting medical condition. Men who have male erectile disorder often are anxious, fear failure, and doubt their sexual performance. These psychological concerns often result in lack of sexual excitement and pleasure, avoidance of sexual intercourse, and disturbance in sexual and marital relationships.

Isolated episodes of inability to obtain an erection are almost universal among men. The reasons include, among others, stress, fatigue, overindulgence of food or drink, and adjusting to a new partner (Masters et al., 1999).

Orgasmic Disorders

Orgasmic disorders are dysfunctions related to the orgasm phase of sexual response. These disorders center on the inability of men and women to release pent-up sexual tension through orgasm. These people are interested in sexual relations and are able to become sexually aroused. Their problems relate to their inability to move to the next stage of sexual response, orgasm.

Female Orgasmic Disorder   Formerly known as *inhibited female orgasm*, female orgasmic disorder is a persistent or recurring delay in or absence of orgasm following a typical excitement phase. Three specific APA criteria must be met to di-

Orgasmic disorders
Dysfunctions related to the orgasm phase of sexual response

agnose this condition: (a) the absence of orgasm following a "normal" excitement phase, (b) accompanying marked distress or interpersonal difficulty, and (c) not the result of another medical or psychological condition or direct physiological effects of a substance.

The "normal" excitement phase is highly variable. The clinician has to assess what is a normal excitement phase for any given patient. This assessment takes into account the woman's sexual experience, history, and the level and adequacy of stimulation she receives. A normal excitement phase for one woman may be markedly different from that of another woman.

Because the female capacity for orgasm increases with age, female orgasmic disorder is more prevalent in younger women. As women experience more variety of sexual stimulation, become more knowledgeable about their bodies, and better communicate their needs to their partner, they tend to gain orgasmic facility. Most female orgasmic disorder is lifelong rather than acquired, as women who learn to be orgasmic rarely lose this capacity.

When orgasmic disorders are situational, they often are related to issues such as stress, fatigue, overindulgence of food or drink, or relationship problems such as poor communication and poor technique. Many, if not most, women do not receive enough direct clitoral stimulation through back-and-forth vaginal thrusting. Vaginal intercourse alone does not always provide enough clitoral stimulation for orgasm (Fisher, 1973; Hite, 1975).

Emphasis on intercourse (especially the man-on-top position) as the only acceptable sexual outlet for women can be the root of the problem. Often, women who are unable to achieve an orgasm through vaginal intercourse find that they can achieve it during cunnilingus or masturbation or with additional manual clitoral stimulation during coitus.

Some educators and therapists call women who never have had an orgasm "preorgasmic," implying that all women are inherently capable of achieving orgasm. These professionals prefer to view the inability to orgasm as a developmental learning issue versus a dysfunction (Barbach, 1982; Dodson, 1974).

Emotional Wellness

Emotions are related intimately to sexual response. All phases of the sexual response cycle are subject to the effects of emotions. Sexual interest and desire are fueled by positive emotions such as happiness, love, joy, respect, and trust. Negative emotions (especially directed at a partner), such as anxiety, anger, hate, fear, disgust, and mistrust, make interest and desire difficult at best and impossible for most. For the body to respond properly, the mind must let go and relax. Arousal and orgasm also are affected by our emotions. The ability to prolong and enjoy sex are affected in part by emotions. Relaxing and becoming immersed in the sensuality of the plateau stage are difficult if we are feeling anxious, rushed, fearful, or angry. We just want to hurry up and get it over with. When we can relax, let down our guard, and allow our senses free rein, we can enjoy the plateau.

Orgasm is contingent on the buildup of tension through adequate stimulation. It is triggered when we give up mental control and allow our body to be swept along in the ecstasy of physical pleasuring. This is difficult if we are on guard, tense, angry, or resentful.

Resolution might be considered a thankful end to a resentful experience in which partners uncouple, roll over, and fall asleep. Or the resolution phase can be a special time. Lovers who are emotionally healthy can bask in the afterglow of loving time spent pleasuring each other.

Male Orgasmic Disorder Formerly known as **inhibited male orgasm,** this disorder is a persistent or recurrent delay in or absence of orgasm following a normal excitement phase. As for female orgasmic disorder, the three APA diagnostic criteria that must be met in making this diagnosis are (a) absence of orgasm following a "normal" excitement phase, (b) marked distress or interpersonal difficulty, and (c) not the result of a preexisting medical or psychological condition or physiological effects of a medication or other drug.

Men who have this condition most commonly cannot reach orgasm during intercourse. They usually are able to reach orgasm if intercourse is accompanied by manual or oral stimulation of the penis. In less common manifestations, the men are able to experience orgasm only after a substantial amount of noncoital stimulation. A smaller group of men with male orgasmic disorder are able to ejaculate only through masturbation or upon waking from an erotic dream.

Men who have male orgasmic disorder are able to experience pleasure during the excitement phase of sexual activity and enjoy the beginnings of a sexual encounter but rapidly lose interest. For these men, thrusting and prolonging sexual activity are a chore rather than a pleasure. Many men with male orgasmic disorder have a pattern of paraphiliac sexual arousal and are unable to experience orgasm without the object of their desire.

Another male orgasmic disorder is **premature ejaculation,** the persistent or recurring onset of orgasm and ejaculation shortly after penetration or before the man wishes it. The condition is diagnosed after the following three APA criteria have been met: (a) the clinician must take into account factors that affect the duration of the excitement phase such as age, novelty of the partner or scenario, and the frequency of activity; (b) accompanying marked distress and interpersonal difficulty; and (c) not a result of the effects of a substance.

Sometimes premature ejaculation is related to the level of desire and excitement. An extremely high level of sexual arousal can trigger orgasm prematurely and does not represent the true disorder. Occasional episodes are common and are not a problem if they do not cause marked distress and interpersonal difficulty. Also, specific exercises can be practiced to delay orgasm.

With sexual experience and aging, most men learn to delay orgasm. As with women, this technique is related to learning from experience and better sexual communication. Some men continue to have premature ejaculation under all circumstances. Others incur this disorder only when they are with a new partner. Premature ejaculation can create tension and discord in sexual relationships and deter single men from dating and initiating new relationships because of fear and performance anxiety.

Sexual Pain Disorders

The most common sexual pain disorders are dyspareunia and vaginismus. Medical conditions also can result in pain during sexual intercourse.

Dyspareunia **Dyspareunia** is genital pain associated with sexual intercourse. It may be present before, during, or after sexual intercourse and can affect both men and women. Symptoms range from mild discomfort to sharp pain.

Three APA diagnostic criteria must be met to diagnose this condition: (a) recurrent or persistent pain associated with sexual intercourse; (b) marked accompanying psychological distress or interpersonal difficulty; and (c) not caused exclusively by vaginismus or lack of lubrication, a preexisting psychological or medical condition, or the direct effects of a substance.

Sexual pain disorders are not the result of insufficient excitement (which can account for insufficient lubrication and erection and tense muscles) or poor technique. Nor are they a result of medical conditions that affect sexual functioning

Inhibited male orgasm A persistent or recurrent delay in or absence of orgasm following a normal excitement phase

Premature ejaculation The persistent or recurring early onset of orgasm and ejaculation

Dyspareunia Genital pain associated with sexual intercourse (such as STDs or scar tissue) or substance use. Sexual pain disorder is diagnosed when these other conditions are ruled out and the pain has no clear-cut physiological or medical basis.

Vaginismus Painful, involuntary contractions of the outer third of the vagina during attempted penetration

Vaginismus   **Vaginismus** is the recurrent or persistent involuntary contraction of the perineal muscles surrounding the outer third of the vagina during attempted penetration with a penis, finger, tampon, or speculum. In some cases, even the anticipation of vaginal penetration can cause muscle spasms. Symptoms range from mild discomfort and tightness to severe contractions and cramping.

The three APA diagnostic criteria that must be met to diagnose this condition are (a) recurrent or persistent involuntary spasm of the musculature of the outer third of the vagina upon insertion, (b) accompanying psychological distress or interpersonal difficulty, and (c) not caused by a preexisting psychological or medical condition.

Vaginismus usually is discovered upon first gynecological examination or the onset of sexual intercourse. It is more common in young women than older women but can become chronic if it is not treated. It is a primary contributing factor to unconsummated marriages and can limit the development of relationships. Vaginismus is more common in women who have negative attitudes about sex, as well as females who have a history of sexual abuse or trauma.

Sexual Dysfunction Caused by a General Medical Condition

The essential features of this disorder are pain, hypoactive sexual desire, male erectile dysfunction, or other types of sexual dysfunction that are direct physiological effects of an established medical condition. Medical conditions range from obvious sexual disorders such as sexually transmitted diseases to inapparent conditions such as arteriosclerosis.

The three diagnostic criteria that must be met to establish the presence of this disorder are (a) clinically significant sexual dysfunction resulting in marked distress or interpersonal difficulty; (b) medical history, physical examination, or laboratory findings fully explaining the dysfunction as the direct physiological effect of a general medical condition; and (c) not better accounted for by another mental disorder.

A Survey of Sexual Dysfunction

At a meeting of the Office of Research on Women's Health, National Institutes of Health, the director of the Partnership for Women's Health at Columbia, Marianne Legato (1999), reported that 43 percent of women and 30 percent of men have some sexual dysfunction. Figure 12.1 presents the various problems by gender. Many of these problems respond well to various treatments.

A New Paradigm for Understanding Sexual Dysfunction

As we mentioned in Chapter 7, Basson's theory of sexual response sheds new light on the importance of intimacy in understanding sexual interest, desire, arousal, and satisfaction. It also can be used as the basis for understanding sexual dysfunction and how to treat it (Lieblum, 2001).

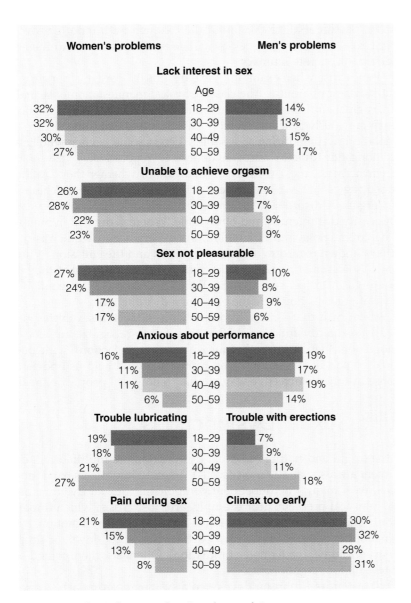

Figure 12.1 *Sexual Dysfunction by Gender and Age*
Source: National Health and Life Survey, 1992.

According to this new paradigm, understanding sexual desire disorders, for instance, requires a deeper emphasis on examining the role of intimacy in relationships. Since Basson et al. (2000) found that intimacy seeking is often the motivation for sexual desire in women, sexual desire disorders may in fact be more related to lack of intimacy than lack of desire. Desire in women often springs out of intimacy with a partner. Women diagnosed with "low sexual desire" may in fact have normal levels of desire for sexual activity but inadequate intimacy in their relationships. Insufficient intimacy can manifest itself as "low sexual desire" because the two are interrelated. For these women, sexual desire (physical sexual release) is not the starting point in their sexual response; the desire for intimacy is (Lieblum, 2001).

For example, if someone asked his or her female partner, "Do you want to have sex?" the answer might be "No, let's snuggle." The person initiating might interpret this as his or her partner not wanting to have sex, while the female partner might view this as a prelude to sexual activity or as a *big* part of her sexual activity.

Additionally, Basson et al. (2000) found that women with reported low internal feelings of sexual desire might seek to initiate sexual activity with their partners out of a desire to generate intimacy.

Similar issues arise when examining sexual arousal disorders. In men, erection is a clear-cut indicator of arousal. The classic physical manifestation of sexual arousal in women, vaginal lubrication, has been found to be a much less reliable indicator of arousal than previously believed. Lieblum (2001) reports that some victims of sexual assault report lubricating during an assault, whereas some women who have an absence of lubrication due to estrogen deficiency report being "psychologically" aroused. Furthermore, most women are unaware of whether they are lubricating and experiencing genital swelling associated with vasocongestion (Lieblum, 2001).

Female orgasmic disorder relies on a very male-oriented view that orgasm is something easily documented and observable. Whereas orgasm in men is distinguished by contractions and ejaculation, the experience in women is much less clear. Little is known regarding female ejaculation and the emission of fluid other than urine. As Basson et al. (2000) note, many women report that they need not experience orgasm to feel sexually satisfied. This leads one to wonder whether the absence of orgasm should be the basis for a dysfunction.

Lief (1985) argued that a major problem with models of sexual response (and consequently sexual dysfunction) is that they fail to recognize any end point to the phenomenon. Lief believes that measures of "satisfaction" with the experience should be part of any model. This approach would help us understand sexual response in a more subjective way, similar to how real people define it.

Treating Sexual Dysfunctions

Because the origin and nature of sexual dysfunction are multifaceted, diagnosis and treatment are also usually multifaceted. Treating impaired sexual functioning is complex, with many interdependent components. Sexual dysfunction can be caused by physical problems (for example, arteriosclerosis, which impairs vasocongestion), emotional disorders (excessive stress or negative emotions), spiritual distress (no longer being in love with a partner, lack of self-love), or simple ignorance (poor technique, inadequate stimulation). Often, sex therapy and enhancement involve all four components.

In 1959, Masters and Johnson developed a systematic approach to sex therapy that incorporated an extensive physical examination (to root out organic causes) and individual and couple counseling in the treatment of sexual dysfunction. Most sex therapists take an extensive medical history, and many incorporate a physical examination as part of the diagnostic work-up of their patients. The individual and couple approaches to counseling and treatment have many variations.

Treating Sexual Dysfunction Related to Medical Conditions

The first step in treating medically related sexual dysfunction is to properly diagnose the condition. A thorough medical examination, combined with a detailed sexual/medical history, guides the therapist in diagnosis. The overwhelming majority of cases of erectile disorder are caused by medical conditions and respond to medical treatment.

Viagra The drug sildenafil, prescribed for the treatment of erectile disorder

Viagra and Levitra   **Viagra,** the trade name for sildenafil, a drug that went on the market in the United States in April 1998, is revolutionizing the treatment of erectile disorder. The response to the drug by men who have erectile disorder has been staggering. After 3 weeks on the market, Viagra was being prescribed at a rate of at least 10,000 prescriptions a day (Handy, 1998).

Much of the appeal of Viagra is its ease of use. Doctors recommend taking Viagra 1 hour before intercourse is desired. Unlike injectable drugs that produce an erection regardless of context, Viagra paves the way for the possibility of one. Viagra works with sexual desire in triggering erections. Once a user feels desire for his partner, Viagra allows erections to proceed.

The muscular and vascular changes of erection are controlled by a chemical called **guanosine triphosphate** (GMP). During sexual arousal, if the man feels sexual desire, GMP is released from cells in the penis that are stimulated by the brain and nervous system. The GMP triggers receptor cells in the spongy erectile tissue, allowing muscles there to relax and penile arteries to dilate. As the erectile tissue expands, it squeezes shut the veins responsible for removing the blood to the area. After orgasm, GMP is broken down by a normally occurring enzyme called *phosphodiesterase 5* (PDE5).

Most men with erectile disorder don't produce enough GMP to override the ever-present PDE5. Their erectile tissue doesn't expand enough to squeeze the veins shut, and consequently the penis does not attain complete erection. Viagra works by suppressing the effects of PDE5, allowing even a limited amount of GMP to cause erections.

Viagra does not increase sexual desire. If a man is not interested in sex or has little sexual desire for a partner, Viagra will not increase his desire. Viagra works for men who desire sex but can't get erections because they produce limited amounts of GMP.

Another important thing to know about Viagra is that more is not better. Viagra is prescribed in either 50- or 100-milligram tablets. The correct dose is the smallest needed to create the desired effect. The penis has a limited number of receptors for GMP, and the body can process only so much of it. Taking a bigger dose of Viagra will not allow more GMP to be processed than the body can handle. Men who are not having problems with GMP production will not obtain any enhanced erectile effects from taking the drug because the body is already processing as much GMP as it can handle. Any enhanced erectile response reported probably is placebo effect rather than an effect of Viagra (Handy, 1998).

Viagra has been tried with women, too, resulting in increased blood flow to the genital area, as in men. It may help a small group of women, such as those with nerve damage from multiple sclerosis (Berman, Berman, & Goldstein, 1999).

The main reason that Viagra seems to be less of a breakthrough for women than for men is that for most women with a sexual dysfunction, vasocongestion is already occurring. For the majority of women seeking sex therapy, vasocongestion is not the issue (Basson et al., 2000). As we mentioned earlier, Viagra does not enhance sexual desire. As we've seen in Basson et al.'s (2000) work, sexual interest, sexual desire, and sexual arousal are all very interrelated and thrive on intimacy. Because Viagra doesn't influence intimacy directly, its utility as anything other than a placebo is limited to those women with problems related to blood flow and engorgement of genital tissue (Boschert, 2001).

Recently, two new drugs, Levitra (vardanafil) and Cialis (tedalafil), have become available for the treatment of erectile disorder in addition to Viagra. Both work exactly the same way as Viagra by blocking PDE5. As we go to press, Cialis was just approved by the Food and Drug Administration for sale in the United States (Stief, Porst, Saenz de Tejada, Uckert, & Hedulund, 2003).

Although Viagra and Levitra work almost identically, there are some differences between the two. The recommended time to take Levitra prior to sex is 25 to 45 minutes, while it is recommended to take Viagra 60 minutes prior to sex. In one clinical study of Levitra, some subjects were able to obtain erections that were suitable for intercourse as early as 16 minutes after dosing (Padma-Nathan, Kaufman, & Taylor, 2003). Both last about the same time in the body (Levitra works for up to 6 hours and Viagra up to 5). The most common side effects of both are headache and facial flushing. Viagra use has been associated with altered or

Guanosine triphosphate A chemical that controls the muscular and vascular changes of erection bluish vision, whereas Levitra has not been found to produce these vision-related side effects. Levitra can be taken with food; Viagra is taken on an empty stomach. Viagra comes in two primary dosages, while Levitra has three (WallCann, 2003). Because the two drugs are so similar, we recommend discussing each drug with your doctor before deciding on which is most appropriate.

Drug Injections   Prior to Viagra, most medically caused erectile disorder was treated with self-injections of a drug (alprostadil, a synthetic prostaglandin, is a common one) directly into the penis. The drug works by relaxing the muscles of the spongy erectile tissue, allowing the arteries to dilate and engorgement to occur. Men (and often their partners) were taught how to administer the injections using tiny needles similar to the ones diabetics use to inject insulin. The injections produce a pinprick sensation that patients usually tolerate well.

Unlike Viagra, injection treatment produces an erection without requiring the brain to initiate it through sexual desire. The injections lead to erections in approximately 15 minutes. The medication is premeasured in doses that will produce erections that last for approximately an hour (Parrish, 1997).

Another method of delivering alprostadil involves inserting tiny pellets of the drug directly into the urethra. A small plastic tube containing a plunger product is inserted about 1 inch into the urethra. When the plunger is pushed, it releases the drug, which resembles tiny rabbit food pellets, into the urethra. Within 10 minutes the drug begins to take effect.

Vacuum Pumps   Prior to Viagra and injectable drug therapy, vacuum pumps and surgical implants were used to treat erectile disorder. The vacuum pump is a flexible plastic sleeve that is placed over the penis and secured at the base of the lubricated penis with an elastic band. Suction is applied to the sleeve, by mouth or a small hand pump, through a tube that connects at the other end. The pump draws blood into the penis, filling the erectile tissue and thereby causing an erection. Once the man achieves a sufficient erection, the sleeve is removed and the band is kept in place to trap the blood for about half an hour.

Implants and Other Surgery   Implant treatment involves the surgical implantation of an inflatable penile prosthesis. The device consists of two hollow cylinders connected to a fluid-filled reservoir and a pump. The cylinders are implanted in the shaft of the penis, the reservoir in the abdomen, and the pump in the scrotum. When the man desires an erection, he activates the pump, which fills the cylinders and causes erection. After intercourse, he turns a valve, which empties the cylinders back into the reservoir. Figure 12.2 depicts a penis pump.

Implant surgery is considered radical treatment and should be considered only if other forms of treatment fail. It can lead to permanent damage that could make a natural erection impossible.

Finally, some structural problems in sexual anatomy may have to be corrected with surgery. Examples are removing scar tissue and freeing adhesions that cause pain during intercourse.

Figure 12.2 *Penis Pump* The penis pump uses a closed system consisting of a hydraulic pump (hidden in the testes), a fluid reservoir (concealed in the abdominal cavity), and expandable chambers (hidden in the penis). To produce an erection, fluid is pumped from the reservoir to the chambers.

Hormone Treatments   Certain medical conditions, particularly those of the endocrine system, respond to medication or hormone replacement therapy. Correcting a hormonal imbalance that might affect disorders of sexual arousal might best be treated through the oral administration of hormone replacement therapy. Sometimes endocrine glands need help in being stimulated to begin producing adequate amounts of sex hormones. Medications are available that activate endocrine glands to release their hormones.

Although testosterone is often considered a male hormone, both men and women have testosterone, and it is believed to play an important role in libido. As levels of this hormone decline with age, sexual interest may wane. Many women are helped by taking testosterone, in low enough doses to prevent any male secondary characteristics to develop. Also, estrogen improves vaginal lubrication in postmenopausal women.

Other Medical Treatments   Still other sexual dysfunctions are related to a disease that can be treated or cured with medication. Sexual pain disorders associated with sexually transmitted infection, for instance, respond quite well to treatment or cure of the underlying disease condition. Sexual arousal disorders related to cardiovascular problems such as arteriosclerosis often can be improved through medication designed to change blood biochemistry and improve the flow of blood and blood pressure.

Treating Drug-Induced Sexual Dysfunction

Similar to treating organic-based sexual dysfunction, the treatment of drug-induced sexual dysfunction begins with a thorough sexual/medical history and medical examination. The assessment includes current drug use (licit and illicit). The specific drugs are analyzed for possible side effects and interactions to assess their role in the sexual dysfunction. The therapist examines the onset of the sexual dysfunction in relation to the onset of drug use.

Many commonly prescribed medications, alone or in combination with other prescription or over-the-counter medications or psychoactive substances, have potential negative side effects related to sexual response. Sometimes treatment is as simple as changing the dosage of the medication or switching to a similar drug with different side effects. An example is provided by medication for controlling high blood pressure.

A common side effect of certain hypertension medications is erectile dysfunction. Changing the medication often relieves the erectile problem and still controls the patient's high blood pressure. In other cases, treatment consists of avoiding additional medications or substances that, when taken with the prescribed drug, result in sexual dysfunction. Patients often are unaware of the potentially troubling side effects of combining substances.

Treating Psychosocially Based Sexual Dysfunction

Several different sex therapy approaches can be applied when the origin of the dysfunction is psychosocial in nature. The therapeutic approach has four main variables:

- The therapist's theoretical framework
- Duration and schedule of treatment
- Individual versus couple or group approach
- Use of surrogates

Sex therapists come from a variety of backgrounds. Some are physicians with advanced training in psychiatry, sex therapy, psychoanalysis, or counseling. Others are psychologists, psychoanalysts, counselors, and social workers. No uniform credentials are required for sex therapists across the United States; credentialing requirements vary from state to state.

Each of these professionals has a philosophical and theoretical framework regarding sex therapy that guides his or her work. Psychoanalysts, for instance, take a psychodynamic approach to treatment that is grounded in the work of Freud. A basic element in their approach is helping the client gain insight into the origin of his or her problem.

Counselors using a behaviorist approach, in contrast, do not believe it is necessary to delve deeply into their clients' past to help them gain insight into the origin of their problem. Rather, the behaviorist focuses on the here and now and examines the nature of the problem, how the client perceives it, and how it directly affects the person's quality of life.

The therapist's theoretical framework is intimately related to the duration and schedule of therapy. A psychoanalyst might spend several sessions just getting to know the client and establishing trust while beginning to look back into his or her past. A Masters and Johnson–trained therapist team would be finished with therapy by that time because the approach is to get right down to the business of treating the presenting problem in an intensive 2-week program.

Some sex therapists work only with individuals. Most however, believe that sexual dysfunction can be understood and treated only within the context of the relationship. Couples are seen together and individually, and treatment involves treating the couple as well as the individual. Others incorporate group therapy to help couples view their problems in a broader context.

Finally, some sex therapists provide explicit help by using trained **sex surrogate** partners. Although these surrogates are sexually responsive trained professionals who serve as partners for clients, the American Association of Sex Educators, Counselors and Therapists (AASECT, 1998), one of the leading professional groups charged with certifying sex therapists, does not recommend their use in the treatment of sexual dysfunctions.

Most sex therapy is eclectic, combining elements from various forms of psychotherapy, education, and medicine. Six common threads that seem to underlie the practice of sex therapy, regardless of the therapist's theoretical framework, are (a) permission giving, (b) limited information, (c) specific suggestions, (d) self-awareness, (e) communication training, and (f) use of masturbation.

Sex surrogate A person who acts as a substitute sex partner during therapy

Permission Giving

Permission giving is the unconditional support the therapist offers for becoming a fully self-actualized sexual being. Clients are given permission to explore any thoughts, feelings, desires, fantasies, and behaviors that might enhance their sexual pleasure. They also are given permission not to engage in behaviors and relationships that undermine their sexual and other well-being.

Information Giving

Information giving or education is a key element in all forms of sex therapy. Because most people receive little or no formal sex education, they often are misinformed about simple issues that can undermine their sexual enjoyment, such as penis size, level of sexual activity, and effects of aging. Often, providing information, along with permission giving, is liberating enough to help people work their way out of some sexual dysfunctions.

Information giving can include didactic sessions with the therapist related to the individual's specific concerns, guided reading (reading a prescribed set of materials), and viewing instructional videotapes. Providing limited information helps change negative attitudes, open lines of communication, and develop sexual skills necessary for enhancing performance and pleasure.

Specific Suggestions

Each person or couple has unique problems and needs that can be addressed through specific suggestions. The main technique in this regard is "homework as-

A Great Sex Life

personal exploration activity

Unfortunately, many of us have just a few sexual issues and hang-ups that may cause our sex life to be less than great. However, there are many things we can do to increase our enjoyment and physical response so that we can have a better sex life. Your task is to find one or more methods to incorporate that would improve your sexual response.

While reading this chapter, compare your sexual response to various sexual disorders. Your goal is to find one that is similar to an issue that you may have experienced. Then choose a sexual therapy that you can try to see whether it improves the way you respond. You may choose one to do alone or with a partner. If you cannot find anything you need to improve, try one of the therapies just for fun. You may find something like sensate focus increases the enjoyment you already experience and may decide to incorporate it in your routine sexual activities. Look for some therapy that would increase pleasure or skill and give it a try. Hopefully, you will find the results worth the work.

signments" with one's partner. The range of specific suggestions varies depending on the nature of the problem and the specific individual or couple involved. Usually these homework assignments require the couple to practice activities and techniques that the therapist has discussed with them. These often are coupled with communication activities designed to help couples open up and share their feelings with each other.

Intellectual Wellness

Many sexual problems are based on ignorance, illogical thinking and irrational expectations, and poor technique. Intellectual wellness is fostered through knowledge, logical thinking, rational expectations, and improved sexual technique. Much of sex therapy revolves around relearning what good sex is and what being a good lover means. These things can be taught. You can learn about sexual response and what to expect during lovemaking. You can learn to understand the factors that influence interest, desire, plateau, orgasm, and resolution and begin to set more realistic and logical expectations about lovemaking. You can learn techniques and practice your skills (by yourself or with your partner) and become a better lover.

Self-Awareness

Increased self-awareness is a natural outgrowth of permission and information giving. Many of the specific suggestions prescribed as homework help individuals and couples focus on their sensual/sexual response. This is the first time many clients have spent focusing on their sexual response and specific techniques related to sensual and sexual arousal.

One commonly used activity is called **sensate focus.** In the early stages of sex therapy, the couple is instructed to refrain from sexual activity involving genital contact. This approach is designed to relieve performance anxiety and other forms of anxiety and to allow the couple to focus on nongenital pleasuring.

During the first phase of sensate focus (Figure 12.3), each partner is given a turn to explore the other's body. The breasts and genitals are off-limits. The intent is not to give sexual pleasure but instead to establish awareness of touch by paying attention to the textures, contours, and temperature of the partner and to attend to what it feels like to touch and be touched.

Sensate focus Nongenital pleasuring used to heighten sensuality without sexual activity

381

Figure 12.3 *Couple Practicing Sensate Focus* During the first stage of sensate focus, couples practice nongenital pleasuring.

The partner doing the touching is in control and is not driven by the needs of the person being touched. The initial stage is supposed to be conducted as silently as possible. The person being touched is allowed to convey (either verbally or nonverbally) when the partner's touch makes him or her uncomfortable.

During the second phase of sensate focus, touch is extended to include the breasts and genitals. The couple receive instructions similar to those in the first phase and are advised to gradually expand the touch to include the genitals. The purpose is still to experience the sensation of touch and to discover what types of touch are most pleasurable.

A simple technique called *handriding* is used during this phase. This involves having one partner place his or her hand over the partner's and to guide it on an exploration of the other's body. The guiding hand nonverbally communicates by increasing or decreasing the pressure, changing the speed or type of motion, and holding the hand to linger. The idea is to help the partner who is doing the touching understand the preferences of the partner being touched without controlling the action. The partner doing the touching is still in control but is guided along.

In the third phase of sensate focus, the couple is asked to explore each other at the same time. Rather than take turns, the couple doubles the amount of sensory input by mutual exploration. This simulates real-life touching and allows the couple the opportunity to get lost in the sensations of touch without the pressure to have intercourse.

In the last stage of sensate focus, the couple shifts to the female-on-top position without attempting full penetration of the penis. In this position, the woman can rub her clitoris directly against her partner and stimulate his penis with her vulva and vaginal opening. This position may or may not result in arousal and full erection in her partner. The purpose is not to cause full arousal and intercourse, but if an erection occurs, she can put the tip of the penis into her vaginal opening. The couple are instructed to continue to explore each other, using full body contact to explore the sensations of touch and arousal.

After the couple has worked through the stages of sensate focus successfully and is comfortable with it, the two of them usually are ready to experience full intercourse without difficulty.

Communication Training Couples can learn how to communicate nonverbally through sensate focus and other awareness-building activities. Often, nonverbal communication—such as placing a hand or other body part in a certain position or holding a partner to linger at what he or she is doing—can transmit information that will help treat sexual problems. Improving verbal communication—in particular, expressing needs and desires and communicating using "I" language instead of blaming one's partner—is integral to all forms of sex therapy. Communication building can occur during sessions with the therapist and as homework assignments.

Use of Masturbation Sex therapy commonly includes masturbation, both individual and mutual. It can be used in sexual arousal disorders to help both partners explore the types, intensity, and duration of stimulation necessary for full arousal. It also can help the couple learn how to delay orgasm in cases of premature ejaculation.

A variation of masturbation used to treat premature ejaculation is the squeeze technique, illustrated in Figure 12.4. During manual stimulation of her partner, the woman is instructed to stop periodically and apply firm pressure for a few seconds to the frenulum and coronal ridge with her thumb and first and second fingers, respectively. This squeezing reduces her partner's urgency to ejaculate. She can continue to masturbate her partner, stopping periodically to squeeze. Through this technique her partner can learn to delay ejaculation.

Masturbation also can be used to treat female and male orgasmic disorder. Often these conditions are related to inadequate sexual stimulation. Through permission giving, sensate focus, and masturbation, men and

During handriding, one person guides the partner's hand in sensual exploration.

Figure 12.4 *Squeeze Technique* During the squeeze technique, the partner's erect penis is periodically squeezed to inhibit ejaculation.

Courtesy of Milex Products, Inc., Chicago, Illinois

Vaginal dilators come in varying sizes and colors.

women can learn the type, intensity, and duration of stimulation necessary for orgasm. Treatment progresses from individual masturbation, to masturbation in the presence of the partner, to being masturbated by the partner, to using masturbation as a prelude to intercourse.

Masturbation, coupled with the use of increasingly larger dilators can be used to treat some cases of vaginismus. Women are taught to use permission giving, self-awareness, and masturbation to initiate sexual arousal and to use the varying sizes of dilators for 10 to 15 minutes at a time to introduce objects into her vagina. The goal is to work up to a penis-size dilator and then make the transition to a real penis.

Your responses to the Personal Assessment, Thought Questions, and Test Yourself! quiz questions can be logged online in your Virtual Workbook at **http://health.wadsworth.com/blonna1.**

Personal Assessment

12.1 Are You an Addict?

Substance abuse is not only a risk factor for sexual dysfunction; it can destroy your life. This assessment is designed to help you assess whether your current drug use is considered addictive.

The following questions were written by recovering addicts in Narcotics Anonymous. Please answer yes or no.

1. Do you ever use alone?
2. Have you ever substituted one drug for another, thinking that one particular drug was the problem?
3. Have you ever manipulated or lied to a doctor to obtain prescription drugs?
4. Have you ever stolen drugs or stolen to obtain drugs?
5. Do you regularly use a drug when you wake up or when you go to bed?
6. Have you ever taken one drug to overcome the effects of another?
7. Do you avoid people or places that do not approve of you using drugs?
8. Have you ever used a drug without knowing what it was or what it would do to you?
9. Has your job or school performance ever suffered from the effects of your drug use?
10. Have you ever been arrested as a result of using drugs?
11. Have you ever lied about what or how much you use?
12. Do you put the purchase of drugs ahead of your financial responsibilities?
13. Have you ever tried to stop or control your using?
14. Have you ever been in a jail, hospital, or drug rehabilitation center because of your using?
15. Does using interfere with your sleeping or eating?
16. Does the thought of running out of drugs terrify you?
17. Do you feel it is impossible for you to live without drugs?
18. Do you ever question your own sanity?
19. Is your drug use making life at home unhappy?
20. Have you ever thought you couldn't fit in or have a good time without using drugs?
21. Have you ever felt defensive, guilty, or ashamed about your using?
22. Do you think a lot about drugs?
23. Have you had irrational or indefinable fears?
24. Has using affected your sexual relationships?
25. Have you ever taken drugs you didn't prefer?
26. Have you ever used drugs because of emotional pain or stress?
27. Have you ever overdosed on any drugs?
28. Do you continue to use despite negative consequences?
29. Do you think you might have a drug problem?

Are you an addict? This is a question only you can answer. Members of Narcotics Anonymous found that they all answered different numbers of these questions yes. The actual number of yes responses isn't as important as how you feel inside and how addiction has affected your life. If you are an addict, you must first admit that you have a problem with drugs before any progress can be made toward recovery.

Source: Reprinted by permission from Narcotics Anonymous, copyright © 1986 by Narcotics Anonymous World Services, Inc. All rights reserved.

12.2 Do You Suffer from Erectile Disorder?

Take the Viagra erectile disorder self-assessment at www.viagara.com/consumer/aboutED/findOutShim.asp, and calculate your score. If the results indicate that you may be suffering from erectile disorder, consult your physician for further assessments.

Thought Questions

1. How do the categories of dysfunctions mesh with the stages of the sexual response cycle? Why are they set up this way?

2. What are two dysfunctions related to sexual desire?

3. When does low interest in sexual activity become a desire disorder?

4. What is the relationship between cardiovascular health and sexual arousal disorders?

5. What does the term *preorgasmic* mean?

6. What are three illness-related causes of sexual dysfunction?

7. What are three medication-related causes of sexual dysfunction?

8. Are isolated episodes of sexual dysfunction normal? If so, why?

Test Yourself!

1. Which of the following best characterizes the relationship between cardiovascular disease and sexual dysfunction?
   a. There is very little relationship between cardiovascular disease and any form of sexual dysfunction.
   b. All forms of high blood pressure medication causes impotence in most men and women.
   c. The majority of cases of erectile dysfunction are related to cardiovascular disease.
   d. A small percentage of cases of erectile dysfunction are related to cardiovascular disease.

2. Damage to the blood vessels of the underside of the penis causing erectile dysfunction
   a. can be minimized by using protective athletic cups and contoured bicycle seats.
   b. cannot be minimized by using protective athletic cups and contoured bicycle seats.
   c. is unrelated to sports and other athletic activities.
   d. is grossly overstated.

3. The negative effects of alcohol and other depressant drugs on sexual response begin when
   a. their depressant effects impair good judgment.
   b. their depressant effects move beyond inducing relaxation and reducing anxiety to create paranoia.
   c. their depressant effects move beyond inducing relaxation and reducing anxiety to inhibiting blood flow and other metabolic functions.
   d. their depressant effects put users to sleep.

4. Although stimulant drugs such as cocaine and amphetamines seem to provide energy and increased sexual interest,
   a. they can inhibit orgasm and result in diminished desire.
   b. they do not last long.
   c. their long-term use is misunderstood.
   d. they can cause death due to the strain of orgasm.

5. The use of narcotics such as heroin is associated with
   a. increased sexual interest.
   b. no change in sexual interest.
   c. decreased sexual interest.
   d. distorted sexual interest.

6. Which of the following best describes the relationship between the types of sexual dysfunction categorized by the American Psychiatric Association (APA) and the sexual response cycle?
   a. They are the same thing.
   b. The types of sexual dysfunction correspond to the sexual response cycle.
   c. They are very different from the APA, which takes a very psychiatric approach to this problem.
   d. They are similar but different.

7. What is the difference between sexual disinterest and sexual aversion disorder?
   a. They are the same thing.
   b. People with sexual aversion disorder are anxious about, fear, or are disgusted with sexual activity, whereas those with sexual disinterest are just not very interested in sex.
   c. People with sexual disinterest disorder are anxious about, fear, or are disgusted with sexual activity, whereas those with sexual aversion disorder merely avoid sex.
   d. People with sexual disinterest usually progress to sexual aversion.

8. Which statement best characterizes the use of Viagra in women?
   a. Viagra is an effective treatment for women with female sexual arousal disorder.
   b. Viagra is not an effective treatment for women with female sexual arousal disorder because the condition in women is usually not associated with vascular problems.
   c. Viagra is more effective in women than in men.
   d. Viagra is a very effective treatment for women with female sexual arousal disorder because the condition in women is usually associated with vascular problems.

9. Viagra works in the treatment of male erectile disorder by
   a. increasing sexual desire.
   b. increasing testosterone levels.
   c. relaxing stress associated with performance.
   d. relaxing erectile tissue, allowing penile arteries to dilate.

10. Which of the following is not commonly used in eclectic sex therapy?
    a. Surrogate sex partners
    b. Communication training
    c. Specific suggestions
    d. Masturbation

Media Menu

You can link to the following online tools by visiting
http://health.wadsworth.com/blonna1.

Face to Face Video

Dr. Lisa McIntosh discusses sexual dysfunction.

Film

Erectile Dysfunction

 InfoTrac Activity

Elash, A. (2000, July). Venus envy: Women using Viagra. *Chatelaine, 73*(7), 93–96.

 Web Resources

Viagra Home Page

www.viagra.com

This site is a comprehensive resource for the drug and has had nearly 10 million visits.

Network for Excellence in Women's Sexual Health (NewSHE)

www.newshe.com

A Web site for women and men seeking help in dealing with sexual function problems such as lack of desire, arousal, lubrication, orgasm, and pain. This site provides unique resources, special links, information about clinics, and the latest medical news in this area.

National Foundation for Sexual Health Medicine (NFSHM)

www.nfshm.org/default.asp

A nonprofit organization dedicated to educating the medical community and the public about sexual health. NFSHM addresses the growing need for current information on sexual health by offering information and training to clinicians and the general public. Click the "Resources" link on the top of their page for access to their journals and other resources.

Mental Health Net

http://mentalhelp.net/poc/center/_index.php?id=10

Net guide to mental health, psychology, and psychiatry; addresses the symptoms, online resources, and organizations concerning sexual problems of dyspareunia, exhibitionism, female and male orgasmic disorders, female sexual arousal disorder, fetishism, frotteurism, gender identity disorder, male erectile disorder, premature ejaculation, sexual masochism and sadism, transvestic fetishism, vaginismus, and voyeurism.

References

American Association of Sex Educators, Counselors, and Therapists. (1998). *Ethical guidelines for sex therapists.* Washington, DC: Author.

American Psychiatric Association. (2000). *Diagnostic and statistical manual of mental illness* (4th ed., text revision). Washington, DC: Author.

Barbach, L. (1982). *For each other: Sharing sexual intimacy.* Garden City, NY: Doubleday.

Basson, R., Berman, J., Burnett, A., Derogatis, L., Ferguson, D., Fourcoy, J., Goldstein, L., Graziotto, A., Heiman, J., Laan, E., Lieblum, S., Padma-Nathan, H., Rosen, R., Seagraves, K., Shabsigh, R., Sipsk, M., Wagner, G., & Whipple, B. (2000). Report of the International Consensus Development Conference on Female Sexual Dysfunction: Definitions and classifications. *Journal of Urology, 163,* 888–893.

Berman, J., Berman L, & Goldstein I. (1999). Female sexual dysfunction: Incidence, pathophysiology, evaluation, and treatment options. *Urology, 54,* 385–391.

Boschert, S. (2000, July). Women don't get a rise out of taking Viagra. *Ob Gyn News, 35*(13), 23–24.

Buvat, J., Buvat-Herbaut, M., Lemaire, A., Marcolin, G., & Quittelier, R. (1990). Recent developments in the clinical assessment and diagnosis of erectile dysfunction. *Annual Review of Sex Research, 1,* 265–308.

Dodson, B. (1974). *Liberating masturbation.* New York: Dodson.

Drug Week. (2001, August 24). Viagra-type drugs unlikely to solve many women's sexual response problems [Online]. Article A78895438. Available: NewsRX.net.

Fisher, S. (1973). *The female orgasm.* New York: Bantam.

Goldberg, R. (1997). *Drugs across the spectrum.* Englewood, CO: Morton.

Gutfield, G. (1994). The prescription for male potency. *Prevention, 46*(11), 78–82.

Handy, B. (1998). The Viagra craze. *Time, 151*(17), 50–53.

Heapes, T. (1994). Smoking your sex life away. *Muscle & Fitness, 55*(4), 42.

Hite, S. (1977). *The Hite report.* New York: Dell.

Horvitz, L. A. (1997). Can better sex come with a pill? The nineties impotence cure. *Insight on the News, 13*(46), 38–40.

Hyde, J. S. (1994). *Understanding human sexuality* (5th ed.). New York: McGraw-Hill.

Jones, H. B., & Jones, H. (1977). *Sensual drugs: Deprivation and rehabilitation of the mind.* London: Cambridge University Press.

Kinsey, A. E. (1953). *Sexual behavior in the human female.* Philadelphia: Saunders.

Kita, J. (2001, November). The sex crusaders. *Men's Health, 16*(9), 98–106.

Kobilinsky, S., & Palmeter, J. (1984). Sex role orientation, mother's expression of affection toward spouse and college women's attitudes towards sexual behaviors. *Journal of Sex Research, 20,* 32–43.

Legato, M. (1999). *Summary: U.S. Department of Health and Human Services, Public Health Service, National Institutes of Health: A report of the task force on the NIH Women's Health Research Agenda for the 21st century. Vol. 1: Executive summary* [Online]. Available: www4.od.nih.gov/orwh/report.pdf. Leland, J. (1997). A pill for impotence? *Newsweek, 130*(20), 62–68.

Lieblum, S. R. (2000, November). Redefining female sexual response. *Contemporary ObGyn, 45*(11), 120–131.

Lief, H. (1985). Evaluation of inhibited sexual desire: Relationship aspects. In H. S. Kaplan (Ed.), *Comprehensive evaluation of disorders of sexual desire* (pp. 59–76). Washington, DC: American Psychiatric Press.

Lowinson, J. H., Ruiz, P., Millman, R. B., & Langrod, J. G. (1992). *Substance abuse: A comprehensive textbook* (2nd ed.). Baltimore: Williams & Wilkinson.

Masters, W. H, & Johnson, V. E. (1970). *Human sexual inadequacy.* Boston: Little, Brown.

Masters, W. H., Johnson, V. E., & Kolodny, R. (1996). *Human sexuality* (5th ed.). New York: HarperCollins.

Montague, A. (1977). *Touching: The human significance of the skin.* New York: Harper & Row.

O'Donohue, W., & Geer, J. H. (1993). *Handbook of sexual dysfunctions: Assessment and treatment.* Needham Heights, MA: Allyn & Bacon.

Padma-Nathan, H., Kaufman, J., & Taylor, T. (2003, June 28–July 1). *Earliest time of onset of erections with vardenafil determined in an at-home setting.* Paper presented at the Second International Consultation on Erectile and Sexual Dysfunctions, Paris.

Parrish, M. (1997). Up, up, and away. *Playboy, 44*(6), 92–99.

Purcell, S. (1985, August 25). *The relationship between religious orthodoxy and marital sexual functioning.* Paper presented at annual meeting of American Psychological Association.

Richardson, J. D. (1991). Medical causes of sexual dysfunction. *Medical Journal of Australia, 155,* 29–33.

Rosen, R. G. (1991). Alcohol and drug effects on sexual response. *Annual Reviews of Sex Research, 2,* 119–129.

Singer-Kaplan, H. (1974). *The new sex therapy.* New York: Brunner/Mazel.

Stevenson, R. W. D. (2002, January). Sexual dysfunction: Attending to the mind–body continuum. *Medical Aspects of Human Sexuality, 2,* 7–9.

Stief, C., Porst, H., Saenz de Tejada, I., Uckert, S., & Hedulund, E. (2003, June 28–July 1). *Sustained efficacy and tolerability of vardenafil over two years in men with erectile dysfunction.* Paper presented at the Second International Consultation on Erectile and Sexual Dysfunctions, Paris.

WallCann. (2003). Comparing Viagra, Levitra, and Cialis [Online].

Available: www.vardenafil-viagra-cialis.com/compare-cialis-levitra-viagra.htm.

Witters, W., Venturelli, P., & Hanson, P. (1992). *Drugs and society.* 3rd ed. Boston: Jones & Bartlett.

Zilbergeld, B. (1992). *The new male sexuality.* New York: Bantam.

chapter *thirteen*

Human Reproduction

Student Learning Objectives

After reading this chapter, students will be able to

- Describe the dynamics of conception.

- Describe normal developmental characteristics during the three trimesters of pregnancy.

- Assess the influence of a variety of negative personal behaviors (such as alcohol use) on prenatal development.

- Describe personal health behaviors that enhance pregnancy outcomes.

- Identify a variety of alternatives to traditional conception and parenting.

- Describe a variety of factors related to infertility.

- Identify options available to enhance fertility.

- Describe the process of childbirth.

- Evaluate options for labor and delivery.

- Identify areas where health policies affect individual choices.

Test your understanding of these objectives by taking the end-of-chapter quiz, available online at ***http://health.wadsworth.com/blonna1.***

activity teaser: *Are you ready to be a parent? Find out with the Personal Exploration Activity on page 391.*

case study 13.1

Ana, Then and Now

Ana, 24, identifies as Dominican American.

Critical Thinking

If Ana's family had not been supportive at the time of her first pregnancy, what kinds of decisions may she have had to make at that time? What impact might those decisions have had in contrast to how she is living now?

Use your Virtual Workbook to explore your answers to these questions at **http://health.wadsworth.com/blonna1.**

One day in class, Ana shared with her peers that she had had a child at the age of 15. Her boyfriend at the time was a senior in high school. They seldom used any method of birth control; he told her not to worry, and she figured that since she had been a virgin up until then, there really was not much to worry about. He knew what he was doing.

Ana was not particularly aware of when she got her period, didn't understand fertility too well, and when she hadn't had her period for 3 months, realized that she may be pregnant. She was able to do a pregnancy test, and when it came up positive, she felt so confused. Eventually, she told her mother, who was upset yet very supportive. They went to the local hospital that had a teen clinic, and from that point of 16 weeks' pregnant forward, she received the prenatal care she needed. The birth was hard, but the baby was healthy.

Finishing high school and going on to college was always a part of Ana's dreams. And she followed that dream. What she didn't do then, she admits, was be a very good mother. Her mother "mothered" her son, and they all continued living at her home. The father of the baby hasn't had too much to do with them, although occasionally he visits or sends some money.

Today, Ana is a 24-year-old college senior, married and pregnant again. She laughs as she recounts how the baby's due date is 2 weeks after graduation. She planned this pregnancy, has been receiving prenatal care all along, and knows what to expect during delivery. Her sonogram let her know that she is having another boy, and from all reports he is developing normally. She feels so lucky that her husband is an active father to her older son and has been so involved with her pregnancy. He actively participates at the birthing classes and has his camera ready for the delivery. This time around, Ana knows she can be the parent she needs to be.

As a child, learning the "facts of life" or about "the birds and the bees"—getting an answer to "Where did I come from?"—may have made parents squirm a bit. Words might have been carefully chosen, offering vague descriptions of sexual intercourse, followed by a brief summary of gestation, and ending with the birth at a hospital. Children asking this question today may receive answers that are far more complicated, as the ways in which babies are "made" and "born" have become more varied.

Imagine that a child asks her parents, "Where did I come from?" and gets the following answer:

> *Mom and Dad weren't able to have a child in the typical way, but we very much wanted to become parents. Because Mom's ovaries didn't work quite right, we went to the fertility bank, where we found an ova donor who was a lot like Mom. Her skin and hair color were like mine, and we seemed to like to do the same things. She seemed a good match for me.*
>
> *Dad found out that his body didn't make enough sperm, so he used the sperm directory and also found a good match. The laboratory was able to join the donated ova with the donated sperm, and then a very kind lady carried you as you grew inside her uterus. Nine months later we watched your birth and took you home!*

Even though one couple would not likely utilize all of this technology, each facet is possible today. Not even the U.S. legal system has been able to keep up with the rapid changes in reproductive technologies, with some very modern and difficult questions posed to the courts.

The World's Greatest Parent

Taking care of a baby before it is born is essential to the well-being of the child. However, the hard work has just begun. Parenting is complex and challenging, and often we are totally unprepared for the job. The following interview activity will help you begin the process of determining what you will need to do to be an effective, loving parent.

It is time to put your friends to work again to help you gather some ideas about healthy and unhealthy parenting. Interview five of your friends or acquaintances using the following questions, recording all of their answers in a journal.

1. What are the characteristics of a good parent?
2. What are the characteristics of a poor parent?
3. What are some things your parents or friend's parents did that you would like to do with your children?
4. What are some things your parents or friend's parents did that you will not do with your children?
5. How did your parents or friends' parents handle sexuality that you will also do with your children?
6. How did your parents or friends' parents handle sexuality that you will not do with your children?
7. In what activities will you encourage your children to participate?
8. What activities will you discourage your children from participating in?

When you have finished interviewing, review your list and add ideas you have about each question. Can you incorporate the ideas you gathered so you can be "the world's greatest parent"?

To date, individuals and couples alike have turned to the legal system for what sometimes seem Solomonesque decisions concerning their fertility and reproductive rights. In one divorce case, the wife wanted the embryos as her only chance at a pregnancy, and the husband wanted them destroyed. The court found that the frozen embryos were part of the property to be split in a divorce. The wife was awarded custody of the embryos. On appeal, the husband got "custody" of the embryos—and he destroyed them. Other cases have focused on unhealthy babies born from donors and large amounts of money having exchanged hands, leaving the "buyer" unhappy with his or her "purchase." Indeed, having babies has moved from the bedroom and out into the medical, technological, legal, and business worlds.

To Parent or Not to Parent

The decision about whether or not to have children is one that individuals in the United States are free to make. As will be discussed in greater detail in Chapter 14, the term **family planning** refers to the conscious act of planning a family. Prospective parents can decide whether to have children, how many to have, when to have them, and how far apart to space them. With reproductive technologies becoming more familiar and accessible, prenatal screenings more widespread, and better prenatal care more available, prospective parents have the opportunity to improve the health and welfare of their babies. In addition, if biological parenthood is not possible, adoption opportunities—albeit at great personal, emotional, and financial expense—exist both within and outside the United States.

Family planning The conscious effort of deciding to have a family, including when to have children, how many, and how far apart to space them

sex in society 13.1

Who Makes Appropriate Parents?

Society makes judgments about who would make appropriate parents, with the ideal not matching up well to the diverse realities of American families. Income, age, marital status, and sexual orientation become a few of the focal points for commentary and public policy.

Young teens who become parents are part of the "teen pregnancy problem" in the United States. School dropout rates and teen parenthood often intersect with poverty, lack of academic achievement, and a focus biased in the direction of the girl (Cassell, 2002). Compared to living with two parents, research indicates that a child growing up in a household headed by a young, poor teen mother is twice as likely to drop out of high school, 2.5 times as likely to become a teen mother, and 1.4 times as likely to be out of school and unemployed (Cassell, 2002). There is a growing and perhaps long overdue need to address the sexual and reproductive rights of males. For males, age at first intercourse, early fatherhood and living apart from their biological children, higher rates of infection, and marriage and divorce rates all seem to be exacerbated by poverty (Alan Guttmacher Institute, 2002). The development of policies to promote healthier families requires addressing the experiences of both males and females.

In 1997, a woman who had "tricked" a fertility program by claiming to be in her early 50s when she actually was in her early 60s subsequently gave birth to her first child at age 62. This prompted numerous editorials and angry letters to editors in newspapers across the country. How selfish for a woman to become a mother at that age! In contrast, when actor Tony Randall fathered his first child in his mid-70s, he was not subject to as much ridicule or outrage.

Nonetheless, waiting until older to become a parent has its drawbacks. Although it is no longer unusual to see "gray-haired parents " at PTA meetings of elementary-aged children, women in particular still struggle with their "biological clocks." Sylvia Ann Hewlett (2002), in the book *Creating a Life: Professional Women and the Quest for Children*, reported on a national survey of high-achieving women. She found that 42 percent of these

women working in corporate America still did not have children at age 40. Although admittedly some women in the group chose a professional career with no thoughts of having children, others found themselves childless by circumstance. The decision to become a parent after age 35 for women can mean greater reliance on infertility programs, with or without success, not to mention great financial expense. The concept of a "ticking biological clock" does not affect men in the same way. At the same time, being close to two generations older than a child can impact family dynamics.

When lesbian and gay couples choose to parent, they often find themselves being judged by a culture that traditionally has defined parenthood as a heterosexual right. Psychological studies have shown that good parenting is the key ingredient to raising healthy children, not the sexual orientation of the parents. The concern that having gay or lesbian parents will deprive a child of the opposite sex's influence is common yet without a scientific basis. Apart from the realities that children are exposed to many individuals throughout their schooling, play, neighborhoods, and media, the key to good development is to have a caring, consistent adult with good parenting skills. A comprehensive report conducted by the American Psychological Association concluded that there is no evidence to suggest that gay and lesbian parents are unfit to parent or that their children's healthy development is compromised in any way (Patterson, 1995).

The American Academy of Pediatrics issued a statement in 2002 supporting coparent and second-parent adoptions by same-sex couples: "There is a considerable body of professional literature that suggest children with parents who are homosexual have the same advantages and the same expectations for health, adjustment, and development as children whose parents are heterosexual." In addition to adoption, lesbian couples may choose to use artificial insemination with donor sperm to create their families. As described in Case Study 13.2, lesbian couples today have more options for bearing children and sharing in the joys of parenthood.

case study 13.2

The Joy of Matthew

Elizabeth, 37, is white.

I remember when I came out as a lesbian to my family and friends—it took a little while to live openly and share my life with those closest to me. I also thought that as a lesbian I had to give up my dreams of owning a home, getting married, and having kids. Then I met Maria, and everything changed. Maria and I have been together for 6 years now and have built a really fulfilling life together. We have a home. We had a commitment ceremony and would have married if that had been an option. And we have our wonderful son, Matthew.

Maria and I were together 3 years before we decided to begin building our family. We know gay and lesbian couples who have adopted children, others who have children from previous marriages, and those who had a child biologically together. After a lot of discussions, we decided to have our own biological child. There we were with all those eggs, but no sperm. We needed a donor.

After even more discussion—and I mean lots of talking and soul searching—we decided that Maria would be the biological mother. I know that many couples "plan" their children, but for two prospective parents of the same gender, the planning is more complicated and takes on a lot of the same issues faced by infertile heterosexual couples. We had to know when Maria was fertile and then inseminate her at the right time. And as with all couples trying to create a pregnancy, success does not necessarily happen right away. It took nearly 9 months before Maria became pregnant. Believe me, this baby was planned and so very wanted!

Luckily, we had found our way to a gay-friendly health clinic that referred us to a helpful physician. With donor sperm, insemination took place at home. We're not quite sure yet what we're going to tell Matthew about how he was conceived, but since he's a baby, we have time to figure out how best to explain things. Even though friends may be curious about the donor, they've been really understanding and respect our privacy.

For now we're just basking in the joys (and challenges!) of parenthood. Maria is breastfeeding Matthew, but all other parenting roles we share. Our son has a hyphenated last name representing both of us, and I have legally adopted him to ensure I have the same parental rights as Maria. Maria is "Mama" to Matthew, and I'm "E-Mom" for "Elizabeth Mom." But the other night, he pointed at Maria and said, "Mama," then pointed at me and said, "Mama." He gets it. Smart kid.

Almost as wonderful as Matthew himself has been the growing awareness that people see and accept us as the loving family we are. While there is certainly much more that needs to happen when it comes to lesbian and gay rights, we feel very lucky to live at a time where there is so much more acceptance and understanding. We have a great support network of family and friends. We always had great support from our doctor, and the birthing experience at the hospital was totally positive. We haven't experienced any homophobia as we meet other families, and we have families with all different structures in our life. All we hear over and over again is what a great kid Matthew is. People could care less that he's got two moms instead of a mom and a dad. That's pretty neat.

Matthew is safe, secure, and totally loved by his two moms and the wonderful people we're lucky enough to have in our lives.

Critical Thinking

What do you see as unique child-rearing issues for gay and lesbian parents? Do you think there are unique "growing-up" issues for children of lesbian and gay parents? If so, what are they?

Use your Virtual Workbook to explore your answers to these questions at **http://health.wadsworth.com/blonna1.**

Intellectual and Emotional Wellness

Becoming a parent has many intellectual challenges. Individuals find themselves thinking about their values, what is important, and how best to rear a child. College students may find that the challenges of college preclude time to take care of children. Particularly with young children, little time may be available to attend classes, read, study, and prepare papers. More and more colleges and universities are providing child care facilities, yet comprehensive care, including infant care, is limited.

Becoming a parent requires emotional readiness. Some individuals know "I'm just not ready to do this now." The role of mother or father has been so idealized that reality comes as a major shock to many new parents. Finding no time for oneself, with another person so totally dependent on the parent, is a new experience. The lack of sleep that accompanies new parenthood also takes its toll. When babies have colic and cry for what seems like months, can you be the patient, adoring parent that you envisioned being? How well are you able to put another's needs above your own?

The emotional/mental illnesses of the parents certainly have an impact on the welfare of the children. Television and newspapers often highlight the worst cases— stories of children physically and mentally abused or killed by parents who could not cope. In the 1990s, a case that made national news involved two college students from Wyckoff, New Jersey, who were convicted of killing their newborn baby and leaving him in a motel dumpster. Parenthood and the care of a baby are not always "natural," positive experiences for which everyone is ready.

Not everyone wants to be a parent. Not everyone has the physical capability to become a parent. And, certainly, plenty of evidence shows that not everyone is able to be a good parent. Too often, individuals are asked, "When are you going to settle down and get married?" and once in a committed relationship, "When are you two going to have children?" If individuals or couples respond that they don't want children, some people are taken aback, as if an offense has been committed. Only recently has the language changed to become less judgmental. Couples without children now are referred to as *childfree* rather than *childless.* In any case, planning to become a parent rather than stumbling on impending parenthood has clear advantages. The wellness model provides a useful framework for assessing readiness for parenting.

The Menstrual Cycle and Ovulation

Fertilization/conception Union of the sperm and ovum

Ovulation The release of an egg from the ovary

A pregnancy begins with the union of an ovum (or ova) and a sperm, a process called **fertilization** or **conception.** For conception to take place, the sperm must get to the ovum within a 24-hour period after its release from the ovary, a process known as **ovulation.** Ovulation occurs about 14 days before a woman's next menstrual cycle. Consequently, a woman who understands her menstrual cycle can predict when ovulation is most likely to occur. Although most women ovulate within 14 to 16 days from the beginning of the menstrual cycle, the timing depends on the length of the cycle itself—a piece of information not available until the cycle is over.

Couples have to try to predict when fertility is most likely. Women who have cycles that are 25 days long will ovulate closer to the first day of menstruation (the first day of the cycle). Women whose cycles are 31 days in duration will ovulate farther from the first date of the cycle. (See Chapter 2, Figure 2.9, which illustrates the menstrual cycle and timing of ovulation.) Understanding when a woman is fertile allows us to know when conception can take place.

Women who pay close attention to their body changes throughout the menstrual cycle may be more successful at predicting ovulation. The cervical mucus goes through changes: At ovulation it is clear and thin—sort of like egg white. Sometimes a discharge signals ovulation.

Changes in body temperature can be used to monitor ovulation. Women use a basal body temperature thermometer to determine slight fluctuations in temperature. Ovulation is marked by a few tenths of a degree drop, followed by an increase, in which the body temperature remains slightly elevated until the next menstrual cycle. The temperature must be taken first thing in the morning, before any activity, tooth brushing, or drinking of hot or cold beverages. Careful charting over a period of months is necessary to see individual patterns (see Figure 14.1, the basal body temperature chart, in Chapter 14).

In recent years, the pharmaceutical industry has been producing ovulation kits, which purport to detect critical hormonal changes signaling that ovulation will occur within 1 to 2 days. The kits can be helpful, although frequent use could become costly. Couples who develop difficulties in conceiving should consult a medical specialist.

healthy sex hints 13.1

Consumer Reports Ratings of Ovulation Kits

The Consumers Union tested and evaluated various ovulation test kits on the market. Their chart shows the highest-rated product at top, down to the lowest-rated one at the bottom.

Overall Ratings — In performance order

Excellent ● Very good ◕ Good ○ Fair ◔ Poor ●

BRAND & MODEL	PRICE/ NO. TESTS	OVERALL SCORE (0–100, P F G VG E)	LH SENSITIVITY	RECOMMENDATIONS & NOTES
ClearPlan Easy Ovulation Test Pack[1]	$30.32/5		●	Wick-type stick. The most sensitive product by far, but will not detect the LH surge of approximately 12 percent of women. Easier to read than most.
ClearPlan Easy Fertility Monitor[2]	195.01/20		◕	Reusable electronic meter with wick-type sticks. Also measures estradiol level. Easier to read than most. 30-stick test replacement packs available for $49.99. Permits only one reading per day.
CVS One Step Ovulation Predictor	13.57/5		○	Wick-type stick.
Eckerd One Step Ovulation Predictor	17.18/5		○	Wick-type stick.
Inverness Medical Early Ovulation Predictor[3]	21.57/5		○	Cassette.
Inverness Medical Early Ovulation Predictor[3]	17.29/5		○	Wick-type stick.
Rite Aid One Step Ovulation Predictor	14.48/7		○	Wick-type stick.
Target Brand One Step Ovulation Predictor	12.59/5		○	Wick-type stick.
Walgreens One Step Ovulation Predictor	14.99/5		○	Wick-type stick.
First Response Pregnancy Planning Kit	32.76/7		◕	Wick-type stick.
Answer Quick & Simple One-Step Ovulation Test	16.89/5		●	Wick-type stick. No protective cap; may be somewhat messy to use. May not work for many women.

[1] Renamed ClearBlue Easy Ovulation Test Pack in March 2003.
[2] Renamed ClearBlue Easy Fertility Monitor in March 2003.
[3] Renamed Accu-Clear Early Ovulation Predictor in March 2003.

Notes: Overall score is based mainly on the lowest level of LH the test could detect, with added points given for ease of reading and use. LH sensitivity was measured by adding progressively higher concentrations of LH to female urine. The lower the concentration the test could detect, the higher the score. Price is a national average based on a survey of prices paid in supermarkets and drug stores.

Source: Consumers Union (2003a, p. 49).

Conception

Fallopian tubes Conduits
connected to the uterus
through which the egg
passes into the uterus
during ovulation.
Fertilization usually takes
place at the outer third of
the tube.

Allurin A chemical released
by a mature ovum that
attracts a sperm to enable
conception

Fertilin A protein on the
plasma membrane of the
sperm that enables it to
bind with the ovum

Implantation The
attachment of a fertilized
egg to lining of uterus

Embryo A fertilized egg up
to 8 weeks gestation

Fetus A fertilized egg from
8 weeks after conception to
birth

Amniotic fluid The
transparent liquid contained
in the amniotic sac that
protects the fetus from
injury and helps maintain an
even temperature

Placenta An organ that
attaches to the uterine wall
and serves as a conduit for
oxygen and nutrients to
pass to the developing
fetus

Conception results from the successful journey of a group of sperm to the outer third of the **fallopian tube.** After being deposited in the vagina, ideally close to the cervix, sperm must make their way into the uterus, over to and up the fallopian tube where the ovum is waiting. Some argue that conception is enhanced when sperm arrive "early" and wait for the ova to be released.

A normal ejaculation usually contains between 250 and 500 million sperm. Although only one penetrates the membrane of the ovum at conception, millions are needed for conception. For a male to be considered fertile, the sperm count must be 20 million/milliliter of semen (Sherwood, 2004). Sperm survive best in an alkaline environment, and many die when confronting the acidity of the male urethra and female vagina. Continued losses result from sperm not heading toward the correct tube (the two tubes alternate in egg production each month). Finally, the much smaller group reaches the ovum. Consequently, though the sperm count starts at millions, only a few thousand make it to the fallopian tube, and a couple hundred get close to the ovum.

Descriptions of conception have often left mental images of the valiant, strong, surviving sperm successfully attacking and breaking through the membrane of the ovum. Research has demonstrated that the process is more complicated. A mature ovum will release the chemical **allurin,** which attracts the sperm. The sperm that ultimately penetrates the outer membrane of the ovum is able to do so because of **fertilin,** a protein on its plasma membrane (Sherwood, 2004). The ovum extends microvilli up from its surface, which hold down the sperm and push other sperm away. Finally, the egg pulls the sperm inside toward its nucleus. This process and its aftermath are depicted in Figure 13.1.

The fertilized egg, beginning a process of rapid cell division, travels down the fallopian tube over 3 to 4 days and sometimes longer, reaching the uterus, where it will attach to the uterine wall in a process called **implantation.** During this time, cell division is occurring constantly. Once implanted, the fertilized egg, now referred to as an **embryo,** will be nourished through the remaining term of the pregnancy. After 8 weeks, the structure is referred to as a **fetus.**

The environment within the uterus is highly protected. The fetus floats in, and is protected by, **amniotic fluid.** The **placenta,** an organ of interchange that attaches to the uterine wall, passes oxygen and nutrients through the umbilical cord to the fetus and passes waste products and carbon dioxide back to the mother. Unfortunately, as will be discussed later, numerous toxins may also cross the placenta and damage the fetus in a variety of ways.

Infertility

Infertility The inability to
conceive after 1 year of
unprotected intercourse

Although pregnancy and childbirth are "natural" occurrences, they don't occur easily for all couples. One in every five to six couples in the United States is infertile (Black, 1995; Burns, 1990). Based on surveys conducted by the National Center for Health Statistics (NCHS) in 1995, 6.1 million women between ages 15 and 44 had an impaired ability to have children; the number of infertile married couples was reported to be 2.1 million (Centers for Disease Control [CDC], 1995).

Infertility is the inability to conceive or impregnate after 1 year of regularly engaging in sexual intercourse without the use of birth control. In approximately 40 percent of cases, the problem centers on the woman's body, in 40 percent of cases on the male's body, and the remaining 20 percent of unknown origin. On occasion, individuals may know or suspect that they may have difficulty or be unable to reproduce. For others the knowledge comes as a painful reality. In recent years, reproductive technologies have greatly expanded to enable couples to biologically

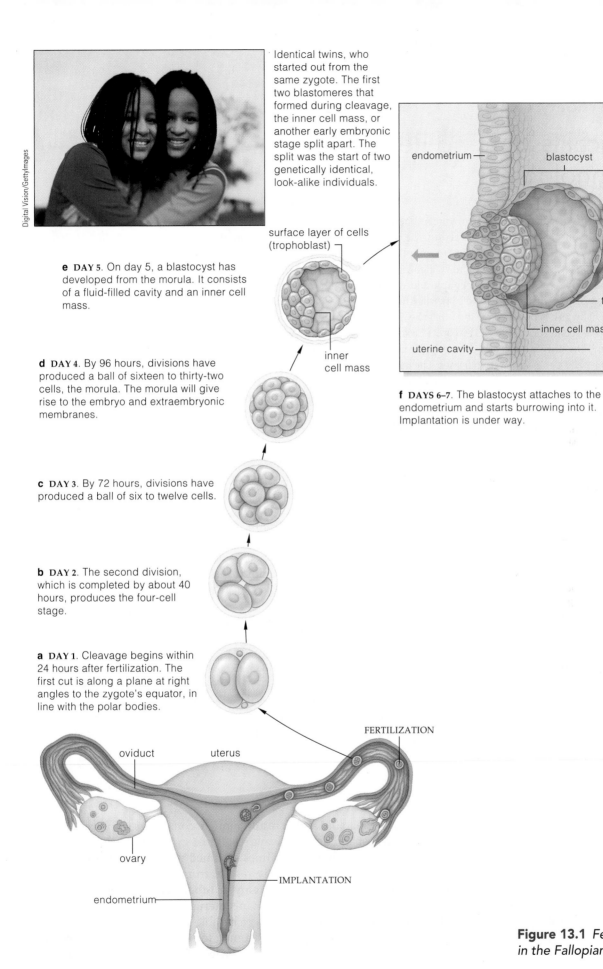

Identical twins, who started out from the same zygote. The first two blastomeres that formed during cleavage, the inner cell mass, or another early embryonic stage split apart. The split was the start of two genetically identical, look-alike individuals.

endometrium

blastocyst

surface layer of cells (trophoblast)

trophoblast

inner cell mass

uterine cavity

e DAY 5. On day 5, a blastocyst has developed from the morula. It consists of a fluid-filled cavity and an inner cell mass.

inner cell mass

d DAY 4. By 96 hours, divisions have produced a ball of sixteen to thirty-two cells, the morula. The morula will give rise to the embryo and extraembryonic membranes.

f DAYS 6–7. The blastocyst attaches to the endometrium and starts burrowing into it. Implantation is under way.

actual size

c DAY 3. By 72 hours, divisions have produced a ball of six to twelve cells.

b DAY 2. The second division, which is completed by about 40 hours, produces the four-cell stage.

a DAY 1. Cleavage begins within 24 hours after fertilization. The first cut is along a plane at right angles to the zygote's equator, in line with the polar bodies.

FERTILIZATION

oviduct   uterus

ovary

IMPLANTATION

endometrium

Figure 13.1 *Fertilization in the Fallopian Tube*

sex in society 13.2

Ethical Issues and Reproductive Technologies

Among attempts to have a child, surrogate motherhood remains an option—albeit a controversial one. The case of Mary Beth Whitehead in 1986 brought the complicated issues of surrogacy to national attention. Whitehead had signed a contract with a New Jersey couple and was artificially inseminated with the husband's sperm. After giving birth to a baby girl, Whitehead decided that she didn't want to give up the child for adoption. The courts became involved, and the story spread across the popular media. For a while the baby girl even had two names. The outcome of the court case was that the child was given to the adoptive parents, with Whitehead being granted visitation rights.

As a result of this case, a number of legal and ethical issues were brought to national attention. To some people, the use of surrogate mothers extends the array of reproductive options for infertile couples. It represents a choice that is both private and not much different from traditional adoption. To others, it represents exploitation of women's bodies. Those who are able to pay hire women whose need of income may be paramount. The contractual elements, fees involved, and possible legal challenges all contribute to the debate over surrogate mothering.

Another public case had to do with John and Luanne Buzzanca. After 6 years of infertility treatments, the couple turned to a laboratory that supplied donor sperm and ova, paid a surrogate, and finally became parents in San Francisco in April 1995. Shortly after the birth, John filed for divorce and refused to make child support payments on the grounds that he wasn't the baby's father in any true legal sense, despite having earlier signed a contract agreeing to the child's birth. The Superior Court agreed, claiming that baby Jaycee had been conceived in a petri dish, from anonymous donors, and carried and delivered by a surrogate mother with no genetic ties to her. Consequently, according to California law, not only was John not the father, but Luanne was not the legal mother. By California law, the child had no parents.

A petition filed with the California Court of Appeals for the Fourth Circuit (March 1998), however, resulted in the determination that both John and Luanne Buzzanca were the legal parents of Jaycee (Vorzimer, O'Hara, & Shafton, 1998). As a result of that ruling, individuals who use assisted reproductive technologies and intend to be considered the parents can finalize their parental rights before the child is born, regardless of whether they use a traditional or a gestational surrogate. Specific to this case, because John Buzzanca initially had consented to using donor sperm and a surrogate to produce a child, he was viewed as the father and, therefore, has financial responsibilities to Jaycee.

A more recent case involved an infertile woman from Staten Island, New York, who with the help of in vitro fertilization found out she was carrying twins. To her surprise at the birth, one child was white and one black. She and her husband are white yet were using the same fertility clinic as another couple from New Jersey, who were African American. Upon investigation, it was determined that the lab "accidentally" had forwarded one embryo for transplant that belonged to the New Jersey couple. To complicate matters further, the African American couple from New Jersey had been unsuccessful in their pregnancy attempts.

Despite litigation and an eventual resolution of each child staying with his biological parents, fundamental fertility questions remain. Were the boys twins? Should the gestational mother be entitled to visitation rights? Was the woman from Staten Island forced into surrogacy without compensation?

Sterility The permanent inability to reproduce

Vasectomy The surgical sterilization of the male that involves cutting and tying off the vas deferens

become parents. The pregnancies that result, though, come at great physical, emotional, and financial cost and do not always result in a successful birth.

Individuals and couples have sometimes assumed mistakenly that they were infertile or even sterile. **Sterility** usually results from the purposeful action of being surgically sterilized through **vasectomy** or **tubal ligation.** Sterility also can result from disease. For example, if a woman's uterus is removed because of cancer or extensive fibroids, she will no longer be able to become pregnant. When chemotherapy is prescribed for men and women for the treatment of cancer, one common aftereffect is damage to the ovaries or testicles, impairing the ability to produce ova and sperm. We have sometimes heard young people describe themselves as "sterile" or "infertile." The explanation given is "I've been having sex for years, and I never use birth control. Since I never got pregnant, I just assume I'm sterile." Just because a couple has been lax in the use of contraception and has avoided unintended pregnancy, they should not assume infertility or sterility.

Individuals should not initially suspect infertility unless they are aware of specific health problems, congenital abnormalities, or environmental exposures that could impair the reproductive system. In women, infertility can be attributable to lack of ovulation, hormonal imbalances that impair endometrial functioning, scar tissue in the uterus and fallopian tubes resulting from advanced pelvic infections, endometriosis, habitual miscarriage, and production of antisperm antibodies. Other factors cited as causes of infertility include advanced age, cigarette smoking, drug use, and excessive dieting and exercise. The last two factors are related to body fat levels and the ability of the female body to store estrogen.

Male infertility focuses primarily on sperm production. Inadequate sperm production can be related to structural deformities, hormonal deficiencies, lifestyle habits including drug use, and sexual dysfunction. Problems generally focus on sperm being too few or none at all, slow movement of sperm present, or misshapen sperm. The cause of any problem has to be determined.

Numerous tests, with varying degrees of invasiveness, have been developed to determine the cause(s) of infertility. Males and females alike initially will have complete physical assessments, including a detailed medical and lifestyle history. The man will be asked to ejaculate into a sterile cup, after which his sperm will be tested for viability and motility. If problems are found with the sperm, correct diagnosis and treatment follow. These might consist of lifestyle changes, hormone treatment, surgery to remove a **varicocele** (an enlarged vein in the scrotum impairing blood flow), and artificial insemination with his sperm.

Tests for the female typically begin after months of first charting her menstrual cycle by taking her basal body temperature. Follow-up blood work can help determine whether she is ovulating. Endometrial biopsies can be performed to assess the readiness of the uterus to accept a fertilized egg. **Hysterosalpingograms** are tests that determine whether the fallopian tubes are open. Laparoscopy and hysteroscopy are two tests that allow physicians to see any evidence of endometriosis and scar tissue. A postcoital test uses cervical mucus removed after intercourse to determine its interaction with sperm (Carlson, Eisenstat, & Ziporyn, 1996).

If the infertility is suspected to result from absence of ovulation, women can be treated hormonally. Two common drugs are clomid and pergonal. One problem with medications is the increased possibility of multiple births—some of which receive a lot of media coverage and attention. Multiple-birth babies, however, are almost always premature and frequently have health problems. Whereas normal gestation takes place over a 40-week period, multiple births usually do not go to term. Each additional fetus shortens the gestation period. When babies are born around the 32nd week of a pregnancy, for example, they weigh little more than 2 pounds and require weeks of treatment in a neonatal intensive care unit. Decades ago, these babies would not have survived. Today, more drugs and technology are available to keep these infants alive. The costs on many levels—physical, social, emotional, and financial—can be staggering. In 2000, it was estimated to cost over $58,000 to deliver twins and close to $282,000 for quadruplets (Wright, Schieve, Reynolds, & Jeng, 2003). Case Study 13.3 describes some of the emotions and experiences typically associated with infertility.

Some women first undergo pelvic surgery to conceive and carry a pregnancy. Endometriosis, a condition in which endometrial tissue grows outside the uterus and in some cases literally wraps around and blocks off the fallopian tubes, can be treated with surgery. Myomectomy, a surgical procedure used to remove fibroid growths but preserve the uterus, can help women as well.

Tubal ligation The surgical sterilization of the female that involves cutting and tying off the fallopian tubes

Varicocele An enlarged vein in the scrotum impairing blood flow

Hysterosalpingograms Tests that determine whether the fallopian tubes are open

case study 13.3

Anthony's Story of Infertility

Anthony, 40, identifies as Italian American.

Critical Thinking

Anthony's case highlights the lengths couples may go to in their attempts to reproduce. With health care so costly, should limits be placed on what options individuals and couples can exercise?

Use your Virtual Workbook to explore your answer to this question at **http://health.wadsworth.com/blonna1.**

Looking back on it now, it all seems so distant. My wife and I married in September of 1989. We planned a perfect life together, filled with love and joy. We thought that most of this joy would come from the children we planned on having.

I don't know whether it was the combination of my going back to college full-time and the pressures of conceiving or whether it just wasn't "God's time" (a phrase we held to that kept our faith), but getting pregnant just wasn't happening. At first we kidded about it. Then we decided to pay more attention to having sex around my wife's ovulation date. Purchasing and using the special thermometer that allowed us to take her basal body temperature was the beginning of a host of infertility treatments. We came to hate that word infertility as much as the constant advice to "relax."

One year passed, and no pregnancy. I thought about how my brother's infertility was remedied by an operation to remove a varicocele. Six months after his surgery, his wife became pregnant. The operation had helped his sperm count, which had been both low and with slow-motility sperm.

Now it was my turn. I delivered more sperm samples to a variety of medical centers than I care to remember! I had such anxiety as I tried to ejaculate into cups, being in public medical facilities with what seemed to be everyone knowing what I was doing. It was determined that I was a candidate for varicocele surgery. Finally our problems would be solved! I had the surgery and hoped to become a father soon. No such luck.

My wife was given two fertility drugs to improve our chances of children. Clomid didn't work. Serephene didn't work. She was then scheduled for a laparoscopy to allow the doctors to see what was going on. It turned out that she had endometriosis, cysts on her ovaries, and one of her fallopian tubes was smaller than the other. All these problems were described as "fixable" and, paired with my problem, could have explained why we weren't getting pregnant. After the necessary surgery, we regained our hope.

Months and months of trying came and went. Negative pregnancy tests . . . trying again . . . waiting and hoping that she wouldn't get her period. Anger and sadness when her period came. And trying again. Lovemaking became a job. We were so upset that we were often no-shows at family christenings and children's birthday parties.

In vitro fertilization (IVF) A procedure in which ova are removed from the woman's body and fertilized with sperm in a laboratory; the embryo is surgically implanted into her uterus.

Blastocysts Spherical clusters of cells, also known as *preembryos*, that form shortly after conception

When a woman's fallopian tubes remain blocked, **in vitro fertilization (IVF)** becomes an option. Her ovaries are first stimulated using hormones, so that more than one ovum matures each month. After surgically "harvesting" the eggs, they are joined with sperm in a laboratory. Often three or four **blastocysts** (preembryos) then will be placed directly into the woman's uterus. Generally, the more embryos that are transplanted, the higher the rate of success. Researchers are also finding that the age of the woman impacts the success of the procedure. Nationally, live-birth rates ranged from 38 percent for women under 35 years to 6 percent for women over 42 (Wright et al., 2003). As women age, it can become more difficult for them to become pregnant for a variety of reasons, including quality of the ova and blockage of the fallopian tubes.

Some couples confront the reality that a pregnancy will result only from the use of donor sperm or donor ova. Fertility clinics can provide information to couples that allow them to choose donors who match them in physical appearance, background, and interests. Because college students are considered young and healthy, they may be approached as possible donors. For women in particular, the money offered is enticing and intended to compensate for the health risks involved. High doses of hormones are prescribed, which stimulate multiple ovula-

Anthony's triplet girls.

After a period of time, the doctor suggested artificial insemination with my sperm. My wife would be put on fertility drugs to increase her chances of ovulation. I would provide a sample—legal masturbation, as I called it—and the sperm would be injected into my wife using a long syringe. We agreed to the procedures. Each time we prayed and prayed yet continued to get negative results.

Not being ready to consider adoption—people were kindly suggesting that to us—we enrolled at the reproductive clinic at a local hospital, known for its successes with infertile couples. I was now 33 years old, finished with college, and fortunately employed at a place with good health benefits. The doctors there suggested in vitro fertilization. We agreed. I had to inject fertility drugs into my wife's buttocks for 21 straight days prior to "the day." Prayer got me through that. Retrieval of the eggs was successful, and we were told that there were seven excellent embryos. The doctors would put three back into my wife's uterus.

My wife had to be monitored daily at the hospital, giving blood and having ultrasounds. The egg retrieval was done on March 17, Saint Patrick's Day. The embryos were put back on March 20, the first day of spring. We would have to wait 14 days for the results. Those were the longest 14 days of our lives.

On Easter Sunday we received the exciting news that she was pregnant! Tests conducted 2 weeks later confirmed that she was carrying triplets. We were grateful . . . scared . . . overwhelmed. There was never a question that, despite the high risks associated with multiple births, we would keep all three babies.

After 20 weeks of bed rest and daily monitoring, my wife gave birth, with me at her side, to three beautiful girls. The road was long and bumpy. It took almost 6 years of trying. Although we had been angry, sad, and frustrated, we never lost our faith. We supported each other from start to finish. And now I live with the four most beautiful women in the world, all coming in "God's time."

tions. The ova are harvested and then retrieved surgically. Both hormone ingestion and surgery carry some risk to the woman's health.

The **assisted reproductive technology (ART)** refers to fertility treatments in which both eggs and sperm are handled by a laboratory. The federal government requires all medical centers in the United States that use ART to report data to the CDC on an annual basis. Assisted reproduction can stem from a couple's fresh eggs and sperm, donor eggs and sperm, "thawed" embryos, and so forth. For 2000, there were 99,629 ART procedures attempted, with 25,228 live-birth deliveries and 35,025 infants born (Wright et al., 2003). Infertile couples come to learn that attempts do not mean automatic success and that multiple births with their concomitant issues are a risk.

Couples spend varying amounts of time, money, and certainly emotional energy being tested and evaluated for the causes of the infertility. Those who consider IVF can expect to pay more than $7,000 for each attempt. Class differences become readily apparent, as those with financial resources and better health insurance plans clearly have an advantage. When all the time and resources result in a healthy baby, however, those efforts pale in comparison to the joy of new parenthood.

Assisted reproductive technology (ART) Infertility interventions in which a laboratory is involved with the union of the sperm and egg

Pregnancy

Human chorionic gonadotropin (hCG) A hormone secreted during pregnancy that shows up in the urine of pregnant women; the basis for determining pregnancy using home kits

Confirming a pregnancy used to mean that a woman had to see her physician, have a urine test, and wait for days for the results. Today, determining whether a woman is pregnant is as simple as purchasing a home pregnancy kit at the local pharmacy. Home pregnancy kits are designed to detect the presence of **human chorionic gonadotropin (hCG)**, a hormone present in the urine of pregnant women. Because this hormone is secreted as the fertilized egg implants in the uterus, early testing can confirm a pregnancy. Many kits can be used reliably within a day or two of a

healthy sex hints 13.2
Ratings of Home Pregnancy Tests

The Consumers Union tested 18 pregnancy test kits for their performance, including average cost, ease of use, and sensitivity. The most highly recommended kit is listed first, down to the worst performer listed at the bottom of the chart.

Excellent ● Very good ◖ Good ○ Fair ◔ Poor ●

BRAND & MODEL	PRICE/ NO. TESTS	OVERALL SCORE	HCG SENSITIVITY	EASE OF READING	10-MINUTE HCG SENSITIVITY	RECOMMENDATIONS & NOTES
First Response Early Result Pregnancy Test	$18.09/2		●	○	●	Wick-type stick. Best combination of sensitivity and reliability.
Answer Quick & Simple One-Step Pregnancy Test	15.22/2		◖	○	◖	Wick-type stick. No wick protection; possibly messy to use.
Answer Pregnancy Test	8.14/1		◖	◔	●	Wick-type stick must be dipped in a cup. No wick protection; possibly messy to use.
ClearBlue Easy One Minute Pregnancy Test[1]	16.02/2		○	○	●	Wick-type stick. Easier to read than most.
Clear Choice At Home Pregnancy Test	9.11/1		●	◔	●	Jar. Some samples failed to work.
e.p.t. Pregnancy Test	16.72/2		○	●	●	Wick-type stick.
ClearPlan Easy Pregnancy Test Pack	17.61/3		○	◔	◖	Wick-type stick.
Inverness Medical Early Pregnancy Test[2]	10.77/2		◔	◔	●	Cassette type.
American Fare (Kmart) Easy to Read Pregnancy Test[1]	9.35/2		◔	●	●	Wick-type stick.
CVS Pregnancy Test	10.86/2		◔	●	○	Wick-type stick.
Target Brand One Step Pregnancy Test	7.99/2		◔	●	○	Wick-type stick.
Walgreens One Step Pregnancy Tests	12.99/2		◔	●	◖	Wick-type stick.
Sav-On Osco (Albertson's) One Step Pregnancy Test	12.99/2		◔	●	○	Wick-type stick.
Inverness Medical Early Pregnancy Test[2]	12.56/2		◔	●	○	Wick-type stick.
Rite Aid One Step Pregnancy Test	7.23/1		◔	●	○	Wick-type stick.
Eckerd One Step Pregnancy Test	12.67/2		◔	●	◔	Wick-type stick.
Equate (Wal-Mart) Pregnancy Test[1]	7.92/2		◔	●	●	Wick-type stick. Some samples failed to work.
Confirm Pregnancy Test	11.19/2		◔	●	◔	Wick-type stick. Some samples failed to work.

Overall Score scale: 0 [P F G VG E] 100

[1] *Reformulation in progress.*

[2] *Renamed Accu-Clear Early Pregnancy Test in March 2003.*

Notes: Except as noted, all the tests came packaged in pairs. *Overall score* is based on the test's hCG sensitivity, both at the recommended reading time and after 10 minutes; and on the ease of reading the result. *hCG sensitivity* was measured by adding progressively higher concentrations of hCG to female urine, then conducting the test according to package instructions. The higher the level of hCG it took to produce a positive result, the lower the sensitivity score.

Ease of reading was based on the intensity of the line signifying a positive result; the more intense the line, the higher the score. None of the products tested had consistently intense lines at all the hCG concentration levels they detected. *10-minute hCG sensitivity* was evaluated by reading the results at the maximum allowable reading time of 10 minutes. *Price* is a national average based on a survey of prices paid in supermarkets and drugstores.

Source: Consumers Union (2003b, p. 47).

missed period, although reliability improves if used a week after a period is missed (Consumers Union, 2003b). Overall, a woman must be aware that her period was due to have early feedback that she is pregnant.

With slight variations in procedures, home pregnancy tests involve dipping an absorbent wick coated with monoclonal antibodies sensitive to hCG into a small amount of morning urine (which has the highest concentration of hCG). If the concentration of hCG is high enough, the woman will test positive for pregnancy. If the test is done too early into the pregnancy, the test result could be a "false negative." That means the woman is pregnant, but, because of too little hCG, the test showed her not to be pregnant. Increasingly, manufacturers are marketing multiple-test kits, so that a negative test can be repeated a week later.

Although home pregnancy tests are 85 to 95 percent accurate, medical laboratory tests are most accurate. False positives are extremely rare. When a woman has given birth recently, had a miscarriage, or is taking certain fertility drugs, a test may show that she is pregnant when she is not.

In all cases, the woman should follow up with a visit to a physician. A pelvic exam will indicate an enlarged uterus associated with pregnancy and also will allow the physician to estimate the duration of the pregnancy and project a birth date.

Gestation

A pregnancy is measured from the first day of a woman's last menstrual period, with the expected period of **gestation** averaging 40 weeks. A normal birth will take place between the 38th and 42nd week. Deliveries before 38 weeks are considered premature, and after 42 weeks, the extended time may threaten the health of the baby, so labor may be induced. A mathematical calculation called the *Nagele rule* is used by obstetricians, nurse midwives, and other health care providers to help estimate the expected date of birth (McCloskey & Bulecheck, 1996). When a woman's menstrual cycle is regular and she hasn't been on oral contraceptives, the measurement is useful; nonetheless, many babies are actually born before or after their "due date." To calculate the estimated due date, take the first day of the last menstrual period, subtract 3 months, and then add 7 days. (Women need to keep track of their menstrual cycles as a general health practice, but especially around pregnancy.) For example: Jessica's last period began on February 2. Subtracting 3 months brings her to November 2, and adding 7 days makes her estimated due date November 9.

Pregnancies are divided into trimesters, each having unique characteristics. Figure 13.2 is a time line showing features of each.

First Trimester   During the first trimester of the pregnancy, all structures and systems develop in rudimentary form. At the end of 3 months, the fetus has arms, legs, feet, toes, fingers, and the vital organs and body systems are functioning.

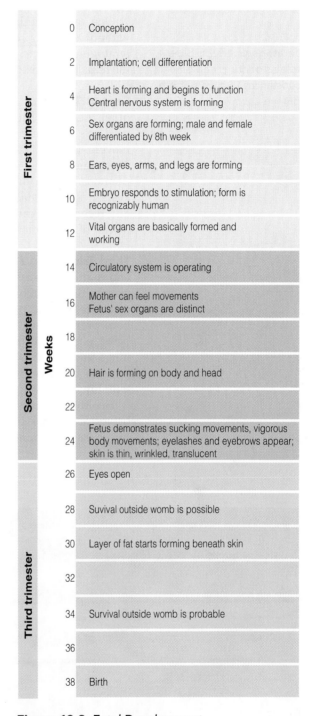

Fetal development

	Weeks	
First trimester	0	Conception
	2	Implantation; cell differentiation
	4	Heart is forming and begins to function Central nervous system is forming
	6	Sex organs are forming; male and female differentiated by 8th week
	8	Ears, eyes, arms, and legs are forming
	10	Embryo responds to stimulation; form is recognizably human
	12	Vital organs are basically formed and working
Second trimester	14	Circulatory system is operating
	16	Mother can feel movements Fetus' sex organs are distinct
	18	
	20	Hair is forming on body and head
	22	
	24	Fetus demonstrates sucking movements, vigorous body movements; eyelashes and eyebrows appear; skin is thin, wrinkled, translucent
Third trimester	26	Eyes open
	28	Suvival outside womb is possible
	30	Layer of fat starts forming beneath skin
	32	
	34	Survival outside womb is probable
	36	
	38	Birth

Figure 13.2 *Fetal Development*

Gestation The period of time representing pregnancy and development of fetus from conception to birth

The mother's taking drugs during the first trimester can have a particularly damaging effect on the fetus.

One overpowering argument for planning a pregnancy lies in the fact that without planning, the mother unintentionally may be taking medications with **teratogenic effects,** causing fetal malformations. At the end of the first trimester, the fetus is approximately 4 inches in length and weighs approximately 1 ounce.

Teratogenic effects Side effects of drugs and other substances that cause birth defects

Second Trimester   The second trimester is marked by growth and maturation of all the fetal systems. As the fetus grows in size and the uterus stretches, the mother's pregnancy becomes evident. During the fifth month of pregnancy, fetal movement is usually active enough for the mother to feel. By the end of the second trimester, the fetus is close to 12 inches long and weighs between 1 and 1.5 pounds. The sex organs are apparent, as is body hair, including eyebrows and eyelashes. Neonatal intensive care units, equipped with the proper medications and technology, can help some babies born prematurely at the end of the sixth month of pregnancy to survive.

Third Trimester   During the third trimester, the fetal systems continue to grow and mature. The last system to develop fully is the respiratory system. Without proper lung function, the blood is not fully oxygenated, which can inflict damage to the fetus. The pharmaceutical industry has advanced treatments for babies born prematurely. Drugs such as survanta, which help the lungs expand and is being used for extremely tiny preemies, and pheophylline, which relaxes the lungs and prevents bronchiospasms, are being used in neonatal intensive care units to improve lung function and reduce the congenital problems associated with low-birth-weight babies (D. Devine, personal communication, 1998).

Health care costs associated with prematurity are high, and low-birth-weight babies are at risk for lasting health problems. At birth, most babies weigh between 6 and 9 pounds and are approximately 20 inches in length.

Lennart Nilsson

At four weeks, the embryo is approximately 1/4 inch in length.

At the end of 8 weeks the developing embryo is now referred to as a fetus, and is approximately 1.5 inches long.

Physical, Psychological, and Social Effects of Pregnancy

Clearly, pregnancy has a powerful impact on health. The woman experiences a number of physical changes as her body responds to the physical demands of the pregnancy. Carrying an ever larger baby in the front of one's body puts demands on all the systems.

Physical Wellness

Pregnancy and childbirth clearly have an impact on a woman's health, and parenting affects the health of all caregivers. The mere fact that pregnant women are advised to gain between 25 and 35 pounds to have a healthy baby can put a strain on many body systems. Blood pressure may increase. Respiration becomes more labored. Muscles and ligaments must stretch. Throughout pregnancy, women report varying degrees of fatigue, shortness of breath, heartburn, indigestion, nausea, gas, constipation, headaches, leg cramps, backaches, water retention, varicose veins, and difficulty sleeping. Nerves may be impinged upon by the developing fetus; sciatica is a common complaint. Maintaining a healthy pregnancy requires good prenatal care, focusing on nutrition, exercise, and monitored use of medication. Any problems that develop can then hopefully be managed without harm to the developing fetus.

As part of prenatal care, discussed later, the mother should be monitored for signs of hypertension and gestational diabetes. Pregnancy and childbirth may well be the greatest physical challenges in a woman's life.

Emotionally, fathers and mothers both respond to pregnancy in various ways. A planned pregnancy should connect to positive feelings—happiness, joy, excitement. Even so, periods of anxiety and fear about pending parenthood are normal. The high hormone levels in pregnancy affect women's moods and may result in being weepy, irritable, and upset. As the projected date of birth gets closer and closer, pending parenthood, or the addition of another child to the family, becomes all the more real. Couples might have difficulty concentrating on anything but the soon-to-arrive baby.

Pregnancy may affect social relationships as well. Because the birth of a child, and having children, changes our lives in so many ways, some people report feeling awkward around those who have not had the experience of pregnancy. Once children are born, relationships may go through periods of additional strain. Couples with children are talking about their baby's smallest accomplishment or where to buy diapers at the lowest expense, whereas childfree couples may be discussing their latest vacation. Continuing to be able to relate to each other's lifestyle can test the bounds of friendship.

Relationships with family members also may change. Excited grandparents can be a tremendous source of support. Relations between adult children and their parents may improve as the new parents come to better understand the roles of mother and father. In some situations, however, grandparents offer unsolicited advice and become controlling. Something as basic as naming a child and honoring relatives can be a source of tension.

placenta

At 16 weeks, the fetus is approximately 6.5 inches long and weighs approximately 7 ounces. In contrast, a full term baby is 19 to 21 inches long and weighs approximately 7.5 pounds.

Lennart Nilsson

Couples can manage the stresses associated with pregnancy, and later child rearing itself, by communicating openly. Private time to share what can be an intensely spiritual event becomes important.

Lovemaking During Pregnancy

Lovemaking can continue throughout a pregnancy, although males and females report changes in sexual desire at various stages. Many women have a progressive decline in sexual interest and activity, particularly by the third trimester (Bogren, 1991). Some women feel less attractive as their body becomes larger and larger and their nipples become darker and ultrasensitive, with stretch marks possibly forming. Other women feel sexy, attractive, and responsive throughout the pregnancy. Some males respond positively to their pregnant partners, and others fear hurting the developing fetus.

Many couples find massage and holding to be important sensual experiences during this time. Oral sex may be continued, although air should not be blown into the vagina. Couples do find the need to adjust positions when engaging in intercourse. The man-on-top position can be uncomfortable, if not difficult, as the pregnancy progresses.

If a pregnancy has been determined to be high-risk, a physician may advise modifications in lovemaking patterns. Women who are spotting, bleeding, at risk for premature labor, or in pain may be advised against sexual intercourse.

Prenatal Care

Creating a healthy environment for both the mother and developing fetus is the focus of prenatal care. Good prenatal care enhances the health of the mother and developing baby and reduces the possibility of congenital birth defects. The basic components of prenatal care are proper nutrition, exercise, medical monitoring, and, when medications are necessary for the mother's health, careful monitoring of those medications. Table 13.1 shows both birthrates and prenatal care rates analyzed by race and ethnicity.

Getting good prenatal care is tied to making an early connection with a health care provider. Traditionally, women have relied on physicians who specialize in obstetrics and gynecology (ob-gyn) for care and delivery. Gynecologists specialize in reproductive health, yet not all will also provide obstetrical care, which focuses on pregnancy and childbirth. Increased malpractice insurance rates and the lifestyle associated with "being on call" have led to physicians reducing and/or eliminating obstetric services (W. Warren, personal communication, 2003). The American College of Obstetricians and Gynecologists (2003), the certifying organization, reported that one in four ob-gyns were experiencing dissatisfaction with their profession, and although the number of residency positions had remained the same, only 68 percent were filled by medical schools in 2003.

Family practitioners, nurse midwives, and lay midwives may also provide care. Overall, services vary around the United States, and options, in turn, may be limited. It has been projected that it will be increasingly difficult for couples to find a physician nearby who will be available to deliver their baby.

Nutrition   During pregnancy, the mother should consume the proper amount of nutrient-dense foods. She must pay attention to her intake of all nutrients—protein, carbohydrates, fats, vitamins, minerals, fiber, and water. Pregnancy requires more calories and more protein. Because pregnant women also require more folic acid, iron, and calcium, a physician's prescription for vitamins and minerals may be needed (Boston Women's Health Book Collective, 1998).

Table 13.1 Registered Births to Teens, Unmarried Mothers, and Prenatal Care: 1990 to 1999

Characteristics	1990	1994	1995	1996	1997	1998	1999
Percent of births to teenage mothers	**12.8**	**13.1**	**13.1**	**12.9**	**12.7**	**12.5**	**12.3**
White	10.9	11.3	11.5	11.3	11.2	11.1	10.9
Black	23.1	23.2	23.1	22.8	22.2	21.5	20.7
American Indian, Eskimo, Aleut	19.5	21.0	21.4	20.9	20.8	20.9	20.2
Asian and Pacific Islander[1]	5.7	5.7	5.6	5.3	5.2	5.4	5.1
Filipino	6.1	6.0	6.2	6.1	5.9	6.2	5.9
Chinese	1.2	1.0	0.9	0.9	0.9	0.9	0.9
Japanese	2.9	2.8	2.5	2.5	2.2	2.4	2.1
Hawaiian	18.4	19.6	19.1	18.4	18.6	18.8	18.2
Other	(NA)	6.4	6.3	5.8	5.7	5.8	5.5
Hispanic origin[2]	16.8	17.8	17.9	17.4	17.0	16.9	16.7
Mexican	17.7	18.6	18.8	18.1	17.7	17.5	17.4
Puerto Rican	21.7	23.2	23.5	23.1	22.3	21.9	21.1
Cuban	7.7	7.3	7.7	7.6	7.4	6.9	7.7
Central and South American	9.0	10.4	10.6	10.5	10.5	10.3	10.0
Other and unknown Hispanic	(NA)	20.8	20.1	19.8	19.8	20.2	19.5
Percent births to unmarried mothers	**26.6**	**32.6**	**32.2**	**32.4**	**32.4**	**32.8**	**33.0**
White	16.9	25.4	25.3	25.7	25.8	26.3	26.8
Black	66.7	70.4	69.9	69.8	69.2	69.1	68.9
American Indian, Eskimo, Aleut	53.6	57.0	57.2	58.0	58.7	59.3	58.9
Asian and Pacific Islander[1]	(NA)	16.2	16.3	16.7	15.6	15.6	15.4
Filipino	15.9	18.5	19.5	19.4	19.5	19.7	21.1
Chinese	5.0	7.2	7.9	9.2	6.5	6.4	6.9
Japanese	9.6	11.2	10.8	11.4	10.1	9.7	9.9
Hawaiian	45.0	48.6	49.0	49.9	49.1	51.1	50.4
Hispanic origin[2]	36.7	43.1	40.8	40.7	40.9	41.6	42.2
Mexican	33.3	40.8	38.1	37.9	38.9	39.6	40.1
Puerto Rican	55.9	60.2	60.0	60.7	59.4	59.5	59.6
Cuban	18.2	22.9	23.8	24.7	24.4	24.8	26.4
Central and South American	41.2	45.9	44.1	44.7	41.8	42.0	43.7
Percent of mothers beginning prenatal care 1st trimester	**74.2**	**80.2**	**81.3**	**81.9**	**82.5**	**82.8**	**83.2**
White	77.7	82.8	83.6	84.0	84.7	84.8	85.1
Black	60.7	68.3	70.4	71.4	72.3	73.3	74.1
American Indian, Eskimo, Aleut	57.9	65.2	66.7	67.7	68.1	68.8	69.5
Asian and Pacific Islander[1]	(NA)	79.7	79.9	81.2	82.1	83.1	83.7
Filipino	77.1	81.3	80.9	82.5	83.3	84.2	84.2
Chinese	81.3	86.2	85.7	86.8	87.4	88.5	88.5
Japanese	87.0	89.2	89.7	89.3	89.3	90.2	90.7
Hawaiian	65.8	77.0	75.9	78.5	78.0	78.8	79.6
Hispanic origin[2]	60.2	68.9	70.8	72.2	73.7	74.3	74.4
Mexican	57.8	67.3	69.1	70.7	72.1	72.8	73.1
Puerto Rican	63.5	71.7	74.0	75.0	76.5	76.9	77.7
Cuban	84.8	90.1	89.2	89.2	90.4	91.8	91.4
Central and South American	61.5	71.2	73.2	75.0	76.9	78.0	77.6

(continued)

Table 13.1 Registered Births to Teens, Unmarried Mothers, and Prenatal Care: 1990 to 1999 *(continued)*

Characteristics	1990	1994	1995	1996	1997	1998	1999
Percent of mothers beginning							
prenatal care 3d trimester or no care	**6.0**	**4.4**	**4.2**	**4.0**	**3.9**	**3.9**	**3.8**
White	4.9	3.6	3.5	3.3	3.2	3.3	3.2
Black	10.9	8.2	7.6	7.3	7.3	7.0	6.6
American Indian, Eskimo, Aleut	12.9	9.8	9.5	8.6	8.6	8.5	8.2
Asian and Pacific Islander[1]	(NA)	4.1	4.3	3.9	3.8	3.6	3.5
Filipino	4.5	3.6	4.1	3.3	3.3	3.1	2.8
Chinese	3.4	2.7	3.0	2.5	2.4	2.2	2.0
Japanese	2.9	1.9	2.3	2.2	2.7	2.1	2.1
Hawaiian	8.7	4.7	5.1	5.0	5.4	4.7	4.0
Hispanic origin[2]	12.0	7.6	7.4	6.7	6.2	6.3	6.3
Mexican	13.2	8.3	8.1	7.2	6.7	6.8	6.7
Puerto Rican	10.6	6.5	5.5	5.7	5.4	5.1	5.0
Cuban	2.8	1.6	2.1	1.6	1.5	1.2	1.4
Central and South American	10.9	6.5	6.1	5.5	5.0	4.9	5.2
Percent of births with low birth weight[3]	**7.0**	**7.3**	**7.3**	**7.4**	**7.5**	**7.6**	**7.6**
White	5.7	6.1	6.2	6.3	6.5	6.5	6.6
Black	13.3	13.2	13.1	13.0	13.0	13.0	13.1
American Indian, Eskimo, Aleut	6.1	6.4	6.6	6.5	6.8	6.8	7.1
Asian and Pacific Islander[1]	(NA)	6.8	6.9	7.1	7.2	7.4	7.4
Filipino	7.3	7.8	7.8	7.9	8.3	8.2	8.3
Chinese	4.7	4.8	5.3	5.0	5.1	5.3	5.2
Japanese	6.2	6.9	7.3	7.3	6.8	7.5	7.9
Hawaiian	7.2	7.2	6.8	6.8	7.2	7.2	7.7
Hispanic origin[2]	6.1	6.2	6.3	7.4	6.4	6.4	6.4
Mexican	5.5	5.8	5.8	5.9	6.0	6.0	5.9
Puerto Rican	9.0	9.1	9.4	9.2	9.4	9.7	9.3
Cuban	5.7	6.3	6.5	6.5	6.8	6.5	6.8
Central and South American	5.8	6.0	6.2	6.0	6.3	6.5	6.4

Notes: NA-Not available.

[1]Includes other races not shown separately.

[2]Hispanic persons may be of any race. Includes other types, not shown separately.

[3]Births less than 2,500 grams (5 lb.-8.oz).

Source: U.S. National Center for Health Statistics (2001, p. 63).

Appropriate weight gain for the mother remains controversial. The general recommendation is that women who begin at a normal weight should gain between 25 and 35 pounds over the course of their pregnancy. Women who are overweight should gain 15 to 25 pounds; those who are underweight should gain between 28 and 40 pounds (March of Dimes, 2003). Researchers have been examining the type of weight gained rather than the precise amount; weight from fat and weight from fluid can have a different impact on the health of the baby. Other researchers are looking at the time within the pregnancy when the weight is gained, rather than the actual amount gained.

Weight gains during pregnancy can range from less than 15 pounds to 50 pounds or more and still produce a healthy baby. What is certain is that women should gain weight and should not engage in a weight loss diet during a pregnancy. Figure 13.3 shows the breakdown of weight for a 30-pound weight gain. Actual weight gain will be reflected in the weight of the baby and the other variables cited.

Exercise   Exercise during pregnancy is important, although that area has been controversial as well. Exercise has been associated with fewer cesarean births. A woman's exercise routine should be consistent with her prepregnancy exercise levels, and she should not begin a vigorous program to get in shape once she is pregnant. The American College of Obstetrics and Gynecology recommends that pregnant women not exercise strenuously for more than 15 minutes at a time. The body temperature should not rise above 100 degrees Fahrenheit, and the heart rate should not rise above 140 beats per minute.

That too much exercise may cause miscarriage or harm the fetus is a myth (Sizer & Whitney, 1997). Moderate exercise during pregnancy has the benefits of improving muscle tone and alleviating pregnancy-related discomforts such as backache, bloating, constipation, and swollen hands and feet. Whether pregnant or not, exercise relieves stress, gives the woman a sense of control of her body, and promotes relaxation (Planned Parenthood, 1997).

Drug Use During Pregnancy

Because so many substances can cross the placenta, pregnant women are advised not to take any drug without first consulting a physician. Table 13.2 highlights safety concerns related to various drugs as categorized by the Food and Drug Administration. In practical terms, however, that may not be possible, particularly given inadequate health care services for many women. Public health messages have been created to make women aware of the dangers of consuming alcohol and smoking during pregnancy. Increasing awareness is the first strategy. Actually getting women to stop drinking and smoking is more difficult.

Smoking cigarettes and inhaling secondhand smoke both affect the health of the fetus negatively. Cigarette smoke reduces the amount of oxygen in the bloodstream, adversely affecting fetal growth. Babies born to smokers tend to have a lower birth weight and more breathing problems. Exposure to cigarette smoke also has been associated with spontaneous abortion/miscarriages (Ostrea, Knapp, Romero, Montes, & Ostrea, 1994).

Baby	**7.5**	pounds
Placenta	**1.5**	pounds
Amniotic fluid	**2**	pounds
Uterine enlargement	**2**	pounds
Maternal breast tissue	**2**	pounds
Maternal blood volume	**4**	pounds
Fluids in maternal tissue	**4**	pounds
Maternal fat	**7**	pounds
Average total:	**30**	pounds

Note: Based on a 30-pound weight gain

Figure 13.3 *Breakdown of Weight Gain During Pregnancy*

Source: *What to Expect When You're Expecting,* Murkoff, H., Eisenberg, A., and Hathaway, S. (New York: Workman Publishing, 2002).

healthy sex hints 13.3

For Pregnant Women

To reduce complications during pregnancy, at delivery, and after delivery:

1. Begin prenatal care as soon as you know you are pregnant. If you cannot afford prenatal care from a private physician, it is available through your local public health department. Prenatal care is important for
   a. consistent monitoring of the status of the mother and fetus;
   b. consistent monitoring of the mother's weight gain;
   c. consistent monitoring of the mother's nutritional needs.

2. Do not use any psychoactive substances, including tobacco and alcohol, during pregnancy. Drug use may cause problems in the pregnancy and damage the unborn baby.
3. Do not become pregnant without being certain that you have been immunized against German measles.
4. Schedule any of the fetal tests suggested by your health provider.

Table 13.2 Safety of Selected Drugs During Pregnancy

Food and Drug Administration Ratings	Safety Concerns
Category A Folic Acid Vitamin B_6 Thyroid Medication	These drugs have been tested and found to be safe during pregnancy.
Category B Antibiotics Acetaminophen (Tylenol) Aspartame (sweetener) Benadryl (antihistamine) Famotidine (Pepcid) Prednisone Insulin (for diabetes) Ibuprofen (Advil, Motrin)	Drugs that have been used a lot during pregnancy and have not been found to cause major birth defects or problems. Ibuprofen should not be taken during the last 3 months of the pregnancy.
Category C Celecoxib (Celebrex) Prochlorperzaine (Compazine) Sudafed Fluticasone (Flonase) Fluconazole (Diflucan) Ciprofloxacin (Cipro) Some antidepressants Methylphenidate (Ritalin) Aspirin	Drugs that are more likely to cause problems for the mother or fetus, and some which do not have safety studies. The drugs often are packaged with a warning to consult the physician, with usage related to benefits outweighing risks.
Category D Lithium (for manic depression) Phenytoin (Dilantin) Chemotherapy drugs (for cancer) Alcohol	These drugs have clear risks to the development of the fetus.
Category X Accutane (for acne) Tegison, Soriatane (for psoriasis) Thalidomide	These drugs cause birth defects and should never be taken by pregnant women.
Herbal remedies Echinacea Gingko biloba St. John's wort	Few studies have been made to determine the safety and effectiveness of herbal remedies. Women should consult with their physicians.

Sources: Office on Women's Health (2002); Sullivan (2001).

According to the Centers for Disease Control and Prevention, more than 8,000 babies are born every year with evidence of damage from alcohol. Because it is not known whether there is a "safe" level of drinking, pregnant women are encouraged to abstain totally. The blood alcohol concentration (BAC) of the mother is the same as that of the fetus, so the impact to the fetus is greater. Some evidence indicates that binge drinking is the critical behavior to avoid, as it raises the BAC to dangerous levels. An occasional glass of wine or a beer will not have the same impact. Yet, the risk may not be worth taking.

As of a report in 2002, there were 34 states with policies related to substance abuse by pregnant women. Some states terminate parental rights, some require health care providers to report the drug use, and some, albeit a very few, give the pregnant woman priority access to treatment (Bowen, 2002).

Fetal alcohol syndrome (FAS) is a cluster of effects found in babies as a result of their mother's drinking. Children born with FAS have a small head, abnormal facial features, sleep disorders, short stature, a wide space between the eyes and between the nose and upper lip, hyperactivity, and mental retardation.

Women who abuse cocaine, heroin, and other opiates risk having babies addicted to the abused substance. What is less well known is that many other drugs can have damaging effects.

Fetal alcohol syndrome Effects on embryo and fetus of pregnant woman's alcohol consumption; symptoms include facial abnormalities, mental retardation, and nervous system damage

Environmental/Occupational Wellness

When women become pregnant, they need to determine whether their work surroundings are free of toxins and other pollutants that may affect the fetus. For example, exposure to radiation can damage the fetus. Some women who were smokers stop during their pregnancies but unfortunately return to smoking once the baby is born. Not only are they then harming themselves, but the quality of the air is unhealthy for the baby.

Ideally, new parents should be given support by their employers. Some companies are considered "family-friendly" and provide leave to new parents, birth parents, and adoptive parents. On-site day care is available at some private and public institutions. Flexible work schedules are recognized as valuable to the ever-increasing number of working parents. Overall, however, the United States is not in the forefront of providing quality day care and family support compared to other industrialized nations.

Prenatal Screening

Various screening procedures are available to help determine the health of the fetus. Certain diseases are hereditary—thalassemia and cystic fibrosis, among many others—and some prospective parents want to know whether they are carriers of a disease and their specific risks for having a baby with the disease.

For example, Jews of Eastern European descent are at risk for passing on the gene for Tay Sach's disease, an incurable neurological disorder that results in the degeneration of what appears to be a healthy baby and death by age 5. Knowledge that the parents are carriers may influence their decision to reproduce or terminate a pregnancy that bears the fatal illness.

Common screenings during pregnancy include the following:

1. *Chorionic villus sampling (CVS).* CVS is conducted between the 9th and 11th week of gestation. Cells from the chorionic membrane are removed, usually through the cervix, to screen for genetic abnormalities. Because of the early timing of the test, structural deformities—to legs, arms, and so on—cannot be detected. (An ultrasound can be conducted during the second trimester to identify structural anomalies.)

2. *Ultrasound.* Ultrasound uses high-frequency soundwaves to create a **sonogram,** a picture of the fetus. With advances in technology, more obstetricians are keeping the necessary equipment in their offices and doing this test themselves. The sonogram outlines all structures in the fetus, showing the heart, kidneys, and liver as well as the full skeleton. At 18 to 20 weeks of pregnancy, the ultrasound can detect structural abnormalities in the skull, brain, spine, heart and other

Sonogram The picture of the fetus produced by an ultrasound screening

Amniocentesis Removal of
the amniotic fluid

organs as well as cleft lip, incomplete development of the diaphragm, and so forth (Marks & Miller, 2002). For the couple receiving such feedback, there is emotional upset and difficult questions to be answered. Sometimes surgical corrections can be made during pregnancy or shortly thereafter. Other couples choose to terminate the pregnancy, which would be a second-trimester procedure.

3. *Amniocentesis.* **Amniocentesis** involves removing some of the amniotic fluid and culturing the fetal cells that have sloughed off and are in the fluid. A complete genetic analysis then can be performed, identifying a number of potential diseases and conditions. The genetic analysis also yields the sex of the offspring, but couples are not given that information unless they want it. The test usually is conducted between the 14th and 18th week of gestation. Because an ultrasound is conducted prior to doing an amniocentesis, couples learn of the structural health of the fetus as well.

   Amniocentesis is recommended particularly for women who become pregnant after age 35, because the rate of birth defects related to chromosomal abnormalities rises as women get older. Particular attention has been given to babies born with Down syndrome. At age 20, the risk of Down syndrome is 1 in 1,667; at age 30, it is 1 in 952; and at age 35, it is 1 in 378. Rates associated with other chromosomal abnormalities also increase with maternal age.

4. *Alpha-fetoprotein (AFP) screening.* The AFP test involves taking a blood sample from the pregnant woman between the 15th and 18th week of pregnancy. The fetal liver produces alpha-fetoprotein, and high levels in the mother's blood indicate neural tube defects. These defects include anencephaly, in which the upper portion of the brain and head is missing or underdeveloped, and spina bifida, in which the spinal cord is pushing through the spine. Most babies with anencephaly are stillborn or die shortly after birth, whereas babies with spina bifida, depending on the extent of the disability, can live fairly functional lives.

5. *Blood work.* The woman's blood may be tested at varying points throughout pregnancy. Blood testing has been encouraged especially to detect HIV-positive mothers. The rates of transmission of the virus from mother to fetus are variable. Not all children born to HIV-positive women become HIV-positive themselves. Treating women with the antiviral drug AZT has been shown to reduce the infant's chances of becoming HIV-positive (Dole, 1995).

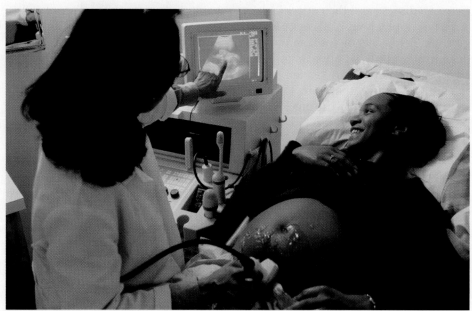

Ultrasound testing can determine position of the baby, abnormalities, and often the sex.

Keith Brofsky/GettyImages

6. *Other tests.* Women with good prenatal care visit their obstetrician or nurse midwife monthly to ensure that the pregnancy is progressing normally and that no health problems are developing. A urine test is conducted at each visit. The presence of sugar in the urine may indicate gestational diabetes. A glucose tolerance test is needed for confirmation.

At each visit, the uterus is measured to ensure that the organ is expanding according to average measurements. The obstetrician or nurse midwife estimates growth of the fetus partly by measuring expansion of the uterus. Also, the woman's blood pressure is taken to watch for signs of hypertension. Each visit includes a weight measurement.

Some individuals and groups are opposed to prenatal screenings on religious and personal grounds. The implication is that results of a screening have to lead to action. Sometimes action is medical intervention during the pregnancy. Sometimes action means ending the pregnancy. Ethical, physical, financial, social, and emotional aspects have to be considered. At what point should decisions be made, and by whom?

Pregnancy, Disability, and Disease

For women with a variety of health conditions, becoming pregnant and getting through the pregnancy itself can pose additional challenges. Greater infertility has been found among women whose own mothers took the drug diethylstilbestrol (DES) during their pregnancies. When able to conceive, DES daughters have an estimated 30 percent risk of miscarriage in the first trimester and are three to four times more likely than women never exposed to DES to losing their pregnancies in the second trimester, having a preterm birth, or having an ectopic pregnancy (Hollander, 2001).

Women, more than men, are susceptible to rheumatoid arthritis, an autoimmune disease that causes terrible joint pain with long-term disabling effects. Ironically, the disease can improve while pregnant, yet women often relapse after pregnancy (Dorssaers-Bakkers, Zwinderman, Van Zeben, Breedveld, & Hazes, 2002). Similar patterns of feeling better while pregnant yet relapsing postpartum are also found in women with multiple sclerosis ("Multiple Sclerosis in Pregnancy," 1998).

Men and women who are spinal cord injured (SCI) are capable of having children, with the location of the cord injury determining special needs. Men with SCI often experience difficulty with erectile and ejaculatory functioning, and the quality of their semen may reduce chances of impregnating a partner through sexual intercourse. With the use of electrical stimulation, however, semen can be obtained and then assisted reproductive techniques employed to inseminate the female (Brackett, Nash, & Lynnes, 1996).

For women, critical concerns focus on weight gain, issues related to bladder and bowel management, and their ability to recognize symptoms of labor (Estill, 2002). In addition, women with SCI may have an increased incidence of early labor or babies with low birth weight (Brackett et al., 1996).

Childbirth

Childbirth encompasses labor and delivery. Although the baby is born from the mother's body, the experience is increasingly viewed as one to be shared by the couple. Stories of experiences with childbirth vary from couple to couple, woman to woman, and birth to birth, even for the same woman.

For much of history, women helped women birth their babies. With the advent of "modern medicine," obstetricians began to deliver babies. Mothers left their

Childbirth Labor and delivery

other children at home, went to a hospital, and gave birth, while the fathers waited in the expectant fathers' waiting room. By the end of the 20th century, birthing became an extended family event with much greater support and participation from partners, family, and friends.

Depending to some extent on geography and the availability of health care providers, couples do have choices as to where and how their baby is born. Most babies in the United States are born in hospitals. Establishing a relationship with a private gynecologist/obstetrician, hospital clinic, or birthing center will determine where the baby is born. Although facilities share some fundamental aspects of delivery, they can have philosophical differences in practice and procedures. Being informed about the staff, facilities, and philosophy will enhance the birth experience. The type of health insurance, if any, that the couple has may be the driving force in making a choice.

The Childbirth Process

Childbirth is a three-phase process, shown in Figure 13.4, occurring over a 12- to 14-hour period on average. Some women have a rapid labor, delivering even before they can make it to the hospital. Others report long labors of 30 or more hours. Partly because of an appreciation of these women's exhaustion and partly because of the fear of malpractice, women today seldom are left to labor beyond 24 hours.

The first stage of labor is the longest; it also tends to be longer for a first delivery than subsequent births. A number of signs indicate that labor is beginning:

- The uterus begins to contract. As labor progresses, these contractions become more regular, closer together in time, and more intense.
- The thick mucous plug that has been covering the cervix, protecting the pregnancy, is dislodged. Because this mucus can be stained with blood, it sometimes is referred to as a "bloody show."
- Rupture of the amniotic membranes releases much of the amniotic fluid in the uterus that has protected the baby, and it trickles or gushes from the vagina. Not all women experience loss of amniotic fluid early in labor; it may happen later in the process. Other women may think their membranes have ruptured but actually may be experiencing urinary incontinence from all the pressure. Because the risk of infection increases after the rupture of membranes, women who think their "water has burst" should get in touch with their health care provider.

First Stage The first stage of labor is marked by dilation of the cervix to 10 centimeters (4 inches)—the diameter needed for safe passage of the baby's head. **Effacement,** the thinning of the cervix, also takes place during this phase. The end of the first stage of labor, called *transition*, is marked by the most intense contractions, and some women experience chills, vomiting, and irritability. Women sometimes request medication during the first stage of labor.

Effacement Thinning of the cervix during first stage of labor

Second Stage The second stage of labor involves the actual birth. This is a short stage for some women—one to three pushes and the baby is out. Other women push for 1 or 2 hours and end up not only with a baby but also hemorrhoids, which aggravate the postpartum experience. Traditionally, women are given an **episiotomy** to make more room for the birth. Nurse midwives have lower rates of episiotomies than physicians do, as the former use massage prior to and during labor to stretch the perineal tissues (Locke, 1996).

Episiotomy The surgical cutting of the perineum to facilitate childbirth

Afterbirth The placenta, umbilical cord, which has been cut at the baby's abdomen but attached to the placenta, and membranes expelled after the birth of a child

Third Stage The third stage of labor consists of delivery of the **afterbirth.** This includes the placenta, which had been attached to the uterine wall, and the umbilical cord, which has been cut at the baby's abdomen but remains attached to

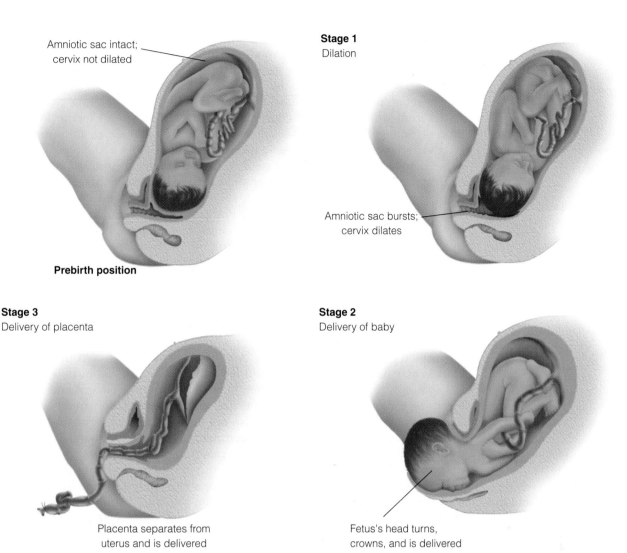

Amniotic sac intact;
cervix not dilated

Stage 1
Dilation

Prebirth position

Amniotic sac bursts;
cervix dilates

Stage 3
Delivery of placenta

Stage 2
Delivery of baby

Placenta separates from
uterus and is delivered

Fetus's head turns,
crowns, and is delivered

Figure 13.4 *Stages of Childbirth*

the placenta at the other end. Delivery of the afterbirth takes approximately 15 minutes. During the third stage, women may experience the rush of emotions associated with the birth itself and holding their newborn.

Delivery Options

Nowadays, delivery options include not only the traditional method but also birthing centers, home births, and cesarean deliveries.

Traditional Delivery   What has come to be viewed as traditional today is different from the traditional delivery of years ago. Both mother and father are often present at the delivery, which takes place in a hospital. Some fathers videotape and photograph their child's first minutes. Prior to that, couples attend prepared childbirth classes that teach about pregnancy and childbirth. Learning Lamaze techniques helps a woman reduce the fear and pain often associated with labor. Key strategies involve controlled deep breathing, light massage of the abdomen, and concentration on a focal point.

   Some women come to their deliveries with a "coach," who may not necessarily be the father of the child. For lesbian couples, the partner helps with the birth.

Some women want their own mothers or sisters to be present. Whatever the circumstance, most hospitals have modified their obstetrical practices to allow for one or more family members or designated friends to participate in the birth.

Hospitals have revamped the labor room/delivery room/recovery room/patient room/nursery arrangement in a variety of ways. Some of the changes resulted from women's voiced concerns for less of a "hospital" feel to the birth process. Some of the changes resulted from research that showed an improved labor experience as a result of being prepared, being flexible, and having support. Other changes undoubtedly have resulted from economic considerations.

Hospital births afford both mother and baby the availability of technology and monitoring. Some facilities also are known for their neonatal intensive care units, which become particularly important if the baby is at high risk—premature, physical deformities, infant in other than head-first position, blood incompatibility between mother and fetus, **toxemia,** multiple births, and so on.

Toxemia A highly dangerous condition during pregnancy when high blood pressure occurs

Hospitals are set up to give women a lot of attention, with specialized nurses to care for the mother and the baby. During labor, women can be monitored with fetal heart monitors to detect fetal distress. Although this attention is comforting to some patients and is required by some physicians, it does limit the woman's movement during labor, requiring her to stay in bed. By contrast, walking around may reduce the length of labor.

Hospital births give women more options for managing pain. Although individuals may have decided beforehand what their philosophy of birth is, the true test comes during labor. Some women manage their pain well and find that the breathing techniques they learned in their childbirth classes prepared them well. Relaxation techniques and hypnosis also can be helpful in managing the discomfort associated with labor. Other women request a shot of demoral, a narcotic, that quickly reduces the pain but also can cross the placenta.

Epidural anesthetic An injection of a drug into the spinal cord during labor to dull pain

Increasingly popular in hospitals is the use of an **epidural anesthetic** during labor. The epidural can be administered once a woman has dilated to 5 centimeters. This numbs her abdominal area, removing pain and discomfort while allowing labor to progress. Women who have an epidural must remain in bed. Its advantage is that the dosage of the drug is monitored in such a way so that the woman regains the capacity to push the baby out at the time of delivery.

Even though hospitals maintain nurseries, the baby spends most of the time in the room with the mother. Hospitals have greatly eased visitation restrictions. Fathers have few limitations on the amount of time they can spend in the room, and some choose to sleep at the hospital. Siblings, too, can visit their newborn brother or sister. Gone are the days when the family looked at the new addition briefly behind glass windows.

Birthing Centers   Birthing centers gained in popularity with the growth of the women's movement in the 1970s. Women were taking an increased role in the birth of their own babies and asking for changes to traditional delivery. Birthing centers were operated by nurse midwives who worked under the supervision of obstetricians, in close physical proximity to hospitals.

The unique feature of birthing centers is the belief that the woman, with the support of her partner, should have as much control over the birthing process as possible. They were the first places where the space for deliveries was "homey," utilizing birthing beds, wallpapered rooms, and rocking chairs. They also cut back on the use of fetal heart monitors so the woman could move around more easily during the first stage of labor. Women could take showers, eat lightly, and have family, including their other children, with them.

Women who deliver at birthing centers usually are screened to rule out high-risk cases. Multiple births, health conditions that warrant close medical monitoring—for example, diabetes and heart conditions—and being over 40 years of age are situations in which a hospital birth is encouraged or required.

As hospitals have increasingly embraced some of the offerings of birthing centers—leaving women to labor and deliver in one room, making those rooms more attractive and less stereotypically hospital-like, having nurse midwives on staff—free-standing birthing centers away from hospitals may be a less attractive option now. New Jersey, for example, has one free-standing birthing center and recently closed the birthing center that was housed within a hospital. One explanation for the closing was women's increasing desire to have epidural anesthesia rather than experience the first stage of labor more drug-free.

Home Births   Delivering babies at home may be a personal choice or may result from rapid labor. Lay midwives have delivered many babies at home. In the South, prior to changes resulting from the civil rights movement of the 1960s, segregation in medical care and minimal hospital facilities resulted in many black women delivering their babies at home. Today, the attitude toward home birth is that it puts the life and welfare of both the baby and mother at risk. Because of the risk of charges of medical malpractice, obstetricians do not conduct home births, and only a select number of licensed nurse midwives will do so. In contrast, approximately 80 percent of the world's babies are born at home, particularly in nonindustrialized countries.

Cesarean Deliveries   **Cesarean delivery,** or **c-section,** is a surgical procedure done for a variety of reasons related to the health and survival of either the mother or the baby, or both. The 20 percent rate of cesarean births in the United States is high by contrast to that of other industrialized nations. Some argue that our improved methods of screening and prenatal care identify more problems that require surgical intervention. Others cynically claim that expectations of giving birth to the perfect child and the rise in medical malpractice lawsuits have changed the culture of childbirth to a point at which physicians do not want to take the risk of waiting for the outcome of a vaginal birth.

C-sections are generally done when the baby is in a **breech position**—feet or buttocks presenting first. Other indications for cesarean delivery are incompatibility between the baby's head size and size of the mother's pelvis, signs of fetal distress picked up by fetal heart monitors, weak contractions of the uterus and prolonged labor, or problems with the placenta and identified bleeding. If the surgery is performed under emergency conditions, such as a detached placenta, general anesthesia is administered. In other situations, where time allows, anesthesia can be given with an epidural, which allows the mother to remain awake and, in many hospitals, her partner to be present.

Cesarean delivery (c-section) The surgical form of childbirth in which an incision is made through the abdomen and uterus to deliver the baby

Breech position A birth position in which the buttocks or foot rather than the baby's head presents at the cervix

Postpartum

The *postpartum* period represents the time after the birth, with all its various dimensions of change. First-time mothers and fathers are "new" to parenthood and sometimes overly anxious. Parents having a second, third, or fourth child, by contrast, will find themselves focused on the needs of the baby along with those of their other children. If the baby has health problems and has to stay in the hospital longer than the mother, the emotional feelings at the time are intensified.

Women, whether breastfeeding or bottle feeding, will experience marked changes in their hormone levels, which in turn affect emotions. Levels of estrogen and progesterone drop rapidly within 24 hours and then continue dropping until the body reaches its prepregnancy levels. It is normal to experience unexplained sadness, often termed "baby blues," after birth. For some, the blues last a few hours; for others, they can last for 1 to 2 weeks. Postpartum depression (PPD) can start after the birth and affects approximately 10 to 15 percent of mothers (Wood, Thomas, Droppleman, & Meighan, 1997). Women may have feelings of anxiety, irritability, and sadness. Some may not have any interest in their babies, whereas others become overly worried. Some may not be able to eat, while others overeat.

Although a range of symptoms may occur, prolonged depression warrants therapeutic intervention (Schmidt, 2002).

One of the major adjustments postpartum is the effect of lack of sleep on the body. Some newborns wake to eat every 2 to 3 hours, and for those women who breastfeed, the burden of being available and awake cannot be equally divided. Anthony, in Case Study 13.2, later shared that for the 1st year with his triplets, there was never 1 hour when all three were asleep at the same time! Prolonged sleep deprivation affects mood, energy, interest in socializing, and ability to concentrate.

Adjustment in this period also includes a reassessing of roles—parent, partner, individual. Who comes first? Fatigue for the parents, with the simultaneous constancy of attending to a baby, may interfere with any desire to resume lovemaking. After birth, the uterus produces a bloody discharge called **lochia,** which can be on again/off again for weeks. Incisions from either an episiotomy or cesarean section also need to heal. As a result, physicians will often advise women to wait approximately 6 weeks before resuming sexual intercourse. Overall, any sexual activity can be reintroduced into a couple's lifestyle once the woman feels comfortable.

Lochia The uterine discharge that is released over a period of weeks after childbirth

Breastfeeding

Women today are strongly being encouraged to breastfeed their babies, even for a short period of time. Depending on the length of a woman's maternity leave if working outside the home, the prospect of successfully breastfeeding once back to work can seem daunting. A private space and on-site refrigeration can help those women who want to express breast milk for bottles and then breastfeed directly when home.

Breastfeeding brings numerous health benefits. Breast milk supplies the newborn with the mother's immunity; encourages better mouth and tooth development in the baby; is more affordable and convenient; and is thought to give the baby better control of its intake, thereby reducing later obesity (Carlson et al., 1996). Not all women can or want to breastfeed, and they need to know that improved formulas do provide the essential nutrients needed by the newborn. Women who are HIV-positive, have an active case of tuberculosis, or are on any medication that may be passed through breast milk at dangerous levels should not breastfeed (Carlson et al., 1996).

Social and Spiritual Wellness

Once children become a fact of life, notions of family expand and change. Relationships with parents, employers, and friends take on new dimensions and demands. Caring for children is a 24-hour job, not easily filled by one person. Will parenting responsibilities be shared? Who will take care of this child? What networks of support are in place? Will the mother work? Is child care available? Play groups? Recognizing what is required helps promote social health.

Parenthood can convey a sense of purpose and add meaning to life. Parents often discover new meaning in life/death issues as they become responsible for another human being. Parenthood brings with it an ongoing assessment of the relationship to one's child. Is the child like me? Does that matter? Can I love this child? Can I help him/her grow and be free to live his/her own life? What happens when parents die? If children die?

Although answering some of these questions may be uncomfortable and difficult, doing so is essential to plan for responsible parenthood. Parents need to have a will and designate guardians. Some children know of adults who became their godparents, yet those individuals may or may not assume an active role throughout their lives.

Complications During Pregnancy and Childbirth

Pregnancies that are wanted present a positive emotional experience for couples. Some couples are so excited that they notify friends and relatives as soon as their home pregnancy tests register a positive result. Not all pregnancies go to completion, however, and the sadness and sometimes guilt associated with the loss can be great.

Some women painfully decide to terminate a pregnancy due to the results of a prenatal diagnosis. Because those results come in the second trimester of pregnancy, there has been bonding with the pregnancy as well as increasing numbers of people in one's community and workplace knowing about the pregnancy. The long-term emotional responses are similar to those experienced by women who have late miscarriages or experience early death of a newborn (Salversen, Oyen, Schmidt, Malt, & Eik-Nes, 1997). Individuals and couples may have repeated feelings of grief and sadness as they mark the baby's due date, pregnancy confirmation date, or test notification date.

Infertile couples who may have had repeated miscarriages can share similar feelings. One of the author's students commented how difficult holidays had become, with all the presents at family gatherings, yet no children of their own. Repeated miscarriages and a nagging fear that a successful pregnancy will never occur make being around other's children painful.

Increasingly, hospitals have been setting up support groups for women who have had miscarriages, stillbirths, and infant deaths. The Internet has provided women and couples with other ways to secure the emotional support needed.

Fortunately, many complications that arise during a pregnancy can be monitored and safely treated today as long as they are identified and care is available. That said, not everyone has access to the latest, high-quality, technological treatment. Furthermore, there are those who even when advice and treatments are offered, resist any intervention. Finally, the reality of pregnancy and childbirth is that it is a natural event yet very stressful to a woman's body; not all women have healthy pregnancies and not all babies survive.

Your responses to the Personal Assessment, Thought Questions, and Test Yourself! quiz responses can be logged online in your Virtual Workbook at **http://health.wadsworth.com/blonna1.**

Personal Assessment

13.1 Assessing Readiness for Parenting

Using the wellness model, assess your readiness on each dimension. Issues that focus specifically on the pregnancy itself are weighted more toward the female parent. Nonetheless, for both males and females, parenthood touches on all dimensions of health and wellness.

Physical Wellness

Are you physically healthy? Is your weight, blood pressure, and respiration within a normal range?

Do you have any chronic illnesses that may impact your ability to conceive? Maintain a pregnancy? Experience childbirth?

Are you taking any medications that may affect the normal growth and development of the fetus?

Do you regularly use any drugs recreationally? Are you addicted to any substance? Could you stop using caffeine, alcohol, or other recreational drugs?

What are your sleep patterns? How well do you function with interrupted sleep?

Are you physically fit? Do you exercise regularly?

Do you have any physical disabilities that may affect your ability to maintain a pregnancy? Go through childbirth? Take care of a child? If so, do you have the resources to make pregnancy, childbirth, and caregiving manageable?

Intellectual Wellness

Have you thought about the roles and responsibilities of being a parent?

Have you thought about why you want to become a parent? Do they seem sound?

Have you read any educational material on pregnancy, childbirth, and parenting skills?

Have you assessed your financial readiness for parenthood?

Do you have the financial resources to provide for a child—food, clothing, medical expenses?

Emotional Wellness

Are you excited about becoming a parent?

Are you comfortable with the person you are? Do you love yourself? Are you able to offer love to another?

Do you handle frustration well? Anger?

Are you currently struggling with any emotional problems that could interfere with your becoming a parent?

Have you been diagnosed with any problems or mental conditions for which you take medication? If so, would a pregnancy aggravate your condition? Would parenthood affect your condition in any way?

Social Wellness

Is the quality of your relationship with your partner healthy?

Are you considering being a single parent?

What is the quality of your relationship with your family of origin? Will family members be involved as grandparents, aunts, cousins, uncles? Is that important to you?

What is the quality of your relationship with the family of your partner? Will any of them be involved as grandparents, aunts, cousins, uncles? Is that important to you?

Do you have other social support networks? Neighbors? Friends?

Spiritual Wellness

Have you thought about the impact of parenthood on your life?

Do you feel ready to be responsible for another? Nurture and love another? Put someone else's needs above your own?

Do you and your partner share similar beliefs about religion? Would having a child bring to the surface any tensions and differences?

Environmental/Occupational Wellness

Are you currently living in a place where you can stay?

What kind of living space will you provide for a baby? Is it safe, smoke-free?

What kind of a community will you live in? Is the area safe? Can you easily get around (say, with a stroller)?

Do you have access to medical care? For you? For a baby?

Do you have access to a supermarket or other store for items such as baby food and diapers?

Do you have access to transportation?

Are you currently employed? If so, is your workplace "family-friendly"?

Does your employer have child care facilities?

Do you have family health care coverage through your work?

The answers to these questions can give you a sense of whether or not you are ready for parenthood. Keep in mind that no one is totally prepared for parenthood. It has too many unknowns, and the personal experience far exceeds your imagination and descriptions provided in books. Thinking about the issues, preparing for the possibilities, and being ready on many levels is part of good decision making and planning.

Thought Questions

1. When is the "right" time to have a baby? What are some of the considerations that go into this?

2. What happens in the process of fertilization and conception?

3. What major changes in the fetus are associated with each trimester?

4. What are the basic wellness guidelines to ensure a healthy pregnancy?

5. What tests and other technological advances are available to aid with pregnancy, labor, and delivery? How do these contribute to political debate?

6. What are the differences in hospital versus home (or birth center) births?

7. What is the role of the midwife?

8. What is cesarean birth? What is the rate of c-sections in the United States? What factors contribute to the high rate in the United States?

Test Yourself!

1. Which would be the least helpful to a woman trying to determine whether or not she was fertile?
   a. Using a home pregnancy kit
   b. Looking for the presence of cervical mucous
   c. Taking her morning temperature
   d. Keeping track of her menstrual cycle on the calendar

2. Fertilization of the ovum takes place
   a. at the cervix.
   b. in the vagina.
   c. in the fallopian tube.
   d. in the uterus.

3. Home pregnancy tests look for the presence of _____ in a woman's urine.
   a. increased levels of estrogen
   b. human chorionic gonadotropin (hCG)
   c. increased levels of progesterone
   d. increased levels of testosterone

4. A normal period of gestation takes how long?
   a. 28 weeks
   b. 40 weeks
   c. 36 weeks
   d. 45 weeks

5. Good prenatal care requires that a health care provider monitor all but which of the following?
   a. A woman's nutritional intake
   b. Fetal size and growth
   c. A woman's medication use
   d. A woman's sexual interest

6. Guidelines for recreational alcohol use during pregnancy include which of the following?
   a. Women should only drink beer.
   b. No more than three glasses of wine per week.
   c. No safe limits for alcohol consumption have been established.
   d. No alcohol use until the third trimester of pregnancy.

7. Prenatal screening tests, such as amniocentesis, are primarily designed to
   a. determine whether labor will be normal.
   b. determine whether the fetus is developing normally.
   c. determine health risks to the mother because of pregnancy.
   d. determine whether the fetus is male or female.

8. A woman should suspect that labor is beginning if
   a. she experiences nausea.
   b. she feels some intermittent cramping.
   c. she is 40 weeks pregnant.
   d. she passes a bloody, mucous plug.

9. A cesarean delivery may be performed because
   a. the baby is in a breech position.
   b. the mother is overweight.
   c. the parents have requested it.
   d. the first stage of labor is too short.

10. A baby is born during the _____ stage of labor.
    a. first
    b. second
    c. third
    d. fourth

Media Menu

You can link to the following online tools by visiting
http://health.wadsworth.com/blonna1.

Film

Deciding Whether or Not to Have Children

Animation

In Utero Phases of Development
Formation of Early Embryo
Emergence of Human Features

 InfoTrac Activity

Egg donation on the rise as alternative for women in their 40s and 50s. (2002, April 18). *Women's Health Weekly*, 13.

 Web Resources

International Council on Infertility Information Dissemination (INCIID)

www.inciid.org

A nonprofit organization committed to providing information about diagnosis, treatment, and prevention of infertility and pregnancy loss. The site accesses fact sheets and transcripts of auditoriums with renowned experts, more than 150 referrals and links to nonprofit organizations providing quality, sound infertility information, such as the American Society of Reproductive Medicine and the International Federation of Fertility Societies.

Infertility Resources

www.ihr.com

Offers extensive information about infertility organizations and clinics, IVF, egg donor, financial issues, subject matter experts, sperm banks, Internet newsgroups and mailing lists, research, journals, medications, infertility medical supplies, and adoption. The infertility educational articles offer diagnosis, male factors, treatment, drugs/medication, psychological and social issues, plus financial and legal information.

March of Dimes

www.modimes.org

A nonprofit organization providing information on birth defects, prenatal screening tests, prenatal care guidelines, and other research related to pregnancy.

National SHARE Office

www.nationalshareoffice.com

A national organization with affiliates that provide resources and support for parents who have experienced miscarriage, stillbirth, or death of a baby.

The Fatherhood Project

www.fatherhoodproject.org

An educational resource site distributing information targeted at improving male involvement in child rearing.

Planned Parenthood Federation of America

www.plannedparenthood.org

Provides information and resources related to a full range of reproductive health issues.

References

Alan Guttmacher Institute. (2002, February/March). In their own right is new report addressing the sexual reproductive health needs of American men. *SIECUS Report, 30*(3).

American Academy of Pediatrics. (2002). *Policy on same sex adoption* [Online]. Available: www.aap.org/policy/02008t.htm.

American College of Obstetricians and Gynecologists. (2003, August 29). Dissatisfaction up, residency applications down, in ob-gyn. *ACOG News Release*.

Black, R. (1995, June/July). Conception at any cost? *Child*, 79–81, 83.

Bogren, L. (1991). Changes in sexuality in women and men during pregnancy. *Archives of Sexual Behavior, 20*, 35–46.

Boston Women's Health Book Collective. (1998). *Our bodies, ourselves for the new century.* New York: Simon & Schuster.

Bowen, K. (2002, February/March). Pregnancy and state policies. *SIECUS Report, 30*(3).

Brackett, N., Nash, M., & Lynne, C. (1996, November). Male infertility following spinal cord injury: Facts and fiction. *Physical Therapy, 76*(11), 1221.

Burns, L. H. (1990). An exploratory study of perceptions of parenting after infertility. *Family Systems Medicine, 8*, 177–189.

Carlson, K., Eisenstat, S., & Ziporyn, T. (1996). *The Harvard guide to women's health.* Cambridge, MA: Harvard University Press.

Cassell, C. (2002, February/March). Let it shine: Promoting school success, life aspirations to prevent school-age parenthood. *SIECUS Report, 30*(3).

Centers for Disease Control, National Center for Health Statistics. (1995). *Vital and Health Statistics Series, 23*(19) [Online]. Available: www.cdc.gov/nchs/fastats.

Consumers Union. (2003a, February). The fertility window. *Consumer Reports, 68*, 48–50.

Consumers Union. (2003b, February). When the test really counts. *Consumer Reports, 68*, 45–47.

Dole, V. B. (1995). ACT in pregnant women with HIV: Risks and benefits. *Neonatal Network, 14*(2), 62–63.

Dorssaers-Bakkers, K. W., Zwinderman, A. H., Van Zeben, D., Breedveld, F. C., & Hazes, J. M. W. (2002, May). Pregnancy and oral contraceptive use do not significantly influence outcome in long term rheumatoid arthritis. *Annals of Rheumatic Diseases, 61*(5), 405.

Estill, S. (2002, March). A story of two women: Add pregnancy and parenting to spinal-cord injury and you really have a challenge! *Paraplegia News, 56*(3), 15.

Hewlett, S. A. (2002). *Creating a life: Professional women and the quest for children.* New York: Hyperion.

Hollander, D. (2001, January). Women exposed to DES in utero have elevated risks of fertility impairment and adverse pregnancy outcomes. *Family Planning Perspectives, 33*(1), 43.

Locke, L. (1996). Nurse midwife presentation, St. Joseph's Hospital, Paterson, NJ.

March of Dimes. (2003). Weight gain during pregnancy. *During Your Pregnancy: Weigh to Grow* [Online]. Available: www.marchofdimes.com/pnhec/159_153.asp.

Marks, J., & Miller, M. (2002). Reproductive health technology and genetic counseling. In G. Wingood & R. DiClemente (Eds.), *Handbook of reproductive health.* New York: Kluwer Academic/Plenum.

McCloskey, J., & Bulecheck, G. (1996). *Nursing intervention classification (NIC)* (2nd ed.). St. Louis: Mosby.

Multiple sclerosis in pregnancy. (1998, Winter). *Special Delivery, 21*(4), 10.

Murkoff, H., Eisenberg, A., & Hathaway, S. (2002). *What to expect when you're expecting.* New York: Workman.

Office on Women's Health, Department of Health and Human Services. (2002, November). Pregnancy and medication [Online]. Available: www.4woman.gov/faq/pregmed.htm

Ostrea, E., Knapp, D. Romero, A., Montes, M., & Ostrea, A. (1994). Meconium analysis to assess fetal exposure to nicotine by active and passive maternal smoking. *Journal of Pediatrics, 124*, 471–476.

Patterson, C. (1995). Lesbian and gay parenting. *APA Public Interest Directorate: Research Summary on Lesbian and Gay Parenting,* American Psychological Association [Online]. Available: www.apa.org/pi/parent.html.

Planned Parenthood. (1997). *All about sex: A family resource on sex and sexuality.* New York: Three Rivers Press.

Salversen, K. A., Oyen, L., Schmidt, N. Malt, F., & Eik-Nes, S. (1997). Comparison of long-term psychological responses of women after pregnancy termination due to fetal anomalies and after perinatal loss. *Ultrasound in Obstetrics & Gynecology, 9,* 80–85.

Schmidt, P. (2002, July). Postpartum depression. FAQ from the National Women's Health Information Center [Online]. Available: www.4woman.gov/faq/postpartum.htm.

Sherwood, L. (2004). *Human physiology* (5th ed.). Belmont, CA: Brooks/Cole.

Sizer, F., & Whitney, E. (1997). *Nutrition: Concepts and controversies* (7th ed.). Belmont, CA: West/Wadsworth.

Sullivan, D. L. (2001). The expectant mother's guide to prescription and nonprescription drugs, vitamins, home remedies, and herbal products. New York: St. Martin's Griffin.

U.S. National Center for Health Statistics. (2001). Vital statistics of the United States annual 2001, No. 76. In *Statistical Abstracts of the United States: 2001.* Washington, DC: U.S. Government Printing Office.

Vorzimer, A. W., O'Hara, M. D., & Shafton, L. D. (1998). *Buzzanca v. Buzzanca:* The ruling and ramifications [Online]. Available: www.inciid.org/buzzancaease.

Wood, S., Thomas, D., Droppleman, L., & Meighan, R. (1997) Postpartum depression rates. *Maternal Child Nursing, 22,* 308–316.

Wright, V., Schieve, L., Reynolds, M., & Jeng, G. (2003, August 29). Assisted reproductive technology surveillance—United States, 2000. *Morbidity and Mortality Weekly Report, 52* (SS-9).

chapter *fourteen*

Fertility Control

Student Learning Objectives

After reading this chapter, students will be able to

- Differentiate the following terms: *fertility control, contraception, birth control,* and *family planning.*

- Compare the theoretical effectiveness and the effectiveness of actual use.

- Determine personal level of risk for unintended pregnancy.

- Develop a personal plan for controlling fertility.

- Explain the different mechanisms of fertility control.

- Evaluate a variety of fertility control methods.

- Determine which methods work best for different types of users.

- Describe how fertility control requires change over the life cycle.

- Identify which methods work best in reducing the risks for STD and HIV infection.

- Evaluate the health aspects of various fertility control methods.

*Test your understanding of these objectives by taking the end-of-chapter quiz, available online at **http://health.wadsworth.com/blonna1**.*

activity teaser: *How do you really feel about abortion? Find out in the Personal Exploration Activity on page 458.*

case study 14.1

Joe's Vasectomy

Joe, 34, is white.

The best present I ever gave myself was my vasectomy. I belong to an HMO, and it cost me a dollar to have it done. I'll always feel it was the best dollar I ever spent. I guess I've used almost every method available with my wife and my girlfriends before I got married. All these methods had one problem or another, so I promised myself that after the kids were born, I'd take responsibility and get a vasectomy.

The week after my second son was born, I told my wife I wanted to have it done. She was glad that we could stop using condoms and fertility awareness and supported my decision. The procedure was uneventful. I was in and out in 1 hour. The only glitch was that the anesthesiologist had to give me three shots of painkiller before they could make the incision.

After about 2 weeks, my follow-up tests were negative, and we had sex for the first time without worry of my wife getting pregnant. The first time was in the shower. It was great. I can't remember the last time we made love in the shower. Getting the vasectomy was the biggest boost to our sex life in the past 10 years!

Critical Thinking

Sterilization is often something college students can't envision, yet it remains a very popular form of birth control worldwide. Could you imagine either you or your partner being sterilized after having had the children you wanted?

Use your Virtual Workbook to explore your answer to this question at **http://health.wadsworth.com/blonna1.**

Many people use the terms *birth control, contraception,* and *family planning* interchangeably when referring to controlling fertility. Although the three terms are similar because they refer to strategies for preventing unintended pregnancy, they are vastly different in terms of their nature and scope. Although most people probably agree that avoiding unintended pregnancy is a good idea, how to accomplish this goal generates tremendous disagreement.

Family planning implies the desire to have children at some point in time. Planning a family involves postponing childbearing until it is desired, spacing subsequent births and avoiding pregnancy at other times. As discussed in Chapter 13, family planning may also include all the reproductive technologies available to facilitate a pregnancy as well as adoption. Family planning does not refer to specific methods or techniques to avoid unintended pregnancy.

Contraception refers to all methods designed to prevent conception or fertilization. Contraceptive methods work by preventing the sperm and egg from uniting to cause fertilization. These methods include noninsertive sexual activity, barrier methods, hormonal contraception, withdrawal, fertility awareness, and sterilization. How effective these methods are ranges from "not very" to "almost complete" at the other end of the spectrum.

Birth control is a broad term encompassing all methods designed to prevent pregnancy and birth. It includes all contraceptive methods, what may be considered postconceptive methods, and abortion, which is designed to interrupt an established pregnancy. At its most literal, birth control also includes infanticide, although such a practice is generally viewed with repugnance and considered a crime.

Family planning Postponing children until the optimal point in one's life

Contraception Methods designed to prevent conception

Birth control The broadest term covering all methods designed to prevent the birth of a child

Effectiveness: Theoretical and Actual Use

One of the most important questions regarding any method of fertility control is "How effective is it?" Effectiveness is measured two ways: theoretical use and actual use.

The **theoretical effectiveness** of any fertility control method estimates how it should work if it is used consistently and correctly. It is the ideal effectiveness of the method, determined through laboratory research and experimental studies. Theoretical effectiveness research designs attempt to control for as many variables as possible that may interfere with correct and consistent use. Failure of the method accounts for most of the ineffectiveness. Theoretical effectiveness is the lowest expected percentage of women who will get pregnant while using the method.

The **actual-use effectiveness** of any fertility control method is how it actually works when real people use it under normal circumstances. This is the observed effectiveness of the method, determined by following a group of actual users for 1 year to see how many get pregnant. Actual-use studies are not subject to the same rigorous controls as most theoretical effectiveness studies. Consequently, user failure (failure to use the method consistently and correctly each time a couple has intercourse) largely accounts for the lack of effectiveness. Actual-use effectiveness is a combination of method and user failure, expressed as the percentage of women who get pregnant after 1 year of using the method. Comparison of methods is also done describing *typical-use failure rates* and *perfect-use failure rates*. Current studies base lowest and typical failure rates on the first year of observation. First-year data more accurately represent the risk of getting pregnant for someone using the method for the first time. Here, we will report data from studies that use first-year failure rates.

> **Theoretical effectiveness**
> The lowest expected percentage of women who will get pregnant while using a given contraceptive method
>
> **Actual-use effectiveness**
> The percentage of women who get pregnant while using a contraceptive method for 1 year

Choosing a Method

When contemplating which fertility control method to use, people pose questions ranging from "Is it safe and effective?" "Do I have any health conditions that might make the method particularly risky for me?" to "What is my sexual lifestyle and frequency of activity?" A couple's religious and cultural background may also play a role in decisions about fertility control. No contraceptive method is 100 percent perfect and without risk. Some methods might offer the level of effectiveness you want but lack aesthetic appeal. You may like a method, but your partner hates it. A health care provider might recommend a method that looks ideal on paper, but you might feel squeamish about using it. The self-assessment at the end of the chapter will help you examine your feelings about the various methods.

Given this confusing array of things to consider, what is the best method of fertility control? The best method is the one the person or couple uses consistently and correctly. It is the one that those involved are happy with, that offers the level of protection desired, and that fits the needs of those involved at this point in life. For college students today, choices about fertility control overlap with concerns about STD/HIV risk reduction. Some methods are highly effective in their ability to prevent pregnancy yet offer no protection against infection.

From a public health standpoint, overall costs become a factor in providing services to those least able to pay. Title X of the Public Health Service Act was designed to make comprehensive voluntary family planning services available. Today clinics that are funded through Title X provide services to close to 5 million Americans (Alan Guttmacher Institute, 2003c). As women seek newer, more expensive methods and clinics and programs struggle with smaller budgets, the issue of "choice" and making methods available becomes ever more challenging.

It is important to realize that needs will change over time. Therefore, people would do well to review their fertility control needs periodically and make changes accordingly. Table 14.1 provides a summary of contraceptive methods.

Table 14.1 Comparison of Contraceptives

Method	Typical-Use Effectiveness	Perfect-Use Effectiveness	Protection Against STDs	Accessibility*
Continuous abstinence	0.00	0.00	Complete	Couple communication
Outercourse	N/A	N/A	Good against HIV; reduces risk of others	Couple communication
Sterilization				
Men (vasectomy)	0.15	0.1	None	Requires physician and/or
Women (tubal ligation)	0.5	0.5	None	hospital access
Norplant (not available; being revised to 2 straws)	0.05	0.05	None	Currently being revised to 2 straws; requires physician for insertion
Implanon	0.05	0.05	None	Requires physician for injection
IUD				
ParaGard (Copper T 380A)	0.8	0.6	None	Requires physician for
Mirena (Copper T)	0.1	0.1	None	insertion
Lunelle (injection); taken off the market	N/A	0.05	None	Requires physician for injection
Continuous breastfeeding	2.0	0.5	None	Only useful at early stages of infant feeding
Depo-Provera (injection)	3.0	0.3	None	Requires physician for injection
Combination pills	.5	.1	None	Requires physician for prescription
Progestin-only pill	8.0	0.3	None	Requires physician for prescription
NuvaRing (ring)	N/A	0.3	None	Requires physician for prescription
Ortho Evra Patch	N/A	0.3	None	Requires physician for prescription
Male condom	15.0	2.0	Good against HIV; reduces risk of other STDs	Over-the-counter
Female condom— Reality	21.0	5.0	Reduces risk of vaginal and cervical infection	Over-the-counter
Diaphragm	16.0	6.0	Limited	Requires physician for fitting. Spermicide is purchased independently.
Sponge	14–16	10–11	None	Over-the-counter

Table 14.1 *(continued)*

Method	Typical-Use Effectiveness	Perfect-Use Effectiveness	Protection Against STDs	Accessibility*
Fertility awareness/Periodic abstinence	25.0		None	Requires woman to fully chart menstrual cycle, be aware of probable timing of ovulation, and then abstain from coitus.
Postovulation method		1.0		
Symptothermal method		2.0		
Cervical mucus (ovulation method)		3.0		
Calendar method		9.0		
Withdrawal	27.0	4.0	None	Requires the male to control timing of ejaculation
Spermicide	29.0	15.0	None	Over-the-counter
No method	85.0	85.0	None	
Emergency contraception— Preven and Plan B	Reduces risk of pregnancy by 75–89 percent		None	Requires a prescription; may become over-the-counter

*Reproductive health care services can be provided by private physicians, clinics, nurse practitioners, nurse midwives, and physician's assistants. Costs for methods vary depending on whether the individual has medical insurance, has prescription drug coverage, or must pay out of pocket. For methods bought over the counter, there is some variability in pricing, and overall costs relate to the frequency of using the method.

Sources: Based on information from www.plannedparenthood.org (2003); Nelson, Hatcher, Zieman, Watt, Darney, and Creinin (2003); S. Bernard, personal communication (November 29, 2003).

Physical and Intellectual Wellness

Making good decisions about controlling fertility is a multifaceted process. It is essential that you learn how you and your partner's bodies function. So much information is now accessible on the Internet, making learning about anatomy, physiology, and the biochemistry of the human body and health less of a mystery. Learning about birth control at the time of Margaret Sanger's pioneering efforts in the early 1900s was viewed as obscene, landing her in jail. Today a variety of sources of information are available to help you decide what is available and appropriate.

Fertility control, first, is affected by one's level of physical well-being. Overall physical health influences the fertility methods available to you. For example, physical conditions such as hypertension and diabetes are contraindications for oral contraceptives. Having a history of pelvic inflammatory disease precludes using an IUD. Health status also affects how you use certain methods. For instance, gaining weight necessitates refitting of a diaphragm.

Consistent and proper use of fertility control methods can enhance physical well-being. Practicing fertility control carries less risk to a woman than getting pregnant and having a child. The risk of dying associated with pregnancy and childbirth is much greater than that for using fertility control.

Certain methods impart specific health-enhancing benefits. Hormonal contraception offers protective effects against a variety of diseases including ovarian cancer, along with possible improvement for acne and menstrual cramps. Barrier contraceptives reduce the risk of cervical cancer, as well as some STDs. Fertility awareness can give women a greater understanding of vaginal health and how their bodies work.

Mechanisms of Action

Although birth control methods can be grouped in a variety of ways, we've chosen the following seven categories according to their mechanisms of action.

1. *Provide nonpenetrative sexual pleasure.* This group of methods, sometimes called *outercourse*, provides options for the satisfaction of sexual desire and orgasm that do not involve the penis penetrating the vagina. Methods in this category include kissing, hugging/rubbing, massage, masturbation, use of sex toys, and oral-genital sexual contact.
2. *Prevent sperm from meeting egg.* These methods work either by withdrawing the penis prior to ejaculation or by predicting ovulation and avoiding unprotected intercourse during fertile times.
3. *Provide barrier between sperm and egg.* This group of methods is characterized by putting a mechanical or chemical device between the sperm and the egg (hence the term *barrier*). In either case, these methods prevent the sperm and egg from uniting in the fertilization process. Methods in this group include male condom, female condom, diaphragm, contraceptive sponge, cervical cap, and spermicides.
4. *Prevent release of egg.* Ovulation is suppressed by altering the hormonal balance in the body. This prevents the pituitary gland from stimulating the release of hormones necessary to trigger the release of an egg from the ovary. Methods in this group include oral contraceptives, NuvaRing, and the Evra patch.
5. *Surgically block passage of sperm or egg.* Methods in this category work by sealing off the main egg and sperm transport routes (fallopian tubes and vas deferens, respectively). Female and male sterilization comprise this group.
6. *Prevent implantation.* Methods in this group work by preventing the implantation of a possibly fertilized egg in the uterine lining. These methods encompass the variety of intrauterine devices (IUDs) and emergency contraception. As discussed later, however, evidence seems to suggest that the IUD may prevent sperm from fertilizing the egg.
7. *Terminate an established pregnancy.* This group consists of methods that end an established pregnancy. Methods include abortion, both medical and surgical.

Nonpenetrative Sexual Release

Nonpenetrative activities are sometimes referred to as **outercourse** and include massage, masturbation, manual stimulation of one's partner, and the like. These activities provide sexual release but do not involve vaginal penetration (McDonough, 1995). It is important to understand that there are lots of ways to be sexual without risking pregnancy.

The actual-use effectiveness of sexual activities that do not involve vaginal penetration has not been established. Their effectiveness lies in their theoretical attributes. If vaginal penetration doesn't occur, no mechanism is available for live sperm to reach a mature ovum. Theoretical effectiveness, therefore, should approach 100 percent.

Unprotected anal intercourse is not included in this group because, although it doesn't involve vaginal penetration, the close proximity of the anus could allow migration of fluids across the perineum and into the vagina. Ejaculating near the vagina is discouraged for this reason.

Celibacy/Abstinence   The first category of nonpenetrative methods is celibacy and abstinence. These two terms are often used interchangeably, yet their meanings are distinct. Although the definition of *celibacy* means to avoid sexual relations, the term is often most associated with a religious decision not to marry. Ab-

Outercourse
Nonpenetrative sexual activities such as massage and masturbation

stinence refers to practicing self-restraint and, in the area of fertility control, not having sexual intercourse. People often assume that celibacy and abstinence mean total avoidance of all forms of sexual release. This is not true. A person can be celibate or abstain from sexual intercourse but still masturbate or use other forms of nonpenetrative behaviors to release sexual tension (Norris, 1996).

Haignere (2002) and others (Pinkerton, 2001; Haignere, Gold, & McDanel, 1999) have addressed the issue of failure rates of abstinence, partially in an attempt to counter the rhetoric that only abstinence is 100 percent effective. As with any method, theoretical effectiveness rates differ from actual-use effectiveness rates. User failure rates are connected to how correctly and consistently the method is used. If an individual practices abstinence at a particular point in time, that person will never become pregnant or get a partner pregnant. When abstinence as a method fails, it is because of user failure (Pinkerton, 2001). Haignere et al. (1999) suggest that abstinence failure be thought of as a failure to remain abstinent. For example, in 1999 as part of the Youth Risk Behavior Survey, adolescents in Philadelphia were asked, "Did you ever promise yourself not to have sexual intercourse before marriage?" Overall, 40 percent responded yes, yet of those 45 percent failed to keep the promise and had intercourse. The question then becomes whether their responses represent a 45 percent abstinence user-failure rate (Haignere, 2002).

Outercourse Activities   Couples may choose to touch each other in a variety of ways that do not risk pregnancy. For example, the sucking, licking and rubbing, and tongue probing associated with kissing are pleasurable while imposing no risk for pregnancy. Kissing usually is associated with hugging and rubbing. Once commonly referred to as petting, these activities can take on new meaning when visualized as a viable form of fertility control. Hugging and rubbing, even with the clothes on, can be intensely pleasurable and can be carried to the point of orgasm with no risk of pregnancy. With a little imagination, these safe sex activities can be erotic and provide a satisfying outlet for sexual desire by themselves or when other fertility control methods are unavailable.

Somewhat riskier are activities in which partners are partially clothed or naked. The risk is that further activity not be contemplated and chosen. Nongenital massage is a great sensual delight and can be a stand-alone sensual activity or part of activities culminating with orgasm. Partners can manually stimulate each other to orgasm without worrying about conception. Sex toys also offer a safe, low-pregnancy-risk sexual option (Davis, Blank, Lin, & Bonillas, 1996).

The various forms of oral-genital sexual contact (fellatio, cunnilingus, anilingus) offer a sexual option with low risk for pregnancy. Unlike abstinence and nonpenetrative sexual behavior, however, oral-genital sexual contact can pose risks of disease transmission. We will discuss these risks in detail in Chapter 15.

Preventing Sperm from Reaching Egg (Nonsurgical)

Sperm can be prevented from reaching the ova through coitus interruptus and fertility awareness methods.

Coitus Interruptus (Withdrawal; Pulling Out)   Coitus interruptus is one of the most commonly used and least understood of all the fertility control strategies. *Coitus interruptus* is a Latin term, literally meaning interrupting intercourse by withdrawing the penis prior to ejaculation.

The actual-use effectiveness of coitus interruptus is 65 to 70 percent. Two factors seem to contribute to the relatively low actual-use effectiveness: human error (not withdrawing the penis in time) and use of the method during peak fertility (midcycle versus other times during a woman's menstrual cycle). The commonly held belief that sperm may be present in preejaculatory fluid is without scientific support (Petah Tikva, 2003).

More than half of the couples around the world use coitus interruptus as their primary method of fertility control (Hatcher et al., 1998). Such heavy reliance on what most couples in the United States would characterize as a relatively ineffective method of fertility control is a testament to the effects of poverty and ignorance. Coitus interruptus is free, readily available, and perceived by users as a "natural," "effective" method of fertility control. In a sense, this belief is true. Coitus interruptus is free, it is always available, and it is relatively effective (65 to 70 percent versus 5 percent for "hope and a prayer"). Nonetheless, couples would be much wiser to choose a method with higher reliability and STD protection.

You'll remember from Chapter 3 that orgasm in men is a two-step process. The first step, ejaculatory inevitability, begins with the man feeling the contractions initiating the expulsion of semen that occurs during the next step, emission. Many couples, especially sexually inexperienced ones, overestimate the man's ability to withdraw his penis in time if he waits for ejaculatory inevitability. Timing the removal of the penis so closely sets the stage for method failure. This is difficult for sexually inexperienced men to do. Simultaneously, a woman worried about whether her partner will "pull out" in time cannot fully relax and enjoy the lovemaking. (It is possible for couples to practice the timing of withdrawal by having the female use a backup method of birth control.)

Another way to do coitus interruptus is to withdraw prior to any sense of ejaculatory inevitability and finish with a nonpenetrative sexual method (such as masturbation) or oral-genital sex. This offers more variety in your sexual experience and reduces the risk of unintended pregnancy. You are able to enjoy vaginal intercourse while reducing the risk of pregnancy.

As a man becomes more sexually experienced, he usually develops greater ejaculatory control. He can sense when he is getting excited and beginning to lose control and can slow down (if desired) or remove his penis in time to avoid ejaculating into his partner. Married couples in their 30s and 40s seem to have the lowest failure rates with this method (Hatcher et al., 1998).

The risk of pregnancy using coitus interruptus because of the possibility of live sperm being in preejaculatory fluid seems to be less than originally believed. Studies have demonstrated that the amount of live sperm present in preejaculatory fluid varies from none (Petah Tikva, 2003; Ilaria et al., 1992), to an insignificantly small number (small clumps with a few hundred live sperm) (Prudney, Oneta, Mayer, Seage, & Andersen, 1992). Residual sperm left behind from a prior ejaculation would most likely be washed out by the force of a normal urination (Hatcher et al., 1998). Consequently, the presence of live sperm from a previous ejaculation (unless it was during the same interval of lovemaking) mixing with new preejaculatory fluid would be unlikely.

Two factors influence the presence of live sperm in significant amounts: time since last ejaculation and urination prior to intercourse. The nearer the last ejaculation, the greater is the likelihood of live sperm being present in preejaculatory fluid. Sperm can live for 3 to 5 days. Theoretically, therefore, some still may be present if a man ejaculated within that time. Urinating, however, flushes the urethra with an acidic fluid that generally destroys sperm. If a man has urinated since his last ejaculation, he will flush out his urethra, killing any sperm that may remain.

We suggest that all men who intend to use coitus interruptus urinate before they initiate any sexual activity. Also, we recommend that during sexual arousal and plateau, the couple remove any existing preejaculatory fluid (with a tissue or orally) before intromission of the penis. This will remove some of the fluid.

The last thing to consider with coitus interruptus is your fertility status. One way to increase the effectiveness of coitus interruptus is to limit its use to less fertile times of the menstrual cycle. Avoiding intercourse during peak fertility times will increase its effectiveness.

With an actual-use effectiveness of 82 percent (Hatcher et al., 1998), 18 in 100 women using this method in their first year will get pregnant. It offers no protection against transmission of STDs and HIV. This method usually is recommended for couples in disease-free, monogamous relationships who have greater tolerance for risk of an unintended pregnancy.

Fertility Awareness   **Fertility awareness,** also known as *natural family planning* and the *rhythm method,* is a strategy based on avoiding unprotected intercourse during peak fertility. Peak fertility can be estimated by combining knowledge about an individual woman's menstrual cycle with the latest scientific findings about egg and sperm viability. The four fertility awareness methods are calendar, basal body temperature, cervical mucus, and combined. Each of these methods requires understanding of the specific woman's menstrual cycle and her fertile periods, discussed in Chapter 13. Perfect-use effectiveness data for individual fertility awareness methods are shown in Table 14.1.

Calendar Method. The calendar method of fertility awareness uses the menstrual cycle history to estimate future ovulation. Once a woman can estimate the day she is likely to ovulate, she can build a **safe zone** around this day by factoring in how long an egg (24 hours) and sperm (3 to 5 days) can live. This safe zone represents days prior to and after ovulation when the presence of live sperm could result in fertilization.

Steps involved in the calendar method are as follows:

1. Keep a log of your menstrual cycle for 8 months. The first day of your cycle is the first day of menstrual bleeding. The last day of the cycle is the last day prior to the onset of bleeding.
2. Subtract 18 from your shortest cycle. This represents your first unsafe day.
3. Subtract 11 from your longest cycle. This represents your last unsafe day.
4. Avoid unprotected vaginal intercourse during your unsafe days.

> *Example:*
> *Mary charted her menstrual cycles for 9 months. Her longest cycle was 31 days. Her shortest cycle was 28 days. Thus:*
>
> 28 + 18 = 10   *(Day 10 is her first unsafe day.)*
> 31 + 11 = 20   *(Day 20 is her last unsafe day.)*
>
> *During days 10 to 20, Mary should avoid unprotected vaginal intercourse.*

Cervical Mucus Method. The cervical mucus method works by checking changes in cervical mucus during the menstrual cycle to predict ovulation. Mucus present in the cervix and vagina cause changes described as "wet" or "dry." In general, wet conditions represent fertile, unsafe days, and dry conditions designate infertile, safe days.

Menstruation masks mucus changes. Immediately following menstruation the cycle moves from infertile (dry) to fertile (wet), back to infertile (dry), and into menstruation. During infertile times of the cycle, cervical mucus is scanty, and the vagina and vulva feel dry (some women report an absence of totally dry days). During fertile periods, cervical mucus is abundant, clear, and stringy (it resembles the consistency of egg whites and will stretch if you try to pull it apart), and the vagina and vulva feel wet. Vaginal mucus should be checked a few times a day for a few months to observe how it changes. This can be done by inserting a finger and gathering mucus from the cervix and vaginal walls.

Once you are comfortable with interpreting these changes, you can monitor yourself as follows:

1. Check your cervical/vaginal mucus each time you urinate. Insert a finger and obtain a specimen or wipe a small amount from the vulva and examine it.

Fertility awareness Natural family planning

Safe zone A fertility awareness concept that factors ovulation and length of time sperm and eggs can live as a time to avoid intercourse

2. Record the changes.

3. Once you note the initial wetness, consider yourself fertile. The vagina should feel moist but not distinctly wet. Mucus should be thick, cloudy, and whitish.

4. Notice, a few days later, that your vagina and vulva feel distinctly wet. The mucus becomes more profuse and is stringy and slippery. See if you can stretch a specimen between your thumb and forefinger. If you can do this, you are fertile.

5. Continue checking your mucus. About 4 days after your wettest day, the mucus decreases and is no longer detectable. You should return to a drier state, indicating that ovulation has occurred. It is now safe to resume unprotected intercourse.

As a caution, production of mucus and vaginal/vulval wetness can be altered by antihistamines and other medications, douching, vaginal infection, contraceptive foam, jelly, and lubricants. For maximum effectiveness, this method should be combined with the calendar method to cross-validate the conclusion. For instance, if your calendar indicates that you are approaching midcycle and you don't feel the characteristic wetness, something may have altered your production of mucus. When in doubt, use a backup method.

Basal Body Temperature. To practice this method, you will need a basal body thermometer. This method relies on recognizing the slight, but measurable, change in **basal body temperature (BBT)** associated with ovulation (Hatcher et al., 1998). The procedure is as follows:

1. Each morning, immediately upon rising, take your temperature using the basal body thermometer. Do not eat, shower, smoke, or do anything else before taking your temperature. Do this every day for 3 months.

2. Record your temperature on a special grid, as illustrated in Figure 14.1.

3. After 3 months, note the changes in your cycle. Normally, between 12 to 24 hours prior to ovulation, a woman's basal body temperature will drop (the decrease varies from none to about 0.3 of 1 degree).

Basal body temperature (BBT) The lowest body temperature of a healthy person during waking hours

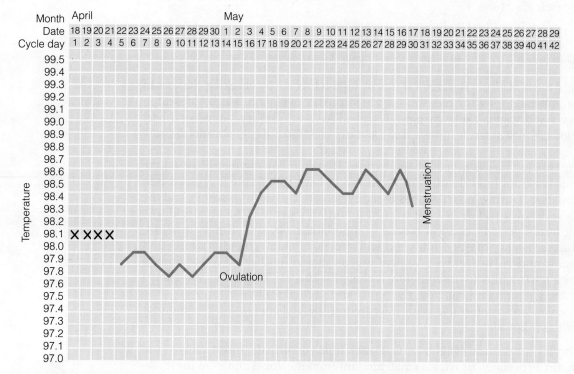

Figure 14.1 *Basal Body Temperature (BBT) Chart*

Lester and Sophia: Making Choices

Lester, 20, identifies as biracial; Sophia, 20, identifies as Latina.

Lester and Sophia are both juniors who have been in a monogamous relationship for 6 months. Lester had two girlfriends in high school and, before Sophia, dated casually at college. Sophia dated casually in high school, and then as a freshman dated a man from her job for a year. The two have been having sex for the past 3 months and sometimes even use nonpenetrative forms of sexual activity as a way to prevent unintended pregnancy.

LESTER: Sophia and I take turns as far as who is responsible for birth control. When we first had sex, I took out a condom . . . my father taught me that the man should always carry a condom. Sophia also had a condom with her! It was uncomfortable at first meeting a female who also had them. We both are comfortable buying condoms, but also like to do other things that don't involve using birth control.

SOPHIA: Right. When I first met Lester, I didn't know how much to trust him and didn't want to rush into a heavy sexual relationship. I had taken the pill when I was a freshman but went off of it when the relationship ended. I have a box of condoms in my dorm room "just in case." As Lester and I got more romantic, we did the "safer sex" things—massages and masturbating each other. And we had fun.

LESTER: Sophia will give me a long massage and then bring me off using her hand. There are times I like that more than having intercourse.

SOPHIA: I feel the same way. Sometimes I'm not in the mood to have sex, but I like to relax and get a massage. Or, I just want to please Lester and don't worry about who's giving and who's getting.

LESTER: Sophia also has this vibrator or massager we use on each other. It's a little kinky, but she uses it and her hand and the sensations are intense.

SOPHIA: It's funny because I bought the vibrator for me before I met Lester. I found that I could have really intense orgasms masturbating with it. I never figured Lester and I would have such a good time with it. It also takes off some of the pressure to always use birth control. Maybe someday I'll go back on the pill. For now switching off suits us fine!

Critical Thinking

Do you feel that Lester and Sophia have made the best decision about a birth control method based on their sexual lifestyle and personal histories? Why or why not?

Use your Virtual Workbook to explore your answers to these questions at **http:// health.wadsworth.com/ blonna1**.

4. Note the subsequent rise in temperature, indicating that ovulation has occurred. The preovulatory drop in temperature is followed by a rise in temperature 0.4 to 0.8 degrees Fahrenheit above your readings for about 6 days preceding the rise.

5. Assume that unprotected intercourse is safe after 3 days of sustained temperature rise.

Because this method does not predict ovulation (it notes when ovulation occurs), sexual activity prior to temperature changes may result in unintended pregnancy. Therefore, this method is best used in combination with either the calendar or the cervical mucus method, which help predict ovulation. The temperature charts should match the calendar charting of safe and unsafe days and the characteristics of wet and dry mucus.

Symptothermal Method. The symptothermal method designates the combination of BBT and mucus methods. It also incorporates some signs indicating that ovulation is imminent or has occurred.

Providing a Barrier Between Sperm and Egg

Barrier methods
Nonsurgical contraceptive measures that prevent the sperm and egg from uniting

Barrier methods are among the oldest and most well known of all methods used to control fertility. They are so named because they work by literally placing a barrier (mechanical, chemical, or a combination) between the sperm and the egg. Although these methods share the same mechanism of action, they differ in terms of how they are applied or inserted.

The mechanical devices use latex and polyurethane barriers to cover the penis (male condom), line the vagina (female condom), or protect the cervix (diaphragm, sponge, cervical cap). The chemical devices either provide a stand-alone spermicidal barrier that covers the cervix (foam, suppositories, film) or are used in combination with a mechanical device (gel/diaphragm or cap, spermicide impregnated in sponge, spermicidal lubricant for condoms.

Male Condom   The male condom is one of the oldest known fertility devices. Three types of condoms are currently available in the United States: latex, polyurethane, and natural lamb membrane (Nelson et al., 2000). As more aggressive efforts were made to reduce the incidence of HIV/AIDS, condom promotion around the world has increased. Along with that has come more creative marketing, packaging, and choices, including colors and a few sizes. Each type is manufactured under stringent quality control, regularly inspected for leaks and other damage. For a batch of condoms to be legally sold, only 4 in 1,000 defects are allowed. If more than one defective condom is found, the entire batch is destroyed (Consumers Union, 1995).

The male condom works by covering the penis and trapping the ejaculate, thereby preventing it from being deposited in the vagina. It offers some protection against STD organisms that might be present in the ejaculate or in lesions on the penis.

Latex Condoms. Latex condoms come in a variety of shapes, colors, and sizes. Latex condoms come individually wrapped in foil or other sealed packets. They are rolled up to the size of a half-dollar or are folded.

Latex condoms can be lubricated (with either a spermicide or a nonspermicidal lubricant) or nonlubricated. Most nonlubricated latex condoms are dusted with powder or cornstarch to facilitate putting them on an erect penis. Latex condoms come in a variety of shapes. The traditional shape is a long, uniform sheath, with a rounded end. Latex condoms also can be scented or unscented. The most recent addition to latex condom accoutrements is flavoring.

A variation of this shape comes with a reservoir tip. It also is a uniformly shaped sheath but has a small nipple that protrudes about 3/4 inch at the sealed end, to catch the ejaculate.

Form-fitting condoms generally mimic the shape of the penis. They are wider at the opening and taper to their narrowest dimension close to the end, where they flare out again in the shape of the glans of the penis. They tend to fit more snugly than traditionally shaped condoms.

The theoretical effectiveness of condoms is 97 percent. Stringent manufacturing standards ensure uniformly high quality. Actual-use effectiveness is 88 percent. The disparity between actual-use and theoretical effectiveness is attributed mostly to human error regarding storage and application. Figure 14.2 describes the steps involved in using a male condom properly.

Some men and women are allergic to latex and itch, become dry, burn, and develop a rash when exposed to it. These people may not be able to use latex condoms (or diaphragms). They are good candidates for natural membrane condoms or the female condom.

Condoms come in different colors and styles.

Charles Thatcher/GettyImages

Pinch or twist the tip of the condom, leaving one-half inch at the tip to catch the semen.

Holding the tip, unroll the condom.

Unroll the condom until it reaches the pubic hairs.

Figure 14.2 *How to Use a Condom*

The marketing of condoms has become creative and diversified over the years. Durex's Performa and Trojan's Extended Pleasure are marketed to help males prolong excitement and delay ejaculation. By placing benzocaine, a mild anesthetic, inside the tip of the condom, the medication can numb the head of the penis yet not be transferred externally to one's partner. Condoms are also produced in flavors such as chocolate and mint, to encourage their usage during oral sex. Other condoms are marketed to the gay community along with messages about their value as part of safer sex practices.

Natural Lamb Membrane Condoms. Unlike their latex cousins, natural lamb membrane condoms are not uniformly manufactured from scratch. They are made from the intestines of commercially slaughtered lambs. They are shipped to the condom manufacturer, where they are cleaned and inspected prior to being cut and sealed at one end. Even though each condom is slightly different from the next, they all must pass safety inspections and are held to the same standards as latex condoms.

Natural membrane condoms tend to fit more loosely than latex condoms. Some secure themselves to the penis with the help of a small elastic band sewn into the base. Others are snugger and grip the penis much like a latex condom. Natural lamb condoms are wet. They are sealed in a foil or other pouch with more liquid than latex condoms to keep them from deteriorating. They are available either with or without spermicides.

Natural lamb condoms offer an entirely different feel than their latex cousins. They simulate human tissue as closely as is possible. The combination of the material (lamb membrane), its wetness, and the loose fit makes natural lamb condoms feel almost like the lining of the vagina or mouth.

As a cautionary note, studies have shown that the surface of natural skin condoms contains small pores that permit the passage of viruses, including the hepatitis B virus, herpes simplex virus, and HIV (Cate & Stone, 1992). Sperm, however, are not able to penetrate these pores because sperm are much larger than viruses.

Female Condom The female condom is a loose-fitting polyurethane pouch that is inserted into the vagina, covering its walls and protruding over the vulva. The female condom works by containing a man's semen after he ejaculates into his partner's vagina. It also offers protection against STD germs that might be in the man's semen or emanating from penile lesions.

Female condoms are made from a polyurethane material that is similar to latex but is less penetrable. The female condom is also lubricated with a spermicide to enhance its fertility control effectiveness. Unlike the male condom, it does not come in different shapes, sizes, colors, or flavors. Female condoms are uniform in size and have a ring at both ends. The rings help with insertion and ensure a proper fit. The ring at the closed end loops around the cervix, anchoring it in place in a way that is similar to a diaphragm (discussed next), although the female condom does not require a prescription. The female condom is inserted like a diaphragm. You first fold the ring in half, then insert it similar to the way a tampon is inserted and feel the inner ring notch against the cervix (see Figure 14.3).

A major advantage of the female condom is that it provides women a reliable source of nonprescription protection against both pregnancy and STDs. A woman does not have to rely on her partner for this protection; she can control the method. A disadvantage of the female condom is that it costs about three times more than a male condom and is not as widely available in stores. Anecdotally, some women have reported that there is noise during thrusting, which can be distracting, embarrassing, and/or humorous depending on one's comfort with one's partner. Like the male condom, it can be used only once. It is considered at least as effective as the male condom in preventing transmission of STDs, including HIV.

healthy sex hints 14.1

Eroticizing Condom Use

Condoms have been making a steady resurgence as a contraceptive method, yet many couples still find condom use unacceptable or not as desirable as making love without one. The following tips on eroticizing condom use might change your thinking about them.

1. It's all in your head (the one on your shoulders).
   - Start to examine your thoughts about condoms.
   - Don't buy into the myth that you can't have great sex if you use a condom.
2. Be prepared.
   - Keep a supply of condoms handy.
   - Distribute packets in the bedroom chest, living room end table, downstairs and upstairs bathrooms, and other places where you might have intercourse.
3. Practice condom use by yourself.
   - Men: Masturbate using a condom (this will help you get used to the feel); practice putting one on under a variety of conditions (in the dark, with lights, one-handed, and so forth)
   - Women: Practice putting a condom on a simulated penis (such as a vibrator); practice putting one on with your mouth.

4. Try several styles/brands.
   - Find a brand and style that feels right for you.
5. Use extra lubrication.
   - Smear some water-soluble lubricating jelly (*not* petroleum-based products) on the head of your penis before putting on the condom.
   - Smear extra jelly on the outside before penetration.
6. Make condom use (and penetration) just one part of lovemaking.
   - Read Chapter 8 about viewing lovemaking as a gourmet meal (you can enjoy a lot of erotic delights before even putting on the condom).
7. Don't rush to remove the condom.
   - Enjoy the afterglow of orgasm. After a while, hold the condom firmly against the base of your penis and pull out.
8. Take turns with birth control.
   - Trade off responsibility every month (condoms this month, spermicides or oral sex the next month, and so on), and you might find using a condom less objectionable.

Applicator

Wrapper

Flex rings

Joel Gordon Photography

Figure 14.3 *Inserting a Female Condom*

The theoretical effectiveness of female condoms is 95 percent; actual-use effectiveness is 79 percent (Hatcher et al., 1998). Researchers found that the female condom rarely breaks, although slippage occurs in approximately 1 in 10 uses, and women may be exposed to semen in up to 1 in 5 uses. Furthermore, a woman is most likely to be exposed to semen if she and her partner experience mechanical problems with the condom, if there is a large disparity between the size of the penis and the size of the woman's vagina, and if intercourse is very active (Alan Guttmacher Institute, 2003b).

Diaphragm   The diaphragm is a spring-loaded rubber or plastic dome that is inserted into the vagina and anchored between the wall of the vagina and the cervix (see Figure 14.4). It is nonlubricated, so before insertion, spermicidal jelly must be placed around the rim and on the inside of the dome for it to work properly. It is not designed to form an impenetrable barrier against the cervix. It works by covering the cervix and thereby blocking access of most sperm to the egg. Any sperm that are able to get around the edge of the diaphragm are immobilized by the spermicide contained in the dome.

A diaphragm must be fitted by an experienced health care professional. This person can determine the proper size to fit into the vagina so the diaphragm will rest comfortably between the cervix and the top portion of the vagina. Diaphragms should be refitted if the woman gains or loses more than 10 pounds, has an abortion, or has a full-term pregnancy (Hatcher et al., 1998).

The theoretical effectiveness of diaphragms is 94 percent. Actual-use effectiveness is 84 percent—slightly lower than the male condom. As with condoms, the dropoff in effectiveness is primarily a result of human error associated with incorrect and inconsistent use. It is recommended that women be given emergency contraception as a backup in advance (Hatcher et al., 2003).

Cream
or jelly

Diaphragm

Squeeze spermicide into
dome of diaphragm and
around the rim.

Squeeze rim together;
insert jelly-side up.

Check placement to make
certain cervix is covered.

Joel Gordon Photography

Figure 14.4 *The Diaphragm and How to Insert It*

The steps in inserting a diaphragm are as follows:

1. Insert the diaphragm up to 6 hours before intercourse.
2. First smear spermicidal jelly (see later discussion for more detail) around the rim, and put about 2 teaspoons inside the dome.
3. Stand with one leg raised, supported on a chair or similar object.
4. Bend the diaphragm in half by moving it with the spring action, and insert it as far into the vagina as possible.
5. Push it the remaining distance with your finger until you feel the rim notch behind your cervix.
6. Leave it in place at least 6 hours (but no more than 24 hours) after intercourse.
7. An additional applicator of contraceptive foam or jelly must be inserted into the vagina for each additional act of intercourse.
8. After 6 hours from the last ejaculation, remove the diaphragm by pulling it out with a finger.
9. Wash it off with clean, soapy water; dry it; dust it with corn starch; and put it into its case.
10. If you are uncomfortable touching yourself or want to get your partner involved, have your lover remove (or insert) the diaphragm.

Cervical Cap The cervical cap is a small, thimble-shaped plastic or rubber cap that fits snugly against the cervix through suction. It is available in four sizes and must be fitted by a health care professional. It works in a fashion similar to the diaphragm, blocking the passage of sperm while utilizing spermicidal jelly as a backup to immobilize sperm that may enter around its rim.

The cervical cap differs from the diaphragm in these ways:

- The cervical cap anchors to the cervix through suction rather than by pressing against the walls of the vagina and the cervix the way the diaphragm does.
- The cap is much smaller and less conspicuous than the diaphragm.
- The cap requires less spermicide (because of its smaller size).
- The cap does not require additional spermicide with additional episodes of intercourse.

The cervical cap fits snugly against the cervix.

Theoretical effectiveness of the cervical cap is comparable to that of other vaginal barrier methods, those being the female condom, diaphragm, and sponge. However, the cervical cap does not work as well for women who have given birth compared to those who have not. The perfect-use failure rate in the first year for parous women (those who have given birth) is 26 percent compared to 9 percent for nulliparous women (those who have not given birth). The typical-use failure rate, by comparison, for parous women is 40 percent in the first year of use, compared to 20 percent for nulliparous women (Nelson et al., 2000). It is advised, therefore, that emergency contraception be kept as a backup at times of possible failure.

The cervical cap may be inserted up to 6 hours prior to intercourse. It must remain in place at least 6 hours but no more than 48 hours after the male ejaculates. To use the cervical cap:

1. Fill the cap with spermicidal jelly.
2. Using the thumb and forefinger, squeeze the cap and push it into the vagina all the way to the cervix. Once it reaches the cervix, release it with a small twist, notching it in place.
3. If multiple acts of intercourse take place, additional spermicide is not needed, but the woman should check that the cap is in place.
4. To remove, insert a finger up the vagina, catch the rim of the cap, and pull it sideways out of the vagina.
5. Wash it out, and store in a dry, cool place.

Vaginal Contraceptive Sponge The vaginal sponge is a soft, white, polyurethane sponge filled with spermicide. It works the same way as the diaphragm and cervical cap: It creates a double barrier (absorbent polyurethane sponge and spermicide) that blocks and absorbs sperm while chemically deactivating them.

Like the diaphragm and cervical cap, the sponge can be inserted up to 6 hours before intercourse. In contrast, however, it can be left in place for 24 hours where no additional applications of spermicide are needed if additional ejaculations occur within that time period. This feature allows greater flexibility in sexual activity without the need for using additional spermicides.

Sex in Society 14.1, "Update on the Sponge," traces the history of this once-popular method. A major advantage of the sponge is that it is a nonprescription device. Sponges typically cost approximately $3. Like the diaphragm and the cervical cap, the vaginal contraceptive sponge provides a protective barrier against the

The sponge provides protection for up to 24 hours.

Update on the Sponge

In March, 1994, Whitehall-Robbins Healthcare in Hammontown, New Jersey, stopped manufacturing the Today Sponge. At that time, Whitehall-Robbins was the only company producing contraceptive sponges. The company stopped production of the sponge after being cited by the Food and Drug Administration (FDA) for unacceptable manufacturing standards. At no point did the FDA cite any problems associated with the sponge itself.

Ironically, many average women learned that the sponge would no longer be available from a now-famous episode of *Seinfeld*. In this storyline, Elaine learns that her chosen method of birth control is being taken off the market. In response, she runs around New York City buying up whatever sponges remain on store shelves. Her need to carefully monitor her supply leads her to wonder whether each prospective date is "sponge-worthy."

Allendale Pharmaceuticals in New Jersey bought the rights to make Today, and it has been distributing it via the Internet with Canada as its distribution base. The company reports that it should again appear on U.S. store shelves sometime in 2004 (Allendale Pharmaceuticals, 2003).

Another sponge, Protectaid, was developed in Canada in 1996 by Axcan Limited, a division of Axcan Pharmaceuticals. It is similar to the Today Sponge in size, shape, use, and instructions. Its manufacturers claim that it offers a major advantage over the Today Sponge in that it has three active spermicidal ingredients: nonoxynol-9, benzalkonium chloride, and sodium cholate. One significant difference, however, is that Protectaid does not have an attached string for easy removal.

World travelers learn that countries have differing laws about what drugs and medical products are available either by prescription or over the counter. The Internet has become a useful resource for information as well as marketing; Allendale Pharmaceuticals has been able to make their product available to women who can order the sponge online. Because neighboring Canada has approved the method, women in the United States can purchase the Today Sponge online and get questions answered at a 24-hour hotline service based in Canada.

cervix. Studies have shown that these female barrier methods also provide limited protection against most STDs (Cate & Stone, 1992; Hatcher et al., 1998).

The vaginal contraceptive sponge is similar in effectiveness to the diaphragm and the cervical cap. Its theoretical effectiveness is 96 percent, and actual-use effectiveness is 84 percent.

To use the contraceptive sponge:

1. Moisten the sponge with 1 to 2 tablespoons of water.
2. Insert it into the vagina up to 6 hours prior to intercourse. Its smaller size makes insertion easier than the diaphragm.
3. Leave the sponge in place for at least 6 hours after the last ejaculation. (Once in place, a woman can have multiple episodes of intercourse without the need for additional spermicides.)
4. Remove the sponge by slipping a finger through the sewn-in loop and pulling out of the vagina.
5. Dispose with regular trash. (Do not flush down toilet.)

Chemical Spermicides   A wide variety of chemical spermicides are available as stand-alone fertility control methods or to be used in conjunction with mechanical barriers as previously discussed. They all work by immobilizing and killing sperm, though they vary in form and method of application. They are available as nonprescription fertility control devices at most drug stores. It was previously thought that nonoxynol-9 was also effective in killing the organisms that cause syphilis, gonorrhea, and genital herpes, HIV/AIDS, and other STDs. To the contrary, the FDA has proposed a warning that nonoxynol-9 may actually increase the prospects of infection transmission due to irritating the skin (Hatcher et al., 2003).

Selected spermacide products

Spermacide products are placed deep in the vagina, either using one's fingers or an applicator depending on the product. One application must be used for each act of intercourse.

Figure 14.5 *Selected Spermicides and How to Insert Them*

The best-known spermicides are foams, gels, and creams. These work by creating a chemical barrier suspended in a shaving-cream-like foam, clear gel, or smooth cream. All three are inserted into the vagina, near the cervix, using a cylindrical applicator (see Figure 14.5). They create an immediate, effective chemical barrier against sperm. These spermicides may be inserted no more than 1 hour prior to intercourse.

Spermicidal film is different, however, because it is not immediately effective. It takes about 15 minutes to transform from its original shape into an effervescent liquid once inserted into the vagina (American Health Consultants, 1992).

Spermicidal suppositories are waxlike cylinders about the size of earplugs. They are applied in the same way as rectal suppositories, except into the vagina. Like film, the suppository requires about 15 minutes to liquefy after insertion into the vagina.

General instructions for using spermicides are as follows:

1. Fill the applicator with the product.
2. While lying down, insert the applicator deep into the vagina, near the cervix.
3. Push the plunger until the contents are completely released against the cervix.
4. If intercourse proceeds longer than 30 minutes, stop and insert another applicator full of spermicide.
5. Insert a new application for each episode of intercourse.

The effectiveness of vaginal spermicides is similar regardless of the specific type. Foam, gel, cream, film, and suppositories are much the same in outcome. The theoretical effectiveness of spermicides is 97 percent. Actual-use effectiveness is much lower, at 79 percent. This figure presumably is mostly a result of incorrect and inconsistent use.

Preventing Implantation of Fertilized Egg

Intrauterine Devices   The intrauterine device (IUD) is designed to prevent implantation, and as such, it had been technically thought of as a postconceptive method of fertility control. Recent studies show, however, that IUDs work primarily by preventing the sperm from fertilizing the egg (Hatcher et al., 1998). IUDs are pieces of plastic that are inserted into the uterus by a gynecologist or other trained reproductive health care professional. The three models currently

sex in society 14.2

Intrauterine Devices Here and Abroad

When teaching undergraduates about intrauterine devices, faculty may get met with blank faces from those who have never heard of such an item nor could imagine having one inserted into the uterus. Some of the original IUDs on the market were responsible for a variety of painful and deadly complications for early users. Although new designs have improved effectiveness and minimized side effects, the method received a lot of "bad press," became impossible to get in the United States for a brief period of time, and lost favor among many women.

In the 1970s, the Dalkon Shield was a commonly prescribed IUD. A significant number of users did not tolerate it. Because of its irregular shape and large size, the Dalkon Shield triggered strong uterine contractions as the body attempted to expel it from the uterus. The contractions often resulted in the shield penetrating the uterus and creating other problems, including severe infection that resulted in pain, hemorrhage, and sometimes death. The company that made the Dalkon Shield lost a civil lawsuit brought by users and their families and subsequently took the product off the market and went out of business. In practice, health care providers would advise this method for women who had been pregnant and had children. It also gave no protection against STDs, and HIV in particular, making it even less popular in the late 20th century.

Many safe IUDs were discontinued because of the costs involved in litigation, even though the companies that produced these products were found innocent of any liability claims. Consumer fears and the costs of litigation had driven most IUDs from the market. At the present time, the Mirena, Progestasert, and ParaGard IUDs are available in the United States.

By contrast, a number of IUDs have been available abroad. Family Health International (FHI; 1996) reports that the IUD is the most widely used reversible contraceptive used worldwide, with approximately 100 million users. Rates of IUD use vary from country to country, with the highest rates reported to be in China. FHI reports that obstacles to greater use involve better training of health care professionals and educational efforts needed to overcome misinformation. A study in Kenya found resistance to the copper in IUDs, which may have tarnished in the package; women were afraid of the greenish color. Professional training in the Philippines had to focus on the myth that the IUD was too big for Filipino women and their accompanying fears that it traveled around the body (FHI, 1996). Overall, the IUD is a cost-effective method of birth control, particularly in nations with large populations of people without large numbers of health care providers.

Figure 14.6 *An Inserted IUD*

available for use in the United States are ParaGard, Progestasert, and the Mirena IUD. Each is T shaped and covered with either a layer of synthetic progesterone or copper. Prior to 1990, several types of IUDs were available. Most were taken off the market after the Dalkon Shield was found to be associated with several serious side effects (Klitsch, 1995).

The IUD is generally believed to control fertility by causing an inflammatory response within the uterus that prevents implantation and by initiating an immune response that mobilizes white blood cells, which attack and immobilize sperm. Figure 14.6 shows an inserted IUD.

Once inside the uterus, the IUD irritates and inflames the endometrial lining and slowly releases either copper or synthetic progesterone depending on the type of device. Both Progestasert and Mirena, with their releasing of synthetic progestin, cause the cervical mucus to thicken, preventing sperm from reaching the ova (Nelson et al., 2000). Once inserted, the IUD provides continuous protection with no further need for the user to do anything except to check the strings daily to be sure they are in place. The user can insert one or two fingers into the vagina and feel for the string. If she feels the string, the IUD is in place. If she doesn't, she should see her health care provider immediately and consider herself fertile.

Intrauterine devices have the advantage of providing long-term effectiveness. Once inserted, the ParaGard, also known as the Copper T, can be worn for up to 10 years. The Mirena, the newest IUD on the market, releases the hormone levonorgestrel, a synthetic progestin. It has the advantage of preventing ectopic pregnancy, lessens menstrual cramping, and decreases the amount of menstrual blood (Advocates for Youth, 2003). Mirena can be worn for up to 7 years, whereas Progestasert, which also releases some progesterone, must be replaced annually.

The IUD is best suited for a woman who already has had at least one child, as the uterus seems to tolerate it better than the uterus of a woman who has never experienced pregnancy or childbirth. Women who have never been pregnant have more severe cramping, as the uterus becomes accustomed to the presence of this device. Women who have never been pregnant, however, can still use the device and achieve the same high actual-use effectiveness as women who have had children.

Many IUD users report heavier than normal menstrual flow. The IUD is not recommended for women with a history of **pelvic inflammatory disease (PID)**, as they are eight times more likely than women who have never had PID to experience a second episode if they use an IUD. Also, women with a history of STDs or who have high-risk sexual lifestyles for STDs are discouraged from using the IUD. If they become infected with an STD, they are four to eight times more likely than low risk-women to develop PID while using the IUD. Because PID can cause infertility, women who desire to have children should be cautious about using the IUD.

Theoretical effectiveness and actual-use effectiveness of IUDs are similar. Theoretical-use effectiveness is approximately 99 percent. Actual-use effectiveness is 97 percent. Most of the failure associated with IUD use has to do with the body's attempt to reject the device through uterine contractions. Proper screening of potential users and vigilance in checking for strings can help reduce the failure rate ("On the Needless Hounding," 1995).

Women who are considering using an IUD should visit a health care provider experienced in inserting IUDs. The provider will measure the size and depth of the uterus by dilating the cervix and using special probes to measure it. This procedure, called *sounding,* is necessary for the safe insertion of any IUD.

If the woman decides to use the IUD, the provider will insert the IUD using an insertion device. Once inserted, the provider pushes the IUD into place and removes the device. The provider locates the strings attached to the end of the IUD and trims them to a shorter length. These strings will pass through the cervix and hang into the vagina. The woman has to demonstrate that she can find these strings, as they let her know whether the IUD is still in place. If the woman experiences bleeding or extreme cramping or cannot find the strings, she must go back to the provider immediately.

Preventing Release of Ova

The methods that prevent the release of an egg are hormonal. Focusing on managing a woman's ovulation has been extremely popular over the years, with the newest methods of birth control emerging in that area. Hormones can be taken orally, by injection, by vaginal insertion, and via a patch. Newer, varied, and hopefully less problematic methods of hormone distribution have been developed, tried, and, in some cases, removed from the market. In 2002 alone, Norplant, which relied on time-released straws inserted into a woman's arm, was

Pelvic inflammatory disease (PID) A catch-all term used to describe infection of the uterus, fallopian tubes, or ovaries resulting in fever, malaise, pain, and other symptoms removed from the market. The hormone injection Lunelle was also recalled in 2002. Evra, the birth control patch, received FDA approval and was aggressively marketed via magazines and television commercials in 2002. Birth control pills used on a 91-day cycle were marketed as Seasonale in 2003.

Environmental/Occupational Wellness

Fertility control does not take place within a vacuum. On a national level, personal fertility control is influenced by legislation that ensures the availability of safe, tested contraceptive methods and unrestricted access to these methods for all users. In December 2000, the U.S. Equal Employment Opportunity Commission (EEOC) argued that for employers' prescription plans to deny coverage for contraception was a violation of Title VII of the Civil Rights Act of 1964, as amended by the Pregnancy Discrimination Act (National Abortion and Reproductive Rights Action League [NARAL] & NARAL Foundation, 2001). By contrast, prescription plans had been covering the costs to men of Viagra, the drug developed to treat erectile dysfunction. In 2002, when a female student at George Washington University complained, the university revised the student health insurance plan to include prescription contraceptives. Since 1998, 26 states have some legislation that gives women financial support from their insurance companies. As of this writing, however, no federal legislation has been enacted to mandate insurance coverage for contraception (NARAL, 2003).

At the local level, users must feel safe in procuring medical care and fertility control. Medical and health care providers, clinics, drug stores, schools, and other outlets for fertility control information and services should be safe and accessible for all, yet in practice they are not.

Oral Contraceptives Oral contraceptives are formulated as combination pills of synthetic estrogen and progesterone, or progestin-only pills (POPs), commonly referred to as minipills. Combination pills are the most commonly used oral contraceptives. The combinations and levels of hormones contained in birth control pills have been changing constantly since their introduction in the early 1960s. Pills that are currently available contain the minimum levels of hormones necessary to carry out their intended functions and are much lower than the original formulations. This has resulted in a safer pill with fewer side effects (Glusker, 1995). In fact, using the birth control pill is safer than carrying a pregnancy to term.

Combination birth control pills work in several ways. The main action is to suppress ovulation by elevating estrogen levels within the bloodstream. An abnormally high level of estrogen inhibits the secretion of follicle stimulating hormone (FSH), which is necessary for the release of a mature ovum.

Normally, levels of estrogen, FSH, and leutinizing hormone (LH) are low during the initial phases of the menstrual cycle. The hypothalamus senses this and triggers the pituitary gland to secrete estrogen, FSH, and LH just prior to midcycle. If there is no surge of these substances, there is no release of a mature ovum. Birth control pills create an artificially high level of estrogen, which floods the hypothalamus, keeping it from releasing more into the bloodstream and thereby preventing ovulation.

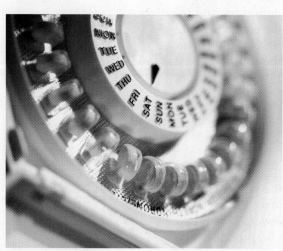

Peter Ardito/Index Stock Imagery

Birth control pills come in containers that are easy to use and allow you to see if you've missed any.

Progestin, the artificial progesterone in combination pills, provides additional protection by keeping the cervical mucus thick. This makes it harder for sperm to penetrate the cervix. In addition, progestin alters the composition of the endometrium, reducing the likelihood of implantation if the effects of estrogen fail and fertilization occurs.

Oral contraceptives are highly effective in controlling fertility. The theoretical effectiveness is over 99 percent. Actual-use effectiveness is 97 percent. The dropoff is associated with human error in failing to take pills consistently and correctly.

Birth control pills come packaged in either 21- or 28-pill containers. In the 28-pill packages, the last seven pills are placebos designed to help keep the woman on schedule and not to produce any contraceptive effect. With either prescription, the woman begins taking the pills on the fifth day of the menstrual cycle or on the first Sunday following the beginning of her period. If you remember from Chapter 2, the first day of bleeding is considered the first day of the cycle.

The woman takes a pill each day until she has consumed them all. With the 21-pill package, she will not take any pills for the last 7 days of the cycle and will begin the new package of pills on the fifth day of bleeding. With the 28-pill package, she takes one pill every day. When she runs out after the 28th day, she begins her new package of pills.

All women taking birth control pills are regulated automatically to a 28-day menstrual cycle. The presence of constant levels of estrogen and progesterone will standardize the cycle (even if the woman has been irregular in the past). Birth control pills frequently are prescribed for women with irregular periods to regulate them as well as to provide fertility control protection.

Consistent use is crucial for maximum effectiveness. The woman should try to take the pill at the same time each day. This will help develop the habit of taking one pill each day, keep the same amount of hormones in the blood level, and ensure consistent use. Some women prefer to take the pill each morning as part of their ritual for getting ready for school or work. Others take it at night as part of a night-time sleep ritual. The time is up to her. Taking the birth control pill should become part of the lifestyle, just like brushing the teeth. The woman doesn't even have to think about it.

If a pill is missed, the woman should take two the next day. Missing one pill will not compromise the effectiveness of the method. Missing two pills, however, does reduce the effectiveness of oral contraceptives, and a backup fertility control method will be necessary. If she misses two pills, she should take two immediately and two the next day. After that, she should continue to take one each day until they are all gone.

Long-Acting Combination Pills. In 2003, the FDA approved an oral contraceptive called Seasonale. Women take tablets with combination hormones for 84 days, followed by 1 week of placebo tablets, making a 91-day regimen. Women using Seasonale will get their periods four times per year, rather than the monthly periods associated with traditional birth control pills. Both rates of effectiveness as well as risks and side effects match those of traditional birth control pills. Similarly, there is no protection against sexually transmitted infections (FDA, 2003).

Progestin-Only Pills. Also referred to as *minipills*, progestin-only pills are to be taken every day. The same precautions and instructions for missed combination pills apply to the minipill. Progestin, the same artificial progesterone used in combination pills, is taken by itself. Its action is identical to the way it works in the combination pill: It keeps cervical mucus thick and alters the composition of the endometrium, reducing the likelihood of fertilization and implantation.

Side Effects and Risks. Some women experience side effects when taking oral contraceptives. The most common side effects mimic symptoms attributed to pregnancy: nausea, breast tenderness, constipation, mild swelling, and skin rashes.

Other common, mild side effects include weight gain or loss, increased vaginal secretions, and increased susceptibility to vaginal infections such as monilia (yeast).

Many of these effects can be minimized or eliminated by changing the formula or brand of pill. Combination pills differ slightly by manufacturer in the amounts of estrogen and progesterone. If the combination of these hormones in the present pill is causing unacceptable side effects, the health care provider can change the prescription and the woman can try a different formulation.

The birth control pill also can interact with other medications. In some cases, oral contraceptives lessen the effectiveness of the other medications. Or other medications can lessen the effectiveness of the pill. Table 14.2 details some of these interactions.

Although the risks associated with oral contraceptives are serious and have to be considered, most of them can be reduced through proper screening of the woman by a health care professional. The benefits far outweigh the risks. Furthermore, many of the side effects are protective and reduce other disease risks. Some of the health benefits of the pill include decreased menstrual cramping and pain associated with ovulation, lowered risk of ovarian and endometrial cancer, reduction in benign breast disease, and decreased risk of pelvic inflammatory disease. Also known is its beneficial use in the treatment of acne (Nelson et al., 2000).

Another way to view the risks associated with use of the pill is to put them into a broader perspective. Most of us assume many risks in the course of a day without even thinking about them. A taken-for-granted activity such as driving a car puts us at a much higher risk of dying than does using the pill or other fertility control techniques. We accept the risk because it is worth assuming. The activity (driving a car, for instance) adds so much to our daily quality of life that we accept the risk it entails. We also do whatever we can to decrease the risks associated with driving. We use seat belts, obey speed limits and other traffic laws, don't drink and drive, and so on. Nonetheless, high blood pressure, migraine headaches, blood clots, and stroke have been associated with the use of birth control pills by selected groups of women.

Oral contraceptives are contraindicated for women who have a history of cardiovascular disease (high blood pressure, heart attack, stroke); diabetes in themselves or in family members; heart attack in family members (particularly women) under 50 years of age; blood clots or a history of blood clots; cancer (breast, vagina, uterus); diseases of the liver, kidney, or gall bladder; and women who smoke.

Ortho Evra Patch The Ortho Evra Patch administers hormones through the skin, and it is reported to be as effective as birth control pills. The patch is thin, beige in color, and measures 1.75 inches on each side. A woman wears a patch for 1 week, replaces it on the same day for 3 consecutive weeks, and is "patch-free" during the fourth week (Ortho-McNeil Pharmaceutical, 2003). Like birth control pills, Evra may impact the cardiovascular system with a risk for clots, stroke, or heart attack; cigarette smoking can increase that risk. Side effects include breast symptoms, headache, skin reactions at the site of application, menstrual cramps, and abdominal pain. As with all the forms of hormonal contraception, the effectiveness for pregnancy prevention is high (99 percent theoretical effectiveness), but there is no protection against STDs (Ortho-McNeil Pharmaceutical, 2003).

Reuters/CORBIS

The patch can be placed on the shoulder, arm, or abdomen, but never on the breast.

Table 14.2 Effects of Common Medications on the Pill

Interacting Drugs	Adverse Effects (Probable Mechanism)	Comments and Recommendations
Acetaminophen (Tylenol and others)	Possible decreased pain-relieving effect (increased metabolism)	Monitor pain-relieving response.
Alcohol	Possible increased effect of alcohol	Use with caution.
Anticoagulants (oral)	Decreased anticoagulant effect	Use alternative contraceptive.
Antidepressants (Elavil, Norpramin, Tofranil, others)	Possible increased antidepressant effect	Monitor antidepressant effect.
Barbiturates (Phenobarbital and others)	Decreased contraceptive effect	Avoid simultaneous use; use alternative contraceptive for epileptics.
Benzodiazepine tranquilizers (Ativan, Librium, Serax, Tranxene, Valium, Xanax, and others)	Possible increased or decreased tranquilizer effects including psychomotor impairments	Use with caution. Greatest impairment occurs during menstrual pause in oral contraceptive dosage.
Beta-blockers (Corgard, Inderal, Lopressor, Tenormin)	Possible increased blocker effect	Monitor cardiovascular status.
Carbamazepine (Tegretol)	Possible decreased contraceptive effect	Use alternative contraceptive.
Corticosteroids (cortisone)	Possible increased corticosteroid toxicity	Clinical significance not established.
Griseofulvin (Fulvicin, GrifulvinV, and others)	Decreased contraceptive effect	Use alternative contraceptive.
Guanethidine (Esimil, Ismelin)	Decreased guanethidine effect (mechanism not established)	Avoid simultaneous use.
Hypoglycemics (Tolbutamide, Diabinese, Orinase, Tolinase)	Possible decreased hypoglycemic effect	Monitor blood glucose.
Methyldopa (Aldoclor, Aldoment, and others)	Decreased hypertensive effect	Avoid simultaneous use.
Penicillin	Decreased contraceptive effect with ampicillin	Low but unpredictable incidence; use alternative contraceptive.
Phenytoin (Dilantin)	Decreased contraceptive effect; possible increased phenytoin effect	Use alternative contraceptive. Monitor phenytoin concentration.
Primidone (Mysoline)	Decreased contraceptive effect	Use alternative contraceptive.
Rifampin	Decreased contraceptive effect	Use alternative contraceptive.
Tetracycline	Decreased contraceptive effect	Use alternative contraceptive.
Theophylline (Bronkotabs, Marax, Primatene, Quibron Tedral, TheorDur, and others)	Increased theophylline effect	Monitor theophylline concentration.
Troleandomycin (TAO)	Jaundice (additive)	Avoid simultaneous use.
Vitamin C	Increased serum concentration and possible increased adverse effects of estrogens with 1 gram or more per day of vitamin C	Decrease vitamin C to 100 milligrams per day.

Source: Contraceptive Technology (16th ed.) by R. Hatcher et al. (New York: Irvington, 1993). Used with permission.

Michael Newman/PhotoEdit, Inc.

The NuvaRing dispenses hormones through the vagina.

To help women remember which day the patch is changed, a Sunday start is advised but not required. Women can apply the patch to the buttocks, abdomen, upper torso, or arm. *The patch may not be applied to the breasts.* The manufacturer advises that the patch not be put where makeup, lotions, or creams are applied. The adhesive on the patch is designed to last the week, regardless of showering or bathing, swimming, exercise, or humidity.

NuvaRing   The NuvaRing, like all oral contraceptives, works on the principle of a woman having a 28-day cycle: 3 weeks of hormonal control followed by 1 week when the reduced endometrium is shed. The NuvaRing appears similar to the plastic ring at the end of the female condom, and it is inserted by the woman deep into the vagina, where it remains for 3 weeks. Although insertion is relatively simple, involving folding the ring and pushing it up the vagina, a woman must be comfortable touching that part of her body in order for this method to work. At the end of the 3-week period, the ring is removed by hooking the index finger under the ring and pulling it out. Kits come with a timer, yet a woman needs to remember to take out the ring, wait a week, and put in a new one. If the ring is left in longer than 4 weeks, a woman may lose her birth control protection. Couples do not feel the ring, and it rarely falls out.

Again, as with other hormonal methods of birth control, NuvaRing's risks include increased risk of blood clots, stroke, and heart attack. Women who smoke cigarettes should not use NuvaRing. Some women report experiencing headache, vaginitis, sinus infections, and nausea (Organon, 2003).

Emergency Contraception Pill   Commonly called the "morning-after pill," emergency contraception (EC) is being marketed in the United States as Preven and Plan B. Although other pills can be used, these two hormonal packages have specifically been designed for postcoital use. Preven is a combination of synthetic estrogen and progestin; Plan B is only progestin. Approved by the FDA, they are designed to be administered under medical supervision within 72 hours after unprotected intercourse. Debate has continued over the critical role of timing and the value of making emergency contraception an over-the-counter product. The early administration of the pills works to prevent the release of an ovum, slow the movement of the ovum, or prevent implantation (Hatcher et al., 1998).

EC works better when started within 24 hours of unprotected intercourse yet can be administered up to 120 hours later. A woman takes the first pill and then 12 hours later takes the second. Some women may report nausea with EC, and taking antinausea medication is permissable (Hatcher et al., 1998). If a woman does not get her menstrual period within 3 weeks, she must take a pregnancy test. Overall, the rate of effectiveness is between 75 and 89 percent, although research conducted by the World Health Organization found only 1.1 percent of women who used progestin-only emergency contraception went on to become pregnant (Nelson et al., 2000).

According to research conducted by the Henry J. Kaiser Family Foundation, 73 percent of women ages 18 to 44 have never heard of EC, with another two-thirds in that group not realizing that it is available in the United States (Murphy & Allina, 2003, p. 1). Whereas availability is often known on college campuses and when needed distributed by campus health centers, such is not the case around the United States. During 2002, the Reproductive Health Technologies Project and a group of medical and women's policy groups began a Back Up Your Birth Control campaign to better inform the public ("Women Often Unaware," 2002).

Depo-Provera Depo-Provera is a progestin-only hormonal contraceptive. Its action is the same as the minipill. A major advantage of Depo-Provera over these other methods is the way in which it is administered: by injection every 3 months. The injections can be administered in either the arm or the buttocks. A single injection provides 3 months' worth of protection.

Depo-Provera has one of the highest actual-use effectiveness rates of all fertility control methods, at 97 percent. This rate can be attributed mostly to the nature of administering the product. There is no room for actual-use error. Once the shot is administered, the user doesn't have to remember to do anything.

Because Depo-Provera does not contain estrogen, it does not produce many of the side effects associated with combination pills. Nevertheless, it does produce two noticeable side effects: weight gain and very light periods. Many women discontinue Depo-Provera because of predictable weight gain (5.4 pounds average during the first year; some women gain three times that). It also produces scanty menstrual flow and **amenorrhea** in some women (Hatcher et al., 1998).

Amenorrhea Absence of menstruation at some time after a female has reached menses

Other Hormonal Methods

Lunelle Lunelle had been available to women until its voluntary recall by Pharmacia, its manufacturer. A clinician had to inject the drug, a combination of estradiol cypionate and medroxyprogesterone acetate, into a woman's arm, buttocks, or thigh, on a monthly basis. Due to syringes being manufactured and distributed with possible inadequate levels of the drug, a voluntary recall was enforced in 2002 (Planned Parenthood, 2002d).

Like other forms of hormonal contraception, Lunelle regulated the menstrual cycle and prevented ovulation. Although it was touted as being convenient, its use required seeing a health care provider on a monthly basis for the injection.

Norplant Norplant, no longer available, was a system of six, thin plastic implants of hormones, medically inserted into a woman's upper arm. It contained the progestin levonorgestrel, which worked to inhibit ovulation, thicken the cervical mucus, and possibly alter the endometrium. It was especially attractive as a new method due to its being effective for a 5-year period, yet it offered no protection against sexually transmitted infections.

Although the average cost made it comparable or less than other hormonal methods, the up-front costs could range from $500 to $750, which included the medical exam, pregnancy test, implants, and cost of insertion (Planned Parenthood, 2000). For some, the mechanism for paying for the method could be a deterrent.

Implanon Implanon is a single rod approximately 4 centimeters long, which is designed to provide hormonally controlled protection for up to 3 years (Baylor College of Medicine, 2002). It releases progestin and within 24 hours of insertion is thought to be reliable. Similar to birth control pills, it works by thickening cervical mucus so that sperm are inhibited in their travel, inhibiting ovulation, and altering the endometrium so that it wouldn't support a fertilized egg (Nelson et al., 2000). Like other hormonal forms of birth control, it offers no protection against sexually transmitted infection. Irregular bleeding and headaches are the most reported side effects.

Table 14.3 compares some of the newer contraceptive methods.

Table 14.3 Comparison of Newer Contraceptive Methods

	Monthly Injectable	Implant	Intrauterine System	Ring	Patch
Office visits	Once/month	Insertion/removal	Insertion/removal	Prescription	Prescription
Easily reversible	Yes	Yes	Yes	Yes	Yes
Dosing frequency*	Once/month	3–5 years	1–10 years	Every 4 weeks	Weekly
User controlled	No	No	No	Yes	Yes
Discreet	Yes	Sometimes	Yes	Yes	Sometimes

*The type of hormonal implant and intrauterine device/system will determine the dosing frequency.
Sources: Adapted from Baylor College of Medicine (2002) and Planned Parenthood Federation of America (2003a).

Future Methods for Males

It should be obvious that the hormonal discussion so far focuses solely on the female body. Over the years, the research question has been posited as to whether hormonal control of male sperm production would be possible. Giving synthetic androgens to men, whether orally, by injection, or by implant, could theoretically reduce sperm production. Finding the right reduction in testosterone without affecting a man's sex drive is the challenge. A clinical study of a contraceptive pill that reduces sperm count is being tested in Italy; additional testosterone injections must be used in conjunction with the pill.

The World Health Organization is testing a weekly injection treatment of a form of testosterone that also reduces sperm count. A combination of testosterone and progesterone is being tested as a once-a-month injection. Subdermal implants, with one rod of gonadotropin-releasing hormone (GnRH) and a second containing an androgen (MENT), are also being studied. Battery-powered capsules, which would be implanted into each vas deferens, are being designed to emit a low-level current that would immobilize sperm as they passed by (Planned Parenthood, 2003b).

Preventing Sperm from Reaching Egg (Surgical)

The surgical methods that prevent sperm from reaching the ova consist of vasectomy and tubal ligation, both **sterilization** techniques. Sterilization does not prevent sperm and ova from being released. It works by blocking the path of either the sperm or the egg as a result of surgical removal of a small section of the vas deferens (vasectomy) in the male or fallopian tubes (minilaparotomy and tubal ligation) in the female. The ends of the vas deferens and fallopian tubes are either folded back and sewn shut or cauterized.

Sterilization Techniques (vasectomy and tubal ligation) that prevent sperm from reaching ova

All sterilization procedures should be viewed as permanent, because once these structures have been surgically altered, there is no guarantee that they can be rejoined. Ova or sperm that are produced after sterilization cannot continue their journey, so they die, break down, and are excreted from the body as waste products.

Both male and female sterilization have theoretical and actual-use effectiveness rates of higher than 99 percent. Once the surgery has been performed, the user has to do nothing more to ensure safe, effective fertility control.

Of the two procedures, vasectomy is the simplest and less costly. Most vasectomies are performed as outpatient visits and last no longer than 20 or 30 minutes.

Female sterilization often requires an overnight stay in the hospital, although some are performed as outpatient procedures. Female sterilization (minilaparotomy and tubal ligation) is relatively simple and usually takes under an hour to perform.

Both procedures require a presurgical conference with the husband and wife and the surgeon, to ensure that the couple understands the permanence of the procedure. Many physicians will not sterilize younger (under age 30) or single persons because of the possibility that they will desire children sometime later in life.

Vasectomy No major preoperative testing procedures are done for a **vasectomy.** During the initial consultation, patients are advised to bring an athletic supporter to wear home after the procedure.

The patient disrobes and lies on his back on the examination table. He is given a local anesthetic in the vas deferens and remains awake throughout the entire procedure (see Figure 14.7). The physician locates the vas deferens and makes a small incision in the scrotal sac. The physician isolates the vas deferens and cuts out a small piece. He or she then cauterizes or ties back the ends of the tubes and sutures the incision. The physician then performs the same procedure on the other vas deferens. The patient is instructed to rest for a short time and is then free to leave. The entire outpatient stay is usually no more than an hour.

Patients normally are cleared to go back to work the next day but are advised to avoid strenuous activity. Often, patients rest the day following surgery as local soreness or swelling makes walking around uncomfortable. Patients can resume intercourse after a couple of days but are cautioned that the procedure is not considered complete until they have a negative sperm sample. If they have intercourse before then, they are advised to use a backup fertility control method.

Because live sperm can still exist after 6 to 10 ejaculations, patients are instructed to bring a semen sample after that time to test for live sperm. If the test is negative, they can resume intercourse without a backup method.

Side effects of a vasectomy are relatively mild; the most common are pain and tenderness. A small percentage of patients (about 5 percent) report swelling of the vas deferens or epididymis. This is related to the surgery and usually is easy to control with ice or heat, support, and rest, in some combination.

A small percentage of men report psychological problems after having a vasectomy. This reaction seems to be a gender identity issue linking virility and potency to sex pleasure and performance. Counseling can help resolve these issues. On the other hand, many men report an increase in sexual desire after being freed from the burden of birth control.

Female Sterilization The two sterilization procedures used most often with women are minilaparotomy and tubal ligation. **Minilaparotomy,** the simpler of the two, usually can be performed under local anesthesia as an outpatient procedure. **Tubal ligation** usually is done under general anesthesia and requires an overnight hospital stay.

Minilaparotomy The patient lies on her back on the examination table and receives an injection of anesthetic into her abdomen. Once the anesthesia has been administered and takes effect, a small incision is made in the abdomen, and a fallopian tube is pulled out. The tube is either cut and tied back or clipped and allowed to slip back into place. The incision is sutured. The same procedure is repeated with the other fallopian tube.

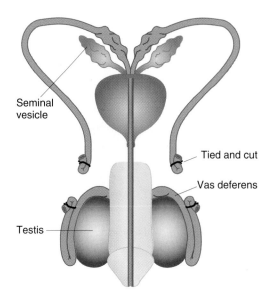

Seminal vesicle

Tied and cut

Vas deferens

Testis

Figure 14.7 *Vasectomy*

Vasectomy A male sterilization procedure in which the vas deferens are cut and tied to block the transport of sperm

Minilaparotomy A female sterilization procedure in which the fallopian tubes are cut to block transport of the egg

Tubal ligation A female sterilization procedure in which a surgical instrument is used to cut and tie back the fallopian tubes to block passage of the ova and thereby prevent fertilization

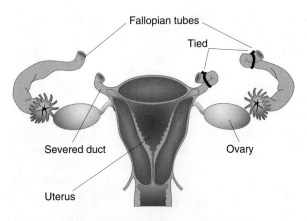

Figure 14.8 *Tubal Ligation*

Laparoscope A flexible surgical instrument with a cameralike attachment that can be inserted into the abdomen to view the fallopian tubes and other organs

Tubal Ligation Once anesthesia is administered and has taken effect, a small incision is made near the navel, and a **laparoscope** is inserted to locate the fallopian tubes. A surgical instrument is threaded through the laparoscope. It is used to cut and tie back the tube (see Figure 14.8). In some cases, the end of each tube is cauterized or plugged before being tied back. The same procedure is repeated with the other fallopian tube.

In 2002, Essure received FDA approval as a new method of sterilization for women. The advantage to the method is that it can be performed as an outpatient procedure without the use of general anesthesia. A physician inserts a small metal spring into each fallopian tube. The coils lead to the development of scar tissue in the tube, which effectively blocks the passageway. Because it takes approximately 3 months for the fallopian tubes to become blocked, women are advised to use a backup method for that period of time (Planned Parenthood, 2002d). Because access to sterilization has been compromised by the restructuring of the hospital system, with more hospital affiliations falling under the auspices and philosophy of the Catholic Church, a method that can be potentially performed in a physician's office or free-standing clinic becomes attractive.

Side Effects Both procedures require several days to a week to heal. Mild abdominal pain or tenderness is common. Intercourse may be resumed when the sutures heal and pain subsides.

As with a vasectomy, side effects are relatively rare. Minor complications may include infection and healing of the incision. As with any surgery, women confront risks related to anesthesia (Hatcher et al., 2003).

Terminating an Established Pregnancy

Abortion Termination of an established pregnancy through surgical or nonsurgical techniques

Viability A gestational weight of the fetus of at least 500 grams and/or age of 24 weeks of age

Established pregnancies can be terminated through surgical and medical means. **Abortion** is defined as the termination, spontaneous or induced, of an established pregnancy and relates to **viability.** A viable fetus has attained a weight of at least 500 grams and/or an age of 24 weeks (gestational age starting at conception). Because of improved reproductive technologies, fetuses have technically been viable earlier than 24 weeks, yet their health is often compromised.

About one-third of all abortions are *spontaneous abortions,* or miscarriages. They result from a variety of conditions ranging from physical trauma to a breakdown of the uterine lining. *Induced abortions* account for the remaining two-thirds. Induced abortions involve purposely ending an established pregnancy. The endometrium, placenta, and embryo or fetus are removed from the uterus. Abortion procedures are of several types, related to the length of the pregnancy and other extenuating circumstances.

Induced abortions have been legal in the United States since 1973, when two U.S. Supreme Court decisions, *Roe v. Wade* and *Doe v. Bolton,* determined that the decision to have a first-trimester abortion need concern only a woman and her physician. States could not use legislation to deny a woman's choice of first-trimester abortions. The ruling did allow states the ability to set standards for second- and third-trimester abortions. The overwhelming majority of women (88 percent) who terminate their pregnancies do so in the first trimester (Alan Guttmacher Institute, 2003a). For women who have had prenatal screenings and receive information about serious health problems in the fetus, a second-trimester

case study 14.3

Mindy's Experience with Abortion

Mindy, 29, is white.

Mindy is a successful small business owner, she has been married to Bob about 5 years, and they have a 2-year-old daughter. This is the account of her decision to have an abortion.

I grew up in a small town and was raised to think that abortion was killing. I remember seeing those films about little babies being tossed out in the garbage after their mothers had abortions and all the posters and billboards with pictures of fully developed fetuses and the headings "Abortion is murder." I couldn't imagine anyone ever having an abortion. But then I got pregnant and began to look at things differently.

I was away at college. I was a 19-year-old sophomore and had been having sex with my boyfriend, Michael, for about 6 months. We were using my diaphragm for birth control, and, to tell you the truth, I don't ever remember having any problems with it. I used it faithfully, every time we had sex.

I couldn't believe I was pregnant. I was frantic. I must have had five pregnancy tests until I finally accepted the fact. I couldn't have this baby! I cried for 2 days, and Michael was very supportive. Sometimes we cried together as we tried to figure out what to do. I knew in my heart that I wasn't ready to be a mother. I still had 3 years of school left, plus graduate school. I had no job, no time, and psychologically just couldn't handle it.

I went to a local abortion clinic. The people were great. They gave me all the information I needed, I took tests, and they assured me that because I was only 6 weeks pregnant, the procedure they would use was safe and relatively simple. I scheduled an appointment and went home to think about it.

It wasn't an easy decision, but I felt I had no acceptable choice. I didn't think I could handle being pregnant, having a baby, and then give it up for adoption or foster care. I didn't want to tell my parents. I wasn't sure how they'd react and didn't want to jeopardize my being away at school. They were paying for everything, and I wasn't sure if they'd force me to drop out.

I felt sad for a few weeks after my abortion. I wished I hadn't gotten pregnant and didn't have to make the decision, but sometimes life doesn't always work out the way you plan. I got over it gradually, finished out the school year, and graduated on time 2 years later. Now, 10 years later and the mother of a 2-year-old girl, I know I never could have been the mom I am now. Although it was a tough decision, it was the right one for me.

Critical Thinking

How do you feel about the decision that Mindy and Michael made about the pregnancy? What if they hadn't agreed to the same resolution to the unplanned pregnancy? How do you think you would have handled the same situation?

Use your Virtual Workbook to explore your answers to these questions at **http://health.wadsworth.com/blonna1.**

abortion becomes an option, particularly since amniocentesis results are not returned until the 18th week of gestation or later.

Third-trimester abortions remain very rare yet are extremely controversial and have been the focus of much legal wrangling and debate. The term *late-term abortion* is applied to cases where the viability of the fetus is not possible, and an attempted birth will leave serious health problems for the mother, resulting in termination during the third trimester. Opponents of the procedure refer to it as "partial birth abortion," a term that has worked its way into media and legislative discussions. In 2003, President George W. Bush signed the Partial Birth Abortion Ban Act, yet three federal courts issued temporary restraining orders against its enactment, claiming the language was vague and did not include preserving the mother's life.

Surgical Methods

Surgical methods include vacuum aspiration, dilation and curettage (D&C), dilation and evacuation (D&E), and hysterotomy.

Vacuum aspiration An induced abortion procedure in which uterine contents are removed by suction; used for early abortions

Suction curettage A surgical abortion procedure that removes the embryo and placenta from the uterus through suction and use of a curette

Cannula A tapered, strawlike tube used in the vacuum aspiration method of abortion

Vacuum Aspiration   **Vacuum aspiration** is the most widely used procedure for early abortions. It can be performed in a medical office or clinic for pregnancies less than 14 weeks gestation (Hatcher et al., 1998). It can be performed as outpatient surgery under local anesthesia and does not require an overnight stay in a hospital. The cost for the procedure varies between $225 and $575.

One form called *manual vacuum aspiration* (MVA) can be done up to 10 weeks and relies on suction alone. **Suction curettage** is performed from the end of the first month throughout the first trimester. It relies on both suction and the use of a *currette*, a narrow metal loop, to clean the walls of the uterus (Planned Parenthood, 2002a).

A vacuum aspiration abortion usually can be performed in approximately 10 minutes. It is safe and usually causes few side effects. The cervix is dilated, and a vacuum tube is inserted into the cervix. At the end of the tube is a **cannula,** which is attached to a vacuum pump (aspirator) used to suction off the contents of the wall of the uterus (endometrium, fetus/embryo, and placenta). Figure 14.9 (see page 458) shows this procedure.

Emotional and Spiritual Wellness

Spirituality plays a big role in how people evaluate fertility control methods and which ones they ultimately choose. Religions have various beliefs regarding fertility control, with variations from division to division, and sometimes region to region. From a broad perspective, all decisions about pregnancy relate to the underlying theme of interconnectedness. The decision to create a new life or to prevent the unintended creation of life is fundamentally a spiritual issue.

The decision to end a pregnancy is not made lightly. Some women don't even tell the male involved, choosing only to seek support from close friends. Deciding to have an abortion may be kept secret from parents and siblings as well. Both males and females may need counseling to deal with the emotional aspects of the decisions they've made.

When couples confront second-trimester abortions, they may find privacy not an option. Family, friends, and coworkers may have been aware of a planned pregnancy. Explanations about deciding to have a second-trimester abortion can be very difficult to share. Again, counseling and support groups can be very helpful.

Dilation and evacuation (D&E) A second-trimester abortion procedure in which the cervix is first dilated, and then the fetus removed by suction and curretage

Dilation and Evacuation (D&E)   **Dilation and evacuation (D&E)** combines the two previously described techniques and can be used in abortions up to the fifth month of gestation. The cervix is dilated, and most of the contents of the uterus are removed through suction. In preparation for the procedure, practitioners may insert a laminaria 6 to 24 hours prior; the laminaria is made of dried seaweed that expands and gently dilates the woman's cervix. Two other synthetic dilators, Lamicel and Dilapan, have also been used. They have the advantage of producing faster cervical dilation (Hatcher et al., 1998).

Like first-trimester abortions, women seek to terminate pregnancies in the second trimester for a variety of reasons. As discussed in Chapter 13, couples do not get the results of prenatal screening tests such as amniocentesis or chorionic villus sampling until the second trimester.

Because of the more advanced stage of fetal development, not all of the uterine contents can be removed through aspiration. A curette is inserted, and the remaining uterine contents are scraped out. General anesthesia or a paracervical block is required for the procedure.

Where Do I Really Stand on Abortion?

The issue of abortion elicits really strong reactions from many people. However, because it is such an emotional issue, many of us do not really examine how we think and feel about abortion. The following questions will help you reflect on your views and stand on abortion.

For the following statements, rank where you stand between the numbers 1 (strongly agree) to 10 (strongly disagree). If you are neutral, you could be a 5; you could be a 3 if you do not quite strongly agree, and so forth.

1. Even if a mother's life is at risk, she should not abort.
2. Married or unmarried, if the father does not agree to an abortion, the mother should not abort.
3. An unloved, unwanted, abused child would have been better off if his or her mother had chosen to abort.
4. Politicians do not have the right to say if a woman can or cannot have an abortion.
5. Abortions should be paid for through Medicaid for the poor who cannot afford an abortion.

Once you have taken your stand, ask some of your friends the same questions and see if they have the same views as you.

Hysterotomy **Hysterotomy** is a major surgical procedure used in second-trimester pregnancies. The procedure is similar to a cesarean section. An incision is made through the abdomen and uterus, and the fetus is removed and destroyed. This procedure is considered major surgery and requires general anesthesia and a hospital stay of several days. It is not used very often.

Surgical abortions are very safe procedures. They have a lower death rate (4 per 100,000 women) than carrying a pregnancy to full term (14 deaths per 100,000) women. Since the legalization of abortion in 1973, the death rate for the procedure has dropped steadily.

Medical Abortions

Medical abortions are those that do not involve surgical intervention but rather the use of medications to terminate a pregnancy. Figure 14.9 illustrates this method. Abortions can be induced by administering agents that work two ways: (a) by causing the uterus to contract and expel its contents or (b) by initiating the breakdown of the endometrium, making it impossible to sustain the pregnancy. Although some physicians use methotrexate, a drug more commonly associated with the treatment of cancer and rheumatic diseases, to induce abortion, the politics around nonsurgical abortion has focused primarily on the release of RU-486 in the United States.

RU-486 is the drug mifepristone and was marketed in 2000 as Mifeprex. It is an antiprogesterone drug that works by blocking the absorption of progesterone, the hormone necessary for continued viability of the endometrium. If progesterone is blocked, the uterine lining will no longer support fetal development. A second drug, misoprostol (a type of prostaglandin), is administered 3 to 7 days later, causing uterine contractions. These contractions cause the uterine lining and products of conception to be sloughed off within 24 hours (Nelson et al., 2000). Medical abortions can be performed up to the 9th week of pregnancy.

Hysterotomy A surgical procedure in which the fetus and placenta are removed surgically through an abdominal incision

RU-486 Known as the "abortion pill"; mifepristone, a drug used to induce menstruation by blocking the absorption of progesterone and thereby preventing the uterine lining from supporting an embryo

Medical abortion

Fallopian tube

Uterus

Ovary

Progesterone

Cervix

Fertilized egg

Progesterone, a hormone produced by the ovaries, is necessary for the implantation and development of a fertilized egg.

Progesterone

Mifepristone

Taken early in pregnancy mifepristone blocks the action of progesterone and makes the body react as if it isn't pregnant.

Prostaglandins

Prostaglandins, taken two days later, cause the uterus to contract and the cervix to soften and dilate. As a result, the fertilized egg is expelled in 97% of the cases.

Figure 14.9 *Abortion Methods Used in Early Gestation*

Vacuum aspiration

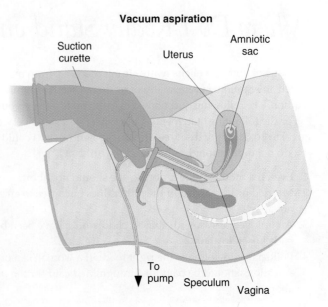

Suction curette

Uterus

Amniotic sac

To pump   Speculum   Vagina

sex in society 14.2

Some Facts About Abortion

Despite abortion being legal in the United States since *Roe v. Wade* in 1973, many women hesitate to talk openly about a procedure that an estimated 46 million women worldwide experience annually. Consider the following facts:

- Forty-nine percent of pregnancies among women in the United States are unintended, with half of them ending in abortion.
- Fifty-two percent of U.S. women obtaining abortions are under 25 years of age, with teens representing 19 percent of those seeking abortions.
- Black women are more than 3 times as likely as white women to have an abortion, and Hispanic women 2½ times as likely.
- Over 60 percent of abortions are among women who already have at least one child.
- About 13,000 women each year have abortions as a result of rape or incest.
- Fifty-four percent of women having abortions used a contraceptive method during the month they became pregnant.

- Eight percent of women having abortions have never used a method of birth control, with nonuse greatest among those who are young, unmarried, poor, black, Hispanic, or poorly educated.
- As much as 43 percent of the decline in abortion between 1994 and 2000 can be attributed to the availability of emergency contraception.
- The U.S. Congress has barred the use of federal Medicaid funds to pay for abortion except when the woman's life would be endangered by a full-term pregnancy or if the pregnancy resulted from rape or incest. Seventeen states do use public funds to pay for abortions for some women (Alaska, Arizona, California, Connecticut, Hawaii, Illinois, Massachusetts, Maryland, Maine, Montana, New Jersey, New Mexico, New York, Oregon, Vermont, Washington, and Wyoming).

Source: Alan Guttmacher Institute (2003a).

The Alan Guttmacher Institute reports that physicians use RU-486 and similar medications in about 6 percent of abortions performed during the first trimester (Associated Press, 2003). The expectation that women would prefer the medical procedure over a surgical one does not seem to be the case. Having to wait the longer amount of time for the procedure to be complete, along with having to expel the embryo possibly at home, makes the medical abortion in some ways more difficult. Most women whose first phase of treatment was with mifepristone will complete the abortion within hours of taking misoprostol. For those who first took methotrexate, about half have the abortion the same day; for others, completion could take days (Planned Parenthood, 2002a).

Prostaglandins Prostaglandins, discussed in Chapter 2, are responsible for causing the uterus to contract during menstruation. They also can be used to induce an abortion. Prostaglandins can be administered either by injection into the amniotic fluid or by insertion as vaginal suppositories. The prostaglandins initiate strong contractions, which dislodge the uterine lining and expel its contents.

Saline Solution Saline solution or urea acid is also used to induce nonsurgical abortion. Either can be injected into the amniotic fluid. These substances are toxic to the fetus and cause fetal death. This triggers the uterus to induce contractions, slough off the uterine lining, and expel its contents.

Table 14.4 gives the relative risks of death for activities including fertility control methods. This puts contraception into perspective.

Table 14.4 Relative Risks for Death from Various Activities Including the Prevention of Pregnancy

Activity	Chance of Death in a Year
Risks per year for men and women of all ages who participate in	
Motorcycling	1 in 1,000
Automobile driving	1 in 5,900
Power boating	1 in 5,900
Rock climbing	1 in 7,200
Playing football	1 in 25,000
Canoeing	1 in 100,000
Risks per year for women 15 to 44 years of age	
Using tampons	1 in 350,000
Having sexual intercourse (PID)	1 in 50,000
Risks for women preventing pregnancy	
Using oral contraceptives (per year)	
Nonsmoker	1 in 66,700
Age younger than 35 years	1 in 200,000
Ages 35–44	1 in 28,600
Heavy smoker (25 or more cigarettes per day)	1 in 1,700
Age younger than 35 years	1 in 5,300
Ages 35–44	1 in 700
Using IUDs (per year)	1 in 10,000,000
Using diaphragm, condom, or spermicides	None
Using fertility awareness methods	None
Undergoing sterilization:	
Laparoscopic tubal ligation	1 in 38,500
Hysterectomy	1 in 1,600
Vasectomy	1 in 1,000,000
Risk per pregnancy from continuing pregnancy	1 in 10,000
Risk from terminating pregnancy	
Legal abortion	
Before 9 weeks	1 in 262,800
Between 9 and 12 weeks	1 in 100,100
Between 13 and 15 weeks	1 in 34,400
After 15 weeks	1 in 10,200

Source: Contraceptive Technology (17th ed.), by Robert A. Hatcher et al., p. 230. © 1998 Ardent Media, Inc., New York. Used with permission.

Reactions to the Abortion Experience

Deciding to terminate a pregnancy is a decision women, often along with their partners, make with great thought. The reasons for having an abortion are varied. They include concerns for the physical and mental health of the mother, discovery of serious birth defects in the fetus, economic concerns of a couple regarding their ability to take care of another child, the break-up of a relationship and inability or desire to be a single parent, and concerns related to a pregnancy that resulted from rape or incest. The reasons are many, yet the one similarity for all is that *this* pregnancy is unwanted. Most women report the immediate feeling of relief, with the abortion representing the end to a crisis pregnancy.

Postabortion syndrome (PAS) is a term used to characterize the suggested long-term negative psychological effects of abortion. According to the National Right to Life Committee, "Post-abortion syndrome is a pattern of denial that may last for 5 to 10 years before emotional difficulties surface" (Levathes, 1995, p. 86). Women who have PAS may experience the following psychosocial effects: drug and alcohol abuse, personal relationship disorders, nightmares, sexual dysfunction, difficulty with communication, damaged self-esteem, and even suicide.

PAS activists are especially concerned about the possible negative psychological effects of RU-486. Unlike other abortion methods, which distance the woman from her aborted fetus, using RU-486 often results in the abortion occurring in a home setting in which the woman is confronted with having to dispose of fetal remains (Levathes, 1995).

The American Psychiatric Association (2000) does not recognize PAS, and PAS is not included in the most recent *Diagnostic and Statistical Manual*, which characterizes recognized psychological illnesses. Critics claim that much of the available data on the purported syndrome has come from "expert witnesses" in congressional hearings and anecdotal reports from physicians, clinicians, and women who have incurred ill effects after having abortions.

Abortion follow-up includes referral for postabortion counseling and group therapy for women who need these services to cope with their distress. Postabortion counseling and support groups are viable options for women who have emotional distress related to their abortions.

The decision to have an abortion is not an easy one to make. It is a complex moral and ethical decision that most women (and men) take seriously. The decision has both immediate- and long-term consequences that need to be taken into account. Overall, the decision to terminate an unwanted pregnancy becomes one of the many decisions couples make over the course of their reproductive years.

Postabortion syndrome (PAS) A controversial term referring to supposed long-term negative psychological effects of abortion

Your responses to the Personal Assessment, Thought Questions, and Test Yourself! quiz questions can be logged online in your Virtual Workbook at **http://health.wadsworth.com/blonna1.**

Personal Assessment

14.1 Is This the Right Method for Me?

It is important to choose a method of birth control that works well to prevent pregnancy. It is also important to choose a method you will like! Ask yourself these questions so you can judge carefully.

What type of birth control are you thinking about? _____

Have you ever used it before? _____ yes _____ no

If yes, how long did you use it? _____

_____

Circle your answer:

Are you afraid of using this method?	yes	no	don't know
Would you rather not use this method?	yes	no	don't know
Will you have trouble remembering to use this method?	yes	no	don't know
Have you ever become pregnant while using this method?	yes	no	don't know
Will you have trouble using this method carefully?	yes	no	don't know
Do you have unanswered questions about this method?	yes	no	don't know
Does this method make menstrual periods longer or more painful?	yes	no	don't know
Does this method cost more than you can afford?	yes	no	don't know
Does this method ever cause serious health problems?	yes	no	don't know
Do you object to this method because of religious beliefs?	yes	no	don't know
Have you already had problems using this method?	yes	no	don't know
Is your partner opposed to this method?	yes	no	don't know
Are you using this method without your partner's knowledge?	yes	no	don't know
Will using this method embarrass you?	yes	no	don't know
Will using this method embarrass your partner?	yes	no	don't know
Will you enjoy intercourse less because of this method?	yes	no	don't know
Will this method interrupt lovemaking?	yes	no	don't know
Has a nurse or doctor ever told you *not* to use this method?	yes	no	don't know

Do you have any "don't know" answers? Ask your instructor or physician to help you with more information.

Do you have any "yes" answers? "Yes" answers mean you may not like this method. If you have several "yes" answers, chances go up that you might not like this method; you may need to think about another method.

Source: Contraceptive Technology (17th ed.), by Robert A. Hatcher et al. © 1998 Ardent Media, Inc., New York. Used with permission.

Thought Questions

1. What are the differences among birth control, contraception, and family planning?

2. What are the five mechanisms of action for fertility control methods?

3. What is an acceptable level of risk of pregnancy for a fertility control method? Why?

4. What are the risks associated with pregnancy and childbirth for the various fertility control methods?

5. What category of fertility control methods offers the best protection against STDs? What are differences in STD protection among the methods in this category?

6. How do hormonal contraception measures work?

7. What risks are associated with the pill?

8. How do a person's (or couple's) fertility control needs change over the course of a lifetime?

9. What key questions should you ask yourself when evaluating any fertility control method?

Test Yourself!

1. Birth control methods are best described as techniques that enable couples to
   a. prevent births.
   b. prevent conception.
   c. prevent families.
   d. prevent implantation.

2. When couples choose a method of birth control, which issue is most critical to preventing a pregnancy?
   a. The theoretical effectiveness rate associated with the method
   b. Their willingness to use the method correctly and consistently
   c. Whether the method is prescriptive or over-the-counter
   d. Whether the method is hormonal or a barrier method

3. To practice natural family planning effectively, a woman must
   a. be able to communicate with her physician.
   b. purchase an ovulation kit.
   c. understand her menstrual cycle and fertile periods.
   d. abstain from any sexual contact for 6 to 8 days per month.

4. All but which of the following are considered barrier methods of birth control?
   a. Condom
   b. Diaphragm
   c. Vaginal sponge
   d. IUD

5. A woman who has trouble remembering dates and time periods would be wisest to choose which of the following methods of birth control?
   a. IUD
   b. Evra
   c. Birth control pill
   d. NuvaRing

6. Students who are concerned with protection against pregnancy and STDs would be wisest to use which form of birth control?
   a. The Evra patch
   b. NuvaRing
   c. Vaginal sponge
   d. Condom

7. Emergency contraception is effective up to _____ days after unprotected sexual intercourse.
   a. 3
   b. 5
   c. 1
   d. 10

8. A tubal ligation as a method of birth control might be an attractive choice to
   a. a single woman under 30 without children.
   b. a lesbian in a long-term relationship.
   c. a woman over 35 with children.
   d. a woman conflicted about motherhood.

9. Men who have had a vasectomy
   a. no longer ejaculate.
   b. no longer get erections.
   c. no longer have sperm in the ejaculate.
   d. no longer produce sperm.

10. The majority of women who terminate their pregnancies
    a. go on to experience posttraumatic stress disorders.
    b. do so in the first trimester of their pregnancies.
    c. rely on nonsurgical techniques such as oral medications.
    d. make the decision to do so around the 14th week of pregnancy.

Media Menu

You can link to the following online tools by visiting
http://health.wadsworth.com/blonna1.

Animation

Conception Simulator

 InfoTrac Activity

Hollander, D. (2003, January–February). Availability of emergency contraception through student health centers is growing, but gaps remain. *Perspectives on Sexual and Reproductive Health, 35* (1), 54–55.

 Web Resources

Alan Guttmacher Institute

www.guttmacher.org

A nonprofit institute protecting and expanding reproductive choices of women and men, including preventing unintended pregnancies, guaranteeing freedom to terminate unwanted pregnancies, protecting reproductive capacity and promoting wanted pregnancies, fostering women's health throughout pregnancy and childbirth, and promoting the birth of healthy infants. The site provides the latest statistics and the latest policy papers concerning these topics.

Feminist Women's Health Center (FWHC)

www.fwhc.org/homemast.htm

A nonprofit organization that promotes and protects a woman's right to choose and receive reproductive health care, including keeping abortion safe, legal, accessible, and acceptable. Articles are accessible on women's health, birth control, abortion, breast cancer, menopause, and resources.

Birthright International

www.birthright.org

A support organization to girls and women who experience distress from unplanned pregnancy. Provides alternatives to abortion; free pregnancy tests; legal, medical, financial, and legal assistance; referral to social agencies; and maternity and baby clothes.

Successful Contraception

www.arhp.org/success/index.html

A site of the Association of Reproductive Health Professionals, an interdisciplinary group composed of professionals who provide reproductive health services or education and conduct reproductive health research. This site link provides a survey for a profile of birth control options that seem best suited for you, based on your medical history and lifestyle; the survey takes approximately 15 minutes to complete.

NARAL Pro Choice America

www.naral.org

This organization, previously known as NARAL (National Abortion and Reproductive Rights Action League), is a key political action and educational organization designed to promote reproductive freedom. Its specific mission has been to track laws at the federal and state levels, educate voters, and keep legislators and the courts prochoice.

Planned Parenthood Federation of America (PPFA)

www.plannedparenthood.org

Planned Parenthood is both an advocacy group for reproductive rights as well as a major provider of reproductive health care services. It is also committed to providing comprehensive sexuality education.

American College of Obstetricians and Gynecologists

www.acog.com

The certifying organization of physicians who specialize in reproductive health. Its Web site provides information on birth control as well as providers.

References

Advocates for Youth. (2003). Contraceptive choices: Intrauterine device [Online]. Available: www.advocatesforyouth.org/teens/health/contraceptives/iud.htm.

Alan Guttmacher Institute. (2003a). Induced abortion. *Facts in Brief* [Online]. Available: www.guttmacher.org.

Alan Guttmacher Institute. (2003b, July/August). Method-related problems account for most failures of the female condom. *Perspectives on Sexual and Reproductive Health, 35*(4) [Online]. Available: www.agi-usa.org/pubs/journals/3519303.html.

Alan Guttmacher Institute. (2003c, January). Nowhere but up: Rising costs for Title X clinics. *Issues in Brief, 1.*

Allendale Pharmaceuticals. (2003). Today Sponge [Online]. Available: www.allendalepharm.com.

American Health Consultants. (1992, November). VCF: Convenient contraceptive, but it may be hard to find. *Contraceptive Technology Update, 13*(11), 1–2.

American Psychiatric Association. (2000). *Diagnostic and statistical manual* (4th ed., text revision). Washington, DC: Author.

Associated Press. (2003, January 16). Doctors use pills in 6 percent of abortions, group reports. *New York Times,* p. A20.

Baylor College of Medicine. (2002, September). Contraception now: New options, better choices [Online]. Available: www.contraceptiononline.org.

Cate, W., & Stone, K. M. (1992). Family planning, sexually transmitted diseases and contraceptive choice: A literature update—Part 1. *Family Planning Perspectives, 24*(2), 75–84.

Consumers Union. (1995, May). How reliable are condoms? *Consumer Reports,* pp. 320–325.

Davis, C., Blank, J., Lin, H. Y., & Bonillas, C. (1996). Characteristics of vibrator use among women. *Journal of Sex Research, 33*(4), 313–321.

Family Health International. (1996, Winter). Proper IUD use requires training. *Network, 16*(2) [Online]. Available: www.fhi.org.

Food and Drug Administration. (2003, September 5). FDA approves Seasonale oral contraceptive [Online]. FDA Talk Paper, T03-65. Available: www.fda.gov.

Glusker, A. (1995, November/December). The pill: What it's done for us, and to us. *Ms.,* pp. 30–32.

Haignere, C. S. (2002, March 20). *Sexual abstinence education: Is it really 100% effective?* Paper presented at the Advanced Sexuality Education Trainers Retreat, Swarthmore, PA.

Haignere, C. S., Gold, R., & McDanel, H. (1999, February). Adolescent abstinence and condom use: Are we sure we are really teaching what is safe? *Health Education & Behavior, 26*(1), 43–54.

Hatcher, R., Nelson, A. Zieman, M., Darney, P. Creinin, M., Stosur, H., & Cwiak, C. (2003). *Managing contraception.* Tiger, GA: Bridging the Gap Foundation.

Hatcher, R. A., Trussel, J., Stewart, F., Cates, W., Stewart, G., Guest, F., & Kowal, D. (1998). *Contraceptive technology* (17th ed.). New York: Arden Media.

Ilaria, G., Jacobs, J. L., Polsky, B., Koll, B., Baron, P., MacLow, C., Armstrong, D., & Schlegal, P. N. (1992). Detection of HIV-1DNA sequences in pre-ejaculatory fluid. *Lancet, 340*(8833), 1469.

Klitsch, M. (1995). Still waiting for the contraceptive revolution. *Family Planning Perspectives, 27*(6), 246–253.

Levathes, L. (1995, January/February). Listening to RU-486. *Health,* pp. 86–89.

McDonough, P. (1995, September/October). The safest sex. *Psychology Today,* pp. 47–49.

Murphy, R., & Allina, A. (2003, January/February). Improving access to emergency contraception. *Network News.*

NARAL. (2003, January 21). *Insurance coverage for contraception improves the health of women and families* [Online]. Available: www.naral.org.

NARAL & NARAL Foundation. (2001). *Who decides? A state-by-state review of abortion and reproductive rights* (10th ed.). Washington, DC: NARAL.

Nelson, A., Hatcher, R., Zieman, M., Watt, A., Darney, P., & Creinin, M. (2000). *Managing contraception.* Tiger, GA: Bridging the Gap Foundation.

Norris, K. (1996, September). Celibate passion. *Utne Reader,* pp. 51–53.

On the needless hounding of a safe contraceptive. *Economist, 336*(7930), 75–77.

Organon Inc. (2003). NuvaRing FAQs [Online]. Available: www.nuvaring.com/consumer/faqs.

Ortho-McNeil Pharmaceutical. (2003). Ortho Evra [Online]. Available: http://birthcontrol.orthoevra/faqs/faqs.html.

Petah Tikva, I. (2003, April). Does preejaculatory penile secretion originating from Cowper's gland contain sperm? *Journal of Assisted Reproduction and Genetics, 20*(4).

Pinkerton, S. D. (2001, February). A relative risk-based, disease-specific definition of sexual abstinence failure rates. *Health Education & Behavior, 28*(1), 10–20.

Planned Parenthood Federation of America. (2000). Norplant and you [Online]. Available: www.plannedparenthood.org/bc/norplant2.html.

Planned Parenthood Federation of America. (2002a, December). Abortion [Online]. Available: www.plannedparenthood.org/abortion.

Planned Parenthood Federation of America. (2002b, August). Fact sheet: Emergency contraception [Online]. Available: www.ppfa.org/library/Birthcontrol/EC.html.

Planned Parenthood Federation of America. (2003c, November). Facts about birth control [Online]. Available: www.plannedparenthood.org/bc/bcfacts.

Planned Parenthood Federation of America. (2002d, November 4). FDA approves innovative non-incision permanent birth control procedure for women [Online]. Available: www.plannedparenthood.org/About/pr/021105_birthcontrol.html.

Planned Parenthood Federation of America. (2003a). Future birth control methods for men [Online]. Available: www.plannedparenthood.org/articles/bcfuture_m.html.

Planned Parenthood Federation of America. (2003b, October). Planned Parenthood counseling patients about voluntary recall of the once-a-month injectable hormonal contraceptive Lunelle [Online]. Available: www.plannedparenthood.org/about/pr/021010_lunelle.html.

Prudney, J., Oneta, M., Mayer, K., Seage, G., & Andersen, D. (1992). Pre-ejaculatory fluid as a potential vector for the transmission of HIV-1. *Lancet, 340*(8833), 1470.

Women often unaware of emergency contraception. (2002, March). *SIECUS Report.*

chapter *fifteen*

Sexually Transmitted Diseases (STDs)

Student Learning Objectives

After reading this chapter, students will be able to

- Describe the major STD trends of the past decade.
- Diagram and describe the Pyramid of Risk for STD/HIV infection.
- Explain how demographic variables are related to STD/HIV risk.
- Describe how sexual orientation affects STD/HIV risk.
- Describe the characteristics of core transmitters of STD, including HIV.
- Evaluate the relationship between sexual/medical history and STD/HIV risk.
- Assess a variety of sexual lifestyles and the continuum of risk for STD that they represent.
- Evaluate the risks inherent in a variety of sexual behaviors.
- Develop a personal plan for reducing the risk for STD/HIV infection.
- Describe the major modes of STD/HIV transmission.
- Describe the major symptoms associated with STD/HIV infection.
- Describe the epidemiology of a variety of STDs.

Test your understanding of these objectives by taking the end-of-chapter quiz, available online at **http://health.wadsworth.com/blonna1.**

activity teaser: *Why should you wait to have sex? Find out with the Personal Exploration Activity on page 481.*

case study 15.1

Yolanda: Assessing the Risk

Yolanda, 22, single, identifies as Latina.

Yolanda, a student in a human sexuality class, expressed the following concerns about finding out about her sex partners' medical histories:

It looks like I'm going to have to spend a lot more time getting to know my sex partners before I take a chance of having sex with them without condoms. Up until today I thought I was a responsible lady because I'm on the pill and take responsibility for my sexuality. I always thought the pill would protect me against STDs. Boy, was I wrong. I never realized that there was so much to find out about a guy before you could tell if he was a threat to you.

I used to try to sneak a look to see if he had any symptoms, but now you're saying there are lots of other things that are important about his sexual past that I need to know about. I'm not sure what I'm going to do, but I know I'll never let any guy in there bareback until I can answer all those questions about him.

Critical Thinking

How does one actually acquire from a potential sex partner the type of detailed sexual/medical information necessary to make an informed decision about the STD risks posed by that individual?

Use your Virtual Workbook to explore your answer to this question at **http://health.wadsworth.com/blonna1.**

Sexually transmitted diseases (STDs) Diseases that are spread from person to person through sexual contact

Sexually transmitted diseases (STDs), also known as sexually transmitted infections (STIs), are infections that are almost always contracted through sexual contact. We will continue to use the term *STDs* because it is the term of choice used by the Centers for Disease Control, the lead agency in the United States for the control of infectious diseases. Although STDs theoretically can be transmitted via any form of sexual contact, vaginal and anal intercourse are much more *efficient* modes of transmission than is oral-genital sexual contact. Some STDs, such as HIV and hepatitis B, also are transmitted by contaminated blood through needle sharing associated with injection drug use (Eng & Butler, 1997).

More than 65 million people in the United States are currently infected with an incurable sexually transmitted disease, and each year an additional 15 million people develop new cases of one or more of the 25 diseases categorized as STDs. Of these new cases, roughly half are incurable, lifelong infections (Division of STD Prevention [DSTD], 2000; Cates et al., 1999). STDs represent 87 percent of the cases of the diseases reported to the Centers for Disease Control and Prevention. Five of the top 10 most frequently reported diseases in the United States are STDs (DSTD, 2002). The STD **epidemic** is really a series of epidemics since we are really talking about over two dozen different types of infections, many of which are asymptomatic (without symptoms). Because of the asymptomatic nature of many STDs, many of those who are infected go undiagnosed. This situation has led public health officials to refer to the problem as the "hidden epidemic" (DSTD, 2000).

Epidemic Levels of infection in populations that exceed those normally expected for that population

Tracking the hidden epidemic is difficult to do because individuals with asymptomatic diseases do not even know they are infected. Their infections go undiagnosed as they continue to infect others. For a variety of public health reasons, not all STDs are reportable by law. Consequently, surveillance of these diseases by public health officials requires periodic surveys of health care providers to assess the full magnitude of the problem. Often, STDs and other communicable diseases present trends that help enable us to understand who is at greatest risk and what the key risk factors are.

Table 15.1 Estimated Incidence and Prevalence of Common STDs

STD	Incidence (estimated new cases every year)	Prevalence (estimated number of people currently infected)
Chlamydia	3 million	2 million
Gonorrhea	650,000	Not available
Syphilis	70,000	Not available
Herpes	1 million	45 million
Human papilloma virus (HPV)	5.5 million	20 million
Hepatitis B	120,000	417,000
Trichomoniasis	5 million	Not available
Bacterial vaginosis	Not available	Not available

Source: DSTD (2000).

Besides the asymptomatic nature of some STDs, another problem associated with understanding and tracking STD trends relates to how they are tabulated and reported. STD statistics are generally presented as **rates.** There are two types of rates: (a) **incidence rates,** which measure new cases and assess the risk of the spread of new cases of disease, and (b) **prevalence rates,** which measure the prevailing number of old and new cases and are a good barometer on the full impact of the condition as a public health problem. Acute infections that can be cured with antibiotics, such as syphilis, gonorrhea, and chlamydia, are typically reported and analyzed using incidence rates. Chronic diseases that can be treated but not cured such as HIV/AIDS, genital herpes, and human papilloma virus (HPV) are often reported and analyzed using prevalence rates. Table 15.1 shows the incidence and prevalence rates of commons STDs.

Epidemiological Synergy

Wasserheit (1992) coined the term **epidemiological synergy** to refer to the effects of infection with one STD on the transmission and development of complications of another. Generally this works two ways:

- Infection with one STD provides an entry point where other STD pathogens can invade.
- Infection with one form of STD could weaken the body's immune system, making exposure to another infection more risky.

An example of the former is the synergistic effect between genital ulcer diseases such as chancroid, genital herpes, and syphilis and increased susceptibility to HIV infection. The ulcerative lesions caused by chancroid, genital herpes, and syphilis literally provide an entry point for HIV.

Someone who has a genital ulcer and has sex with a person who is infected with HIV is more likely to become infected as a result. The epidemic of syphilis among men who have sex with men (MSM) in six major U.S. cities (discussed later) illustrates this phenomenon. Twenty to 73 percent of these men had coexisting HIV infection (MMWR [Morbidity and Mortality Weekly Report], 2002b).

Rates Statistics calculated by dividing the number of cases of disease by the population at risk of infection

Incidence rates Rates of new infection used to measure the likelihood of becoming infected

Prevalence rates Rates of prevailing infection used to measure the extent of the overall threat faced by the public

Epidemiological synergy The distribution of disease caused by the effects of infection with more than one condition

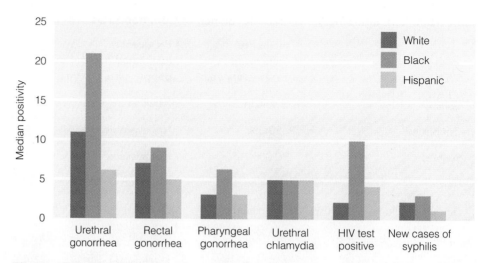

Figure 15.1 *Men Who Have Sex with Men* Health officials are alarmed at the dramatic rise in the numbers of cases of STDs among select groups of men who have sex with other men.
Source: DSTD (2002).

Genital ulcer disease may increase the risk of transmission per exposure 10 to 50 times in male-to-female transmission, and 50 to 300 times in female-to-male exposure (Hayes, Schulz, & Plummer, 1995). Figure 15.1 shows the high percentage of MSM attending public STD clinics who are infected with various STDs.

In comparison, consider infection with tuberculosis. Tuberculosis (TB), a communicable disease, has dropped 10-fold (from 53 to 5.6 cases per 100,000 people) since 1953. Although not a sexually transmitted disease, TB is an opportunistic infection among people with HIV and must be followed closely in this population (Division of TB Elimination [DTB], 2001). Infection with HIV weakens the immune system and the body's ability to resist exposure to new disease-causing organisms. A person who is HIV-positive and is exposed to tuberculosis is at greater risk for acquiring the infection than a person who is not HIV-positive (Finelli, Budd, & Spitalny, 1993). The coexistence of HIV with these other conditions also makes diagnosis, treatment, and follow-up much more difficult.

STD Transmission, Signs, and Symptoms

STDs can be grouped in several ways to study their transmission, symptoms, treatment, and prevention. Table 15.2 provides a summary of the transmission, symptoms, diagnosis, and treatment of the most common STDs.

One simple way to group STDs is by the nature of transmission. The main modes of STD transmission are as follows:

- Direct sexual contact (sexual contact with someone's STD symptoms, such as genital ulcers) or sexual contact with someone's infected semen, vaginal lubricant, blood, and other body fluids
- Maternal transfer (mother to fetus during pregnancy or childbirth)
- Sharing contaminated needles through injectable drug use

Minor STDs, such as crabs and scabies, can be passed through direct sexual contact with infected persons or, in rare cases, their contaminated bedding, items of clothing, and similar objects. Some STDs (such as HIV and hepatitis B) can be spread both by sexual contact and by injectable drug use.

Table 15.2 Common STDs, Their Source, Symptoms, Diagnosis, and Treatment

Name	Source	Signs and Symptoms	Diagnosis	Treatment
Chlamydia	Bacterium	Male: Watery discharge; pain when urinating Female: Usually asymptomatic; sometimes a similar discharge to men's; leading cause of pelvic inflammatory disease (PID)	Men: Culture of discharge from urethra Female: Cervical culture	Antibiotics other than penicillin
Gonorrhea (clap)	Bacterium	Male: Pus discharge from urethra; burning during urination Female: Usually asymptomatic; can lead to PID and sterility in both men and women	Male: Culture of discharge Female: Cervical culture	Antibiotics (ceftriaxone)
Genital herpes	Virus	Blisters in genital and rectal area	Presence of blisters and laboratory identification of virus in fluid of blister	Zovirax (acyclovir prescription)
Venereal warts	Virus (HPV)	Cauliflower-like growths in genital and rectal areas	Presence of lesions	Removal of lesions by laser surgery or chemicals
Syphilis	Bacterium (spirochete)	Primary: Chancre Secondary: Rash Latent: Asymptomatic Late: Irreversible damage to central nervous system, cardiovascular system	Blood test	Penicillin or other antibiotic
HIV/AIDS	Virus	Asymptomatic at first; opportunistic infections	Blood test, usually none in initial stages	AZT (now called ZDV; not a cure)
Chancroid	Bacterium (*Bacillus*)	Male: Painful irregular chancre on penis Female: Chancre on labia	Smear/stain and microscopic identification	Tetracycline
Pubic lice (crabs)	Metazoan	Intense itching of areas covered with pubic hair	Presence of lice and nits (eggs) on pubic hair	Prescription or over-the-counter shampoo

During sexual exposure to genital ulcers or other symptoms (such as genital warts), the uninfected person is exposed to infectious organisms that are present in the **serous fluid** of the lesions. During sexual contact, these pathogens are transmitted through the thrusting and grinding of sexual activity. The organisms are introduced into tiny breaks in the skin that commonly occur during sexual activity.

During sexual exposure to semen, vaginal lubricants, blood, and other body fluids, the infected partner passes the infection through unprotected vaginal or

Serous fluid A fluid that has the characteristics of serum anal intercourse or oral sex. During sexual exposure to contaminated blood, STD organisms that live in the blood are passed between individuals as they exchange this body fluid. Blood is exchanged from person to person most commonly through (a) sexual contact with someone who has open lesions or ulcers that bleed during sex or (b) sexual contact that involves unlubricated anal intercourse and some vaginal intercourse.

STD micro-organisms can be passed by maternal transfer two ways:

- During pregnancy, STD micro-organisms in the mother's blood pass through the placenta and enter the bloodstream of the fetus.
- During labor and delivery, the newborn is exposed directly to disease-causing germs present in the birth canal.

Any type of shared injectable drug use is capable of transmitting blood-borne STDs. The transmission could be by an athlete shooting steroids and then passing the unsterilized needle to a friend to use, or it could be by a heroin addict doing the same. The risk is in the sharing, not the drug of choice.

In most cases, infestation with scabies and crabs occurs during sexual contact. A person whose genitals are infected with the lice pass on the crabs or scabies during sexual contact with an uninfected sex partner. Lice also are able to live on clothing and bedding and, in rare cases, can be spread via these inanimate objects.

Prevention and Risk Reduction

Personal health STD/HIV prevention programs focus largely on individual behavior as the basis for risk reduction. Many of these programs emphasize "safer sex" (using condoms consistently and correctly and verifying HIV status through testing) as the primary prevention approach. Others stress abstinence from sexual intercourse as the preferred preventive approach (Howard & McCabe, 1990).

Community health prevention programs emphasize public health interventions designed to stop the diseases from spreading. Examples of activities are political lobbying to establish needle exchange programs, increased funding of STD/HIV services (for example, to allow expanded hours), free and confidential treatment, and sociomarketing to promote condom distribution and family planning services.

The problem with compartmentalizing STD/HIV risks is that it fails to acknowledge that personal and community risks have a synergistic effect. We propose a new way to conceptualize the relationship between community and personal risks as pyramidal in nature, consisting of various public and personal factors that build upon each other. Figure 15.2 illustrates this Pyramid of Risk.

The foundation of the pyramid is made up of demographic variables that influence STD/HIV risk. These are generally beyond our individual control.

The next level of risk revolves around the sexual and medical history of ourselves or our partners. Because these risks are part of a person's past, they also cannot be changed. They are the history that each of us brings to any sexual encounter.

Sexual lifestyle The interaction between types and numbers of current sex partners

The third level of risk represents a person's current **sexual lifestyle,** the interaction between the types and numbers of current sex partners. The last level of risk is the one most educators focus on: personal sexual behavior. Most risk reduction pamphlets provide a laundry list of sexual behaviors that range from low risk to high risk. Although the four levels of factors influence STD/HIV risk independently, the interaction of levels can have a synergistic effect that can increase or reduce personal risk dramatically.

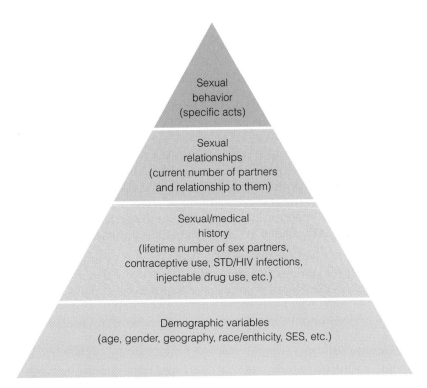

Figure 15.2 *A Pyramid of Risk for STDs* To assess one's true risk of acquiring STDs, demographic and sexual/medical history risks must be combined with behavioral and lifestyle factors.

Demographic Variables and the Distribution of STDs/HIV

Seven major demographic variables that contribute to STD/HIV risk are age, gender, sexual orientation, injecting drug user (IDU; the clustering of injectable drug users in communities), geography, socioeconomic status (SES), and race/ethnicity.

Age There are more cases of STDs distributed throughout people aged 15 to 25 than in any other age group. Because more cases exist in this age group, the risk of acquiring an infection is greater if someone has sex with persons from this age category (versus the 55+ age group, in which STD rates are much lower). The risk is associated with the likelihood that someone will interact sexually with a member of this subpopulation.

Sexually active teenagers have the highest rates of infection with almost all STDs. Trends in gonorrhea infection illustrate this best. Teenage girls had the highest risk of becoming infected. Rates for females in the 15- to 19-year-old age groups were 716 cases per 100,000 people. This was more than five times the national rate (about 132/100,000) (DSTD, 2001). Young women were approximately 20 times more likely to be infected with gonorrhea than females 30 years of age and older (Webster, Berman, & Greenspan, 1993; DSTD, 2000, 2001).

Other age-related STD considerations are as follows:

- The earlier the onset of intercourse (first time a person has sexual intercourse), the greater their potential exposure to different sex partners over their lifetime. There is an association between lifetime number of sex partners and increased risk of acquiring STDs.

- Individuals who initiate sexual activity earlier are more likely to have more sex partners over a lifetime (more than 25 percent of women initiating intercourse by age 15 had more than 10 lifetime sex partners, whereas only 6 percent of women initiating intercourse at age 20 or later had more than 10 sex partners).
- Adolescents and young adults are more likely than older adults to have multiple (sequential or concurrent) sexual partners.
- Adolescents and young adults are more likely than older adults to engage in unprotected sexual intercourse.
- The partners of adolescents and young adults are more likely to be at higher risk for having an STD than the partners of older adults.
- The transformation zone in women (the end of the cervix, where cervical tissue meets vaginal tissue) is most exposed during adolescence, and this tissue is most susceptible to STD infection in general and viral infection (cancer-causing) in particular (DSTD, 2000; Quinn & Cates, 1993; Alan Guttmacher Institute, 1991).

Data from the 2001 National Youth Risk Behavior Survey indicate new positive trends in sexual behavior among adolescents. Analysis of data from 1991 to 2001 shows a decrease in the overall percentage of high school students who have ever had sexual intercourse and who had multiple sex partners. Additionally, the study showed that condom use among students who were sexually active increased during that time period.

Unfortunately, reported condom use has leveled off since 1999. The lone disturbing finding of the study was an increased use, among sexually active teenagers, of alcohol or drugs before their last reported episode of sexual intercourse (MMWR, 2002e).

Gender   The risk for STDs/HIV is different for men and women. Biological gender is a risk factor related to the genetic, anatomical, and physiological differences between men and women (Kennedy, Scarlett, Duer, & Chu, 1995). Women face a greater risk than men for both acquiring a sexually transmitted disease and developing complications for several reasons:

- Heterosexual women are receptive sexually—vaginally, orally, and anally. This greatly increases their risks for initial infection by exposing a greater surface area of mucosal tissue (Quinn & Cates, 1993). Once infected with most STDs, heterosexual women tend to be asymptomatic more often than heterosexual men. Most heterosexual men notice initial symptoms of infection, whereas about half of women are asymptomatic (Morse, Moreland, & Thompson, 1990).
- Because of the asymptomatic nature of STDs in women, more women than men do not seek treatment during the initial stages of infection. This delayed access to treatment results in progression of the disease and a greater likelihood of developing complications. For example, about 15 percent of women develop complications associated with gonorrhea or chlamydia versus less than 1 percent of men (Morse et al., 1990).
- Menstruation plays a role in facilitating the movement of pathogens from the lower reproductive tract (below the cervix) to the upper parts, facilitating the development of complications. Women face the added risk of passing on their infection to their developing fetus during pregnancy or newborn through childbirth (Smeltzer & Whipple, 1991). The likelihood of transmitting infections such as syphilis or HIV is greatly reduced if mothers attend routine prenatal screening and receive treatment.

Sexual Orientation   Risks for STDs are affected by a person's sexual orientation. The risks that heterosexual women face accrue as a result of their anatomy and physiology, which facilitate exposure to disease agents. Sexual exposure results in infection without symptoms, and menstruation facilitates infection.

case study 15.2

Jim

Jim, 24, single, is white.

Jim was a student in Dr. Blonna's human sexuality class. Jim came to see him after class about some concerns regarding STDs.

You've got to help me. I made a mistake, and I'm superparanoid about what's going to happen to me. I was coming back to school last Friday night late, and I was cruising through Paterson [a large city adjacent to the town where the college campus is located]. I don't know what got into me, but I picked up a hitchhiker on Broadway and gave her a ride to the end of Paterson. She was really hot and offered to give me a blow job to thank me.

I said yes, and she went down on me in the parking lot where she lived. I don't know how to describe how I felt afterward—part ashamed, part stupid, part afraid. I'm so worried that I got AIDS from her.

On Monday in class, you talked about demographic risks, and the whole thing got me freaked. My girlfriend wanted to have sex last night, and I used a condom with her. She freaked out. She's on the pill, and we never use condoms. I broke down and had to tell her what I did. Am I going to die of AIDS?

Critical Thinking

What other sexual options did Jim have following his ride with the hitchhiker?

Use your Virtual Workbook to explore your answer to this question at **http://health.wadsworth.com/blonna1.**

Gay and bisexual men have some of the risks that heterosexual women do. They are receptive sexually and tend to have asymptomatic infections. This facilitates the development and spread of disease. In addition, certain diseases, such as HIV and hepatitis B, exist in **endemic** levels in the gay community. These diseases are incurable and capable of causing death (American Medical Association [AMA], 1996; Alter & Margolis, 1990).

Heterosexual men are at less risk than heterosexual women and gay men for a variety of reasons. First, their symptoms tend to be more obvious because these men usually are the insertive sexual partners and develop external symptoms. Early detection facilitates seeking prompt treatment and reducing complications. As an example, fewer than 1 percent of all heterosexual men infected with gonorrhea develop complications such as **epididymitis** (Morse et al., 1990). Also, female-to-male transmission of STDs is more difficult because heterosexual men are not receptive sexually, and vaginal fluids are less likely to transmit infection than is contaminated semen (Eng & Butler, 1997).

Of the four groups, lesbian women have the lowest rates of infection. Lesbian women tend to have fewer sexual partners over the course of their lifetime, and they do not engage in vaginal or anal intercourse (Kennedy et al., 1995).

IDU The risk for STD/HIV is becoming increasingly related to the prevalence of **IDUs** (injectable drug users) in a community. Drug use is associated with increased STD/HIV risk in two ways.

- Psychoactive drugs impair users' ability to make good decisions regarding sexual behavior. Therefore, engaging in safer sex becomes less likely when a person is using psychoactive drugs. And good choice of partner(s) is impaired by psychoactive drug use.
- Injectable drug use often involves needle sharing between users. This facilitates the transmission of blood-borne infections such as HIV and hepatitis B if one of the users is infected.

Endemic A 20 percent level of ongoing infection within a specific population

Epididymitis Inflammation of the small oblong body that rests upon and beside the surface of the testes

IDU The acronym for *injectable drug user*

The drugs most often involved are crack cocaine and injectable heroin. A vicious cycle of drug abuse, exchanging sex for money or other resources, unsafe sex, and infection with a variety of genital ulcer diseases has occurred since the mid-1980s. This cycle is intimately related to the resurgence of syphilis and other diseases in urban America. The effects are most notable among young, urban, black and Hispanic/Latino men and women.

Urban/Rural and Geographic Differences STDs including HIV are disproportionately higher in urban areas than in rural or suburban locations (DSTD, 2002). "Core urban populations" may be a major contributing factor for higher STD rates in urban communities and disproportionately high personal risk, despite individual behavior (Garnett & Anderson, 1996). The rate of acquisition of gonorrhea, for instance, in core urban populations is as much as 300 times higher than in the rest of the population (Rice, Roberts, & Handsfield, 1991). With a high level of infection and prevalence of deadly diseases, any sexual activity (even so-called safer sex) between or with members of this population carries a higher degree of risk than the same behavior with non–core group people.

Social and Environmental Wellness

STDs used to be called "social diseases" because of the nature of sexual transmission. Social wellness is a major preventive strategy against STDs. Being in a mutually exclusive, monogamous, disease-free relationship is the best prevention against STDs. In the United States, the quality of one's social environment seems to be directly proportional to socioeconomic status (SES). As SES rises, most Americans seek out safer, healthier communities, and safe communities carry much lower risk for STDs. High-risk/low-wellness communities should be targeted for STD prevention and treatment services and programs.

Socioeconomic Status (SES) To a large extent, STDs mimic other chronic diseases. SES can either facilitate or hinder access to preventive and interventive STD health care. People of lower SES tend to lack enabling factors related to prevention and treatment of STDs such as health care insurance and access to treatment services. Even though free public clinics are available, they may not be utilized promptly because poor people often lack access to transportation, don't have sick days if they are employed, or are unaware of the availability of free care (Donelan et al., 1996).

Also, people of lower SES often do not perceive themselves to be at great risk for STDs/HIV and tend not to respond to symptoms promptly or consistently practice preventive behavior (Ramos, Shain, & Johnson, 1995). Poverty and lower SES, too, contribute to higher levels of drug use—a major risk factor for STDs/HIV (Potterat, Rothenberg, Woodhouse, Muth, Pratts, & Fogle, 1985).

Race/Ethnicity African Americans and Hispanics continue to have the highest rates of STD infection in the United States. Rates for almost all STDs are substantially higher for these groups than for whites. Risk for certain STDs like gonorrhea and syphilis are as much as 30 times higher for African Americans than for whites (DSTD, 2000). Part of that disparity is attributed to the higher use of public health clinics by African Americans than whites. Public clinics tend to have more complete reporting of STDs than private health care providers (DSTD, 2000).

sex in society 15.1

Core Transmitters of STDs

STDs seem to be much more common in certain pockets of the population. These pockets occur mostly in urban areas among specific subpopulations of sexually active people called *core groups*. People in core groups (mostly urban African American and Latino lower-SES young men and women) have a disproportionate risk for acquiring STDs. The risk of transmission of STDs among a core group is 300 to 600 times greater than among the U.S. population in general. The following factors are related to transmission of STDs in the core population:

Endemic levels of infection (20 percent or more of the population infected) (Eng & Butler, 1997)

High concentrations of infected persons in small geographic areas (DSTD, 2000). Only 5.9 percent of census tracts accounted for 51 percent of cases of STDs, and an additional 9 adjacent census tracts accounted for 72 percent of cases and 74 percent of sexual contacts) (Garnett & Anderson, 1996).

High levels of intergroup sexual activity and socializing (Piot & Islam, 1994). Of those infected with STDs, 51 percent had picked up their sexual partners in the same location (only 2 percent of all the bars and clubs in town) (Webster et al., 1993).

High levels of repeat infections. Small percentages of infected individuals accounted for large percentages of multiple infections (Garnett & Anderson, 1996).

High levels of multiple STD infections (coexisting infection with gonorrhea and chlamydia; syphilis and HIV; HIV and chancroid) (Nakashima et al., 1996).

Longer than average duration of infectivity (because of a delay in seeking treatment) *and rate of asymptomatic infection* among core group members (Garnett & Anderson, 1996)

High levels of substance abuse and *higher levels of sex for drugs* than non–core group patients (Finelli et al., 1993)

Although disease rates in general are higher for blacks and Hispanics than whites, racial/ethnic differences are often markers for social class and poverty (Navarro, 1990). Poverty, especially that which affects the urban poor, is the true risk factor. The increased problem of STDs in minority populations in inner cities may stem in part from the unequal distribution of poverty, not race or ethnicity (Navarro, 1990). A greater proportion of blacks and Hispanics/Latinos live at or below poverty than whites. Socioeconomic differentials (often referred to as *class differentials*) are larger than race differentials in **morbidity.** When studies control for SES differentials, racial differences in disease distribution drop markedly. The problem of STDs in minority populations in inner cities is a result, in part, of the unequal distribution of SES (Navarro, 1990).

Morbidity The relative incidence of a disease

Sexual/Medical History

The next level of risk on the pyramid is sexual medical history. This is something we cannot control because it has occurred in the past. Yet, a person's sexual and medical history can greatly influence the present level of risk for STDs/HIV. The following are sexual/medical factors most associated with the current risk for STDs/HIV:

Lifetime number of sexual partners. In general, the greater the number, the higher the risk. Threshold levels of "safe" sexual activity have been identified (Dan, 1996). Once the threshold number of sexual partners is reached, the risk for disease increases exponentially.

Contraceptive use. Barrier contraceptive users have the lowest rates of infection. They are followed by other contraceptive users and nonusers, who have the highest risk (Rosenberg & Gollub, 1992).

Incidence The number of new cases of a disease during a specific time period

History of IDU. Persons with a history of IDU have an increased **incidence** of infection with blood-borne diseases, particularly HIV and hepatitis B (Alter & Margolis, 1990; Finelli et al., 1993).

Prior STD history. Persons who have been infected with STDs in the past are more likely to become infected again than those who have never been infected (Darrow, Barrett, McPhil, & Young, 1981).

Sexual Relationships

Sexual relationship refers to the connections between people rather then the specific behaviors in which they engage. In general, the risk for STDs/HIV decreases as sexual relationships move away from multiple, anonymous, sexual encounters toward monogamous (with uninfected partner), trusting partnerships. STD/HIV sexual relationship risks are specifically related to overall numbers of partners and the quality of the relationship (trust, understanding, and knowledge of one's partner). Figure 15.3 shows the continuum of risks for sexual relationships.

There are two dimensions of lifestyle of partner risk:

Familiarity risk. Familiarity risk is synonymous with *anonymity.* Laumann, Gagnon, Michael, and Michaels (1994) operationally defined the extent of familiarity along a continuum that measured how long the study subjects knew their partners before having sex with them. Their findings confirmed that the less familiar one is with the sex partner (the greater the anonymity), the greater is the risk. Anonymity is a risk factor because it influences the ability to make an informed choice about the risk for STD/HIV.

Exclusivity risk. Laumann et al. (1994) call the second variable *exclusivity*—the quality of the sexual relationship. Exclusivity, they believe, has to be examined for *both* partners. If one partner is monogamous but the other is not, the benefits of exclusivity are lost. Furthermore, if an uninfected person is monogamous with someone who has an STD, exclusivity can actually increase the risk by increasing the extent of exposure. For exclusivity to work, both partners have to be uninfected and monogamous. Subjects (and partners) who were not sexually exclusive were at increased risk for acquiring an STD (Lauman et al., 1994).

The highest risks were associated with the "interaction of risky partners" (lack of exclusivity and familiarity) and many partners. This sexual lifestyle, which combines multiple partners with anonymous sexual encounters, creates a deadly synergy that increases the risk exponentially (Lauman et al., 1994).

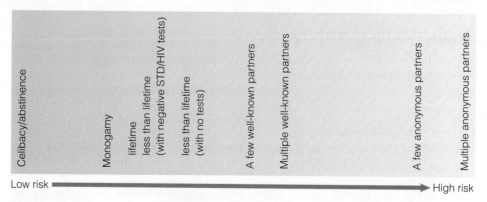

Figure 15.3 *Continuum of Risk for Sexual Relationships* STD risks increase as relationships become less familiar and exclusive.

case study 15.3

Lillie's Risk

Lillie, 43, divorced, is white.

Lillie is a continuing student who made these comments in class:

Thank you! Finally, someone has said what I believed all along: It's not just sexual behavior that's the risk. It's the behavior in the context of a relationship that determines risk. I was always so annoyed and insulted when sex educators told me that I should always insist that my partner wear a condom and that any woman who is sexually active is at equal risk of becoming infected. I always felt that as long as I had one uninfected partner, and the two of us were monogamous, I was at low risk.

It's funny because even though I'm not married, my boyfriend (of 3 years) is less of a threat to me than my husband used to be. My ex-husband was always cheating on me, and I was worried that even though I was monogamous, he'd bring something home to me.

I fully trust my current boyfriend. We've been monogamous (though unmarried) for 3 years, and I've never felt safer. We spent a lot of time building the trust and commitment in our relationship. I have great sex with him because I can fully relax and trust him, even though I've never gone down the list of things I need to know about his sexual past. We did talk about whether either of us ever had a viral STD, because viruses are forever.

Critical Thinking

Do you agree with Lillie's assessment of her STD risk? Why or why not?

Use your Virtual Workbook to explore your answers to these questions at **http:// health.wadsworth.com/ blonna1.**

Sexual Behavior

At the top of the Pyramid of Risk is sexual behavior. In general, as illustrated in Figure 15.4, the risks increase as behaviors incorporate unprotected insertion and ejaculation. The lower-risk behaviors are nonpenetrative and do not involve an exchange of bodily fluids. As we move along the continuum of risk, the behaviors reflect attempts to utilize barrier protection against infectious agents. The highest-risk behavior is receptive anal penetration including ejaculation, which consists of unprotected ejaculation of semen into the delicate, nonlubricated tissue of the rectum. This allows direct access of infectious STD/HIV agents to the bloodstream. Theoretically, as Figure 15.4 illustrates, the risk for STD/HIV is greater for the receptive partner of any sexual activity.

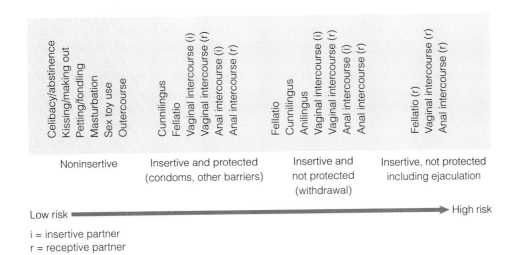

i = insertive partner
r = receptive partner

Figure 15.4 *A Continuum of Risk for Sexual Behaviors* STD risks increase as sexual activities become unprotected and receptive.

A Closer Look at Sexual Behaviors and STD Risk

Much remains to be known about the relative safety of various sexual behaviors. For instance, a wealth of literature documents the degree of protection condoms provide in preventing STDs. Little, however, has been written concerning the effects of nonpenetrative sexual activity and withdrawal. Some of these activities now are included in "safer sex" methods, instead of "safe sex" behaviors because of the lack of adequate documentation on their effectiveness.

The effects of some of the more bizarre techniques haven't been documented at all. Consider the recommendation of some safe sex educators of the use of dental dams and clear plastic food wraps to prevent the transmission of STDs through cunnilingus, fellatio, and vaginal intercourse. We do not advocate these measures because they are untested and not intended for those purposes. No evidence is available to suggest that they work. In fact, the American Dental Association issued a disclaimer concerning using dental dams (square pieces of latex designed to be used over the mouths of dental patients) for any circumstances other than dental hygiene. Clear plastic food wraps are an even more vivid example of safe sex gone mad. The notion of covering one's genitalia with plastic wrap and then having intercourse or oral sex would be comical if the potential results weren't so dangerous.

For those who choose to have sexual intercourse, barrier methods provide the best protection. For those who do not want to have intercourse, a variety of nonpenetrative sexual activities offer close to 100 percent effectiveness against STDs.

Condoms   If worn properly and used consistently, condoms (both male and female) help protect the wearer against some STD infection by preventing direct contact between the penis and cervical, vaginal, rectal, or pharyngeal secretions or lesions. They also protect against exposure to penile lesions, discharges, and infected semen. Proper use for preventing STDs requires putting them on prior to any sexual contact, and they must remain intact throughout sexual activity.

Condoms are more effective against sexually transmitted infections such as gonorrhea, chlamydia, trichomoniasis, and HIV, which are transmitted by fluids from mucosal surfaces and from semen (and therefore captured or blocked by the condom) than STDs transmitted by skin-to-skin contact such as HPV, herpes simplex virus (HSV), syphilis, and chancroid. The organisms of the latter diseases and others live in outcrops of blisters, warts, and lesions that could exist in areas that condoms do not protect (MMWR, 2002f). In laboratory studies, male latex condoms have been shown to block the larger bacterial pathogens (gonorrhea and chlamydia) and, to a lesser extent, smaller viral organisms (such as HIV, HSV, and HPV) (Grimes & Cates, 1990; Conant, Hardy, Sernatinger, Spicer, & Levy, 1986; Minuk, Bohme, & Bowen, 1986). Similar findings have not been found for natural membrane condoms. Although they block the passage of sperm and are similar in their ability to prevent pregnancy, their pores are large enough to allow the passage of some STD organisms. Natural membrane condoms should not be the first choice for the prevention of STDs unless one is allergic to latex (MMWR, 2002f).

In human studies, condoms also have been shown to be effective in reducing the risks for contracting STDs. Studies from all over the world, with diverse populations of users, have consistently documented that condoms reduce the risks for spreading STDs. Research as far back as the 1940s studied the use of condoms by troops in World War II and the Korean and Vietnam conflicts. In all three conflicts, soldiers and seamen using condoms had significantly lower rates of infection than their peers who did not use condoms (Hart, 1974).

More recent studies of college men, men and women attending STD clinics, sex workers in Kenya and Zaire, and many others document that condoms provide some protection against a host of STDs (Darrow, 1989; Cameron et al., 1991; Mann

My Most Persuasive Reasons to Wait to Have Sex

Although there are many great reasons to have sexual intercourse, there are also some really good reasons to wait. One of the best ways to avoid an STD is to limit your sexual partners. This activity will help you practice being assertive about why you want to wait to have sex.

This will be more fun if you can find a friend to role-play this with you. It will be even more fun if you find a friend of the opposite sex. Tell your friend that you would like for him or her to act out the following scenario with you. You are playing the parts of a couple who disagree when to become sexually active. One partner is ready to become sexually intimate, but the other partner wants to stay monogamous and to wait at least 4 months to be tested for HIV/AIDS and STDs before becoming intimate. Your friend will play the role of trying to persuade you to have sex, and your role is to give your friend all of the good reasons that you two should wait. Once you have finished, decide who was the most persuasive and discuss other good arguments you could have used. The more we practice assertively telling a partner what we need, the more likely we are to do it in our "real" relationships.

et al., 1987). Although use of condoms does not provide 100 percent protection against STDs, the studies we have mentioned have reduced risk by 50 to 80 percent in actual users (Cates & Stone, 1992).

Women-Centered Barriers Although the male condom is the most reliable form of barrier protection against STDs/HIV, studies show that the women who stand to benefit the most do not use them consistently and correctly. The least consistent users of the male condom are adolescent women, women with a history of STD infection, and lower-SES women (who generally have less power and equality in their sexual relationships with men and have less negotiating skill) (Rosenberg & Gollub, 1992). This problem could be dramatically lessened, if not eliminated, if more women were to use female barriers consistently and correctly.

Clinical studies of the effectiveness of female condoms in preventing STDs are very limited. Laboratory studies have demonstrated the effectiveness of the female condom in blocking viruses. Female condoms are recommended for use when male condoms cannot be used properly (MMWR, 2002f).

In both laboratory and STD clinic studies, the following rates of effectiveness were reported for the sponge, diaphragm, and spermicides:

- An overall reduced STD infection rate among barrier users compared to nonbarrier users
- Lower STD infection rates (87 percent lower) for women using barriers and attending health maintenance organizations (HMOs) than nonusers
- Lower STD infection rates (61 percent lower than nonusers) for women attending STD clinics who used barriers
- Up to 70 percent effectiveness against gonorrhea when using barriers
- Up to 40 percent effectiveness against chlamydia when using barriers (Rosenberg & Golub, 1992)

Furthermore, in a study of 5,681 STD patients on the effectiveness of various contraceptive methods against STDs, not only was there a lower rate of infection among barrier users, but the lowest rates of infection were among sponge and diaphragm users. These rates were stable across all types of subjects, forms of sexual behavior, and STDs (Rosenberg & Gollub, 1992).

Even though condoms have a higher rate of theoretical effectiveness against STDs, the women who need them the most use them less consistently and correctly. Woman-centered barriers, though theoretically less effective against STDs, provided greater actual effectiveness for women who used them instead of the male condom.

Nonpenetrative Sexual Behaviors   The effectiveness of nonpenetrative sexual activity in preventing STDs is relatively undocumented. Effectiveness in preventing STDs is generalized from the hypothesized ability of these methods to prevent unintended pregnancy by preventing the deposit of live sperm into the vagina. Because these methods exclude penetration and ejaculation, their ability to prevent pregnancy is very high (theoretically close to 100 percent).

Methods such as masturbation, use of sex toys, and even oral-genital sexual contact in preventing the transmission of STDs have not been scientifically studied and documented. Do these methods offer the same protection against STDs?

healthy sex hints 15.1
Reducing the Risk for STDs: Some Basic Guidelines

Although no universal solutions will work equally well for everyone, here are a few guidelines for reducing your risk for acquiring an STD.

1. *Become comfortable with your own sexuality.* Learn as much as you can about your sexuality. This will make you more accepting of who you are and what you need. You will be less likely to give in to doing something risky if you know and respect yourself. This includes choosing to abstain if that's what you desire.
2. *Check yourself for signs and symptoms of STDs.* This goes hand in hand with item 1. If you are comfortable with your body and your sexuality, you will be more aware of changes that signify possible STD infection. If you or your partner has the sores, rashes, discharges, itching, or pain associated with STDs, avoid sex.
3. *Develop a repertoire of low-risk sexual outlets.* Learn how to enjoy a low-risk sexual outlet. It's perfectly OK to say no to unprotected intercourse and yes to masturbation or massage.
4. *Work on your communication skills.* Practice how to initiate a dialogue about STD risk reduction. You'll need to find out a lot about your partner to assess and reduce your personal risk. The only way to do this is to be able to talk openly about your sexual lifestyle. Practice now.

5. *Understand your demographic risks.* Find out about the area in which you live. You can get information about the level of STDs in your community from your local and state health departments.
6. *Know your partner's sexual/medical history.* Take time and care to find out the things you need to know about your partner, or develop the level of trust in the relationship that will allow you to make some judgments about your risk. In the meantime, if you choose to have sex with your partner, use condoms and non-intercourse options to reduce your risk.
7. *If you are at risk, seek regular checkups.* If you have a very high-risk profile, go in for an STD checkup every 3 months. If you are in a lower risk category, go in at least twice a year. Most states have a list of free public clinics in your area.
8. *If you are not in a mutually monogamous, disease-free relationship, protect yourself.* Do not rely on your partner to look out for your health. All forms of sexual activity carry some degree of risk for spreading STDs. Gauge the level of risk you are willing to assume.
9. *Strive to be in a mutually satisfying, disease-free relationship with one person.* If both you and your sex partner are monogamous and disease-free, you will not be at risk for STDs. Two mutually exclusive, uninfected partners can enjoy sex without fear of infection.

No one knows for sure. When theorizing about their ability to prevent STDs, one can say that, because they do not involve penetration and ejaculation, they must offer a high level of protection against STDs as well. We are not as totally convinced of this hypothesis as some other safer sex educators are.

The major difference in the ability of these activities to prevent STDs would be the presence or absence of genital symptoms that potentially could spread pathogens even in the absence of penile penetration and ejaculation. Also, STD organisms, in rare instances, could be passed from genital ulcers to the eyes via contaminated fingers. For instance, if a person who had genital lesions associated with herpes were to engage in mutual masturbation with his or her partner, and then rubbed the eyes, the herpes virus could be spread to this site.

These facts are why we present sexual behaviors on a continuum of risk from low to high. No behavior except celibacy is completely risk-free. Viewing sexual activity in this way will allow you to examine the risk of specific behaviors in the context of other sexual activities. You also must evaluate any behavior within the context of the relationship you have with your partner. The less you know about your partner, the more risky any behavior becomes.

Using the Pyramid to Reduce Risks

The pyramid model presented earlier in the chapter shows that the risk for STDs/HIV combines personal lifestyle and behavior, past sexual history, and demographic factors. Focusing on just one set of factors and ignoring the others

healthy sex hints 15.2

Are You Really Sleeping with Your Partner's Partners?

Probably the most overused myth associated with sexual lifestyle is the notion that when you "sleep with someone, you sleep with everyone they have ever had sex with." We're sure you all have heard this at one point or another during your lives. Here are seven reasons why we disagree with this message:

1. For the most part, it is an antisex, fear-based message. It targets guilt and a sense of helplessness. None of these are part of healthy sexuality.
2. It uses incorrect terminology. You will rarely get any STDs (except maybe crabs or scabies) by merely *sleeping* with someone. You must engage in some kind of sexual activity with the person to acquire an STD.
3. You do not "have sex" with anyone but the *person* you actually come in physical contact with. Any explanation other than this is nonsense (actually, it's a metaphor to induce fear).
4. Most nonviral STDs are cured when a person receives treatment. If your partner had a nonviral STD and was properly treated, the infection stopped there.

5. If your partner's partner was infected with an STD but did not pass it on to your partner, it *cannot infect you* under any circumstances.
6. Even viral STDs such as genital herpes can be controlled with treatment. *You* are not at risk for your partner's partner who had a viral STD unless this person infected your lover, who then passes the infection on to you.
7. Being exposed to your partner's antibodies to past sex partners is *not the same* as being exposed to disease-producing germs (although research shows that people can develop antibodies in response to being exposed to human semen, this is not the same thing as *being infected* with a disease).

Based on the data we just presented, do you still think you are sleeping with everyone your partner has slept with when you have sex with him or her?

Interactions Among Geographic Differences, Sexual Behavior, and Disease Infectivity

Pinkerton, Chesson, and Layde (2002) found that the risk of acquiring STDs varies significantly according to the interaction of four major risk factors: (a) disease infectivity (the ease with which a disease is transmitted through penile-vaginal intercourse), (b) the level of infection within a community, (c) the number of different sex partners, and (d) the number of unprotected sex acts (consistent condom use).

Pinkerton et al. (2002) found that in geographic areas with high morbidity of very infectious diseases such as gonorrhea and chlamydia, the best way to reduce risk was to decrease the overall number of sexual partners. This was found to be more protective than the overall number of protected sex acts. In other words, by decreasing the overall number of different sex partners, one decreased their risk more than by using condoms consistently with multiple sex partners. Because highly infectious diseases are relatively easy to acquire with even one sexual exposure, lowering the number of potential exposures (by decreasing the overall number of partners) was found to be the best way to reduce risk.

In contrast, in geographic areas with high morbidity of less infectious diseases such as HIV, the best way to reduce risk was to increase the number of protected sex acts. Having fewer partners was less protective than using condoms with each sex act.

Because HIV is more difficult to spread through penile-vaginal intercourse than gonorrhea and chlamydia, being exposed to a single episode of intercourse with different partners (most of whom might be uninfected) might pose less of a risk of infection with HIV than being consistently exposed to a single, infected partner. Consistent exposure to a single infectious partner therefore required more consistent condom use (decreasing the overall number of unprotected sex acts).

The same dynamic can hold true for sexual/medical history. If the sex partner has a high-risk past (used injectable drugs and might be HIV-positive, for instance), the other partner's personal behavior might be much different from that of someone whose partner has no history of infection. If the personal history includes a risk such as prior infection with gonococcal pelvic inflammatory disease (PID), for instance, a woman might take extra precautions against becoming infected with gonorrhea again as it could increase the risk for developing PID again. Each individual has to develop a personal plan for STD risk reduction based on his or her (and the partner's) pyramid. Plans will vary according to the individuals involved. Although reducing risks this way takes a little more thought, it also respects individuality.

isn't enough. Though a person can never dismiss personal behavior as crucial to the success of prevention activities, other factors affect personal risk despite the most exemplary personal behavior.

For example, in certain core areas, individuals have 300 times more risk for acquiring infection simply by virtue of community risk factors (Potterat et al., 1985). Even if you are rather conservative in your behavior, if you live and interact sexually in such an area, engaging in any sexual activity carries a higher risk of becoming infected and engaging in risky sexual behavior may be life-threatening. This demographic influence might make risk reduction measures much different from someone who lives in a lower-risk area.

Diagnosis, Treatment, and Epidemiology of Various STDs

Epidemiological Dealing with incidence, distribution, and control, as in STDs

The following sections take a more detailed look at several STDs. Specifically, we'll consider how they are diagnosed and treated and, more generally, look at **epidemiological** issues around each one.

Syphillis

Diagnosis Syphilis is a blood-borne STD caused by infection with *Treponema pallidum*, a corkscrew-shaped bacterium. A **spirochete** type of bacteria, the *T. pallidum* is easily killed by penicillin and other broad-spectrum antibiotics. It is unique among STD organisms because its corkscrew shape and motility facilitate its entry into the bloodstream.

After exposure to the bacterium, it enters the body through breaks in the skin or by penetrating intact skin, and from there passes into the bloodstream. Once in the bloodstream, it can move freely throughout the body. The usual incubation period for syphilis is 3 to 4 weeks, but it can be as short as 10 days or as long as 90 days.

After the incubation period, a **chancre** appears at the spot where the organism entered. The primary chancre is painless and disappears within 1 to 5 weeks without treatment. Often it is internal (inside the vagina, mouth, or rectum). Because of this, many people who become infected with syphilis don't realize it. An infected person's blood test will detect antibodies to the syphilis spirochete a short time after the primary chancre appears. Fluid from chancres can also be used to diagnose early syphilis. A specimen of the fluid can be examined under a darkfield microscope. If infected, the specimen should be teeming with spirochetes, moving in their typical corkscrew motion.

About 6 weeks later a generalized rash appears. The rash varies from being highly noticeable, covering the entire trunk, to a mild eruption on the hands or feet. As with the chancre, the rash disappears without treatment after 2 to 6 weeks.

In about 25 percent of the cases, a second rash appears and also goes away without treatment. At this point, those who are infected enter the latency period, during which time they are infected but have no symptoms. They are capable of transmitting the infection only by donating blood or by a mother passing the infection across the placenta to a developing fetus, resulting in **congenital syphilis.**

All blood in the United States is tested for syphilis, and no cases of disease have been detected this way in decades. Because the symptoms of syphilis can be so mild and varied, it has been dubbed the "great imitator." It can mimic a variety of dermatological conditions and often is mistaken for these less serious infections. In adults, un-

Syphilis An STD caused by the spirochete bacterium *Treponema pallidum*

Spirochete A mobile, flexible, corkscrew-shaped bacterium of the genus *Spirocheta*, one type of which causes syphilis

Chancre A painless, indurated primary lesion of early syphilis

Congenital syphilis The disease acquired by the fetus in the womb and present at birth

The typical chancre of primary syphilis is round with raised edges and painless; it is often internal and goes unobserved.

Centers for Disease Control and Prevention

Centers for Disease Control and Prevention

The typical rash associated with secondary syphilis is bilateral (on both hands or feet instead of just one), discolored, and raised.

treated syphilis takes several years to develop into a serious illness. Because the spirochetes are traveling throughout the body, they can infect any organ or body system and cause major damage.

In the United States, untreated syphilis going undetected for the decades required to develop life-threatening illness is unusual. Most Americans have a blood test for syphilis (for example, for work, marriage, induction into the Armed Forces) at some point in their adult life. This also explains why disenfranchised people who live in poverty and are not in the mainstream are more likely to have undetected syphilis.

Treatment   Treatment of syphilis is relatively straightforward. Injections of penicillin are sufficient to treat most early cases of syphilis. One shot is administered to those who have been infected for less than 1 year. Those having infections more than 1 year are given three injections, each spaced 1 week apart. For individuals who are allergic to penicillin, Doxycycline or tetracycline, taken for a minimum of 14 days, is recommended for the treatment of early syphilis (MMWR, 2002f).

Epidemiology   The incidence of syphilis declined by a dramatic 99 percent from the 1940s to the present, primarily because of (a) the availability and widespread use of penicillin therapy and (b) the public health strategy of aggressive follow-up of sex partners. Public health officials prioritized syphilis control and insisted that all infected persons be interviewed and counseled about their disease. Their sex partners were followed up and given preventive treatment (penicillin unless allergic) for the disease (Dunn & Rolfs, 1991).

The largest recent decline has been in gay men of all ages from 1983 to 1986, partly because of their adoption of safer sex behaviors. From 1986 to 1990, in an epidemic of syphilis throughout the United States, rates increased from 12 cases per 100,000 to 20 per 100,000 (St. Louis & Wasserheit, 1998; Webster & Rolfs, 1993). This represented the highest level in the United States in 40 years.

Figure 15.5 *Primary and Secondary Syphilis Rates by Gender* Primary and secondary syphilis rates for men and women have steadily declined.

Source: DSTD (2002).

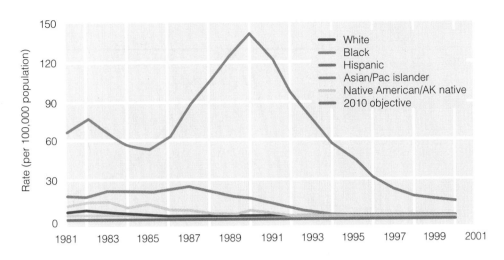

Figure 15.6 *Primary and Secondary Syphilis Rates by Race/Ethnicity* The decline in new cases of syphilis is consistent among all racial and ethnic groups.
Source: DSTD (2002).

Since that time however, syphilis rates have been dropping, reaching an all-time low. In 1999, 79 percent of over 3,000 counties in the United States reported no cases of early syphilis (DSTD 1999, 2001). Figures 15.5 and 15.6 show primary and secondary syphilis rates.

One disturbing contradiction to this trend has been the occurrence of several "miniepidemics" of syphilis within urban populations of men who have sex with men (MSM) in major metropolitan areas across the United States. Since 1977, syphilis outbreaks among MSM have occurred in New York City, Seattle, Chicago, San Francisco, Los Angeles, and Chicago (MMWR, 1999, 2002b; Rutherford, 2002; Bertrami, 2002). These men also demonstrated an increased risk for multiple STDs (Ciesielski, Flynn, & McLean, 2002).

The occurrence of these miniepidemics is generally accepted as secondary evidence of a relaxation of safe sex behavior of MSM in these areas. Many of these men suffer from what experts call "AIDS burnout," the relapsing back to unsafe sexual activity due to years and years of exposure to prevention messages and compliance with safe sex behaviors. This is prompting public health officials and members of the gay community to launch new safe sex campaigns to call attention to this new threat posed by the resurgence of syphilis within their communities (Rutherford, 2002; Bertrami, 2002).

Congenital Syphilis

The epidemic of early syphilis in the 1980s resulted in a dramatic increase in congenital syphilis cases and rates. Reported cases of congenital syphilis increased from 158 in 1983 to 7,219 cases in 1990 (from 4.3 to 174.7 cases per 100,000) (Zenker, 1991). A partial explanation for the dramatic rise in congenital syphilis was the adoption of a new case definition from the CDC. Under this new definition, a *case* is defined as any infant whose mother was determined to be untreated or inadequately treated for syphilis, regardless of the presence/absence of symptoms in the baby. This epidemic hit young, urban, African American and Hispanic people the hardest.

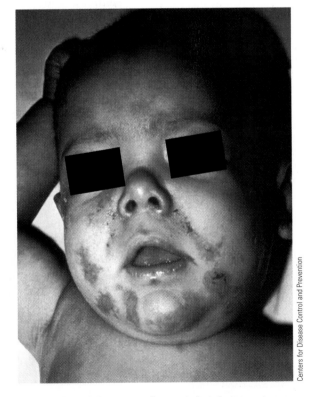

Congenital syphilis occurs when an infected pregnant woman passes the infection to her developing fetus in utero.

Figure 15.7 *Congenital Syphilis Rates* Congenital syphilis rates have declined significantly but are still above the targets sets by Healthy People 2010.
Source: DSTD (2002).

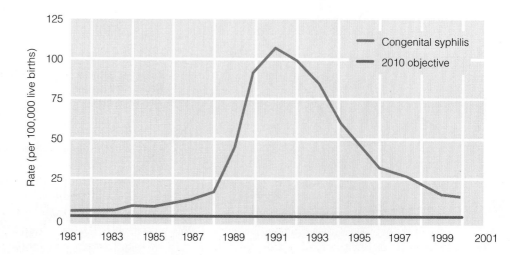

Since 1990, the decline in early syphilis has led to a corresponding decrease in congenital syphilis rates (see Figure 15.7). From 1990 through 2000, the average yearly decrease in congenital syphilis was 220 percent (compared to 21 percent for early syphilis). The current rate of 13.4 cases per 100,000 women is the lowest in a decade (DSTD, 2001).

The risks of congenital syphilis were greatest among young, lower-SES, drug-abusing mothers (Cates & Stone, 1992; Zenker, 1991; Nakashima et al., 1996). These young women are much less likely than their older, more affluent, and better-educated peers to seek and obtain adequate prenatal care. Many of these pregnant women fail to have the recommended three trimester visits with an obstetrician. A requirement of routine prenatal care is a blood test for syphilis. Most adult women with health insurance get this test early in their pregnancies. If it is positive, they can be treated. Treatment of the mother almost always results in treatment of her developing fetus.

Chancroid

Chancroid An STD named for the irregular and painful genital lesions it produces, caused by the bacterium *Haemophilus ducreyi*

Diagnosis   **Chancroid** is often confused with syphilis because both present with an initial genital ulcer as the primary symptom. The ulcers associated with chancroid, however, are irregular in shape and painful (versus symmetrical and painless for syphilis).

The typical incubation period is 4 to 10 days, after which the ulcer appears. After their initial appearance, the ulcers progress to become beefy, granular, painful erosions. The ulcers are accompanied by painful, swollen, lymph glands in the groin.

Like syphilis, chancroid is diagnosed through the presence (or history) of symptoms and the results of a blood test. It is often diagnosed in part, ruling out infection with syphilis. A negative test for syphilis focuses the diagnosis on looking for antibodies to the causative organism, *Haemophilus ducreyi,* or isolating it in a biological culture.

Treatment   Chancroid is easily treated with antibiotics taken either orally or through an intramuscular injection.

Unlike syphilis, the ulcers of chancroid are irregular in shape and painful.

Centers for Disease Control and Prevention

sex in society 15.3

The Tuskegee Study: It Couldn't Happen Here—or Could It?

In 1932, the U.S. Public Health Service (USPHS) embarked on one of the most tragic experiments ever conducted by a government on its own people. From 1932 to 1970, in Macon County, Alabama, the USPHS conducted a study under the guidance of the Tuskegee Institute (which, ironically, is one of the nation's most prestigious black academic institutions) on the history of syphilis in blacks.

Syphilis, it was hypothesized, progressed differently in blacks than whites. The study originally was intended to be a short-term investigation (6 to 9 months' duration) but evolved into a 40-year project that followed the subjects well beyond the initial stages of their disease through latency into complications and ultimately to their deaths. Much of what we know about the disease, how it spreads, its complications, and how it attacks the body and kills comes from the Tuskegee Study.

The study followed 600 black subjects (399 infected men and 201 uninfected controls) for 40 years. Treatment was withheld intentionally from these men, even after they were diagnosed with serious, life-threatening complications of the disease. None of them benefited from penicillin as the effective treatment of choice in 1951. The USPHS devised elaborate plans to keep track of these men (and to continue to withhold treatment) even after they moved from Alabama to other states.

In 1966, Peter Buxtun, an investigator for the USPHS, brought the matter before the then-director of the Division of Venereal Diseases, Peter Brown. Given the moral climate and racial turmoil of the 1960s and the immorality of such an experiment, Buxtun pleaded that something be done. A special committee was impaneled within the USPHS to discuss the study. The committee ruled in favor of continuing the study to its natural end point.

Buxtun's pleas went unheeded, and the experiment continued. Not until Buxtun leaked his story to an Associated Press writer and it broke on the front pages of the *Washington Post* in 1972 was something done. In 1973, a special subcommittee of the U.S. Congress, chaired by Edward Kennedy (D-MA) began to investigate the matter. The committee found the USPHS culpable, the study was terminated, and special regulations concerning conducting government experiments were drawn up. These regulations now serve as guidelines for handling human subjects in any government-financed study. Surviving participants of the Tuskegee Study and their heirs filed a $1.8 billion class action lawsuit. The government settled the suit out of court for $10 million.

How all of this was allowed to happen—the circumstances behind the massive cover-up and the racial bigotry that may have poisoned a legitimate scientific quest for knowledge and understanding—are all chronicled in the work of James Jones's 1993 book *Bad Blood: The Tuskegee Study—A Tragedy of Race and Medicine.*

Epidemiology   Although chancroid is not common in the United States and other developed countries, it is endemic in some Third World countries and is considered a cofactor in the explosion of HIV infection in these nations. In the United States, the incidence of chancroid peaked in 1947 with 10,000 cases nationwide and steadily declined until 1981.

From 1981 to 1987, morbidity increased slightly, with eight distinct outbreaks scattered around the country. These outbreaks all had the following commonalities:

The introduction of infected individuals from outside areas (including merchant seamen and recent immigrants)
Predominance in black and Hispanic males
Linkage to prostitution (Hayes et al., 1995; Cameron et al., 1991; Morse et al., 1990)

Since 1987, chancroid morbidity has decreased steadily. The current level of infection is the lowest in 20 years, with just 78 cases reported in the United States. Of the 12 states reporting infections in 2001, three (New York, South Carolina, and Texas) were responsible for over 70 percent of all cases (DSTD, 2002).

HIV/AIDS

AIDS The acronym for *acquired immunodeficiency syndrome*, the end result of HIV infection

HIV The acronym for *human immunodeficiency virus*, the infection that leads to AIDS

AIDS represents the end stage of **HIV.** Figure 15.8 traces the natural progression of HIV infection. As you can see, AIDS can develop within 2 years of exposure but typically takes longer. HIV infection is caused by person-to-person transmission of the human immunodeficiency virus. The most common modes of transmission are (a) sexual contact (vaginal or anal intercourse are most efficient), (b) sharing contaminated needles (through injecting drug use), and (c) maternal-to-fetal transfer. Once the virus has been transmitted, it enters the bloodstream, where it incubates from 8 weeks to 6 months, when it will show positive on a blood test.

Diagnosis   A person who elects to take a blood test for HIV is given a screening test, called the *ELISA* (enzyme-linked immunosorbent assay), which detects the presence of antibodies to the HIV. If this test is negative, the person is counseled to come back for a second ELISA in a few months, to make sure the maximum incubation period has elapsed. If a person tests positive on the initial ELISA, he or she is given a second test, called the *Western blot,* to confirm infection. If this test comes back positive, the person is diagnosed as having HIV infection.

There are two new tests marketed by OraSure Technologies. OraSure, an oral screening using a swab, tests saliva for HIV antibodies. OraQuick tests blood from a fingerstick sample and provides results in 20 minutes. For either test, a positive result is followed up by a Western blot test.

HIV infection is essentially a disorder of the immune system. The virus weakens the body's immune system, making the person susceptible to other infections and chronic diseases. These are called **opportunistic infections** because they take advantage of the body's weakened state to attack and cause disease. When people with a fully functioning immune system come in contact with opportunistic organisms, they normally repel them.

People with HIV cannot fight off opportunistic infections and eventually die from them. Most people with HIV infection are completely free of symptoms for more than 10 years. Others deteriorate rapidly and develop symptoms and AIDS within 2 to 4 years.

Early symptoms of HIV infection stem from infections that begin to invade the body because of its weakened immune status. When the immune system begins to fail, the following symptoms begin to occur: fatigue, diarrhea, fever, night sweats, skin rashes, sudden weight loss, dry cough, swollen lymph nodes, and vaginal yeast infection. These symptoms can be present for weeks, months, or even years without opportunistic infections taking hold.

With treatment, many people with HIV can prevent these symptoms from ever occurring. And aggressive treatment can return symptomatic individuals to a symptom-free state. Although the medication doesn't kill the virus, it slows or stops viral replication and thereby boosts **immunocompetence.** If an opportunistic infection does take hold, the person moves from being infected with HIV to being diagnosed as having AIDS. In 1993, the CDC broadened the definition of AIDS to include 26 opportunistic infections. Infection with any one of these combined with being HIV-positive leads to a diagnosis of AIDS.

Treatment   HIV/AIDS treatment is not a cure, because viruses have no cure. The multitude of new antiviral drugs and combination drug treatment regimens do not kill all of the HIV, as antibiotics kill bacteria. Antiviral therapy prevents or slows the unchecked replication and growth of HIV, helping the infected person's immune system keep the virus in check. This prevents the person from contracting opportunistic infections. Other treatments focus on killing the opportunistic infections that take hold.

Figure 15.8 *The Natural History of HIV* It may take several years for a person infected with HIV to develop AIDS.

Prior to 1995, most HIV antiviral treatment revolved around drugs that inhibited the activity of reverse transcriptase, an enzyme that HIV requires to transform its RNA (ribonucleic acid) genetic material into DNA (deoxyribonucleic acid)—the first step in viral replication. These drugs prevented the spread of HIV to new cells but did little to stop viral replication in cells that were infected already.

In 1995, the FDA approved a new group of antiviral drugs called **protease inhibitors.** These drugs act against an enzyme, HIV protease, whose function is to break down and reassemble the proteins that infectious viral particles require. When protease is inhibited in infected cells, a noninfectious virus results.

Current treatment regimens called *highly active antiretroviral therapy* (HAART) combine the older reverse transcriptase drugs with the newer protease inhibitors to attack the virus in two ways. HAART is effective, first, in halting the spread of the virus and, second, in reducing viral loads (the amount of HIV RNA in plasma, a direct measure of disease progression) (Division of HIV/AIDS [DHIV/AIDS], 2002b; Ungvarski, 1997).

These advances in treatment have enabled persons infected with HIV to live longer and also have changed the face of the AIDS epidemic. As people live longer with HIV, fewer people develop AIDS and die as a result of HIV infection. In a sense, HIV becomes more of a chronic disease. Nowhere is this more apparent than in the declining death rate for AIDS.

An interesting note regarding HAART relates to its effectiveness in improving the quality of life of people with AIDS. HAART is responsible for increasing not only the life span of AIDS patients but also their daily activity level. Patients often have enough energy and feel well enough to resume most of their daily activities (including sexual activity). This increased level of sexual activity among people with AIDS, coupled with a desensitization to prevention messages, has been implicated in the recent increase in syphilis among MSM in major metropolitan areas in the United States discussed earlier in the chapter (MMWR, 2002b).

Epidemiology Tracking HIV and AIDS is complicated by the fact that while AIDS is a reportable disease by law in all states, HIV reporting is not mandated. HIV incidence and prevalence are usually estimated from extrapolating data from selected serologic testing sites. HIV seropositivity data found at these sites is generalized to the United States population as a whole to estimate the extent of the problem in society. Because AIDS reporting is mandatory, AIDS morbidity and **mortality** data are used to track the condition (DHIV/AIDS, 2002b).

> **Opportunistic infection** An infection that is able to develop as a result of the body's weakened immune status
>
> **Immunocompetence** The level of efficiency of the immune system
>
> **Protease inhibitors** A group of antiviral drugs used to prevent replication of HIV-infected cells
>
> **Mortality** The number of deaths during a specific time period

healthy sex hints 15.3
Should You Take the AIDS Test?

The question about whether to get tested for HIV has concerned many individuals. Where HIV infection and AIDS are concerned, clouds of fear, suspicion, and misunderstanding still loom large in many communities. Fears of being ostracized by family and friends, being kicked out of school, or losing a job have kept many people who suspect exposure to HIV from being tested. In some cases, people simply cannot face the possibility of a positive test and do not want to know.

If you are considering having a screening test for HIV, keep these tips in mind:

- Take your test anonymously in an alternative-site facility where you will be given a number and your name will not be used (some facilities do confidential, not anonymous, testing).

- Make sure the testing site does counseling before and after the test.

- Many college health centers offer HIV testing. Students can also get tested through Planned Parenthood, health departments, and other facilities specifically designed for HIV/STD testing.

Figure 15.9 *AIDS Cases by Race/Ethnicity* AIDS cases are not equally distributed among all racial/ethnic groups. *Source:* DHIV/AIDS (2002a).

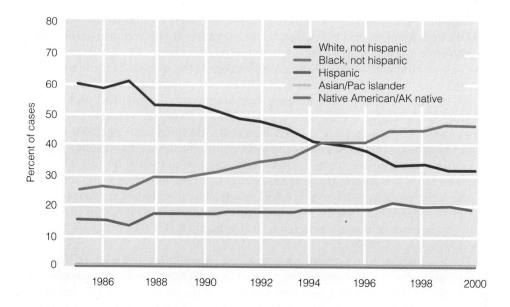

As of December 31, 2002, 816,149 persons had been diagnosed with AIDS in the United States. Of the total, there were 666,026 cases in males and 141,048 cases in females. Of those, 57 percent (467,910) have died (DHIV/AIDS, 2002b). Of the prevailing cases, 50,352 (6 percent) were reported during 1981–1987, 203,217 (25 percent) during 1988–1992, 387,517 (47 percent) during 1992–1997, and the remaining 175,063 (22 percent) have been diagnosed since then (MMWR 1991, 1995a; DHIV/AIDS, 2002b).

Three major trends have occurred regarding HIV and AIDS in the past decade:

- Overall AIDS morbidity is down.
- Overall AIDS mortality is down.
- Overall HIV morbidity is down.

Since 1996, there has been a dramatic decline in the number of cases of AIDS. Morbidity declined among all risk groups from 1996 to 1998 but increased slightly from 1998 to 2001 among persons exposed through heterosexual contact (DHIV/AIDS, 2002a). From 1998 to 1999, AIDS incidence leveled

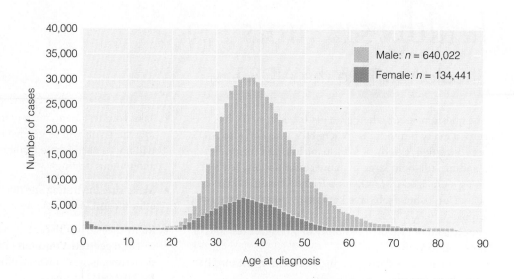

Figure 15.10 *AIDS Cases by Gender* The number of cases of AIDS has dropped dramatically for both men and women. *Source:* DHIV/AIDS (2002).

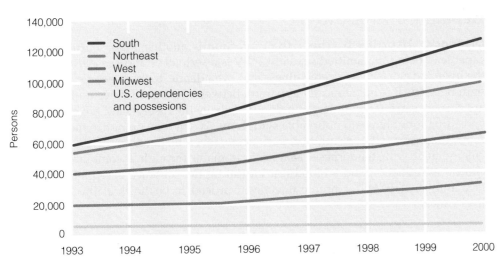

Figure 15.11 *Estimated Number of Persons Living with AIDS* People with AIDS are living longer thanks to more effective treatment regimens.

Source: DHIV/AIDS (2002).

off at around 41,000 cases, and there has been little change in the level of infection since then. AIDS prevalence is estimated at 362,827 persons (see Figures 15.9 and 15.10).

Regionally, AIDS morbidity has mimicked syphilis with all regions except the southern region experiencing a decrease in new cases (see Figure 15.11). AIDS remains a continuing problem of major public health significance, with most new cases occurring among MSM and injectable drug users (Karon, Fleming, Steketee, & DeCock, 2001; DHIV/AIDS, 2002b; MMWR, 2002c).

The number of AIDS deaths also sharply declined in 1996 and has continued to drop every year since then (Figure 15.12). The decline in AIDS deaths is consistent across all regions and all risk groups (DHIV/AIDS, 2002a). This decrease can be attributed mostly to the success of the newest generation of AIDS medications (MMWR, 1995b, 1995c, 1995d). The lowered AIDS death rate has resulted in more people with AIDS surviving the disease than at any time in the past. Lowering the death rate resulted in a slight increase in the prevalence of the condition as more existing cases add into the new cases each year.

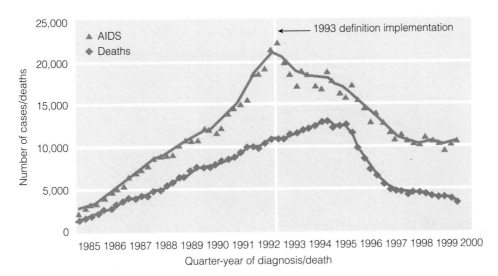

Figure 15.12 *Overall Incidence of AIDS Morbidity and Mortality* Both the number of AIDS cases and the number of AIDS deaths have declined markedly.

Source: DHIV/AIDS (2002).

Hepatitis B Virus (HBV)

Diagnosis   Hepatitis B virus (HBV) infection is another blood-borne disease capable of being transmitted sexually. HBV is a serious viral disease that attacks the liver and can cause extreme illness and even death. To most people, infection with hepatitis B is not clinically apparent. Between 10 and 68 percent of all cases are chronic **carriers;** the infected individuals have the disease and are capable of spreading it but have no noticeable symptoms. When they do notice their symptoms, they usually have jaundice, dark urine, fever, malaise, and moderate liver enlargement with tenderness. Diagnosis is made through a combination of a clinical examination and a blood test indicating the presence of hepatitis B surface antigen (HBsAG). Chronic infection can lead to cirrhosis of the liver and liver cancer.

Treatment   HBV infection has no cure because, like HIV, it is caused by a virus. Treatment consists of boosting the strength of the immune system to help the body keep the virus in check. A vaccine for HBV has been available since 1981. At first, the vaccine was recommended for use by those whose work caused them to come in contact with potentially contaminated blood (such as health care workers and those living with persons infected with HBV). It is now recognized that many other persons are potentially at risk through drug-related behavior and sexual activity with infected persons and should consider becoming vaccinated (MMWR, 2002f).

Epidemiology   An estimated 5 percent of the U.S. population is infected with HBV, with an estimated 200,000 new infections occurring annually. Of those 200,000 cases, 120,000 are thought to have been acquired through sexual activity with an infected partner. Of those, it is estimated that about 25,000 have acute infection acquired sexually (DSTD, 2000).

   The risks associated with HBV infection are gender, age, sexual orientation, IDU status, and race/ethnicity (Figures 15.13 and 15.14). Men have a slightly higher incidence of HBV than women. Part of this is attributed to a higher risk among gay men. Eighteen percent of all HBV cases are among gay men. Hetero-

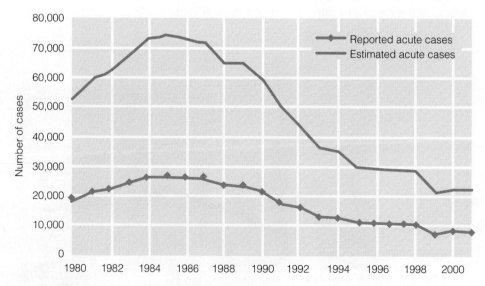

Figure 15.13 *Cases of Hepatitis B* Cases of hepatitis B have steadily declined since the mid-1980s.
Source: NCID (2003).

sexuals (especially those with a history of STDs and multiple sex partners) accounted for 40 percent of all infections. Persons involved with IDU activities accounted for 15 percent of all cases. Health care workers accounted for 2 percent of all cases, and household contact with a person infected with HBV accounted for 3 percent of the cases (National Center for Infectious Disease [NCID], 2003).

Genital Herpes Infection

Diagnosis **Genital herpes** infection is caused by exposure to the herpes simplex virus type 1 (HSV 1) or herpes simplex virus type 2 (HSV 2) through sexual contact. HSV 1 initially was associated with oral infection and HSV 2 with genital infection. Over the past 25 years, however, the increased popularity of oral sex has led to an almost equal probability of contracting either form from the genital area. A 2- to 12-day incubation period follows transmission of the virus.

The initial symptoms (also known as the primary outbreak) start as discrete grouped **vesicles.** After a short time (a few hours to a few days), the vesicles break open, merge with each other, and form painful ulcers, which drain and crust over. The entire first episode takes 15 to 20 days. Often, a systemic, flulike syndrome accompanies the primary outbreak. The symptoms of this syndrome, known as the **prodrome,** include aches, fever, and malaise.

Recurring outbreaks occur in most sufferers on an average of five to eight times per year and last approximately 10 days per episode. Recurrences often are preceded by the same prodromal syndrome that accompanies the primary episode. The frequency and severity of recurring episodes diminish with time. Genital herpes in adults tends to be a self-limiting, albeit painful, STD. It is a much more serious condition among newborns (infected as they pass through the birth canal) and those whose immune systems are compromised because of HIV infection (MMWR, 2002f; Fleming et al., 1997).

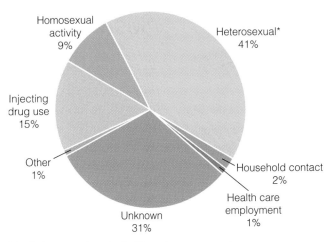

* Includes sexual contact with acute cases, carriers, and multiple partners

Figure 15.14 *Risk Factors for Hepatitis B* The majority of cases of hepatitis B are acquired through injector drug use and sexual activity.
Source: NCID (2003).

Genital herpes An infection caused by exposure to the herpes simplex virus type 1 or type 2 through sexual contact

Vesicles Fluid-filled blisters

Prodrome A systemic, flulike syndrome that accompanies genital herpes infection

The primary symptoms of herpes are fluid-filled vesicles that break open to form painful, highly infectious ulcers.

Centers for Disease Control and Prevention

case study 15.4

Susan, an HSV Sufferer

Susan, 23, single, is white.

Susan was a woman one of the authors met while conducting a self-help group for persons suffering with genital herpes. Susan had just found out that the ulcerative genital infection she had was caused by HSV. She came to the group to learn how to manage her disease.

I was shocked when my doctor told me I had herpes. I couldn't figure out how I got it, since I've been sexually involved with just my boyfriend for the past 6 months and he doesn't have any symptoms.

The doctor explained that my present boyfriend might not even have given it to me. [The doctor] explained that since I had several other sex partners since beginning to have intercourse at 19 years old, any of those guys could have given it to me. He said I might not have had any initial symptoms or might have missed them because they were so mild.

Now, because I've been stressed out—a new job, graduate school, getting engaged, moving into a house—the herpes is coming back. He suggested that I come here and learn about how to cope with it if I keep getting recurrences. I'm so stressed, but I know this is also the worst thing for me if I want to help my body keep it under control. Please help me!

Treatment Genital HSV infection has no cure. Advances in antiviral therapies, such as acyclovir, have made drugs available that shorten the duration of outbreaks and reduce the number and likelihood of recurrent episodes (Morse et al., 1990). Systemic antiviral drugs such as acyclovir can be used as daily suppressive therapy (suppress the likelihood of an outbreak); however, these drugs do not have lasting effects once discontinued (MMWR, 2002f). As with the other viral STDs, most treatment regimens focus on slowing the replication of the virus and boosting the immune system. Treatment also includes techniques to speed drying and healing of the vesicles and blisters associated with the infection.

Epidemiology Initial consultations with private physicians for genital herpes increased from fewer than 25,000 in 1996 to about 175,000 in 1997 (see Figure 15.15). A similar increase in office visits (from 18,000 to 176,000)—a more accurate index of morbidity—was also noted.

Figure 15.15 *Genital Herpes Consultations* The number of visits to physicians for genital herpes has increased significantly over the past 40 years.
Source: DSTD (2002b).

The prevalence of HSV remained relatively stable through the 1990s, with an estimated 45 million people in the United States infected with the virus (DSTD, 2000). The majority of those infected do not have clinical disease. In a broad-based national study, fewer than 10 percent of those who tested positive with the virus knew they were infected (Fleming et al., 1997). Women are at a greater risk than men for acquiring the infection. It is suggested that this is due to the greater efficiency of male to female transmission (DSTD, 2002).

Genital Warts (HPV)

Diagnosis   **Genital warts,** also known as venereal warts, are caused by infection with the **human papilloma virus (HPV).** There are at least 46 known varieties of HPV. Of these, at least 12 types of the virus are associated with genital infection. The virus is spread through direct contact with an infected person's genital warts during sexual contact.

The average incubation period for genital warts is 3 months from the time of exposure. The initial warts can be isolated or appear in clusters on the genitals and perianal area. The warts vary in size from 1/8 inch to considerably larger, and in some cases growths become so large that they cause deformity of genital structures. Growths can **autoinnoculate** adjoining tissue. These "kissing lesions" are often found on the labia or under the foreskin of uncircumcised men. Infection with warts is not painful, but continued growth can cause a painful obstruction of the vaginal, anal, or urethral opening.

Estimates of infection with no symptoms vary from 10 to 45 percent of infected individuals (Cates, 1991). Most HPV infections are temporary, and symptoms resolve by the body's immune response. Although studies have shown that most cases of HPV are undetectable after 2 years, reactivation of the virus can occur (DSTD, 2002; Ho, Bierman, Beardsley, Chang, & Burk, 1998).

Genital warts An STD caused by the HPV or human papilloma virus

Human papilloma virus (HPV) A condition spread through direct contact with an infected person's genital warts during sexual contact

Autoinnoculate To self-inflict the spread of disease from one body part to another

healthy sex hints 15.4

Self-Help for People with Genital Herpes

Most people with genital herpes are able to manage their infections and prevent spreading their infection to others. The following tips will help you do just that.

1. If you are taking acyclovir or other herpes medication on a maintenance schedule and it helps reduce recurring episodes of infection, continue taking the medicine as prescribed.
2. At the first hint of prodromal symptoms, consider yourself infectious and capable of spreading your infection. During this time, abstain from intercourse, engage in nongenital sexual pleasuring, or use condoms.
3. Treat any outbreak as you would the flu (another viral infection), with bed rest and over-the-counter pain relievers.

4. Keep your genitals clean and dry. Take short baths, pat your genitals with a towel, and use a hair dryer to dry the area thoroughly.
5. Avoid pantyhose, tight underwear, and binding clothes until the blisters crust over and dry up. If you can, take a day or two off during the worst symptoms, stay in bed, and avoid wearing clothes.
6. Do not cover the blisters with petroleum jelly or other cream that blocks air from drying the area.
7. Minimize stress, as it delays healing.

The genital warts associated with HPV infection can get large enough to block the openings of the urethra, vagina or anus.

Cervical interepithelial neoplasms (CIN) Tumors or growths within the cervical membrane tissues

The major concern associated with HPV is the increased risk for cancer. Cervical infection with HPV is associated with at least 80 percent of all cervical cancer cases (Schiffman, 1992; Woodman et al., 2001). Women with HPV infection of the cervix are 10 times more likely to develop cervical cancer than women without the infection (Schiffman, 1992). As many as 10 percent of women with cervical HPV infections will develop **cervical interepithelial neoplasms (CINs)** within 1 year. HPV types 16, 18, and 31 have been found in all types of genital cancers. HPV 16 is responsible for more than half of all cases of cervical cancer. Four HPV types, 16, 18, 31, and 45, account for 80 percent of all cervical cancer associated with HPV (Ciaran et al., 2003; DSTD, 2000).

Treatment No medication is available to cure a person of HPV infection, because this is another viral condition. Various forms of treatment, however, are used to remove warts from the skin's surface. Warts do not disappear by themselves. They are removed by applying medications to the warts that dry them out. If this treatment doesn't work, the warts are removed surgically by laser excision, through freezing, or by burning them off.

Epidemiology An estimated 20 million Americans are infected with HPV. Each year approximately 5.5 million new people are infected in the United States (Ciaran et al., 2003; DSTD, 2000). Recent estimates, based on studies of diverse populations ranging from adolescent high school girls and female students attending college health centers to STD clinic patients, indicate that approximately 1 percent of all Americans are infected with HPV (Moscicki et al., 2000; DSTD 2000).

Women and individuals in the 20- to 24-year-old age bracket constitute the bulk of the visits (see Figure 15.16). Routine testing of women for HPV in four locations yielded the following infectivity percentages:

9 percent of women seeking routine Pap smears at ob/gyn facilities across the United States tested positive;

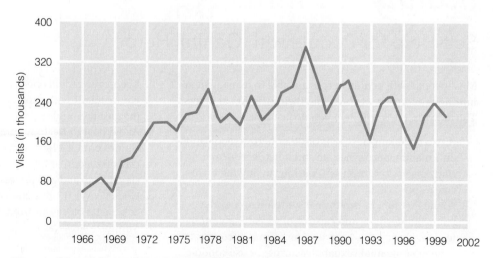

Figure 15.16 *Genital Warts Consultations* The number of visits to physicians for genital warts has leveled off somewhat over the past decade but still remain very high. *Source:* DSTD (2002).

between 9 percent and 45 percent of women attending health services in a university health center had positive test results;

23 percent of women attending family planning clinics were positive;

82 percent of street prostitutes in a select study had the virus (Quinn & Cates, 1993).

Moscicki et al. (2000) found that over 50 percent of adolescent girls who were HIV-positive and over 30 percent of those who were HIV-negative tested positive for HPV. HPV may become an even more serious problem among HIV-infected persons than other groups. These individuals have a greater susceptibility to precancerous lesions on the cervix (among heterosexual women) and anus (among gay men) than their non-HIV-infected peers. In one HIV study of gay men, HPV infection was found in 60 percent of those who were HIV-negative and almost 100 percent of those who were HIV-positive (DSTD, 2000).

Chlamydia

Diagnosis Chlamydia is a sexually transmitted disease caused by the *Chlamydia trachomatis* organism. It is transmitted through contact with infected semen or cervical mucus. It also can be passed through oral contact (usually fellatio) with infected mucus patches in the throat.

During sexual contact, the organisms are passed by person-to-person contact with the infected ejaculate or mucus. Incubation is from 1 to 30 days. The initial symptoms of chlamydia in men are a scanty, clear to milky-white discharge from the penis, and burning upon urination. Some women notice a scanty, clear to milky-white discharge and irritation of the vulva. Seventy-five percent of women and 50 percent of men usually have no symptoms for chlamydia. As previously mentioned, this is why screening sexually active women (and their sex partners) for chlamydia in a variety of health care facilities that serve them is the basis for the government's prevention program for the disease.

Chlamydia trachomatis The most prevalent sexually transmitted bacterial pathogen, causing the STD chlamydia

healthy sex hints 15.5

NAATs: Tests for Chlamydia

A recent advance in chlamydia and gonorrhea testing is the nucleic acid amplification tests (NAATs). These tests detect the presence of chlamydia through DNA testing. They actually identify nucleic acid sequences that are specific to chlamydia. Unlike smear or culture tests, NAATs do not require viable organisms to diagnose the disease. The specimens are easily obtained through urine samples. Patients do not need to be symptomatic to obtain specimens, and samples can be collected anywhere urine collection can be performed. The beauty of NAATs is that it reduces dependence on invasive tests and allows public health programs to expand testing into locations such as schools where other means of testing were unacceptable.

A recent study in a Philadelphia school-based clinic setting demonstrated a yield of more than 20 percent among students tested (Bertrami, 2002).

Another advantage of NAATs is their ability to test for gonorrhea infection at the same time using the same specimen. The same Philadelphia study found that almost half of students infected with chlamydia had coexistent gonorrhea infection. These gonorrhea infections would often go undetected with traditional tests that only checked for chlamydia. The ability to test for both infections simultaneously using an easy-to-obtain urine specimen represents a major breakthrough in STD testing and a major tool in the prevention of gonorrhea and chlamydia (MMWR, 2002d).

In the 1960s and 1970s, chlamydia infection was believed to be a relatively minor problem. Men with the infection were often referred to as having "nonspecific urethritis" and were not counseled extensively regarding the necessity to have their sexual partners examined. Chlamydia, however, was discovered to be a major source of **PID** (pelvic inflammatory disease). Up to 20 percent of all women with *C. trachomatis* infection will develop PID. PID can result in chronic pain, ectopic pregnancy, and sterility, and in rare instances it is fatal. More than half of all PID is caused by *C. trachomatis*. Infection in men rarely leads to major complications. Less than 1 percent of men infected with *C. trachomatis* develop epididymitis (Morse et al., 1990).

Treatment Chlamydia infection is relatively easy to treat. Azithromycin (1 gram, taken orally in a single dose) or doxycycline (100 milligrams, taken orally twice a day for 7 days) are the two recommended treatments. The organism is destroyed by a number of antibiotics and alternative treatments (MMWR, 2002f).

Epidemiology *Chlamydia trachomatis* is the most prevalent sexually transmitted bacterial pathogen in the United States. In 2000, 702,093 cases of chlamydia were reported to the Centers for Disease control from 50 states and the District of Columbia (DSTD, 2001). The chlamydia rate for 2000 was 257.5 cases per 100,000 persons. This represents an increase of 2.3 percent from the rate of 251.6 in 1999. The reported number of chlamydia infections was approximately double the 358,995 reported cases of gonorrhea (DSTD, 2001).

Between 1987 and 2000, the chlamydia rate in the United States increased from 50.8 to 257.5 cases per 100,000 persons (DSTD, 2001). Most experts agree that the continuing increase in reported cases of chlamydia is due to increased screening for this infection and also the development and use of more sensitive screening tests (DSTD, 2001). Figure 15.17 shows the rapid climb in rates during the years 1987–2000.

Although the current estimated incidence is about 3 million cases annually (down from estimates of 4 to 5 million), chlamydia rates continue to rise and represent a serious disease threat because of the asymptomatic nature of infection (Webster et al., 1993). Seventy-five percent of women and 50 percent of men usu-

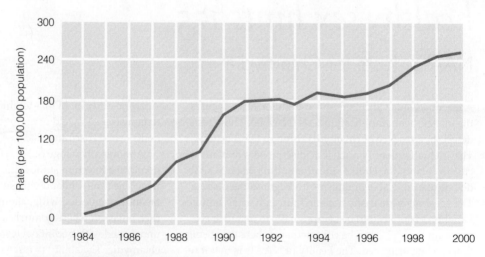

Figure 15.17 *Chlamydia Morbidity* The number of new cases of chlamydia infection continues to rise every year.
Source: DSTD (2002).

ally have no symptoms for chlamydia. This is why screening sexually active women (and their sex partners) for chlamydia in a variety of health care facilities that serve them is the basis for the government's prevention program for the disease. Most public STD and family planning clinics routinely screen all gonorrhea patients for infection with chlamydia trachomatis, since roughly 50 percent of all gonorrhea patients have coexistent infection with chlamydia (Cates et al, 1999).

Reported chlamydia rates in women are much higher because screening programs have typically been directed mostly at women. Most cases of nongonococcal urethritis infection (NGU) are attributed to *C. trachomatis*. Chlamydia exists at endemic levels in young women. More than 40 percent of all cases of chlamydia are among 15- to 19-year-olds. In studies of adolescents, approximately 10 percent of all girls and 5 percent of all boys tested positive for the infection (DSTD, 2000). Chlamydia rates by race/ethnicity show a slightly lower rate for whites than for all other racial/ethnic groups. As with many STDs, rates are highest in the South than in other regions (DSTD, 2002; Karon et al., 2001; Guaschino & DeSeta, 2000).

Gonorrhea

Diagnosis   **Gonorrhea** is similar to *C. trachomatis* clinically. Following sexual exposure, the organism incubates from 1 to 30 days. Most people who develop symptoms notice them within 1 to 3 days. The initial symptoms are the same as those associated with chlamydia. Discharge and burning upon urination are the most common symptoms in men. The difference is in the severity of symptoms. Gonorrhea symptoms usually are more severe—heavy discharge, yellowish-green in color, and severe burning. The symptoms usually are enough to cause men with the infection to seek treatment. Up to 20 percent of men have no symptoms. About 50 percent of women infected with gonorrhea are asymptomatic, and a small percentage will notice a discharge or have irritation of the vulva.

In women, gonorrhea often results in complications, the most common of which is PID (pelvic inflammatory disease)—occurring in approximately 15 percent of all women with untreated gonorrhea. These women, as with those who develop PID from chlamydia, have an increased risk for chronic pain, ectopic pregnancy, sterility, and even death. Less than 1 percent of men with untreated gonorrhea develop disseminated gonococcal infection and/or epididymitis (Morse et al., 1990). Like chlamydia, gonorrhea is easy to treat.

Gonorrhea A sexually transmitted disease caused by the bacteria *Neisseria gonorrheae*

Centers for Disease Control and Prevention

Gonorrhea infection typically produces a profuse, thick, yellow-green discharge, but it can also mimic the milder symptoms of chlamydia. Infection in the cervix, throat, or rectum is often asymptomatic.

Intellectual and Emotional Wellness

High-level intellectual wellness is the cornerstone of effective prevention of STDs. Knowing the risks and how to reduce them is critical to preventing STDs. This knowledge includes information about personal behavior and also about lifestyles and demographic risks. Intellectual wellness also fosters enhanced decision making. Reducing the risks for STD is all about personal choice. Because STDs are sexually transmitted, their prevention and control are more than just a medical matter. STDs involve our most intimate emotions. Knowing about prevention and seeking treatment are one thing. Working through the anxiety, fear, and guilt, and a host of other emotions that interfere with clear thinking about STDs is another thing. Emotional health can help us deal with the emotions that can cloud rational thinking.

Treatment   Recent increases in drug-resistant strains of gonorrhea, particularly those acquired in Asia or the Pacific, including Hawaii, have prompted a change in the recommended treatment for gonorrhea. Single-dose regimens taken either orally or intramuscularly (via a shot) of the following drugs are the recommended treatment: Cefiximine (oral), Ceftriaxone (intramuscularly), Ofloxacin (oral), and Levofloxacin. Because infection with chlamydia often coexists asymptomatically with gonorrhea, the CDC recommends that all persons with gonorrhea who have not had a test to rule out chlamydia be treated for both infections at the time of their gonorrhea diagnosis (MMWR, 2002f).

Epidemiology   Gonorrhea is one of the most common STDs, with more than 350,000 cases reported annually (DSTD, 2002). Because it can be easily diagnosed clinically in a physician's office, public health officials estimate that gonorrhea might be underreported by as much as 50 percent (DSTD, 2000). Between 1975 and 1997 (see Figure 15.18), gonorrhea rates decreased by 72 percent nationally (DSTD, 2002). Of that decline, 22 percent was between 1986 and 1989 and credited largely to safer-sex behaviors by white gay men (Fox, Del Rio, & Holmes, 2001). One of the Healthy People 2010 health status objectives for the nation, reducing gonorrhea rates to 225 cases per 100,000 people, was based on a projection of the continued decline in gonorrhea rates (U.S. Department of Health and Human Services [USDHHS], 2002).

Figure 15.18 *Gonorrhea Rates* Gonorrhea rates seem to have leveled off but still exceed targets set by Healthy People 2010.

Note: The Healthy People 2010 (HP2010) objective for gonorrhea is 19.0 cases per 100,000 population.

Source: DSTD (2002).

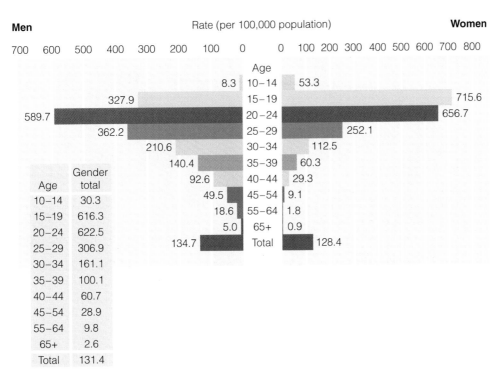

Figure 15.19 *Gonorrhea Rates by Age and Gender* Gonorrhea is endemic among some populations of young men and women.
Source: DSTD (2002).

Since 1997, however, gonorrhea morbidity has been on the rise. Gonorrhea rates have risen 9 percent since 1999 (DSTD, 2002). Experts fear that the 9 percent overall rise in morbidity might actually mask a more serious increase in gonorrhea rates among men who have sex with men. A national program that tracks drug-resistant gonorrhea in 26 major cities across the United States reported that during the period 1994–1999, the proportion of gonorrhea cases among MSM more than doubled, from 6 to 13 percent. In San Francisco, the rate of rectal gonorrhea among men infected with the disease increased from 21 cases per 100,000 to 38 cases per 100,000 for 1994–1997.

These data could indicate a reversal in the adoption of safer-sex practices among this population that spearheaded the dramatic decline in cases a decade ago. It also is an ominous warning of possible changes in HIV morbidity if safe-sex practices among this high-risk group change (DSTD, 2001). Even more alarming is the increase in drug-resistant gonorrhea reported in Hawaii and several clusters within the continental United States (DSTD, 2001).

Figure 15.19 illustrates gonorrhea rates by age and gender. Gonorrhea rates continue to be highest in the 15- to 19- and 20- to 24-year-old age groups for both men and women. The highest rates continue to be among young girls between 15 and 19 years old. Rates among adolescents increased by 13 percent from 1997 to 1999. Rates for these women (regardless of race/ethnicity) are approximately double those of men at this age. Rates for men and women in the 20- to 24-year-old age group are more closely aligned. Rates have increased in all racial/ethnic groups since 1997. The southern states continue to have the highest rates among all regions in the United States (DSTD, 2002).

Nongonococcal Urethritis (NGU)

Diagnosis Nongonococcal urethritis (NGU) is diagnosed when *Neisseria gonorrhea* is ruled out as the causative agent of discharge and burning in a male. In most cases, a negative lab test for gonorrhea and the presence of symptoms is

Nongonococcal urethritis (NGU) An infection in the urethra of males, usually caused by chlamydia bacteria

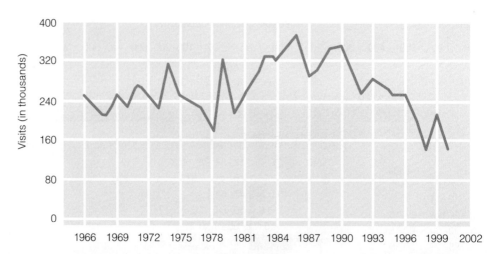

Figure 15.20 *Nongonococcal Urethritis Consultations* The number of visits to private physicians for NGU has dropped in the past decade.
Source: DSTD (2002).

enough to diagnose NGU. NGU is also a surrogate measure of chlamydia in men, as more than half of all cases of NGU are attributable to *C. trachomatis*. In some cases, a test for *C. trachomatis* is done.

Treatment   NGU presents the same symptoms as chlamydia infection in men and is treated using the same treatment schedule recommended for chlamydia.

Epidemiology   Figure 15.20 illustrates visits to physicians' offices for NGU. Visits to physicians for NGU peaked in 1990 and, except for a slight increase in 1999, declined steadily throughout the decade (DSTD, 2002). Annual incidence of NGU is estimated at approximately 3 million cases annually in the United States (DSTD, 2000).

Pubic Lice

Pubic lice *Phthirius pubis;* small insects (metazoan) that infest the host's pubic hair

Diagnosis   Infection with **pubic lice,** commonly called *crabs,* is caused by infestation of *Phthirius pubis.* The lice are transmitted during sexual contact from the infested pubic hair of one person to the other. In rarer instances, the lice are transmitted from contaminated bedding, clothing, and towels that people share. Female lice lay eggs, called *nits,* which attach to the shaft of the pubic hair of the exposed individual. The incubation period for lice is between 24 and 48 hours, at which time the eggs hatch and another batch of lice spread throughout the pubic hair.

Symptoms of pubic lice are (a) visual confirmation of the lice, (b) intense itching of the pubic and perianal area, (c) skin irritation, and (d) secondary sores and erosions from scratching. Although infestation rarely leads to complications, persons with pubic lice sometimes develop secondary infections from their intense scratching.

Treatment   Treatment of lice consists of special shampoos that kill the lice on the skin and hair. The shampoos are applied to the affected areas, allowed to sit for up to 10 minutes, and rinsed off thoroughly. Bedding, clothing, and other contaminated articles must be washed and dried thoroughly under hot settings or dry-cleaned. Fumigation of the person's house is not necessary (MMWR, 2002f).

Scabies

Diagnosis   Like crabs, **scabies** is caused by infestation with a mite. This mite, *Sarcoptes scabies,* is transmitted in the same way as pubic lice. Symptoms are similar with one notable exception: *S. scabies* actually burrows under the skin of an infected person and feeds on cellular matter. Diagnosis usually consists of identifying the mite's burrows under the skin.

Treatment   Because of the burrowing of the mites involved in scabies, treatment involves applying a lotion (similar to the shampoos used in pubic lice) that is left on the skin for 8 to 14 hours before being washed off. More than one application of the lotion may be required (MMWR, 2002f).

Scabies A condition caused by the *Sarcoptes scabiei* parasite, which burrows under the skin and lays eggs

> *Your responses to the Personal Assessment, Thought Questions, and Test Yourself! quiz questions can be logged online in your Virtual Workbook at* **http://health.wadsworth.com/blonna1.**

Personal Assessment

15.1 American College Health Association Risk Assessment Form

Many factors must be considered in assessing your health and fitness. Among these are (a) your risk of acquiring or transmitting any sexually transmitted disease (STD) and (b) your use of psychoactive chemicals in connection with sexual activity, a practice that can increase your risk of acquiring an STD. STDs considered here include, but are not limited to, gonorrhea; syphilis; genital herpes; genital warts; chlamydia; hepatitis B; giardiasis; and infection with HIV, the virus that causes AIDS.

The first two questions are biographical in nature and are not part of the risk assessment score. They are intended to guide your provider in making the best possible appraisal of your health. The remaining 11 are the scored behavioral risk assessment. Please be honest in responding to the questions—we assure you that this document will be handled with the utmost confidentiality by you and your health care provider only. Please feel free to discuss the results with your provider. You may retain the survey for your own reference. *In any event, it will not be placed in your medical record.*

There are 11 questions listed below. Please check the one single answer that best describes your preferences or activities.

A. How long have you been sexually active? _____

B. Your most recent consistent sexual partner experience

  male _____ female _____ both male and female _____

1. How many sexual partners *per month* in the last year?
   3 _____ 5 or more
   2 _____ 2–4
   1 _____ 0–1

2. How many partners *per month* in the year previous?
   3 _____ 5 or more
   2 _____ 2–4
   1 _____ 0–1

3. The kinds of sexual contacts I have are
   3 _____ one-time or anonymous "tricks," "one night stands," groups, or prostitutes
   2 _____ multiple times with two or more partners
   1 _____ exclusively with one partner

4. I have sexual encounters or contacts most frequently
   3 _____ in baths, bookstores, parties, "massage parlors," "spas," public restrooms, autos
   1 _____ in my or my partner's home

5. The frequency with which I use drugs or alcohol to enhance my sexual encounters:
   3 _____ frequently
   2 _____ occasionally
   1 _____ rarely/never

   Please circle drug used: "poppers" (amyl or butyl nitrates), alcohol, marijuana, hallucinogens (LSD, mushrooms), "angel dust" (PCP), amphetamines, barbiturates, Quaaludes, ecstasy, eve, cocaine, crack, or (please fill in others)

6. I have injected myself with one or more of the above drugs in the past 5 years.
   4 _____ yes
   1 _____ no

7. I have sexual encounters most frequently in
   3 _____ New York, Los Angeles, San Francisco, Miami, Washington, Dallas, Houston, Newark, Atlanta
   2 _____ other large urban areas (Boston, Philadelphia, St. Louis, Seattle, San Diego, etc.)
   1 _____ small cities, towns, rural areas

8. Those kinds of sexual activities I practice most frequently are (please circle specific activities)
   4 _____ vaginal or anal intercourse without a condom, oral-anal contact (rimming), direct fecal or urine contact (scat or water sports), or manual anal contact (fisting)
   3 _____ "protected" vaginal or anal intercourse (use of condoms and spermicides)
   2 _____ oral-genital contact (fellatio or cunnilingus)
   1 _____ masturbation, massage, body rubbing, kissing

9. My current sexual partner and I have discussed our previous sexual behavior and experiences with each other.
   4 _____ No
   1 _____ Yes

10. I negotiate with sexual partners for safer sexual practices.
    4 _____ No
    2 _____ Sometimes
    1 _____ Yes

11. I ask potential sexual partners about their use of drugs and steroids, especially their use of needles.
    4 _____ No
    2 _____ Sometimes
    1 _____ Yes

Add up the numbers from each question (1–11) and see the key below to determine your level of risk.

My score is _____.

If you answered "1" (the last option) for question 8, deduct 3 points.

Total Adjusted Score: _____

Key:

17 or more: You appear to be at high risk for developing STDs, including HIV infection, and for possibly developing dependence on psychoactive substances. You should visit your health care provider immediately to discuss your risk of these dangers.

12–16 points: You appear to be at moderate risk for developing either an STD or chemical dependence and are encouraged to lower your overall risk by altering the behaviors that resulted in high scores on some of the questions. See your health care provider for any questions or concerns you may have regarding your risk.

11 points: You are at low risk for problems and are encouraged to continue your healthy behavior. Please feel free to contact your health care provider at any time for updated information regarding safer sex, AIDS, or any other issues.

This scoring system was designed to (a) increase your awareness of STDs and the risk factors associated with acquiring or transmitting STDs, (b) stimulate self-evaluation of your health and your sexual lifestyle, and (c) encourage your taking responsibility for your health and the health of your sexual contacts. **This questionnaire is yours to keep and review. It will not go into your medical record even if you bring it to your health care provider.**

Source: Reprinted from the special report, "AIDS on the College Campus" (no longer in print), by Leland G. Wessell, M.D., M.P.H., with permission from the American College Health Association, PO Box 28937, Baltimore, MD 20840-8937.

Thought Questions

1. What are the various modes of transmission associated with STDs/HIV?

2. What are four major trends associated with STDs over the past two decades?

3. What is the underlying premise of the Pyramid of Risk for STDs?

4. How are demographic variables related to the risk for STD/HIV?

5. What are five important things to know about a potential sex partner's sexual history as related to STD/HIV risk?

6. How do sexual lifestyles and sexual behavior work together to increase or decrease risk?

7. What are the major signs and symptoms of STDs in men and women?

8. Why do gay men and heterosexual women have a similar risk profile?

Test Yourself!

1. Which group is not experiencing an increase in STD morbidity and mortality?
   a. Urban, heterosexual, African Americans
   b. Rural homosexual men
   c. Hispanic adolescents
   d. Female partners of HIV-infected intravenous drug users

2. *Epidemiological synergy* refers to
   a. the proliferation of STDs that cause damage to the epidermis.
   b. a synergestic effect caused by two different germs.
   c. the increased risk for acquiring an STD if already infected with one.
   d. a pattern of rampant disease spread through populations.

3. The Pyramid of Risk for STDs assumes that
   a. there are four levels of STD risk; some can be changed, some cannot.
   b. disease risk is like a pyramid or iceberg.
   c. those at the top of the risk pyramid have the greatest chance of becoming infected.
   d. there are five levels of risk that correspond to demographics.

4. Which best characterizes the risk associated with sexual lifestyle and sexual behaviors?
   a. They are two separate risk categories that do not relate to each other.
   b. The lower your STD lifestyle risk, the less attention you need to pay to specific sexual behaviors.
   c. The higher your STD lifestyle risk, the less attention you need to pay to specific sexual behaviors.
   d. Sexual medical history does not impact sexual lifestyle risk.

5. Which of the following is *not* an STD risk associated with one's sexual medical history?
   a. Number of lifetime sexual partners
   b. History of contraceptive use
   c. Immunization status
   d. Age of onset of sexual intercourse

6. The belief that "when you sleep with someone, you sleep with everyone they have slept with" is inaccurate because
   a. it is a simplistic metaphor.
   b. your partner's sex partners had sex with him or her, not you.
   c. being exposed to antibodies that your partner produced in relation to their sex partners is not the same thing as having sex with those people.
   d. all of the above

7. Which of the following is *not* a viral STD?
   a. Syphilis
   b. HIV
   c. HPV
   d. Genital herpes

8. Why do gay men and heterosexual women share a similar STD risk profile?
   a. They both are sexually attracted to heterosexual men who carry most STDs.
   b. They are insertive sexually.
   c. They are receptive sexually.
   d. Their primary sex partners are men.

9. Which of the following is most responsible for the pattern of decreasing AIDS mortality?
   a. The sexual behavior of HIV high-risk groups has changed.
   b. Cocktail AIDS drugs are used.
   c. Less virulent strains of HIV now predominate.
   d. Most people with AIDS have already died.

10. Which STD is making a comeback in selected major U.S. cities after being on the verge of extinction in the past 5 years?
    a. Smallpox
    b. Syphilis
    c. Scabies
    d. Chancroid

Media Menu

You can link to the following online tools by visiting
http://health.wadsworth.com/blonna1.

Face to Face Video

Debbie shares her experience of living with AIDS.

Film

HIV/AIDS Client Support

 InfoTrac Activity

Levine, H. (2001, August). Should you come clean about your sexual history? *Cosmopolitan, 231*(2), 146–150.

 Web Resources

The Division of STD Prevention

www.cdc.gov/nchstp/dstd/dstdp.html

The Division of STD Prevention, at the Centers for Disease Control and Prevention, provides national leadership through research, policy development, and support of effective services to prevent STDs (including HIV infection) and their complications such as enhanced HIV transmission, infertility, adverse outcomes of pregnancy, and reproductive tract cancer.

The Division of HIV/AIDS Prevention

www.cdc.gov/hiv/dhap.htm

CDC's HIV mission is to prevent HIV infection and reduce the incidence of HIV-related illness and death, in collaboration with community, state, national, and international partners.

University of Pittsburgh Student Health Services

www.studhlth.pitt.edu/about.html

A site that provides a variety of information that encourages healthy lifestyles, including an online self-assessment for STD risk.

American Social Health Association (ASHA)

www.ashastd.org

A nonprofit organization dedicated to stopping sexually transmitted diseases and their consequences. The site offers excellent links and information to other ASHA programs. It provides STD information, facts and questions, sexual health glossary, and support groups sections.

Gay Men's Health Crisis

www.gmhc.org/

A nonprofit organization providing support services to men, women, children, and their families with AIDS in the New York City area, as well as education and advocacy nationwide.

Herpes Resource Center (HRC)

www.ashastd.org/herpes/hrc.html

Accurate information about herpes simplex virus infections. This site offers a wide selection of good herpes links. HRC provides questions and answers, how to tell your partner, when to tell your partner, and issues of herpes and pregnancy.

References

Alan Guttmacher Institute. (1991). *Sex and America's teenagers.* New York: Author.

Alter, M., & Margolis, H. (1990). The emergence of hepatitis B as a sexually transmitted disease. *Medical Clinics of North America, 6,* 1529–1541.

American Medical Association, Council on Scientific Affairs. (1996). Health care needs of gay men and lesbians in the United States. *Journal of American Medical Association, 257,* 1354–1359.

Bertrami, R. (2002, November). *Chlamydia screening in the Philadelphia public schools.* Paper presented at the annual Meeting of the American Public Health Association, Philadelphia.

Cameron, D. W., et al. (1991). Condom use prevents genital ulcers in women working as prostitutes: Influences of human immunodeficiency virus infection. *Sexually Transmitted Diseases, 18,* 188–194.

Cates, W., et al. (1999). Estimates of the incidence and prevalence of sexually transmitted diseases in the United States. *Sexually Transmitted Diseases, 26*(Supplement): S2–S7.

Cates, W., & Stone, K. M. (1992). Family planning, sexually transmitted diseases and contraceptive choice: A literature update—Part I. *Family Planning Perspectives, 24*(2), 75–84.

Ciaran, B. J., Woodman, S. C., Rollason, T. P., Winter, H., Bailey, A., Yates, M., & Young, L. S. (2003, January 4). Human papillomavirus type 18 and rapidly progressing cervical intraepithelial neoplasia: Mechanisms of disease. *The Lancet, 361*(9351), 40.

Ciesielski, C. A., Flynn, J., & McLean, C. (2002, October). *B1B—Sexually transmitted diseases, HIV testing, and HIV risk behaviors among men who have sex with men seeking care at Howard Brown Health Center.* Paper presented at Annual DSTD Meeting.

Conant, M., Hardy, D., Sernatinger, J., Spicer, D., & Levy, J. (1986). Condoms prevent transmission of AIDS-associated retrovirus. *Journal of the American Medical Association, 255,* 1706.

Dan, B. D. (1996). Sex and the singles whirl: The quantum dynamics of hepatitis B. *Journal of the American Medical Association, 256*(10), 1344.

Darrow, W. W. (1989). Condom use and use-effectiveness in high-risk populations. *Sexually Transmitted Diseases, 16,* 157–162.

Darrow, W. W., Barrett, D., McPhil, K. J., & Young, A. (1981). The gay report on sexually transmitted diseases. *American Journal of Public Health, 71*(9), 1004–1011.

Division of HIV/AIDS, Division of STD Prevention. (2002a). Cumulative AIDS cases through 12/02 [Online]. Available: www.cdc.gov/hiv/stats.htm#cumaids.

Division of HIV/AIDS, Division of STD Prevention. (2002b). *Surveillance report, 2001: Year-end edition, 12/01.* Atlanta: Public Health Service.

Division of STD Prevention, Centers for Disease Control and Prevention. (1999). *The national plan to eliminate syphilis from the United States.* Atlanta: Public Health Service.

Division of STD Prevention, Centers for Disease Control and Prevention. (2000). *Tracking the hidden epidemics: Trends in STDs in the United States 2000.* Atlanta: Public Health Service.

Division of STD Prevention, Centers for Disease Control and Prevention. (2001). *Sexually transmitted disease surveillance report 2000.* Atlanta: Public Health Service.

Division of STD Prevention, Centers for Disease Control and Prevention. (2002). *Sexually transmitted disease surveillance report 2001.* Atlanta: Public Health Service.

Division of TB Elimination, Centers for Disease Control. (2001.) *Surveillance report: Executive summary.* Atlanta: Public Health Service.

Donelan, K., Blendon, R. J., Hill, C. A., et al. (1996). Whatever happened to the health insurance crisis in the United States? Voices from a national survey. *Journal of the American Medical Association, 276,* 1346–1350.

Dunn, R. A., & Rolfs, R. T. (1991). The resurgence of syphilis in the United States. *Current Opinions in Infectious Diseases, 4,* 3–11.

Eng, T. R., & Butler, W. T. (Eds.). (1997). *The hidden epidemic: Confronting STDs.* Washington, DC: Academy Press, Institute of Medicine.

Finelli, L., Budd, J., & Spitalny, K. (1993). Early syphilis: Relationships to sex, drugs, and changes in high-risk behavior from 1987–1990. *Sexually Transmitted Diseases, 2,* 89–95.

Fleming, D. T., McQuillan, G. M., Johnson, R. E., Nahmias, A. J., Aral, S. O., Lee, F. K., & St. Louis, M. E. (1997). Herpes simplex virus type 2 in the United States, 1976 to 1994. *New England Journal of Medicine, 337,* 1105–1111.

Fox, K. K., Del Rio, C., & Holmes, K. K. (2001). Gonorrhea in the HIV era: A reversal in trends among men who have sex with men. *American Journal of Public Health, 91,* 907–914.

Garnett, G. P., & Anderson, R. M. (1996). Core-group transmission of STDs. *Sexually Transmitted Diseases, 20*(4), 181–191.

Grimes, D. A., & Cates, W. (1990). Family planning and sexually transmitted diseases. In K. K. Holmes, P. A. Mardh, P. F. Sparling, P. Wiesner, W. Cates, S. M. Lemon, & W. E. Stamm (Eds.), *Sexually transmitted diseases* (2nd ed., pp. 1087–1094). New York: McGraw-Hill.

Guaschino, S., & DeSeta, F. (2000). Update on *Chlamydia trachomatis* [review]. *Annals of the New York Academy of Science, 900,* 293–300.

Hart, G. (1974). Factors influencing venereal infection in a war environment. *British Journal of Venereal Disease, 50,* 68–72.

Hayes, R. J., Schulz, K. F., & Plummer, F. A. (1995). The co-factor effect of genital ulcers on the per-exposure risk of HIV transmission in sub-Sahara Africa. *Journal of Tropical and Medical Hygiene, 98,* 1–8.

Ho, G. Y. F., Bierman, R., Beardsley, L., Chang, C. J., & Burk, R. D. (1998). Natural history of cervicovaginal papilloma virus infection in young women. *New England Journal of Medicine, 338,* 423–428.

Howard, M., & McCabe, J. B. (1990). Helping teenagers postpone sexual involvement. *Family Planning Perspectives, 22,* 21–26.

Karon, J. M., Fleming, P. L., Steketee, R. W., & DeCock, K. M. (2001). HIV in the United States at the turn of the century: An epidemic in transition. *American Journal of Public Health, 91*(7), 1060–1068.

Kennedy, M. B., Scarlett, M. I., Duer, A. C., & Chu, S. Y. (1995). Assessing HIV risk among women who have sex with women: Scientific and communication issues. *Journal of the American Medical Women's Association, 50,* 103–107.

Laumann, E. O., Gagnon, J. H., Michael, R. Y., & Michaels, S. (1994). *The social organization of sexuality: Sexual practices in the United States.* Chicago: University of Chicago Press.

Mann, J., Quinn, T., et al. (1987). Condom use and HIV infection among prostitutes in Zaire [letter]. *New England Journal of Medicine, 316,* 345.

Minuk, G., Bohme, G., & Bowen, T. (1986). Condoms and hepatitis B virus infection. *Annals of Internal Medicine, 104,* 584.

MMWR. (1991). The HIV/AIDS epidemic: The first 10 years. *Mortality and Morbidity Weekly Report, 40,* 22.

MMWR. (1995a, November 24). First 500,000 cases of AIDS—United States. *Mortality and Morbidity Weekly Report, 44.*

MMWR. (1995b, July 14). HIV: Preventing the spread of opportunistic infections. *Mortality and Morbidity Weekly Report, 44.*

MMWR. (1995c, July 7). Preventing HIV infection in women and children. *Mortality and Morbidity Weekly Report.*

MMWR. (1995d, June 2). Update: Trends in AIDS among men who have sex with men—United States, 1989–94. *Morbidity and Mortality Weekly Report, 44.*

MMWR. (1999). Resurgent bacterial sexually transmitted disease among men who have sex with men—King County, Washington, 1997–1999. *Morbidity and Mortality Weekly Report, 48,* 773–777.

MMWR. (2002a). Gonorrhea—United States, 1998. *Morbidity and Mortality Weekly Report, 49,* 538–542.

MMWR. (2002b, September 27). Primary and secondary syphilis among men who have sex with men, NYC 2001. *Morbidity and Mortality Weekly Report, 51*(38), 853–856.

MMWR. (2002c, August 17). Provisional cases of selected notifiable disease. *Morbidity and Mortality Weekly Report, 51,* 746–754.

MMWR. (2002d, October 18). Screening tests to detect chlamydia and gonorrhea infections. *Morbidity and Mortality Weekly Report, 51* (RR-15).

MMWR (2002e, September 27). Trends in sexual risk behaviors among high school students—United States, 1991–2001. *Morbidity and Mortality Weekly Report, 51*(38), 853–856.

MMWR. (2002f, May). 2002: Sexually transmitted disease: Treatment guidelines. *Mortality and Morbidity Weekly Report, 51* (RR-6).

Morse, S., Moreland, A., & Thompson, S. (1990). *Sexually transmitted diseases.* New York: Gower Medical.

Moscicki, A. B., Ellenberg, J. H., Vermund, S. H., Hooland, C. A., Darragh, T., Crowley-Nowick, P. A., et al. (2000, February). Prevalence of and risks for cervical human papillomavirus infection and squamous intraepithelial lesions in adolescent girls. *Archives of Pediatrics & Adolescent Medicine, 154*(2), 127.

Nakashima, A. K., Rolfs, R. T., Flock, M. L., et al. (1996). Epidemiology of syphilis in the United States, 1941–1993. *Sexually Transmitted Diseases, 23*(1), 16–23.

National Center for Infectious Disease. (2003). Hepatitis surveillance 1980–2001 [Online]. Available: www.cdc.gov/ncidod/diseases/hepatitis/resource/dz_burden02.htm.

Navarro, N. (1990). Race or class: Mortality differentials in the United States. *Lancet, 336,* 1238–1240.

Pinkerton, S. T., Chesson, H. W., & Layde, P. M. (2002, September). NIMH prevention trial group: Utility of behavioral changes as markers of STD risk reduction in sexually transmitted disease/HIV prevention trials. *Journal of AIDS, 31*(1), 71–79.

Piot, P., & Islam, M. Q. (1994). Sexually transmitted diseases in the 1990s: Global epidemiology and the challenges for control. *Sexually Transmitted Diseases, 21* (Supplement 2), 7–13.

Potterat, R., Rothenberg, R., Woodhouse, D. E., Muth, J. B., Pratts, C. I., & Fogle, J. S. (1985). Gonorrhea as a social disease. *Sexually Transmitted Diseases, 1,* 25–32.

Quinn, T., & Cates, W. (1993). Epidemiology of STDs in the 1990s. In T. Quinn (Ed.), *Sexually transmitted diseases.* New York: Raven.

Ramos, R., Shain, R. N., & Johnson, L. (1995). Men I mess with don't have anything to do with AIDS: Using ethnotheory to understand sexual risk perception. *Sociology Quarterly, 36,* 483–505.

Rice, R. J., Roberts, P. L., & Handsfield, H. H. (1991). Sociodemographic distribution of gonorrhea incidence: Implications for prevention and behavioral research. *American Journal of Public Health, 10,* 1253–1257.

Rosenberg, M. J., & Gollub, E. L. (1992). Commentary: Methods women can use that may prevent sexually transmitted disease, including HIV. *American Journal of Public Health, 82*(11), 1473–1478.

Rutherford, J. (2002, November). *Rise in syphilis among select groups of men who have sex with men.* Paper presented at the annual Meeting of the American Public Health Association, Philadelphia.

Schiffman, N. H. (1992). Recent progress in defining the epidemiology of human papillomavirus infection and cervical neoplasia. *Journal of National Cancer Institute, 84,* 394–398.

Smeltzer, S., & Whipple, B. (1991). Women & HIV. *Journal of Nursing, 4,* 249–256.

St. Louis, M. E., & Wasserheit, J. N. (1998). Elimination of syphilis in the United States. *Science, 281,* 353–354.

Ungvarski, P. J. (1997). Update on HIV infection. *American Journal of Nursing, 97*(1), 44–51.

U.S. Department of Health and Human Services. (2000, November). *Healthy People 2010: Understanding and improving health* (2nd ed.). Washington, DC: U.S. Government Printing Office.

Wasserheit, J. (1992). Epidemiological synergy. *Sexually Transmitted Diseases, 2,* 61–77.

Webster, L. A., Berman, S. M., & Greenspan, M. (1993), Surveillance for gonorrhea and primary and secondary syphilis among adolescents United States, 1981–1991. *Mortality and Morbidity Weekly Report, 42*(SS-3), 1–10.

Webster, L. A., & Rolfs, R. T. (1993). Surveillance for primary and secondary syphilis, United States, 1991. *Mortality and Morbidity Weekly Report, 42*(SS–3), 13–18.

Woodman, C. B., Collins, S., Winter, H., Barley, A., Ellis, J., Prior, P., et al. (2001). Natural history of cervical human papillomavirus infection in young women: A longitudinal cohort study. *Lancet, 357*(9271), 1831–1836.

Zenker, P. (1991). New case definition for congenital syphilis. *STDs, 1,* 44–45.

chapter *sixteen*

Sexual Coercion

Student Learning Objectives

After reading this chapter, students will be able to

- Define *sexual coercion* and *sexual victimization* and the three forms highlighted in this chapter: harassment, rape, and child sexual abuse.

- Explain and give examples of the three conditions that constitute sexual harassment.

- Describe the dynamic of power over subordinates in determining sexual harassment.

- Define *rape*, and differentiate it from other forms of sexual aggression.

- Describe the typical pattern of rape by a stranger, and develop a personal plan to reduce the risk for this form of rape.

- Define *acquaintance rape* and identify the risks.

- Develop a personal plan for reducing the risk for date rape.

- Describe the risks associated with the major "date rape" drugs.

- Assess the impact of alcohol abuse in coercive sex.

- Describe the characteristics of rapists.

- Evaluate common myths associated with rape and rapists.

- Describe the preconditions of child sexual abuse.

- Evaluate ways to reduce the risks for child sexual abuse.

*Test your understanding of these objectives by taking the end-of-chapter quiz, available online at **http://health.wadsworth.com/blonna1.***

activity teaser: *What is the message in the music? Learn more in the Personal Exploration Activity on page 537.*

Marc: Learning That No Means No

Marc, 23, identifies as Italian American.

Marc, a senior, was a student in one of Dr. Blonna's human sexuality classes. He submitted a written assignment about how he learned the difference between yes and no.

I'm embarrassed to write this, but I think the story needs to be told. I grew up learning that when a woman said no, she really meant yes. My brother and his friends explained it to me by saying that women do this so they can remain ladies but still get laid. It made sense to me then, even though I now realize this kind of thinking is crazy.

I didn't encounter this with the first two women I had sex with. They both willingly went along. I went out with my second girlfriend for almost 2 years. When we broke up, I had to start dating again and didn't get anywhere with the first two girls I went out with. They didn't even let me get to first base.

The third woman was very sexy. I met her at a frat party, and she was hot. We danced a little and had a couple of beers, and then she wanted to leave. I walked her back to her room, and she invited me up. Her roommates had gone home for the weekend, and we started making out on the couch. She was so sexy, and I thought she really wanted to have sex. She let me feel her breasts and put my hand in her pants, but every time I tried to unzip her jeans, she pulled away and said no. I figured she was just teasing and really wanted me to continue, so I kept pushing the limit.

After about 20 minutes of this, she suddenly pushed me off of her and literally dumped me on the floor. She screamed at me, "Look, I told you no five times! I don't want to fuck you. Now get out before I call the campus cops!"

I was shocked and very upset. I really didn't want to rape her, just push her until she gave in. I felt embarrassed and wanted to explain how I felt, but she told me if I didn't leave immediately, she'd call the police. I ran out of there zipping up as I left. I've seen her on campus, but she won't even look at me. I learned that no really means no!

Critical Thinking

Assuming that both Marc and the third woman were really interested in *some form* of sexual encounter, how could this scene have ended differently?

Use your Virtual Workbook to explore your answer to this question at **http://health.wadsworth.com/blonna1.**

Sexual coercion Any nonconsensual sexual behavior that occurs as the result of arguing, pleading, and cajoling and includes, but is not limited to, force

Sexual victimization Depriving a person of free choice and forcing him or her to endure, observe, or comply with sexual acts

Rape Illicit sexual intercourse without consent

As we have seen in the case of Marc, there is a fine line between pursuing sex assertively and sexual coercion. Marc learned firsthand that "No means no," or that line is crossed. **Sexual coercion** is any nonconsensual sexual behavior that occurs as a result of arguing, pleading, and cajoling, in addition to force. **Sexual victimization** occurs when a person is deprived of free choice and is forced to endure, observe, or comply with sexual acts. Coercive sex can take many forms. The commonality is the element of power and victimhood. In this chapter, we focus on three forms: rape (also called sexual assault), sexual harassment, and child sexual abuse. We will start our examination with a look at rape.

Rape

The dictionary definition of **rape** is "sexual intercourse without the consent of the man/woman and effected by force, duress, intimidation or deception as to the nature of the act" (Benton, 1996). The word *rape* comes from the Latin term *rapere*, which means to steal, seize, or carry away. Rape has been a common theme in literature, art, and popular culture throughout history.

Chilling examples of rape occur regularly in cartoons, comic strips, and other "children's entertainment." The caveman, replete with club and knuckles dragging the earth, is out and about to find a mate. When he spies the female he desires, he hits her with the club, knocks her out, and drags her away by her long hair (presumably to make her his wife).

More than 95 percent of rapes are committed by men against women or other men. Although 9 of 10 rapists are men, this does not mean that all men rape, nor are all men potential rapists. If you were to take a sample of 100 rapists, more than 90 would be men. If you were to take a random sample of 100 men, fewer than 10 would be rapists or potential rapists. The statistic does mean, however, that most of the rapes are committed by a small percentage of men who achieve power over women and other men by forced sexual aggression.

Rape is a form **sexual aggression,** a broader term that encompasses all forms of nonconsensual physical sexual activity against men, women, children, and gay people as victims (Cate & Lloyd, 1992). It includes fondling, oral sex, and anal sex, as well as vaginal intercourse. *Sexual coercion,* the broadest term, covers all nonconsensual sexual behavior that results from arguing, pleading, and cajoling, in addition to force.

The term *victim* is gradually being replaced by words such as *target* and *survivor,* in some contexts. This language avoids further degradation of the person who was raped. The new terminology connotes the encouragement for survivors to reclaim control over their lives.

In most states, to be considered rape, the target's body (usually the vagina) has to be penetrated. Forced oral sex and the insertion of fingers and other objects into the vagina, anus, or mouth don't automatically qualify as rape. Although these sexually aggressive acts are still illegal and can result in prosecution, they are tried as less serious offenses than is rape. Rape includes acquaintance rape (also known as date rape), stranger rape, marital rape, gang rape, and statutory rape. A last category of rape, male rape, usually is committed by men against other men but does occur, rarely, with women as the perpetrators.

Sexual aggression Any form of forced sexual contact, including but not limited to intercourse, without the person's consent

Physical Wellness

Men who engage in coercive sex often use their physical strength to intimidate, threaten, and/or overpower their victims. High-level physical wellness may empower women and help prevent becoming victims of coercive sex. Activities such as lifting weights to develop strength and practicing self-defense skills can help women repel would-be attackers. Feeling physically stronger and more prepared to fight might also send nonverbal messages to would-be attackers. Perpetrators are less likely to target women who appear strong, self-assured, and able to defend themselves.

Here are some common myths associated with rape:

Myth: Rape is a sexual act, not a violent one.
Fact: Although the rapist achieves sexual gratification through his actions, the rape is first and foremost an act of violence. If sexual release were all that a rapist desires, he could achieve that by finding a willing partner, masturbating, or paying a prostitute for sex. The rapist seeks to dominate his victim, to exert power, and to humiliate by using threat and violence. In contrast, sex is a consensual act of pleasure, not a violent act of power.
Myth: Women secretly want to be raped.
Fact: Even though many men and women have rape fantasies, there is a world of difference between using fantasy to become sexually aroused and actually desiring to be assaulted, forced to submit to another's sexual onslaught, and humiliated or beaten in the process. In a fantasy, you control the situation, orchestrate the script, and create the happy ending. In a rape, someone assaults you and controls you. Women do *not* want to be raped.

Myth: A woman can't be raped if she really doesn't want to be.

Fact: The logic of this myth revolves around the difficulty surrounding inserting a penis into a vagina that is thrashing to and fro. Men who rape use force to hurt women, to injure them to the point of submission. They have been known to break a woman's hip to stop it from moving. Rape is not about two lovers playfully teasing each other into submission. Rape is about force, domination, and pain.

Myth: Women ask for it by the way they act and dress.

Fact: Women don't dress provocatively to invite rapists. The idea of a woman wanting to attract a man and initiate a sexual liaison by acting in a sexy way is much different from the notion of a woman dressing in revealing clothing because she wants to be raped. If a woman intentionally acts and dresses provocatively to attract a man, that style doesn't give any man the right to rape her.

Myth: *No* really means *yes.*

Fact: Where does the notion that *no* means *yes* come from? Is it a rationalization, made up by men, to justify their domination and overpower women into submission? Or is it a leftover piece of baggage from the Victorian era, reminding women that ladies are not supposed to enjoy sex? In that line of thinking, because a lady can't ask for sex, she has to say no even though she means yes. That way she can have it both ways: maintain her status as a lady and still have sex ("He did it to me"). Wherever this belief came from, it's time to stop it and realize that *no* means *no.* When in doubt, don't continue.

Myth: Rape is justifiable under certain circumstances.

Fact: Rape is never justifiable. No one—husband, lover, boyfriend, father, or any man—ever has the right to force sex on anyone.

Myth: Most rapists are crazy.

Fact: Most rapists are not crazy. They are similar to the average man except for three distinguishing characteristics: (a) They are hostile toward women and have a harder time handling it, (b) they have more traditional beliefs about gender roles, and (c) they are more willing to use force to achieve their ends.

Myth: Women are responsible for preventing rape.

Fact: *Everyone* is responsible for preventing rape.

Posttraumatic Rape Syndrome

An estimated 70 percent of adults in the United States have experienced a traumatic event at least once in their lives, and up to 20 percent of these people go on to develop **posttraumatic stress disorder (PTSD).** PTSD can occur in either victims or witnesses of traumatic events ranging from natural disasters to rape (American Psychiatric Association [APA], 2000). The three main diagnostic criteria for PTSD are (a) reexperiencing the event through dreams, flashbacks, and other means; (b) persistent avoidance of stimuli associated with the event; and (c) persistent symptoms ranging from difficulty falling asleep to irritability and outbursts of anger (APA, 2000).

An estimated 1 out of 10 women will get PTSD at some time in their lives. Women are about twice as likely as men to develop PTSD. This incidence may be due to the fact that women tend to experience interpersonal violence (such as domestic violence, rape, or abuse) more often than men. The estimated risk for developing PTSD for people who have experienced various traumatic events is as follows: rape, 49 percent; severe beating or physical assault, 31.9 percent; other sexual assault, 23.7 percent; serious accident or injury (for example, a car or train accident), 16.8 percent; shooting or stabbing, 15.4 percent; sudden, unexpected death of a family member or friend, 14.3 percent; child's life-threatening illness, 10.4 percent; witness to a killing or serious injury, 7.3 percent.

Posttraumatic stress disorder (PTSD) A syndrome developing after exposure to an extremely traumatic event. Symptoms include anxiety, sleeplessness, eating disorders, depression, and hyperactive nervous system activity.

Burgess and Holmstrom (1974) coined the term *rape trauma syndrome* (RTS) to identify a cluster of emotional responses to the extreme stress experienced by victims of rape. RTS has two phases. The first is the acute (initial) phase, which usually lasts anywhere from a few days to a few weeks after the attack. The next phase is the reorganization phase, which usually lasts anywhere from a few weeks to several days after the attack.

Acquaintance rape, also known as *date rape*, is a form of rape defined as forced sexual intercourse by a dating partner. Many experts consider acquaintance rape to be the most common and least reported of all forms of rape (Cate & Lloyd, 1992). Previous research has shown that college campuses, contrary to public opinion, are not safe havens from sexual coercion. College women are at a greater risk for rape and other forms of sexual assault than women in the general population or in a comparable age group (Fisher, Koss, Gidycz, & Wisnewski, 1987). This is due in part to the nature of the college environment where large concentrations of young women come into contact with young men in a variety of public and private settings at various times on and off their college campuses. Fisher, Cullen, and Turner (2000), in a national study of 4,446 college women, found that almost 3 percent (2.8 percent) of study participants experienced a completed or attempted rape during the academic year. They estimate that women at a college that has 10,000 female students could experience more than 350 rapes a year.

Acquaintance rape Forced intercourse by a person, other than a spouse, whom the victim knows

healthy sex hints 16.1

What to Do If You Are Raped or Sexually Assaulted

What to Do If You Have Been Raped

1. Go to a safe place away from your attacker.
   - Your first concern is your personal safety.
2. Call a friend, family member, or someone else you trust, and ask her or him to stay with you.
3. Go to a hospital emergency department immediately.
   - Preserve all physical evidence of the assault. Do not shower, bathe, douche, brush your teeth, or change your clothes before you go to the hospital.
   - Hospital staff will provide medical care for sexual assault victims.
   - Even if you think that you do not have any physical injuries, you should still have a medical examination and discuss with a health care provider the risk of exposure to sexually transmitted diseases and the possibility of pregnancy resulting from the sexual assault.
4. If you want to report the assault, call your local police department from the hospital.
   - The police department will have trained rape crisis personnel to help you.

- Reporting the crime can help you regain a sense of personal power and control and can also help ensure the safety of other potential victims.
5. If you suspect that you may have been given a rape drug, ask the hospital or clinic where you receive medical care to take a urine sample.
   - The urine sample should be preserved as evidence.
   - Rape drugs, such as Rohypnol and GHB, are more likely to be detected in urine than in blood.
6. Write down as much as you can remember about the circumstances of the assault, including a description of the assailant.
7. Talk with a counselor who is trained to assist rape victims about the emotional and physical impacts of the assault.
   - It will be difficult, but it is important to talk with someone who understands the trauma of rape and knows how to help.

Source: American Academy of Family Physicians (2003).

The Sexual Victimization of College Women

Fischer et al.'s (2000) study, "The National College Women Sexual Victimization Study (NCWSV)," was chartered by the National Institute of Justice, the research arm of the United States Bureau of Justice Statistics. The study is noteworthy for several reasons relating to design, sampling, and questioning methodology.

The NCWSV was designed to overcome the shortcomings of previous studies that attempted to estimate the incidence of sexual victimization of college women. Previous studies were flawed by small sample sizes, nonrandom sampling techniques, delimiting types of sexual victimization studied, and confusing labeling of both the types of sexual victimization under study and the details of the specific incidents reported by subjects.

The study was designed as a telephone survey of 4,446 female college students. Each subject was interviewed over the phone by a trained female interviewer. The study greatly expanded the types of sexual victimization (incidents) under study, including (a) completed rape, (b) attempted rape, (c) completed sexual coercion, (d) attempted sexual coercion, (e) completed sexual contact with force or threat of force, (f) attempted sexual contact with force or threat of force, (g) completed sexual contact without force, (h) attempted sexual contact without force, (i) threat of rape, (j) threat of contact with force or threat of force, (k) threat of penetration with force, and (l) threat of contact with force. These terms are defined in Table 16.1.

The sample for the NCWSV was composed of undergraduate and graduate women attending 2- or 4-year institutions across the United States during the fall 1996 semester. The sample was stratified to include students from all sized institutions (1,000–2,499; 2,500–4,999; 5,000–19,999; and 20,000 or more) and locations (urban, suburban, and rural). Schools were randomly chosen from a probability proportional to total female enrollment. Subjects were then randomly chosen from the institutions picked for the study (Fisher et al., 2000).

A key methodological issue that is credited for the study's success was its use of a two-tiered questioning approach. Subjects were initially queried with a set of "screening" questions that identified whether the subject had experienced a sexual victimization event.

Screening questions were very graphic in their depiction of the potential sexual victimization events. For instance, the first screening question was "Since school began in fall 1996, has anyone made you have sexual intercourse by using force or threatening to harm you or someone close to you? Just so there is no mistake, by *intercourse* I mean putting a penis in your vagina." No previous sexual victimization surveys used such specific screening questions that, in a sense, operationally defined the event under study. Such specific wording left little doubt for subjects regarding the nature of the question being asked and contributed to higher response rates.

If a woman answered yes to the screening question, the interviewer asked a series of "incident report" questions that described in detail the nature of the event. Incident report questions covered all aspects of the event, ranging from the relationship of the perpetrator to the subject, the environment in which the event occurred, whether the victim used force to repel the perpetrator, and additional details.

Key Findings of the NCWSV As previously mentioned, the most startling finding of the study was the overall high incidence of sexual victimization and attempted sexual victimization among college women. Overall, 2.8 percent of the sample had experienced either a completed rape (1.7 percent) or an attempted rape (1.1 percent). This accounts for a rape victimization rate of 27.7 rapes per 1,000 female students (Fisher et al., 2000). The actual rate of the overall incidence

Table 16.1 Descriptions of Types of Victimizations

Type of Victimization	Definition
Completed rape	Unwanted completed penetration by force or the threat of force. Penetration includes penile-vaginal, mouth on your genitals, mouth on someone else's genitals, penile-anal, digital-vaginal, digital-anal, object-vaginal, and object-anal.
Attempted rape	Unwanted attempted penetration by force or the threat of force. Penetration includes penile-vaginal, mouth on your genitals, mouth on someone else's genitals, penile-anal, digital-vaginal, digital-anal, object-vaginal, and object-anal.
Completed sexual coercion	Unwanted completed penetration with the threat of non-physical punishment, promise of reward, or pestering/verbal pressure. Penetration includes penile-vaginal, mouth on your genitals, mouth on someone else's genitals, penile-anal, digital-vaginal, digital-anal, object-vaginal, and object-anal.
Attempted sexual coercion	Unwanted attempted penetration with the threat of non-physical punishment, promise of reward, or pestering/verbal pressure. Penetration includes penile-vaginal, mouth on your genitals, mouth on someone else's genitals, penile-anal, digital-vaginal, digital-anal, object-vaginal, and object-anal.
Completed sexual contact with force or threat of force	Unwanted completed sexual contact (not penetration) with force or the threat of force. Sexual contact includes touching, grabbing or fondling of breasts, buttocks, or genitals, either under or over your clothes; kissing, licking, or sucking; or some other form of unwanted sexual contact.
Completed sexual contact without force	Any type of unwanted completed sexual contact (not penetration) with the threat of nonphysical punishment, promise of reward, or pestering/verbal pressure. Sexual contact includes touching, grabbing or fondling of breasts, buttocks, or genitals, either under or over your clothes; kissing, licking, or sucking; or some other form of unwanted sexual contact.
Attempted sexual contact with force or threat of force	Unwanted attempted sexual contact (not penetration) with force or the threat of force. Sexual contact includes touching, grabbing or fondling of breasts, buttocks, or genitals, either under or over your clothes; kissing, licking, or sucking; or some other form of unwanted sexual contact.
Attempted sexual contact without force	Unwanted attempted sexual contact (not penetration) with the threat of nonphysical punishment, promise or reward, or pestering/verbal pressure. Sexual contact includes touching, grabbing or fondling of breasts, buttocks, or genitals, either under or over your clothes; kissing, licking, or sucking; or some other form of unwanted sexual contact.

(continued)

Table 16.1 Descriptions of Types of Victimizations *(continued)*

Type of Victimization	Definition
Threat of rape	Threat of unwanted penetration with force and threat of force. Penetration includes penile-vaginal, mouth on your genitals, mouth on someone else's genitals, penile-anal, digital-vaginal, digital-anal, object-vaginal, and object-anal.
Threat of contact with force or threat of force	Threat of unwanted sexual contact with force and threat of force. Sexual contact includes touching, grabbing or fondling of breasts, buttocks, or genitals, either under or over your clothes; kissing, licking, or sucking; or some other form of unwanted sexual contact.
Threat of penetration without force	Threat of unwanted penetration with the threat of non-physical punishment, promise of reward, or pestering/verbal pressure. Penetration includes penile-vaginal, mouth on your genitals, mouth on someone else's genitals, penile-anal, digital-vaginal, digital-anal, object-vaginal, and object-anal.
Threat of contact without force	Threat of unwanted sexual contact with the threat of non-physical punishment, promise or reward, or pestering/verbal pressure. Sexual contact includes touching, grabbing or fondling of breasts, buttocks, or genitals, either under or over your clothes; kissing, licking, or sucking; or some other form of unwanted sexual contact.

Source: Fisher, Cullen, and Turner (2000, p. 8).

of rape was actually 35.3 rapes per 1,000 women. This is due to the fact that some women in the study were actually raped or had experienced attempted rape more than one time during the 7-month study period. The 35.3/1,000 rate is what projects out to an estimated 350 rapes per year among 10,000 college women in any given university (Fisher et al., 2000).

Another disturbing finding of the study was the small percentage of women who actually defined their victimization as rape (even though they said yes when asked whether someone had "by force or threat put their penis into your vagina"). Fisher et al. (2000) explain that this reluctance may be due to reasons such as feeling embarrassed, not clearly understanding the legal definition of rape, or being reluctant to label someone they are intimate with and who victimized them as a rapist (Fisher et al., 2000).

A third finding of the study was the overall incidence of other forms of sexual victimization. As Table 16.2 shows, when other forms of sexual victimization were studied, the rates varied from 9.5 to 66.4 cases per 1,000 women. The types of sexual victimization ranged from threats of rape and sexual contact to completed sexual coercion.

Figure 16.1 shows that the overall percentage of women who were sexually victimized in the study exceeded 15 percent (Fisher et al., 2000).

A fourth finding of the study was the relationship of the perpetrator to the victim. For both completed and attempted rape, 9 out of 10 women knew the perpetrator. The relationships most often cited were a boyfriend, ex-boyfriend, classmate, friend, acquaintance, or coworker. College professors were not cited in any of the completed or attempted rapes (Fisher et al., 2000).

Table 16.2 Rates of Sexual Victimization

Type of Victimization	Victims			Incidents	
	Number of Victims in Sample	Percentage of Sample	Rate per 1,000 Female Students	Number of Incidents	Rate per 1,000 Female Students
Completed or attempted					
Completed sexual coercion	74	1.7	16.6	107	24.1
Attempted sexual coercion	60	1.3	13.5	114	25.6
Completed sexual contact with force or threat of force	85	1.9	19.1	130	29.2
Completed sexual contact without force	80	1.8	18.0	132	29.7
Attempted sexual contact with force or threat of force	89	2.0	20.0	166	37.6
Attempted sexual contact without force	133	3.0	29.9	295	66.4
Threats					
Threat of rape	14	0.31	3.2	42	9.5
Threat of contact with force or threat of force	8	0.18	1.8	50	11.3
Threat of penetration without force	10	0.22	2.3	50	11.3
Threat of contact without force	15	0.34	3.4	75	16.9
Total	568			1,161	

Source: Fisher et al. (2000, p. 16).

The vast majority of the rapes occurred after midnight and on campus in the victim's residence, in other living quarters on campus, or at a fraternity house. Risk factors positively associated with rape were (a) frequently drinking to get drunk, (b) being unmarried, (c) having a history of a previous sexual assault, and (d) living on campus. The vast majority of women reported that they did not suffer physical or emotional injuries as a result of the completed or attempted rape. About one in five reported being injured (20 percent). The percentages for other forms of sexual victimization were lower, ranking from 0 percent (completed sexual contact without force) to 17 percent (threatened rape) (Fisher et al., 2000).

Figure 16.1 *Percentage of Women Sexually Victimized*

Source: Fisher et al. (2000, p. 17).

Environmental Wellness

High-level environmental wellness implies safety, security, and respect. A safe home environment includes appropriate parenting, setting boundaries for behavior, and getting help with emotional problems. A neighborhood that offers high-level environmental wellness is well lit and policed, and it has neighbors looking out for one another. The schools are safe and do not tolerate sexual harassment and discrimination. The community has safe playgrounds and parks that are well patrolled and not inviting for sex offenders. A college that offers high-level environmental wellness is a microcosm of any community. It has policies and procedures in place for dealing with harassment and discrimination and offers safety and protection. Its students don't fear walking to their cars after class or attending social functions. In addition, enforcement is swift, fair, and equal for all on campus.

Drinking and Date Rape

Many college students use alcohol and other drugs to "fit in," cope with college stressors, and reduce inhibitions related to dating and sex. Unfortunately, alcohol consumption is often linked to sexual coercion and other forms of violence. The National Advisory Council on Alcohol Abuse and Alcoholism's Report on College Drinking estimates that more than 70,000 students are the victims of alcohol-related sexual victimization (sexual assault and rape) (Task Force, 2002).

Often, this alcohol is consumed in large quantities for the express purpose of getting drunk. Weschler, Davenport, Dowdell, Moeykens, and Castillo (1994) coined the term **binge drinking** to describe such a pattern of alcohol consumption. Binge drinking is operationally defined as "having five or more drinks in a row, at least once during the previous 2 week period" (Weschler et al., 1994, p. 1673). The greatest predictors of binge drinking were living in a fraternity or sorority house, engaging in drinking games, and living a "party-centered" lifestyle (Weschler et al., 1994).

Bingeing on alcohol often becomes part of the social fabric of the college experience. Weschler et al. (1994) studied the binge drinking behavior of more than 17,000 students on 140 four-year college campuses across the United States. About one in six (16 percent) of all the respondents were nondrinkers (15 percent of the men, 16 percent of the women). About two in five (41 percent) were drinkers but did not binge. Almost half (44 percent) of all the students were binge drinkers. About one in five (19 percent) were frequent binge drinkers (17 percent of the women and 23 percent of the men). These students had three or more binge drinking episodes within the past 2 weeks.

Weschler and colleagues found binge drinking to be associated with unplanned and unsafe sexual activity, physical and sexual assault, other criminal violations, physical injury, interpersonal problems, and poor academic performance. Binge drinkers were more likely than nonbinge drinkers and abstainers to engage in unplanned sexual activity, not use protection when having sex, get hurt or injured, damage property, argue with friends, miss classes, get behind in schoolwork, and do something they later regretted. Frequent binge drinkers were 10 times more likely than bingers to have unplanned and unprotected sex, get into trouble with campus police, and get injured or damage property. When asked to evaluate the seriousness of their bingeing and its repercussions, less than 1 percent of the binge drinkers designated themselves as problem drinkers (Weschler et al., 1994).

In a follow-up study, Weschler, Eun, Kuo, Sebring, Nelson, and Lee (2002) found that 1 percent of students living in residence halls or fraternity and sorority

Binge drinking Having four or more drinks at one sitting houses were victims of alcohol-related sexual assault and/or rape. About 20 percent of students experienced alcohol-related threats and and/or attempted sexual contacts.

Despite the overall decline in drinking among all adults in the United States over the past two decades, drinking on college campuses fails to show a corresponding dropoff. Drinking by college students often revolves around its social nature. College women perceive drinking as a way of being around others and seeking the acceptance of peers (Gleason, 1994). Alcohol is consumed more for social than for personal reasons (Montgomery, Benedicto, & Hammerke, 1993). Students reported using alcohol more for the purpose of meeting members of the other sex than for personal reasons, although alcohol did make them feel better about themselves.

Drinking behavior that elsewhere would be characterized as alcohol abuse is often socially acceptable and even desirable behavior on certain college campuses (Weschler et al., 1994). "Party schools" foster reputations and environments in which binge drinking is part of the fabric of college life. Conversely, institutions that do not have alcohol outlets within 1 mile of campus and colleges that prohibit alcohol use for everyone (even those older than 21 years of age) have lower rates of alcohol bingeing.

Other Date Rape Drugs

Many other drugs, used alone or in consort with alcohol have been implicated in sexual victimization. Marijuana, cocaine, gamma hydroxybutyrate (GHB), benzodiazepines, ketamine, barbiturates, chloral hydrate, methaqualone, heroin, morphine, LSD, and other hallucinogens have all been used to facilitate rape (Higher Education Center, 2003). When combined with alcohol (which they often are), many of these drugs cause reduction of inhibitions, weakness, memory loss, and blackout. These incapacitating effects are used by sexual victimization perpetrators to take advantage of their targets (Higher Education Center, 2003).

Two drugs in particular, **Rohypnol** and GHB, have been dubbed "date rape drugs" because of their increased use and association with sexual assault and rape. Rohypnol was the key target in the Drug-Induced Rape Prevention and Punishment Act of 1996. This legislation was developed in response to the threat posed by Rohypnol. The act established harsher penalties for the use of even the smallest quantities of flunitrazepam (the chemical name of Rohypnol) for the purpose of facilitating a violent crime (U.S. Congress, 1996).

Rohypnol—also known as roofies, rophies, Mexican valium, ropies, and the "forget me" drug (to name a few)—is the trade name for flunitrazepam, a benzodiazepine. Benzodiazepines are depressant drugs. Rohypnol is similar to Valium in its effects on the body, only 10 times more powerful. The United Nations Commission on Narcotic Drugs has transferred Rohypnol from a Schedule IV to a Schedule III drug. Several states in the United States have already moved Rohypnol to Schedule I (Office of National Drug Control Policy [ONDCP], 2002b).

Rohypnol is a tasteless, odorless, clear drug available in powder form. It mixes easily in liquids and is virtually undetectable when mixed in alcoholic beverages (its preferred delivery by date rape perpetrators). When swallowed, it takes effect in 15 to 20 minutes, and its effects last for more than 12 hours. Users experience a slowing of psychomotor performance, muscle relaxation, sleepiness, and/or amnesia. Rohypnol leaves the body after 72 hours and is undetectable after that time (ONDCP, 2002b).

Rohypnol and GHB, available in liquid or pill form, are often mixed into the drinks of unsuspecting victims.

Rohypnol A depressant drug also known as the "date rape drug," because it causes loss of memory and makes women vulnerable to uninvited sexual intercourse

Jonathan Nourok/PhotoEdit, Inc.

GHB—also known as cherry meth, liquid X, organic Quaalude, and fantasy, to name a few—is similar in its nature and effects to Rohypnol. It is also a tasteless, odorless, clear, depressant drug. It is available in either powder or liquid form and easily mixes in alcoholic beverages, where it is undetectable. GHB is not produced legally in the United States. It is produced in clandestine laboratories. Users claim it can produce euphoric, hallucinogenic states and act as a growth hormone that stimulates muscle growth. Because of this latter claim, GHB is often marketed through the same channels (gyms, health clubs, rave clubs, and so forth) where anabolic steroids are sold (ONDCP, 2002a).

Both drugs have been implicated in date rape in the United States. Both drugs, besides having classic depressant drug characteristics (slowing central nervous system functioning), can cause memory loss and loss of consciousness. Because of this, women who have been assaulted and raped while under the influence of these drugs are unable to resist the perpetrator or recall any of the details concerning the incident. The assailant mixes the drug into the drink of the unsuspecting woman, allows it to take effect, takes advantage of her, and denies any knowledge of the event if the woman realizes or suspects what has happened. Because both drugs pass through the victim's system within 72 hours, she typically does not have the opportunity to get tested for the drugs (ONDCP 2002a, 2002b).

Stranger Rape

Stranger rape Forced intercourse by a person who is unknown to the target person

Stranger rape is rape by a person whom the target does not know. The overwhelming majority of rapes reported to the police and resulting in prosecution are stranger rapes. Although stranger rape can involve a premeditated assault with an anonymous assailant descending upon the victim totally without warning, statistics prove otherwise. Most cases of stranger rape seem to spring out of

healthy sex hints 16.2

Reducing Risks for Date Rape

The following are specific strategies for women to reduce their risks for date rape:

- Arrange for your first date to be in a public place or as part of a larger group.
- Arrange your own transportation, or go with your friends.
- In the earliest stages of the relationship, suggest paying for yourself. This will derail any notion that your date thinks you owe him something. It also will give you an opportunity to assess his views about women.
- Pay attention to your date's attitudes and behavior. Is he controlling? Does he want to make all of the decisions?
- Avoid using alcohol and other drugs if you don't want to become involved in intimate sexual activities.
- Do not accept *any* drinks from another person. Pour your own drink or only drink from sealed bottles.

- Don't send mixed messages or anything that can be perceived as "teasing." If kissing is acceptable but you don't want to go any farther, state this clearly: "I'd like to hug and kiss, but I don't want to let things go any farther than this."
- If things begin to get out of control, resist. Use more and more emphatic verbal resistance: "I said *no!*" If this doesn't work, use physical force: punch, slap, kick.
- Men are much more likely to believe you if you use physical force when you're saying no. Push him away, stand up, open the door, ask him to stop, or leave. If this doesn't work, say, "This is rape. I'm calling the police."
- Run away. If he persists, escape. Get away. Go to a public place, and call the police.

chance meetings that create the potential for assault. The assailant targets the victim in a park, a shopping mall parking lot, while driving in a car, and so on. The perpetrator initiates contact, appears friendly and "safe," and lulls the victim into relaxing her (usually the victim is female) guard, allowing the perpetrator to strike. The assailant maneuvers the target to one or the other of their cars or lures the victim into an alley, stairwell, or other remote location, then commits the rape.

Stranger rapes are more likely to involve guns, knives, and other weapons than other forms of rape (Rennison, 2001). Older persons are more likely to be

healthy sex hints 16.3
Reducing Risks for Stranger Rape

Personal Preparation

1. *Plan in advance.* Be aware of where you are, areas of possible trouble, and escape routes.
2. *Avoid dark and isolated areas.* Park in well-lit areas, as close to stores as possible. Avoid dark side streets, back roads, and the like, whenever possible. Jog and bicycle only in busy or public places.
3. *Arrange for an escort.* Have someone leave work, school, or an event with you and walk you to your car. Avoid empty stairwells and elevators unless you are accompanied by your escort.
4. *Use technology.* Carry an airhorn or whistle. If you can afford it, install automatic door locks and alarms in your car. Buy a cellular phone and carry it with you. Install your local police department number as a quick-dial memory number.
5. *Take a self-defense course.* Know how to defend yourself. A few simple techniques can make a difference.
6. *Remain vigilant.* Don't let your guard down. You are a potential victim any time you go anywhere by yourself.

What to Do If You Are Attacked

1. *Run away if you can.*
2. *Resist if you can.* Be as active and loud as possible: Scream, curse, yell, and cause a scene. If you have a whistle or horn, blow it.
3. *Fight back.* Kick, punch, bite, scratch, vomit, and spit. Use your keys, umbrellas, rolled-up newspapers, and books to jab for the eyes, throat, and face. There are no rules, and fighting back may reduce the abuse you might sustain without increasing your risk of injury. Carry keys in your hand as a weapon.
4. *Stall for time.* If you can't fight back, talk to your attacker—by name, if you know it. Express "empathy." Get him talking. Try to escape at the first distraction.

In the Car

1. *Always drive with your doors locked.*
2. *Lock your doors immediately after you park.*
3. *Approach your car with your keys in your hand* (have them sticking out like brass knuckles), and check the backseat to make sure no one is hiding there before you let yourself in.
4. *If you break down, do not leave the car.* Leave only to quickly tie a white rag to the antenna, then lock yourself in, and wait for the police. If someone other than the police arrives, ask this person to call the police or a local garage. Don't open the door.
5. *If your car is hit from behind, don't leave the car.* Put your flashers on and wait for the police to arrive.
6. *Buy a cellular phone, if you can afford it.* It will enable you to call the police immediately.

At Home

1. *Don't list your full name in the phone book, over the doorbell, or on the mailbox.*
2. *Install secure locks on all windows and doors.* Change locks if you lose your keys, move, or change your living situation (a roommate, husband, or boyfriend leaves).
3. *Install a peephole and safety chain and bar on your door.*
4. *Don't let people in your home unless you can verify who they are.* All service representatives (gas company, police, and so on) have identification. Request that they hold it in front of the peephole so you can see it. When in doubt, call the agency and verify who they are.
5. *Leave a light on near the entrance* when you know you will be returning home after dark.
6. *Organize or join a neighborhood watch program* for your block, building, or complex.
7. *Get a dog.* Perpetrators are less likely to attack you if you have a dog with you.

case study 16.2

Donna: A Saga of Spousal Abuse

Donna, 33, divorced, identifies as African American.

Critical Thinking

How could Donna's early experiences with her mother and father have resulted in different choices she made in her life after she left home at 18?

Use your Virtual Workbook to explore your answer to this question at **http://health.wadsworth.com/blonna1.**

Donna is a continuing education student and the mother of two daughters, 10 and 11 years of age. She related her story to one of the authors in a diary detailing her sexual development.

My father was an alcoholic. I didn't realize it as a young child, but by the time I was a teenager, I understood why my dad had lost his driver's license a couple of times, had a hard time holding down a steady job, and was so angry all of the time. Of course, by then it was too late. I loved him so much and felt so guilty about admitting to myself that he was an alcoholic. I blamed myself a lot for his behavior. "Maybe it's my fault Daddy drinks so much," I thought. "Maybe if I was a better daughter, he'd be OK."

Often Dad's anger was directed at Mom. He'd come home drunk after stopping off for "a few beers" after work and just be itching for a fight. The least little thing Mom would do would set him off, and he'd smack her with the back of his hand. My sister and I would run for our lives and dive under our bed or lock ourselves in the closet until he'd pass out. We'd hear Mom getting hit but would be too afraid to do anything.

Afterward Mom would try to comfort us by saying that Daddy was really a "good man" and "cared" about her, but he just couldn't hold his liquor. She said that sometimes a woman has to stand by her man even when things weren't going well. I think about those words now, and I shudder.

Sometimes he'd turn on us if we tried to help Mom. He broke my arm once during one of these outbursts, and I had to go to the hospital to have a cast put on. To this day I can't believe that the hospital staff didn't know what was happening and intervene. Not only was my arm broken, but I had black-and-blue marks all over from where Dad hit me with his belt and his hand.

I ran away when I was 18. I guess it wasn't really running away since I was legally an adult, but to me it was because I wasn't leaving—I was escaping (at least I thought I was). I bounced around the country for a couple of years, in and out of jobs as well as relationships with men.

My first real love was a guy who reminded me a lot of my father. I guess I felt like a victim and was attracted to a guy who allowed me to be a victim. I needed to be punished to feel good, and he

raped in their homes than in public places, and the assailant often gains access by overpowering them or by posing as a delivery person, utility representative, and the like (Muram, Miller, & Cutler, 1992). A relatively recent type of stranger rape involves targeting women who are driving by themselves. The perpetrators intentionally rear-end the cars of their potential victims, forcing them to pull off the road, where they are assaulted when they leave their car to investigate the accident. Often the rape is combined with stealing the woman's car.

Marital Rape

For many years, police were reluctant to investigate and prosecute marital rape. In a landmark case from 1978, Greta Rideout of Oregon filed charges against her husband for nonconsensual sex, bringing marital rape to national attention. Approximately 13 percent of married women have been raped by their husbands (Russel, 1990). In most cases, the husband used force (84 percent) or the threat of force (9 percent). The rape was an isolated incident for 31 percent of the victims. Another 31 percent reported being raped more than 20 times, and the rest fell somewhere in the middle (Russel, 1990).

was up to the task. He'd treat me like dirt, constantly tell me I wasn't pretty and was terrible in bed, couldn't do anything right, and on and on. He drank, just like my dad, and beat me just like my dad beat my mom.

Fate saved me from him, however. He was a real bad guy and was arrested for stealing a car and crashing it into a storefront. He was sent to jail for 5 years, and I wasn't into waiting around, so I took off and wound up in a neighboring state.

I met my husband shortly after arriving. I was working as a barmaid, and he came into the bar late one night. I was very attracted to him and wound up going home with him that night. I moved in after about a month and got pregnant with my first child about 6 months later. He liked to drink, but it didn't seem to affect him at first. He was a pretty good guy until times got tough.

After the baby was born, we got married and he lost his job the next week. He couldn't find another job and had to go on unemployment for 6 months. He couldn't handle this and began to take it out on me. I was pregnant with our second child at the time. He started really abusing me for my size (I gained a lot of weight) and began hitting me. I almost miscarried one night after he hit me and knocked me down. When he sobered up, he felt really bad and apologized. He told me he'd never do it again. He said he loved me.

I felt trapped and didn't know what to do. I was pregnant, had a 1-year-old baby, had no education, no real job skills, no money in the bank, and few real friends to turn to. I continued to live with him but began to fear for my safety and that of the kids. I started to try to think of a way out. Something deep within me didn't want to wind up like my mother. He must have sensed it because he got very controlling. He tried to limit my involvement with any friends, checked my mail, scrutinized the phone bills. The beatings were coming more often, and he began to hit the kids more and more.

Things finally came to a head one night. After a particularly savage fight, a neighbor called the police. When the police arrived, they saw what he had done to me and locked him up. My children and I were examined, and I pressed charges for domestic and child abuse. To make a long story short, the kids and I found refuge in a battered women's shelter, and he got 3 years in prison.

As soon as I was able, I filed divorce papers, went back to work, saved a few dollars, and left the state. I located my sister, also divorced with two kids, and we moved in together. We've both been working our way back slowly ever since—caring for each other and our kids, trying to put our lives back together. I'm in a support group for survivors of spousal abuse and have been dating a very nice man for about a year.

Perpetrators of marital rape share some of the same personality traits as other rapists—namely, anger, power, and sadism. Husbands who rape are also more likely to abuse their wives verbally, psychologically, and physically. More than 30 percent of wives who were raped also reported having been targets of physical abuse during their marriage (Frieze, 1983).

Verbal and psychological abuse often prove more damaging than physical abuse. The verbal and psychological abusers create an environment of endless criticism, suspicion, and torment. Abusers often undermine their mates' confidence and self-esteem through constant criticism of everything from the way they look to their level of competence in performing simple household tasks. Abusers are extremely jealous and turn even the most casual remark or involvement with another person into suspicions of flirting or having an affair. This constant flow of criticism, insults, and accusations is tormenting and can result in a host of psychological problems (Marano, 1996).

Survivors of marital rape suffer after-effects that are similar to those of women who have been sexually assaulted by someone they know (date rape). Because they know their assailants intimately and have an established history of trust, they feel especially betrayed, humiliated, and angry.

Statutory Rape

Statutory rape refers to sexual intercourse between a person older than the legal age of consent with a partner who is younger than the legal age of consent. The legal age of consent in the states varies from 12 to 21 years of age. Traditionally, most states' original legal wording of definitions of statutory rape defined perpetrators as males and victims as females. Revised definitions of statutory rape are more gender-neutral and describe adult perpetrators and victims under the legal age of consent.

The recent high-profile case of 34-year-old teacher Mary Kay Letourneau, convicted of the statutory rape of her 12-year-old student/lover, illustrates the importance of these revisions. Letourneau received national attention when the former elementary school teacher was convicted of having sex with (and becoming pregnant by) her former student. Even though the two claimed to be in love and the sex was consensual, the courts convicted her of statutory rape.

In statutory rape cases, consent of the underage partner has little bearing in the case. In the eyes of the law, people under the age of consent are not considered legally capable of making an informed decision concerning their sexual behavior.

Incidence of Rape

The true incidence of rape in the United States is unknown. There are two primary national sources of data regarding rape in the United States: the Federal Bureau of Investigation (FBI) Uniform Crime Reports and the Bureau of Justice's National Crime Victimization Survey.

The FBI collects crime reports sent in on a voluntary basis from the individual states. These crime reports confirm to operational definitions established as part of the FBI's Uniform Crime Reporting (UCR) system. The UCR is a nationwide program that includes over 17,000 city, county, and state law enforcement agencies. It reports crime data that represent about 92 percent of the population of the United States (Rantala & Edwards, 2000).

Traditionally, the UCR has labeled rape as forcible rape and defined it in the following way: "the carnal knowledge of a female forcibly and against her will. Rapes by force and attempts or assaults to rape regardless of the age of the victim are included. Statutory offenses (no force used—victim under the age of consent, are excluded)" (FBI, 2001). Sex crimes other than prostitution were reported under the category "sex offenses."

The UCR underwent major revisions starting in 1982, when the FBI decided to assess and upgrade its crime-reporting system. A new system, the National Incident-Based Reporting System (NIBRS), started phasing in at the end of 1987. NIBRS expanded the number of reportable offenses, revised and refined how these offenses were defined, and collected detailed information surrounding the incidents. Under NIBRS, the FBI not only continued to gather data on forcible rape and sex offenses but added new "group A" offenses: sex offenses—forcible and sex offenses—nonforcible. Currently, 4,192 law enforcement agencies (covering about 17 percent of the U.S. population) submit NIBRS data in addition to UCR crime reports (Rantala & Edwards, 2000).

The Bureau of Justice, National Crime Victimization Survey (NCVS), is a biannual telephone survey of over 89,000 people over the age of 12 conducted by the Census Bureau. It provides an estimate of the volume of violent and nonviolent crime in the United States. It differs from the UCR system because it is a survey and not a tabulation of actual crime reports filed by the police.

The Uniform Crime Reporting (UCR) Program and National Crime Victimization Survey (NCVS) were designed to complement each other. The UCR Program's primary objective is to provide a reliable set of criminal justice statistics for law enforcement administration, operation, and management, as well as to indicate fluctuations in the level of crime in America. The

NCVS was established to obtain and provide previously unavailable information about victims, offenders, and crime (including crime not reported to the police). While the two programs employ different methodologies, they measure a similar subset of serious crimes. (FBI, 2001)

Because studies that use reported incidents as their measure may greatly underestimate the true incidence of rape, independent researchers conduct survey research studies on smaller samples of women and extrapolate the findings to the population as a whole (similar to the NCWSV survey discussed previously). Often these independent studies define rape differently, use differing methodologies, and mix incidence and prevalence measures, making meaningful comparisons of their data almost impossible (Koss, 1996).

In 2001, the FBI's UCR program reported 90,491 cases of rape. This was slightly higher (0.3 percent) than the 90,178 cases reported in 2000 (FBI, 2001). The actual rate of rape was 32 per 100,000 women. This figure is down significantly from the 1992 rate of 70.3 rapes per 100,000 women reported a decade ago (FBI, 2001). The National Crime Victimization Survey reported an estimated 147,000 rapes (92,000 completed and 55,000 attempted) in 2000. This is down significantly from NCVS reports from 1999 of an estimated 201,000 rapes (141,000 completed and 60,000 attempted) (Rennison, 2001).

Although the actual numbers of cases in these two sets of data are greatly disparate, most experts (police and civilian) agree that the actual number of rapes is probably much higher than the reported or estimated numbers that usually show up in reports or in the press. Rape is one of the least reported of all crimes in the United States. Between 10 and 50 percent of all rapes may go unreported to the police (Williams, 1984). If we use the 2000 FBI reported cases as a baseline, that means that as many as 50,000 additional cases went unreported that year. Rape survivors are reluctant to report the crime for several reasons: fear of retaliation by the rapist; embarrassment or shame; fear of rejection by husband, boyfriend, or family; a desire to protect the rapist; and a lack of confidence in the judicial system (Koss, 1992).

In a study of 246 rape victims, the following six variables were found to be related to whether a victim reports a rape (Williams, 1984):

- The relationship between the victim and the rapist
- How the two came together
- Threat of force
- Use of force
- Extent of injury
- Use of medical treatment

Victims were more likely to report when the rapist was a stranger or acquaintance rather than a friend or relative, had broken into her house or had assaulted her in a public place (versus a party or other social situation), had threatened to use force (versus not threatening her), did use force (less likely to report if no actual force), had caused substantial injury (versus little physical harm), and had sought medical care for her injuries (versus not seeking medical care).

A close look at the variables related to a greater likelihood of reporting indicates that women are much more likely to report a rape when evidence of the attack was available. This could consist of observable or clinical evidence of injury and the need for medical attention, when the woman clearly was not at fault (forced entry or a public place, didn't know the perpetrator or didn't know him well), and she felt emotionally distant from the rapist.

The variables found to be unrelated to the reporting of a rape were the victim's age, race, employment, living situation, the rapist's age, race, number of rapists, and place of assault (Williams, 1984). Perhaps more rape victims would come forth if they didn't feel that they were responsible for providing the burden of proof that the crime occurred. This attitude in part stems from the myths associated with rape that persist despite years of efforts to clear up misconceptions about the crime by individuals and organizations concerned about rape.

sex in society 16.1

A Historical Look at Rape

In *Against Our Will*, one of the most definitive works on the subject, author Susan Brownmiller (1975) described the evolution of our current attitudes toward rape and the laws against it. According to Brownmiller, rape has a long, sordid history. In antiquity, women were considered one of the spoils of war, objects to be taken and used in whatever way one wished. After a battle, the conquering army routinely rounded up all female survivors and had free rein to do what they wanted with them. Women who resisted were routinely slaughtered. Women who were spared were often sold off as slaves once their captors became bored with them.

Although rape seems to have been a part of all cultures, it has not always been considered a crime against a person. The earliest statutes against rape were laws related to property. Women were not considered persons. Instead, they were valued as property. They could provide labor and bear children—two important commodities in an agrarian economy dependent on the availability of workers.

Under Hammurabi's Code (a Babylonian law approximately 4,000 years old), a woman was not considered to be a free, independent human being. She was considered to be some man's (father's, husband's) property. Therefore, if someone violated the woman, he committed a crime against that man's property and was prosecuted accordingly.

Women also were categorized according to their marital status and virginity. Virgins were considered purer than nonvirgins in relation to sex-related crimes. The purest of all virgins were those engaged to be married. A man convicted of raping a betrothed virgin was put to death and his victim set free. A man convicted of raping a married woman also was put to death. His victim, however, also was put to death because she was considered a willing victim or accomplice in the crime. Presumably, the feeling was that she somehow led the rapist on or consented to the act.

The two early beliefs briefly described here about women and rape—that a woman is a man's property and that rape cannot occur unless a woman somehow consents—still exist and form the foundation of much of the legislation and belief systems that people share about rape.

Characteristics of Rapists

Most of what we know about men who rape comes from research conducted on convicted rapists. It is estimated that less than 10 percent of all rapists are convicted of this crime. FBI statistics in 1992 on convicted rapists, similar to those for perpetrators of other serious crimes, indicate that most are under 25 years of age, are from single-parent or foster parent homes, are marginally employed, have a low income, and have little formal education.

Because less than 10 percent of all rapists are ever convicted of their crimes, several researchers have studied populations of men who rape who have not been convicted or incarcerated. In one of the most comprehensive reviews of the literature, Cate and Lloyd (1992) identify seven characteristics of men who rape:

1. They are much more likely than their nonrapist peers to hold traditional beliefs about women and women's roles and female stereotypes. These beliefs range from nonsexual views concerning a woman's place (in the home) to sexual beliefs that men are the initiators during sex and that women want men to initiate.

2. They believe in rape-supportive myths—women secretly want to be overpowered during sex; they like it rough; *no* really means *yes*—and other stereotypical beliefs about women.

3. They use exploitative techniques such as coercing women into sex using alcohol and other drugs.

4. They accept the use of violence as a way to solve problems and dominate others.
5. They are more likely to vent their anger and express their need to dominate sexually rather than find other outlets for these feelings.
6. They devalue all that is feminine. They are hostile toward "feminine" personality attributes such as nurturance and collaboration and devalue traditional female pursuits such as child care and homemaking.
7. They are generally more sexually active than their peers who do not rape.

Malamuth, Sockloski, Koss, and Tanaka (1991) studied the sexual behavior of college men. Using a large, representative sample (their sexual histories were unknown) instead of convicted rapists, they found four characteristics of men who rape:

1. *Hostility toward women.* Men who rape have a deep-seated hostility toward women and feminine traits. They devalue traits such as nurturance and equality and value dominance, power, and aggression.
2. *Hostile home environment.* Men who rape grew up in households where violence, battering, sexual abuse, and hostility between family members were the norm.
3. *History of delinquency.* Men who rape associate with peers who are delinquent and reinforce the same hostile, aggressive behaviors that were modeled in their homes and that contributed to their own delinquency.
4. *Sexual **promiscuity.*** Contrary to the perception that men who rape are sexually deprived, rapists generally are more sexually active than nonrapists but report much higher levels of dissatisfaction with their sex lives than their nonraping peers.

Promiscuity Frequent and indiscriminate change in sexual partners

Malamuth et al.'s and Cate and Lloyd's work seems to confirm Sanday's (1987) findings concerning hostility toward women, stereotypical perceptions about women, and the devaluation of women and all things feminine as key attributes of rapists and societies that are "rape-prone."

healthy sex hints 16.4
Helping a Friend Who Has Been Raped

Even though trained rape crisis professionals are available in most communities, the first contact a survivor has is often a friend, roommate, or family member. If someone you care about has been raped, here are some tips to help you support her:

- *Accept her.* Be nonjudgmental about what happened. Tell her she is not to blame for the incident.
- *Listen.* Encourage her to tell you what happened. Listen actively and give her positive feedback.
- *Offer shelter and support.* Tell her you'll be there for her (and be sure you are). Offer her a safe haven until her

ordeal is over. Care for her needs (food, clothing, a shoulder to cry on).
- *Have empathy.* Tell her you're sorry for what happened but glad she's alive and her injuries aren't worse.
- *Encourage action.* Tell her it's important that she report what happened to the police and go to the hospital.
- *Accompany her to the police station and hospital.*
- *Keep your own feelings in check.* She will remain calmer if you do.

Characteristics of Targets

Any female can be the target of rape. The woman can be young or old, attractive or unattractive, dressed provocatively or conservatively. Most targets tend to be under 30 years of age and single. Age and marital status may have more to do with the likelihood that these women travel, shop, walk, and live alone rather than some other factor.

Women who are the targets of rape are no different from nontargets in terms of personality attributes, lifestyle, or behavior. Attempts to characterize targets as being different from other women only serves to blame the victim rather than understand that it is the men who rape through their own actions.

Sexual Harassment

Title VII of the Civil Rights Act of 1964 stipulates that it is an unlawful employment practice for a labor organization to exclude or to expel from its membership or otherwise to discriminate against any individual because of his or her race, color, religion, sex, or national origin. Sexual harassment has been deemed to be a form of discrimination based on sex.

The issue of sexual harassment leaped onto the television screens and front pages of the United States in 1992 with the much-publicized Clarence Thomas–Anita Hill sexual harassment hearings by the U.S. Congress, after President George H. Bush had nominated Thomas to the Supreme Court (see Sex in Society 16.2). Thomas had been Hill's boss at the Equal Employment Opportunity Commission (EEOC). Hill came forward at the time of Thomas's nomination with claims of sexual harassment.

These hearings brought sexual harassment out of the closet and forced people to examine this dark side of human sexual behavior. Since then, the number of sexual harassment complaints filed with the EEOC has increased from 6,000 in 1990 to 15,475 in 2001 (EEOC, 2003). Of the 15,475 charges filed, 7,309 were dropped due to no reasonable cause, 4,628 were closed administratively due to a variety of causes (inability to locate charging party, failure to respond to EEOC communications, and so forth), and 1,389 were withdrawn by the charging party because the claimant received desired benefits. Approximately 4,768 claims merited resolution, with 1,568 settled by the EEOC with the charging party receiving the desired benefits, and the rest being resolved in the charging party's favor through a variety of ways (EEOC, 2003).

U.S. Supreme Court rulings have made it easier to sue (and win) sexual harassment cases because victims no longer have to prove psychological harm, just that sexually inappropriate behavior took place (Kaufman, 1997).

According to the EEOC, sexual harassment consists of unwelcome sexual advances, requests for sexual favors, and other verbal or physical conduct of a sexual nature. These constitute **sexual harassment** when

(1) submission of such conduct is made explicitly, or implicitly a term or condition of an individual's employment or academic advancement, (2) submission or rejection of such conduct by an individual is used as the basis for academic or employment decisions affecting the individual, or (3) such conduct has the purpose or effect of unreasonably interfering with an individual's work or academic performance or creating an intimidating, hostile, or offensive working or educational environment. (EEOC, 2003)

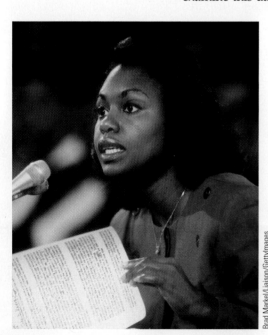

Brad Markel/Liaison/GettyImages

The Thomas–Hill trial brought the subject of sexual harassment out of the closet and into millions of American living rooms, board rooms, and courtrooms.

The Clarence Thomas–Anita Hill Hearings

The Thomas–Hill congressional hearings in 1992 had effects far beyond the matter of deciding whether Clarence Thomas should sit on the U.S. Supreme Court. As a result of these hearings, the issue of sexual harassment came to the fore and led to a whole new zeitgeist of how people are to conduct themselves in the workplace. The hearings were also noteworthy in that this event involved two prominent blacks—Thomas, a judge, and Hill, a law professor at the time of the hearings—with opposing political ideologies.

In her testimony, Hill described her position as an employee of Thomas at the Equal Employment Opportunity Commission (EEOC). She claimed that, beginning in 1982, Thomas had pressured her to go out on dates and that he had made lewd comments to her, including references to a pubic hair on a Coke can and the size of his penis. She stated that, because Thomas was well connected and could help advance her career, she was reluctant to speak out at the time. She produced three witnesses who testified to Hill's having told them that she was being harassed, though they did not recall Hill's having accused Thomas by name.

Hill's critics charged that she waited too long (10 years) to speak of the harassment and that she had agreed to testify to members of committee only under condition of anonymity. Her detractors took this as an indication that she made the charges only to try to derail Thomas's chances to gain a Supreme Court berth. They produced a number of witnesses who had worked for Thomas at the same time as Hill did, and these witnesses testified that they had observed no evidence of harassment and were not harassed themselves. Finally, Hill's critics questioned why she had followed Thomas to another job subsequent to the alleged harassment.

Thomas denounced the charges as completely untrue and a "high-tech lynching." In a close vote, he was confirmed to the Supreme Court. Irrespective of the outcome, the legacy of the hearings was far-reaching and has an enduring symbolic value. Major changes include the recognition of sexual harassment in the workplace, its definition, and enactment of legislation making sexual harassment easier to prove. Monetary awards and settlements also increased dramatically. In 1990, sexual harassment awards handled through the EEOC totaled $7.7 million; by 1996, settlements had reached $27 million.

Awakened by the prospects of costly lawsuits, the public and private sectors alike have gone on the defensive. Sexual harassment training is becoming common. Formal policies now are the rule rather than the exception in the workplace. More women (and men) are filing suit and supporting the victims of harassment. As a result of the Thomas–Hill hearings, public attitudes and actions regarding sexual harassment were irrevocably changed.

Sexual harassment has two facets:

- Unwanted sexual attention or advances
- A hostile environment (work or school) in which the person faces daily stress and oppression because of the unwanted sexual attention

Although the two often go together, they can exist independently.

Sexual harassment relates in part to how males are socialized. Men tend to interpret women's friendliness as a sign of sexual interest, as an invitation to pursue sexual involvement (Johnson, Stockdale, & Saal, 1991; Stockdale, 1993). Men and women perceive sexual harassment differently. Men are much less likely to perceive certain behaviors as harassing than women are (Jones & Remland, 1992). Thus, men have difficulty judging their behavior and its potential for harassment. The courts, too, have trouble determining whether certain actions cross the line between aggressive courting and sexual harassment.

Sexual harassment Unwelcome sexual advances, requests for sexual favors, and other verbal or physical conduct of a sexual nature in the workplace or educational setting

Environmental/Occupational Wellness

A work environment with high-level environmental wellness is a place where workers coexist without fear of abuse, discrimination, or harassment. Policies to guard against harassment and discrimination are in place and are enforced swiftly, fairly, and equally for all levels of workers. Healthy workplaces are environments where people pursue their occupations in a safe and supportive atmosphere. Sexual harassment exists in exactly the opposite environment—one that is hostile, where those in power use their positions to take advantage of others. Each person has the responsibility to report coworkers and bosses who abuse the work site and thus turn it into a hostile environment for everyone.

Conditions of Sexual Harassment

Sexual harassment has three attributes that transcend individual perception and set the context for any interaction between individuals:

- A power differential in the relationship
- Inappropriate approach
- Pressure after expression of disinterest

A hallmark of sexual harassment is the use and abuse of power to secure sexual favors. Power differentials exist in the workplace and the classroom based on roles and responsibilities. The boss, supervisor, and professor have power over workers and students by the nature of their roles and authority. A boss or supervisor is responsible for evaluating work performance, giving assignments, and the like. A professor evaluates papers, tests, and exams and ultimately assigns a grade to students in the class.

When someone holds power over another by virtue of a "superior" role, the subordinate person has a harder time refusing the advances. The subordinates fear reprisal—in a poor performance review, no raise, undesirable work assignments, even termination. In a school environment, the students fear a less objective review of their work and lower grades. Also, being approached in a respectful, inquiring way is vastly different from being approached in a harassing way.

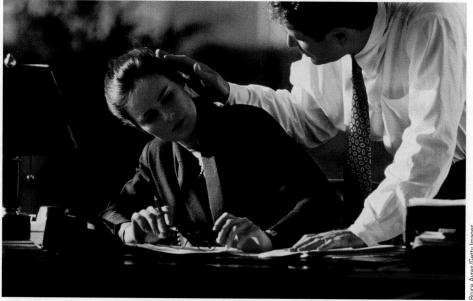

Physical intimidation often plays a big part in creating a hostile environment.

Bruce Ayres/Getty Images

Linda and Beth:
Sexual Harassment Victims

Linda, 27, married, identifies as Filipino; Beth, 33, single, is white.

Linda, a secretary for a medium-sized trucking company, is being harassed by her boss, John. He takes every opportunity to position himself around Linda to maximize the opportunity for physical contact. John leans over her desk, puts his arm around her chair, places himself in a doorway through which she must pass, and uses these opportunities to brush against Linda.

He has made comments about the size of her breasts, her shapely legs, and how he could really show her a good time in bed. Both John and Linda are married, and she has told him she is not interested in having an affair with him.

Beth is a driver for a local bus company, one of two women who drive for this company. The other 48 drivers are men. All drivers report to the local garage, where the buses are parked. The garage has two locker rooms, restrooms, a cafeteria, and administrative offices. Beth has complained to her supervisor (a man) that the work environment is not conducive to her well-being and may even be hostile. The male drivers are fond of soft- and hard-core pornography and have pinned-up pictures of naked women on the walls of the garage. They also leave these magazines out on the tables in the cafeteria.

Besides the print materials, the male drivers congregate in the cafeteria and tell sexually degrading jokes about women. They generally refer to women in derogatory terms when Beth is alone with them and when the other female driver is there. Although no one has made any direct advances toward her (she is living with her boyfriend and uninterested), she feels the work environment is hostile to women.

Both of these women are victims of sexual harassment—Linda, who is the victim of unwanted sexual advances from her boss, and Beth, who hasn't been personally confronted but is forced to work in a hostile environment created by her coworkers.

Critical Thinking

When does one worker's sexually open workplace become another's hostile environment?

Use your Virtual Workbook to explore your answer to this question at **http://health.wadsworth.com/blonna1.**

Finally, if the pursuing person stops the pursuit once the subordinate has expressed noninterest or displeasure, it's not harassment. Persistence and an attempt to pressure the other person into responding, however, are more likely to be considered harassment, especially if the first two criteria are also present.

Sexual Harassment Among Gay People

The original language of the Civil Rights Act of 1964 that governs the EEOC's handling of sexual harassment cases was directed at discrimination based on sex. It was never intended to provide similar protections based on sexual orientation. Quittner (2002) identifies several recent court cases where the plaintiffs filed sexual harassment charges with the EEOC against their employers for discrimination based on sexual orientation.

In all of the cases, convincing cases were made for portraying work sites that were indeed hostile environments and denial of promotions based on sexual orientation. In one case, a butler at a prestigious Las Vegas hotel was subjected to taunts, catcalls, physical assaults (grabbing his crotch, poking his genitals, and so forth), and threats. He became afraid to go to work and was eventually fired from the job. He filed a sexual harassment suit against the hotel. He lost his case, the courts citing that while the law clearly prohibits a gay man or woman from sexually harassing a heterosexual (that is, an opposite-sex) coworker, there were no protections for same-sex sexual harassment in the workplace.

Quittner (2002) cites another case of a male correctional officer in New York state being forced to leave his job after repeated incidents of verbal abuse from fellow heterosexual officers escalated into physical violence. The officer was denied by the District of New York federal court from suing his employer for same-sex sexual harassment. Such cases highlight the need for additional legislation to protect against harassment. In some states and cities, harassment based on sexual orientation is protected under broader antidiscrimination statutes.

Sexual Harassment Involving Children and Teens

One of the outcomes of the Thomas–Hill hearings and subsequent legislation is an attempt to define and prevent harassment at all levels. This has extended into all segments of society, including the elementary school.

Sexual Harassment in Elementary Schools   Sexual harassment in the schools goes way beyond mere teasing. Although poking fun and teasing can be emotionally painful and stressful, they do not constitute sexual harassment. In childhood, teasing peers of the other sex is a developmentally appropriate form of gender validation and, if not carried to an extreme, actually can strengthen the bonds

healthy sex hints 16.5

Sexual Harassment: How to Fight Back

The following guidelines may be helpful in fighting back if you think you have been the victim of sexual harassment on campus or at work.

1. If the harassment includes rape or attempted rape, file criminal charges against the perpetrator.
2. If the act does not include rape or attempted rape, confront the person who is harassing you. Write a letter to the offender, and follow up with a meeting. Be as clear and specific about the offender's actions as possible.
   - Be specific about the incidents, times, and dates. A history and pattern of events are important. Most harassers are repeat offenders.
   - Describe exactly what happened, your feelings about the incidents, and how you reacted. Include a short statement indicating your desire for the harasser to stop.
   - Sign and date the letter, and make duplicate copies.
   - Send a copy to the perpetrator, and indicate that if the behavior doesn't stop immediately, you will press charges using the letter as evidence.
3. Seek support. Don't hide what happened.
   - Talk to coworkers, fellow students, and people identified with the issue. This may help put pressure on the offender to stop.

- Contact a local support group, and talk to others who have experienced the same problem.
- Relate your incidents to your significant other.
4. If the behavior doesn't stop, meet with the offender's supervisor. Discuss the incidents and give a copy of your letter to the supervisor.
   - In a work setting, this is the offender's immediate supervisor.
   - In a college setting, this person may be the department chairperson, the student center director, a member of the sexual harassment panel, or the dean of students.
5. Know your rights. Sexual harassment is against the law. You do not have to put up with it.
   - Obtain the company's/school's sexual harassment policy. Read it thoroughly, and make sure you follow its guidelines for handling your case.
   - Identify the administrative office and person responsible for handling sexual harassment violations in your workplace or school.

Although it may seem frightening, it's better to act quickly than to wait and see what happens. Harassers rarely stop their activities if they are not challenged.

Coercive Sex in the Media

We all know that it is immoral to push, coax, or force someone to have a sexual interaction when they do not want to be sexual. However, this type of behavior is fairly common in today's music. The music we listen to may influence the way we think and act, so it is important to recognize the messages we are receiving. This activity will help you start to critically analyze the impact of the music in your life.

For the next week, list all the songs you hear on a sheet of paper in two columns: sexually coercive lyrics and nonsexual or healthy sexual lyrics. To really analyze the songs, you will have to listen closely to the lyrics. If you cannot understand the words, try looking on the group's Web site for the lyrics. You may be quite surprised at the song's message when you see the actual words. At the end of the week, evaluate your choices of music. Is your favorite music reflecting a healthy, positive view of sexuality or a negative, destructive one? Are you willing to reduce or eliminate the songs that reinforce the idea that sex is to be gotten at all cost and replace these with songs that reflect a healthy, positive approach to sexuality?

little boys and girls have with their friends. Most of it is innocent and not discriminatory.

When the teasing is sexual in nature, it is a different matter. Uninvited sexual advances, lewd comments, ogling, and catcalls are different from simple put-downs ("Boys are better than girls," and vice versa) and nonsexual teasing. Even if they are not outright sexual acts directed at a child, they are capable of creating a climate of hostility that characterizes sexual harassment.

Often the focus of childhood teasing is sexual orientation. Children sometimes tease same- or opposite-sex peers with taunts of "queer," "homo," "fag," "lesbo," "dyke," and the like. Whether the perception is accurate or not, it creates a hostile environment for these children, making daily interactions with peers painful.

Several noteworthy court rulings have been made regarding sexual harassment by elementary school students (LeLand, 1996). In Lexington, North Carolina, in 1966, 6-year-old Jonathan Prevette was suspended for kissing a classmate in an incident that the court ruled was sexual harassment. In response, the boy's parents threatened to sue if their son was not reinstated and the policy changed. The school board reviewed the case and agreed that the incident wasn't sexual harassment and that the policy required retooling.

In another case, in New York, 7-year-old De'Andre Dearinge was charged with sexual harassment for kissing a student against her will and pulling a button off her skirt. Again, the school board intervened and reinstated the child.

What both of these examples illustrate is the difficulty in determining whether specific incidents involving students constitute sexual harassment or represent something else. Obviously, singular, isolated incidents have to be evaluated differently from repeated acts that are more in keeping with creating a hostile climate and failing to stop when the other person expresses a desire to halt the sexual overtures or remarks.

Some child development authorities think that most 6- and 7-year-olds like the ones publicized in North Carolina and New York are too young to understand the concept of sexual harassment. Their behavior might be better labeled as a form of bullying in which they use power over another inappropriately. Some child development experts view this as a sort of testing the waters, and children (both perpetrator and victim) need to be educated about how to handle the situation rather than take it out of their hands. By having the proper authorities (such as school officials) step in, the victim relinquishes the ability to develop a repertoire of assertive behavior that could be used to fend off future would-be harassers (Leland, 1996).

case study 16.4

Bethany: A Proposition from Her Professor

Critical Thinking

Have you ever been in a situation where a grade was so important you said, "I'd do anything to get a better grade in this class?" What makes class grades this important?

Use your Virtual Workbook to explore your answers to these questions at **http://health.wadsworth.com/blonna1.**

Bethany, 23, lesbian, is white.

Bethany, a college senior, was having trouble with one of her classes and went to see her professor, a 35-year-old married man.

When I went to see him, I was a little surprised that he shut the door. It was after our late-afternoon class, and there wasn't anybody around in his department. He had this weird little smile on his face when he asked me to sit down. I sensed something was wrong and should have left then, but I didn't. When I sat down, his first remark was about how good I smelled. I smiled and thanked him but thought to myself that the comment was totally inappropriate.

I explained to him that I was there because I was worried about my grade for the semester. I had gotten a D on the last test and didn't want to lower my grade below a B–. He told me not to worry; he didn't like to see me so sad. Again I smiled but thought that this remark was also inappropriate. He said he'd take care of me, that I was one of his favorite students. With that, he slid his hand over the table and began rubbing my hand with his.

I was getting very uncomfortable by now and moved my hand away. He said, "Don't be so tense; let me rub your shoulders." He started to get up, but I stood up and said, "I don't think that's necessary. I must be going." He said, "Sit down. I thought you wanted to talk about your grade."

I sat back down, and he proceeded to explain to me that he'd had his eye on me all semester and was hoping I'd come to visit him. He explained that other female students in the past had worked out "special arrangements" to boost their grades. I asked him, "What kind of special arrangements?" He said, "Come on now, Beth, don't be so naive. You're a very sexy girl. We could have lots of fun together."

At this point, I was so flustered that I got up quickly and excused myself. I had to beat him to the door because he got up as if to block my exit, but I already had opened the door. He smiled and told me not to do anything foolish. I didn't tell anyone because I was afraid he'd flunk me. He kind of ignored me the rest of the semester but did wind up giving me a higher grade than I thought I earned.

Prosecutors would counter this defense by claiming that abuse of power is the first step in harassment. If a 6- or 7-year-old thinks he or she can kiss or pull a button off a skirt of a classmate, the next act might be more overtly sexual in nature. Also, by stepping in quickly, school officials are bringing the issue to the students' (and parents') awareness.

In response to these and a host of other lawsuits being filed around the country, the U.S. Department of Education's Office for Civil Rights issued a new policy entitled "Sexual Harassment Guidance: Harassment of Students by School Employees, Other Students, and Third Parties." The document attempts to bring standards for determining sexual harassment in line with the guidelines used for evaluating adult cases. The policy defines the same two types of sexual harassment used in adult rulings: quid pro quo (say, sexual favors for advancement) and hostile environment (Chmielewski, 1997).

Sexual Harassment in College

Over the past decade, many colleges have instituted sexual harassment policies, in response to concerns of students, faculty members, and administrators. Most sexual harassment in college is between male professors and female students. Although the reverse (female professor harassing a male student) or same-sex harassment can happen, both are much less common.

Between 15 and 50 percent of undergraduate and graduate-level college women report having been the victim of sexual harassment by a professor. Furthermore, between 10 and 20 percent of male undergraduates have been the victims of sexual harassment (Benson & Thomson, 1990). This behavior encompasses either unwanted sexual advances or the creation of a hostile environment. In a study at the University of California–Berkeley, approximately one-third of female students reported at least one incident of sexual harassment on campus (Benson & Thomson, 1990).

The NCWSV, although not designed to measure sexual harassment per se, found that approximately 11 percent of the 4,446 women studied had been sexually victimized (other than rape). These incidents included sexual coercion, sexual contact with or without force, threats of rape, sexual contact, and penetration. About 10 percent of the women had also been victimized in the past. Even more startling is the percentage of women who reported being stalked in the previous academic year. The NCWSV defined stalked as "repeatedly followed, watched, phoned, e-mailed, or communicated with in some way that seemed obsessive to you and made you afraid or concerned for your safety." Fully 13.1 percent of the women, using these criteria, reported being stalked in the previous academic year. Although none of these NCWSV data meet the classic criteria for sexual harassment, many would argue that this scenario could represent a hostile environment for some campus women (Fisher et al., 2000).

Child Sexual Abuse

Child sexual abuse is any sexual contact between an adult and a child under 18 years of age. Child sexual abuse runs the gamut from inappropriate fondling and touching, to masturbation, to oral sex, to penetration of the anus or vagina with fingers or a penis. These and other forms of sexual behavior are considered evidence of child sexual abuse despite the child's consent or sexual precociousness. Often sexual abuse starts off as normal hugging, kissing, and playful behavior. It then progresses to more intimate touching, manual and oral stimulation, and finally intercourse. The perpetrator often tells the child that he or she is not doing anything wrong but "Don't tell anyone because they might not understand." The perpetrator often uses bribes and rewards to get the child to conceal the illicit behavior. Or, physical threats or threats of desertion scare the child into silence. Children also may not report abuse because of fear and guilt. They sense that something is wrong but can't bear the shame of others finding out. Often, fear of reprisals from the perpetrator or other family member stands in the way of the victim's reporting abuse. In many cases, even when children report the behavior to a parent, they are not believed.

Child sexual abuse involving nonfamily members is generally referred to as **child molestation.** Child sexual abuse involving genetically related family members is called **incest.** Often, the perpetrators are adults who fall between the two forms, such as steprelatives, the mother's boyfriend, or a caregiver brought into the house to watch the children. As we discussed in Chapter 9, a *pedophile* is an adult who is sexually aroused by children and initiates contact with them out of sexual desire. A nonpedophilic **child molester** is not motivated by sexual desire but, rather, by power, the desire to control, or out of affection.

Child sexual abuse Any sexual contact between an adult and a child who is under 18 years of age

Child molestation Abuse of a child by nonfamily members

Incest Child sexual abuse involving genetically related family members

Child molester One who makes indecent sexual advances to children

Intellectual and Emotional Wellness

As adults, we have the intellectual and emotional maturity to make informed choices regarding when and with whom we want to be sexual. Although "age of consent" is a gray area chronologically, theoretically it is the age where intellect and emotion work together in the mature person to make informed choices regarding their behavior. Society has long believed that children must be "protected" sexually from sexual predators until they are mature enough to make informed decisions regarding their behavior. Sexual predators are often very smart and develop elaborate plans for deceiving, luring, and trapping their victims. They observe and note their victim's behavior, patterns, and weaknesses. Their cognitive abilities, although they may be high-level, are without the self-regulating moral/ethical controls that most of us have.

Preconditions Related to Child Sexual Abuse

Child sexual abusers tend to be shy and lonely, and they have poor interpersonal skills with other adults (Bauman, Kasper, & Alford, 1984). They are conservative in their political and sexual beliefs, tend to be religious, and lack knowledge about sex (Segal & Marshall, 1985). **Child molesters** are more likely to be victims of child sexual molestation themselves, alcoholics, and have severe marital difficulties (Johnston, 1987). Preconditions related to child sexual abuse have been identified (Finkelhor, 1984); these are explored in the following sections.

Motivation to Abuse Three key variables influence the perpetrator's motivation to abuse: (a) emotional congruence, (b) sexual arousal, and (c) blockage of alternative forms of sexual arousal. Whereas adults typically are attracted to, and seek emotional connections with, other adults in emotional congruence, pedophiles are drawn to children for this fulfillment. This may be a result of the perpetrator's arrested emotional development, a need to feel powerful and in control, or a reenactment of his own childhood abuse.

Typically, adults are sexually aroused by other adults and find children's bodies immature and nonarousing. Pedophiles feel the opposite. They are sexually aroused by children and not by adults. In addition to the perpetrators' own modeling of sexual relations experienced in their youth or their own childhood trauma, it may be influenced by erotic portrayals of children in advertising and media or exposure to child pornography.

A subgroup of child sexual abusers is **sociopaths** who have **psychoses** or other forms of mental illness. These abusers obtain gratification not only from sexual activity but also from inflicting pain and suffering on their victims.

Blockage refers to child sexual abusers' inability to use other forms of sexual release and gratification. The abusers may be unable to form adult sexual relationships and be sexually naive. Their strict upbringing and sexual values may block their ability to use masturbation and fantasy as outlets for their sexual desire.

Internal Inhibitions Against Abuse Child sexual abusers find ways to overcome **internal inhibitions** against adult–child sexual relations. Whereas other adults may be curious or fantasize about this activity, they stop short of actually doing it because of the strong cultural and social restrictions against such behavior. They have well-developed impulse control. Child sexual abusers, however, lack these inhibitions. Furthermore, they are more likely to use alcohol and drugs to overcome any inhibitions they do have.

Sociopath A manifestly antisocial psychopath

Psychosis A severe form of mental disorder or disease affecting the total personality

Internal inhibitions Natural impulse control against adult–child sexual relations

External Inhibitions Against Abuse External inhibitions against abuse include influences of family members, neighbors, friends, social connections, and household privacy. The greatest inhibitor of sexual abuse is the mother. Child sexual abuse is much more likely to occur in households where the mother is absent or neglectful, has emotional or physical problems, or is a victim of marital abuse.

In cases where the mother herself was a victim of child sexual abuse or is disengaged from her husband, she will turn her back on, or even use, her daughter as a buffer between herself and her husband (Browning & Boatman, 1977). This behavior clears the way for the father, stepfather, mother's boyfriend, or other dominant man to gain access to the child.

Children who are socially isolated (having few close friends or neighbors) also are more likely to be victimized. Household sleeping arrangements and crowding, too, may create opportunities for abusers to gain ready access to victims.

> **External inhibitions** Impulse control against abusing children, as influenced by surrounding people and environment

Social Wellness

As we have just described, sexual predators do not have strong social relationships. Starting with their dysfunctional relationships with their own parents, sexual predators have not developed mature, egalitarian relationships based on caring, respect, and tolerance. From those who harass, to those who rape, to those who abuse children, a common thread is immature, dysfunctional, unsatisfying social relationships. Those who engage in coercive sex often have limited experience with relationships based on love and caring, trust, respect, mutuality, sharing, and commitment. Their relationships are exploitive, self-centered, and destructive. They use power differentials in relationships to take advantage and inflict pain and suffering. Their relationships are really not relationships at all. They are artificial arrangements set up to trap and abuse.

Children's Resistance Child sexual abusers prey on any perceived child weaknesses. They are canny in using coercion, threat, punishment, or force to overcome any resistance a child may use. Children who are emotionally insecure, deprived, needy, and unsupported are prime victims for the abuser's offers, pleas, bribes, and threats. Children who lack education about sexual abuse and do not have good communication skills and caring adult support systems are easier for the abuser to manipulate.

Risks for Child Sexual Abuse

In a study of approximately 800 college students conducted in 1984, eight risk factors were related to an increased likelihood of childhood sexual abuse (Finkelhor, 1984):

1. Have a stepfather
2. Ever lived with mother alone
3. Not close to mother
4. Mother never finished high school
5. Sex-punitive mother
6. No physical affection from father
7. Income under $10,000 a year (although low income by itself is not a risk)
8. Two friends or fewer in childhood

The incidence of childhood sexual abuse was virtually nonexistent in subjects who did not have any of these risk factors. In contrast, two-thirds of the subjects reporting five or more of the risk factors were victims of childhood sexual abuse. The risk factor that was the greatest predictor of child sexual abuse was having a stepfather. This doubled a woman's risk of ever being abused. These findings confirmed those of Russel (1990), who found that 1 in 40 victims of child sexual victims were abused by their biological fathers versus 1 in 6 by stepfathers.

The second greatest predictor was having a sex-punitive mother. This type of mother was likely to scold or punish her daughter for asking questions about sex or engaging in behavior such as masturbation.

Hyde (1994) has speculated about child abuse being related to male psychosexual development. She asserts that men are socialized to be sexually attracted to partners who are smaller and younger than they are, whereas women receive the opposite messages. Women usually are sexually involved with, and attracted to, partners who are larger and older than them.

Incidence of Child Sexual Abuse

The actual number of cases of child sexual abuse is unknown. Like rape, child sexual abuse is often unreported for many reasons. However, following a sustained 15-year increase from 1977 to 1992, reported cases of child sexual abuse have been decreasing since then (Jones & Finkelhor, 2001). Numbers of cases of reported child sexual abuse reached an estimated peak of 149,800 in 1992. Since that time, cases declined 2 to 11 percent each year through 1998 (Jones & Finkelhor, 2001). In 1998, estimated cases of child sexual abuse reached a low of approximately 103,600, which represents a total decline of 31 percent over that 6-year period (Jones & Finkelhor, 2001). This sustained decline in the number of cases contrasts significantly with the 1980s, when the United States experienced 10 percent annual increases in the number of cases of child sexual abuse (Jones & Finkelhor, 2001).

Explanations for the Decline   Wilson (2001), reporting in the Office of Juvenile Justice bulletin, identifies several reasons for the decline in child sexual abuse cases. The past two decades have seen a dramatic increase in public information and information about child sexual abuse. There has been an increase in child abuse prevention programs. The increase in awareness and prevention has led to the arrest and incarceration of more sex offenders. With the onset of Megan's Law (which we will discuss in detail later), new laws have been passed in many states to increase and improve the monitoring of sex offenders (Jones & Finkelhor, 2001).

The decline in child sexual abuse parallels declines in other criminal offenses that may be related to victimizing children. As we mentioned previously, the number of cases of all violent crime, rape, sexual assault, and other types of female victimization are down nationally. Factors that may be related to the declines in these crimes could also be related to the declines in child sexual abuse (Jones & Finkelhor, 2001).

Effects of Child Sexual Abuse

Several factors have an impact on the future well-being of the victim. Four factors are related to the need for long-term treatment and the prognosis for the child (Krugman, Bays, Chadwick, Levitt, McMugh, & Whitworth, 1991). The closer the victim's relationship to the perpetrator, the longer the abuse, the more violent the contact, and the more intrusive the relationship, the greater is the need for treatment and the poorer the hope for an effective outcome.

As adults, child sexual abuse victims report extremely sad, pain-filled childhoods. They recollect feelings of betrayal, fear, and loss of innocence, painting a

case study 16.5

Lucy: A Victim of Child Abuse

Lucy, 16, single, identifies as Latina.

A 16-year-old girl was referred to the STD clinic by her high school nurse. The report showed a classic macular/papular rash on her hands and feet and a blood test confirming secondary syphilis. This girl, Lucy, probably used drugs, had a few boyfriends, and was a dropout candidate. Dr. Blonna saw these kids all the time. Here he relates Lucy's case.

When I first interviewed Lucy, I knew from the start that this was not a cut-and-dried case. She was young, fresh-faced, and preppy-looking in her Catholic schoolgirl's pleated skirt and white socks.

Lucy was quiet, almost sunken in her posture. She averted eye contact, obviously embarrassed. After my usual introduction, explaining why I needed to talk to her, I began to explain the nitty-gritty of sexually transmitted diseases and how they are spread. By the time I got around to asking her about her sexual contacts, she was on the verge of tears.

Lucy's initial response to my asking for the names of her sexual contacts was "There's only one—my boyfriend, Hector." When pressed for Hector's address and telephone number, Lucy hemmed and hawed, said she didn't know where he lived or went to school, and tried to move the interview along. Finally, I had enough and said, "Look, I know you're lying to me. What's going on here?"

It took but a second for Lucy to break down and the floodgates to open up, her tears pouring forth in a torrent followed by shakes, sobs, and near hyperventilation. She couldn't contain herself any longer. Between gasps of air and body-wracking sobs, she told her story. There was no boyfriend Hector. Rather, there was a 45-year-old man, Luis. Luis was the boyfriend of her mother, Maria. He mostly lived with them and had free rein to come and go. It seemed that he liked to come around when Maria was still at work and Lucy and her younger sister were home from school.

Luis had started sexually abusing Lucy about 5 years ago. It started out with her sitting on his lap and his fondling her. It progressed to his exposing himself to her, demanding fellatio, and, for the past couple of years, vaginal intercourse. When it began, Lucy was confused, but Luis told her not to say anything to her mother. Lucy thought her mother knew what was going on because there were times when Lucy didn't want to be left home with Luis, but her mom made excuses for him and didn't let Lucy leave.

When Luis began to force fellatio and intercourse on Lucy, he warned her not to tell her mother or he'd leave them or, worse, hurt her mother and little sister. Lucy was beginning to worry about her little sister. She'd seen the way Luis was eyeing her sister lately, and Lucy didn't want her to have to go through the same thing that she did.

I'm not sure how the story ended. I brought Lucy downtown to the child welfare agency that afternoon. I had to fill out forms and was still there when they returned with her little sister, afraid but unmolested. The social worker told me that they were removing Lucy and her sister from the home, arresting Luis and probably Maria, and would find a safe home for the girls. The last image I have of Lucy is her sitting on the wooden bench in the child welfare office, her arm around her little sister, smoothing the pleats on her school uniform, looking much older and more tired than her 16 years.

Critical Thinking

Social workers and other mental health professionals are trained to pick up on cues like the ones Lucy presented. Should these people be held liable for missing the same cues? Why?

Use your Virtual Workbook to explore your answers to these questions at **http://health.wadsworth.com/blonna1.**

picture of a lost childhood (Felitti, 1991). Victims of child sexual abuse often have difficulty forming intimate relationships as adults. They have feelings of shame and guilt, depression, a lack of trust, and revulsion at being touched, and they often are alcohol and other drug abusers (Frazier & Cohen, 1992). When victims are able to form relationships, they are often characterized by a lack of emotion and sexual interest and gratification (Jackson, Calhoun, Amick, Maddeve, & Habif, 1990).

Megan's Law

On October 31, 1994, the New Jersey State Legislature enacted the Registration
and Community Notification Laws (RCNL), also known as **Megan's Law.** The
law is named after Megan Kanka, who was lured into the house of a neighbor,
whose son, a convicted sex offender, raped and murdered her. Only one family,
neighbors of the perpetrator, had any knowledge of him living on the block.
Megan's Law requires that certain convicted sexual offenders must register with
law enforcement authorities and provide for community notification depending
on the degree of risk that they represent to the community. The law applies to
those who have been convicted of specified sexual offenses and has a grandfa-
ther's clause that includes offenders who were convicted of similar offenses prior
to the passage of the law.

The degree of risk that offenders pose to the community is measured by a
"tiered system" (Brooks, 1996, p. 54).

Tier 1 applies where the risk of reoffense is low. Under Tier 1, all law enforcement
agencies likely to encounter the offender must be notified as well as the vic-
tim(s) and his or her family.

Tier 2 applies where the risk of reoffense is moderate. Under Tier 2, all law enforcement agencies and schools (public and private) likely to encounter the offender
must be notified as well as the victim(s) and his or her family. The statute also
requires notification to organizations in the community, including religious and
youth organizations, likely to encounter the offender. Under the court's decision, individual determinations must be made concerning which institutions or
organizations own or operate an establishment where children or women are
cared for and are "likely to encounter" the offender. The notice to all such organizations must specifically direct them not to notify anyone else.

Tier 3 applies where the risk of reoffense is high. The statute requires that, in addition to the individuals, organizations, and institutions required to be notified
by Tier 2, notification as to Tier 3 offenders must be sufficient to reach members of the public likely to encounter the person registered (individuals residing within a half-mile radius of the offender's home).

Over 40 states rushed to enact Megan's Laws of their own, and in May 1996,
President Bill Clinton signed into law a federal version of the legislation. The federal version of Megan's Law was a revision of the Federal Violent Crimes and
Law Enforcement Act of 1994. The revised law, entitled Megan's Law, required all
states wishing to continue to receive federal funding for law enforcement to comply with its identification and notification of sex offenders criteria (*Economist*,
1997). The law came under intense scrutiny from civil libertarian groups, who
claimed it denies convicted sex offenders their constitutional rights to privacy
and protection (Brooks, 1996).

The various versions of Megan's Law all contain provisions for identifying
convicted sex offenders and ranking them on the aforementioned three-tiered
scale according to their likelihood to offend again. The level of community notification varies according to the offender's level. Tier 1 offenders must register with
local authorities, but their status is not released to the community (Webby, 2003).
High-risk residents (all day care center operators; supervisors of Boy Scouts, Big
Brothers, Big Sisters; and the like) are notified of Tier 2 offenders. All immediate
neighbors and others likely to come in contact with Tier 3 offenders are sent registered letters notifying them of the presence of the offender in their neighborhood
(*Economist*, 2002). In addition to registered letters, other means of community notification include posting of pictures and descriptions of sex offenders; mailings
to families, community groups, and organizations deemed at risk by local authorities; and postings on Internet bulletin boards.

Critics of Megan's Law legislation claim that, in addition to being unconstitutional, it does not work. Just knowing that a sex offender lives on your street is not sufficient to protect your children (Webby, 2003; Bai, 1997). Neighbors of Megan Kanka, for instance, knew that at least one sex offender (the roommate of Megan's killer) already lived on their street (Knight Ridder/Tribune Services, 2003).

Other critics cite that the placement of convicted sex offenders on the tiers often arbitrarily places many people convicted of sex offenses other than child sexual abuse in the highest-risk tiers (Tiers 2 and 3) unnecessarily. Countless lawsuits have been brought against states because of the nature of the tiering and notification processes.

As we go to press, two cases are being reviewed by the United States Supreme Court. In the first case, *The Connecticut Department of Safety v. Doe*, John Doe, a convicted sex offender, successfully sued the state of Connecticut for labeling him at risk for committing a reoffense and posting his name and personal information on the Internet. The lower court in Connecticut ruled in Doe's favor by stating that he had a right to a hearing to determine his risk of becoming a reoffender before being posted on the Internet (National Conference of State Legislators [NCSL], 2002).

The second case, *Otte v. Doe*, is from Alaska and revolves around similar issues. This case attempts to resolve the issue of whether a state has to conduct individualized risk assessments of individuals before their names and personal information are posted on the Internet (Rushkin, 2002).

The resolution of these two cases should help clear up some of the confusion associated with assessing the risks that sex offenders pose to a community and how that risk should be categorized (tiered) and disseminated (community notification) (NCSL, 2002).

In New Jersey, sex offenders are allowed to challenge their tiering. They have 14 days from being notified of their tier designation to challenge it in court. There have been 1,620 cases involving 3,515 specific objections of tier designations since passage of Megan's Law in New Jersey. These 1,620 cases have resulted in 672 tier changes. In 528 cases, a Tier 2 or Tier 3 placement was downgraded to a Tier 1, eliminating the need for community notification (New Jersey Law Network, 2003).

There is no way to identify potential child abusers and isolate them from children. Preventing child sexual abuse must revolve around empowering children by teaching them the warning signs of inappropriate adult sexual behavior and the escape and communication skills necessary to protect themselves. Parents and other adult caregivers must convey to their children a sense of approachability. Children must feel free to discuss their concerns without fear of reprisal.

Strategies to Prevent Child Sexual Abuse

Parents, teachers, and other helpful adults might use the following strategies to help prevent child sexual abuse:

1. *Provide sex education.* One of the cornerstones of any good school-based sexuality education program is a child sexual abuse prevention component. The unit should be comprehensive and cover issues including self-esteem, communication skills, inappropriate adult physical contact, refusal skills, and escape skills. This unit should be presented early in the child's curriculum, as most sexual abuse begins before 8 years of age.
2. *Become an approachable parent.* Open lines of communication early with your children. Continually underscore the fact that your children can come to you with any question involving sex. Do not punish your children for asking questions.

3. *Discuss inappropriate sexual behavior with your children.* Let your children know that you do not approve of any adult–child sexual contact (explain kissing, hugging, and so forth). Tell them that you would never punish them for telling on another adult (no matter how close their relationship—stepfather, baby-sitter, coach). Differentiate "good touch" and "bad touch" while letting your children know that they have the right to want "no touch."

4. *Let your children know they can decide how, when, and by whom they want to be touched.* Do not force them to hug, kiss, or be affectionate with adults with whom they do not want to behave this way. This reinforces their trust in their intuition about other people's sexual behavior.

5. *Discuss refusal skills.* Have your children practice how to say no in an assertive way. Teach them how to refuse an offer to engage in any behavior in which they do not want to be involved.

6. *Discuss escape skills.* Teach your children how to escape from potentially dangerous or abusive situations. Tell them it is OK to yell, scream, hit, and run away from any adult who does not stop touching them when asked to. Help children identify trusted friends, neighbors, and family members with whom they can seek shelter.

7. *Discuss telling.* Your children have to understand that they absolutely must tell you if they have been approached or touched inappropriately by any adult, no matter how close that person's relationship is with you. Children need to understand that this isn't tattle-telling and is the best way to deal with the situation.

Your responses to the Personal Assessment, Thought Questions, and Test Yourself! quiz questions can be logged online in your Virtual Workbook at **http://health.wadsworth.com/blonna1.**

Personal Assessment

16.1 Temper Test

Directions: A number of statements that people have used to describe themselves are given here. Read each statement and then circle the appropriate number to indicate how you generally feel.

	Almost Never	Sometimes	Often	Almost Always
1. I am quick-tempered.	1	2	3	4
2. I get annoyed when I don't receive recognition for doing good work.	1	2	3	4
3. I have a fiery temper.	1	2	3	4
4. I feel infuriated when I do a good job or study hard and get a poor evaluation or test score.	1	2	3	4
5. I am a hot-headed person.	1	2	3	4
6. I get furious when I'm criticized in front of others.	1	2	3	4
7. I get angry when others' mistakes slow me down.	1	2	3	4
8. I fly off the handle easily.	1	2	3	4
9. When I get angry, I say nasty things to anyone around me.	1	2	3	4
10. When I get frustrated, I feel like hitting someone.	1	2	3	4

Total Points: _____

Scoring:

Add the points (1–4) from each item together to get your total score, somewhere between 10 and 40. A man who scores 17 or a woman who scores 18 is just about average. If you score below 13, you're well down in the safe zone. A score above 20 means you may be a hothead—scoring higher than three-quarters of those tested. If these tendencies cause you to take out your anger on anyone else, professional help is advised.

16.2 Personal Alcohol Use

Go to www.intox.com. Click on the "Drink Wheel" on the right side of the screen. Complete the test using the amount and the type of alcohol you usually drink when partying. If you do not drink, use a friend's drinking behavior to complete the assignment.

What were your BAC (blood/breath alcohol concentration) results?

Scroll down and click on "Pharmacology and Disposition of Alcohol in Humans" and "Stages of Alcohol Intoxication." Read the information contained in these links.

What did you learn from this activity?

Thought Questions

1. What sexual acts are covered by the umbrella term *coercive sex*?

2. What conditions are necessary to meet sexual harassment criteria?

3. What is a "hostile environment" in a sexual harassment case? Give an example of a hostile environment.

4. How does power over a subordinate factor into sexual harassment?

5. What are three variations of rape? Is it considered a sexual act? Why or why not?

6. What are three risk factors for acquaintance rape?

7. What are three ways to reduce the risk for acquaintance rape?

8. What are some personality characteristics of a typical child molester?

9. What is the difference between a child molester and a pedophile?

10. What is Megan's Law?

Test Yourself!

1. *Coercive sex* is best defined as
   a. another name for rape.
   b. begging and pleading for sex.
   c. any nonconsensual sexual behavior.
   d. using coercion to set up sexual liaisons.

2. The Sexual Victimization of College Women study found that
   a. date rape is very rare among college women.
   b. about 35 out of every 1,000 college women were rape victims during the time of the study.
   c. about 3.5 out of every 1,000 college women were rape victims last year.
   d. about 3.5 out of every 10,000 college women were rape victims last year.

3. College women are most often raped
   a. in off-campus residences by strangers.
   b. in on-campus residences by strangers.
   c. in off-campus residences by intimate partners.
   d. in on-campus residences by intimate partners.

4. Under Rohypnol, a central nervous system depressant, victims
   a. relax, pass out, are sexually victimized, and suffer from amnesia.
   b. relax, lose their inhibitions, and want sex.
   c. relax, become sexually aroused, and solicit sex.
   d. relax, pass out, and are usually left alone.

5. Under the 1996 Drug-Induced Rape Prevention and Punishment Act,
   a. penalties for Rohypnol and GHB use were made much harsher.
   b. penalties for Rohypnol and GHB use were brought into line with other drugs such as marijuana.
   c. penalties for Rohypnol and GHB use were lessened since they are most often taken for personal use, not major distribution like other drugs such as marijuana or cocaine.
   d. penalties for Rohypnol and GHB use were left unchanged.

6. Which behavior should you avoid if you find yourself the victim of an attempted stranger rape?
   a. Run away if you can.
   b. Try to reason with the perpetrator.
   c. Fight back
   d. Scream, yell, curse.

7. The two criteria needed to prove work site–based sexual harassment are
   a. a hostile environment and unwanted sexual attention.
   b. sex is made a condition for employment.
   c. sex is made a condition of promotion.
   d. hostile sex is part of the work environment.

8. Recent EEOC rulings governing sexual harassment have omitted which of the following groups?
   a. Hispanic women
   b. Homosexuals
   c. White males
   d. African American women

9. Most adults are attracted to, and seek emotional and sexual connections to, other adults. Pedophiles
   a. are attracted to, and seek emotional and sexual connections to, other adults and children.
   b. are attracted to adults but seek emotional and sexual connections to children.
   c. are attracted to, and seek emotional and sexual connections to, children.
   d. neither are attracted to nor seek emotional connections to the children they desire sexually.

10. Megan's Law was recently
    a. struck down in Alaska and Connecticut.
    b. watered down due to cases in Alaska and Connecticut.
    c. upheld due to ruling related to cases in Alaska and Connecticut.
    d. overturned due to cases in Alaska and Connecticut.

Media Menu

You can link to the following online tools by visiting
http://health.wadsworth.com/blonna1.

 InfoTrac Activity

Quittner, J. (2002, December 10). Left out of the law: In the eyes of the court, just about everyone can be a victim of sexual harassment—except, perhaps, out gay men and lesbians. *The Advocate*, pp. 26–30.

 Web Resources

National Center for Victims of Crime

www.ncvc.org

A nonprofit organization providing resources and advocacy to victims of crime. The site offers safety strategies for victims of domestic violence and stalking, highlights of laws and public policy impacting crime victims at state and federal levels, information on crime victims, and finding a lawyer. Access to a virtual library with full-text publications, a directory of publications, recommended reading, bibliographies and a book review, plus links to victim-related sites.

National Organization on Male Sexual Victimization

www.malesurvivor.org

A group started in 1988 by mental health providers who wanted to better understand and treat adult male survivors of childhood sexual abuse. A section on prevention and education talks about how to prevent abused boys from becoming abusive men.

Rape Abuse and Incest National Network (RAINN)

www.rainn.org

A nonprofit organization's hotline providing 24-hour counseling service to survivors of sexual assault. This site also offers information, statistics, and a list of local crisis centers.

Sexual Assault Prevention

www.cc.ysu.edu/rape-prev-info

A site sponsored by the University Counseling Center, Youngstown State University, Youngstown, Ohio. It provides information on prevalence, aftereffects, and treatment of rape and sexual assault and links with a specific focus on higher education.

University of Illinois at Urbana-Champaign, Counseling Center

www.odos.uiuc.edu/Counseling_Center/friends.htm

A site that provides a guide for friends, family, and partners of sexual assault and abuse survivors. Articles address statistics, responses to recent sexual assault/abuse, phases, how to help the survivor, additional suggestions for the romantic partner of a survivor, feelings a victim may experience, how to help oneself, books to read, and other resources.

References

American Academy of Family Physicians. (2003). What to do if you are raped [Online]. Available: http://familydoctor.org/x1976.xml.

American Psychiatric Association. (2000). *Diagnostic and statistical manual of mental disorders* (4th ed., text revision). Washington, DC: Author.

Bai, M. (1997). A report from the front in the war on predators: Years after Megan's murder, her law is still on trial. *Newsweek, 129*(20), 67.

Bauman, R., Kasper, C., & Alford, J. (1984). The child sex abusers. *Corrective and Social Psychiatry, 30*, 76–81.

Benson, D., & Thomson, G. (1990). Sexual harassment on a university campus: The confluence of authority relations, sexual interest, and gender stratification. *Society for the Study of Social Problems, 29*(3), 236–251.

Benton, W. (Ed.). (1996). *Webster's new international dictionary.* Toronto: Encyclopedia Britannica.

Brooks, A. (1996). Megan's Law: Constitutionality and policy. *Criminal Justice Ethics, 15*(56), 51.

Browning, D., & Boatman, B. (1977). Incest: Children at risk. *American Journal of Psychiatry, 134*(1977), 69–72.

Brownmiller, S. (1975). *Against our will.* New York: Simon & Schuster.

Burgess, A. W., & Holmstrom, L. L. (1974). Rape trauma syndrome. *American Journal of Psychiatry, 131*, 981–985.

Cate, R. M., & Lloyd, S. A. (1992). *Courtship.* Newbury Park, Calif.: Sage.

Chmielewski, C. M. (1997). Sexual harassment meets Title IX: New federal rules to combat sexual harassment and place schools at the battlefront. *NEA Today, 16*(2), 25.

The Economist. (1997). Pointing the finger at Megan's Law. *342*(8004), 27–29.

The Economist. (2002, November 16). A scarlet letter: Megan's Law, changing the law for sex offenders. *365*(8299).

Equal Employment Opportunity Commission. (2003). Sexual harassment charges: EEOC and fair employment practices agencies (FEPA) combined, FY 1002-FY 2001 [Online]. Available: www.eeoc.gov/stats/harass.html.

Federal Bureau of Investigation. (2001). *Crime in the United States, 2000.* Washington, DC: U.S. Department of Justice.

Felitti, V. (1991). Long-term medical consequences of incest, rape, and molestation. *Southern Medical Journal, 84,* 328–331.

Finkelhor, D. (1984). *Child sexual abuse: New theory and research.* New York: Free Press.

Fisher, B. S., Cullen, F. T., & Turner, M. G. (2000). *The sexual victimization of college women.* Washington, DC: U.S. Department of Justice.

Fisher, B., Koss, M. P., Gidycz, C. A., & Wisnewski, N. (1987). The scope of rape: Incidence and prevalence of sexual aggression and victimization in a national sample of higher education students. *Journal of Counseling and Clinical Psychology, 55,* 162–170.

Frazier, P., & Cohen, B. (1992). Research on the sexual victimization of women. *Counseling Psychologist, 20,* 141–158.

Frieze, I. H. (1983). Causes and consequences of marital rape. *Signs, 8,* 532–553.

Gleason, N. A. (1994, May). College women and alcohol: A relational perspective. *Journal of American College Health, 42*(6), 279–289.

Higher Education Center. (2003). Sexual assault: Alcohol and other drugs [Online]. Available: www.edc.org/hec/pubs/factsheets/fact_sheet1.html.

Hyde, J. S. (1994). *Understanding human sexuality* (5th ed.). New York: McGraw-Hill.

Jackson, I., Calhoun, K., Amick, A., Maddever, H., & Habif, V. (1990). Young adult women who report childhood intrafamilial sexual abuse: Subsequent adjustment. *Archives of Sexual Behavior, 19,* 211–221.

Johnson, C. B., Stockdale, M. S., & Saal, F. E. (1991). Persistence of men's misperceptions of friendly cues across a variety of interpersonal encounters. *Psychology of Women Quarterly, 15*(3), 463–375.

Johnston, S. (1987, February). The mind of the molester. *Psychology Today,* 60–63.

Jones, L. M., & Finkelhor, D. (2001, January). The decline in child sexual abuse cases. *Juvenile Justice Bulletin.* Washington, DC: Bureau of Justice Statistics, Office of Juvenile Justice and Delinquency Prevention.

Jones, T. S., & Remland, M. S. (1992). Sources of variability in perceptions of and responses to sexual harassment. *Sex Roles, 27*(3–4), 121–142.

Kaufman, L. (1997). A report from the front: Why it's gotten easier to sue for sexual harassment. *Newsweek, 129*(2), 32.

Knight-Ridder/Tribune Services. (2003, January 13). Public must be involved to make Megan's law work. *San Jose Mercury News,* p. 7485.

Koss, M. P. (1992). The underdetection of rape: Methodological choices influence incidental estimates. *Journal of Social Issues, 48,* 61–75.

Koss, M. P. (1996). The measurement of rape victimization in crime surveys. *Criminal Justice and Behavior, 23*(1), 55–69.

Krugman, R., Bays, J., Chadwick, D., Levitt, C., McMugh, M., & Whitworth, J. (1991). Guidelines for evaluation of sexual abuse of children. *Pediatrics, 87,* 254–260.

LeLand, J. (1996). A kiss is just a kiss: Where should schools draw the line between normal childhood behavior and sexual harassment? *Newsweek, 128*(17), 71–72.

Malamuth, N. M., Sockloski, R. J., Koss, M. P., & Tanaka, J. S. (1991). Characteristics of aggressors against women: Testing a model using a national sample of college students. *Journal of Consulting and Clinical Psychology, 59,* 670–781.

Marano, H. E. (1996). Why they stay: A saga of spouse abuse. *Psychology Today, 29*(3), 56–66.

Montgomery, R. L., Benedicto, J. A., & Hammerke, F. M. (1993, December). Personal U.S. social motivation of undergraduates in using alcohol. *Psychological Reports,* 960–962.

Muram, D., Miller, K., & Cutler, A. (1992). Sexual assault of the elderly victim. *Journal of Interpersonal Violence, 791,* 70–76.

National Conference of State Legislators. (2002, July 16). *Connecticut Department of Public Safety vs. Doe.* Law & Justice Committee [Online]. Available: www.ncsl.org/statefed/doe.htm.

New Jersey Law Network. (2003, February 18). New Jersey law [Online]. Available: www.njlawnet.com/megan.html.

Office of National Drug Control Policy. (2002a). Gamma hydrobutyrate (GHB) [Online]. Available: www.whitehousedrugpolicy.gov/publications/factsh/tgamma/index.html.

Office of National Drug Control Policy. (2002b). Rohypnol [Online]. Available: www.whitehousedrugpolicy.gov/publications/factsht/rohypnol/index.html.

Quittner, J. (2002, December 10). Left out of the law: In the eyes of the court, just about everyone can be a victim of sexual harassment—except, perhaps, out gay men and lesbians. *The Advocate,* pp. 26–29.

Rantala, R. R., & Edwards, T. J. (2000, July). *Effects of the NIBRS on crime statistics.* Bureau of Justice Statistics Special Report (NJC 178890). Washington, DC: U.S. Department of Justice, Office of Justice Programs.

Rennison, C. M. (2001). *Criminal victimization 2000: Changes 1999–2000 with trends 1993–2000.* Bureau of Justice Statistics, National Crime Victimization Survey. Washington, DC: U.S. Department of Justice.

Ruskin, L. (2002, November 12). Sex registry goes to court; John Doe: Alaskans say law amounts to retroactive punishment. *Anchorage Daily News.*

Russel, D. E. H. (1990). *Rape in marriage.* Bloomington: Indiana University Press.

Sanday, P. (1987). The socio-cultural context of rape: A cross-cultural study. *Journal of Social Issues, 37*(4), 5–27.

Segal, Z., & Marshall, W. (1985). Heterosexual social skills in a population of rapists and child molesters. *Journal of Consulting and Clinical Psychology, 53,* 55–63.

Stockdale, M. S. (1993). The role of sexual misperceptions of women's friendliness in an emerging theory of sexual harassment. *Journal of Vocational Behavior, 42*(1), 84–101.

Task Force of the National Advisory Council on Alcohol Abuse and Alcoholism. (2002). *A call to action: Changing the culture of drinking at US colleges.* NIH Publication 02-5010. Washington, DC: National Institute on Alcohol Abuse and Alcoholism.

United States Congress. (1996). The Drug-Induced Rape Prevention and Punishment Act of 1996. 21 USC 841(b)(7).

Webby, S. (2003, January 13). Lack of funding, personnel hinder enforcement of Megan's Law. *San Jose Mercury News,* p. 1058.

Wechsler, H., Davenport, A., Dowdell, G., Moeykens, B., & Castillo, S. (1994). Health and behavioral consequences of binge drinking in college. *Journal of American Medical Association, 272*(21), 1672–1677.

Weschler, H., Eun, L. J., Kuo, M., Sebring, M., Nelson, T. F., & Lee, H. (2002). Trends in college binge drinking during a period of increased prevention efforts: Findings from four Harvard School of Public Health college alcohol study surveys, 1993–2001. *Journal of American College Health, 50*(5), 203–217.

Williams, L. (1984). The classic rape: When do victims report? *Social Problems, 31,* 459–467.

Wilson, J. J. (2001, January). Explanation for the decline in child sexual abuse cases. *Juvenile Justice Bulletin.* Washington, DC: Bureau of Justice Statistics, Office of Juvenile Justice and Delinquency Prevention.

chapter *seventeen*

The Business of Sex

Student Learning Objectives

After reading this chapter, students will be able to

- Explain the major historical events that have shaped current attitudes and practices related to sex for sale over the past three decades.

- Describe the significance of Madonna, Calvin Klein, Gary Hart, and Matt Drudge in shaping the sexual climate of today.

- Differentiate pornography, erotica, and obscenity.

- Discuss how technological advances have combined with other historical trends to create a new commercialization of sex.

- Describe some of the problems inherent in policing the Internet for sexual victimization and exploitation.

- Evaluate the effectiveness of blocking tools that parents can use to limit children's access to Internet- or television-based sexual material.

- Evaluate the effects of sexually explicit materials on sexual behavior.

Test your understanding of these objectives by taking the end-of-chapter quiz, available online at **http://health.wadsworth.com/blonna1.**

activity teaser: *Is sex being sold to you? Find out with the Personal Exploration Activity on page 572.*

case study 17.1

Lisa: Addicted to Cybersex

Lisa, 42, married, is white.

Critical Thinking

What are your thoughts about cybersex being *real* sex or just fantasy sex?

Use your Virtual Workbook to explore your answer to this question at **http://health.wadsworth.com/blonna1.**

Lisa is a continuing education student. She has been married for 22 years and is the mother of a 14-year-old daughter and 13-year-old son. She works part-time and is taking one of the author's human sexuality classes for personal enrichment.

I had a real problem with computer sex. I had to see a therapist because I was really addicted. My telephone and Internet bills were getting huge, and I was spending about 3 hours a night online. I've been in counseling for a couple of months and actually took this class to try to understand my sexuality a little better. I think my marriage was in jeopardy, and that scared me.

My addiction began innocently enough. I had a lot of time on my hands. My husband, whom I love very much, travels about half of the time. As the national sales manager for a small company, he is off on business at least 2 weeks a month. He earns a fabulous salary, and I don't have to work. The kids are both grown up and don't need me much except to drive them around. Other than my exercise class, I had no real time commitments.

We bought my son a new, powerful computer with Internet access, and he showed me how to go online and get into these chat rooms. I started to log on and chat with people. Before long, I found my way into a couple of chat rooms that were sexually oriented. I mean, the primary purpose was to discuss sexual fantasies. It was quite a turn-on. I was getting into these intimate discussions with all kinds of men. It started out as kind of generic. We talked about our sex lives and what we liked to do in bed. Then it got personal—what we'd like to do to each other.

At first I didn't think it was a problem, and I didn't feel guilty, but after a while I found that I was getting really worked up about these calls. I'd masturbate after hanging up. Sometimes I'd even make myself come while online. That's when I started to worry. I never wanted to meet these guys face-to-face, but I started to feel like I was still having sex with them. I was also worried about my kids walking in and seeing me playing with myself.

It all came to a head when my husband saw one of the Internet bills. It seems as though I used a toll number instead of one of the toll-free access ones, and the bill was over $550 for the month. I had to explain the whole thing to him, and he freaked out. He felt like I cheated on him, and he considered separation. It took several weeks to restore his trust and convince him that I still loved him. We moved the computer into my son's room, and I promised not to go online again. We started seeing a family therapist, and I got a part-time job to get me out of the house a little. I'm taking this class to try to learn a little about my sexuality.

As the case study points out, sex is definitely for sale on the Internet. The last 50 years have seen technology play an increasingly more significant role in selling sex. Prior to the 1960s, sexual themes in mainstream advertising were mostly covert and reflected the mores of the times. Advertisers were subjected to much more stringent controls concerning issues such as the verbal content of advertisements, overt pictorial displays of nudity, and implied sexual themes. Modesty prevailed, as cleavage, bare midriffs, and other examples of exposing the human body were not allowed. Using sex in advertising was limited to full-bosomed "sweater girls" to promote cigarettes, appliances, and cars.

Besides the lack of overt sexuality in advertising, it was noticeably absent from other forms of entertainment and media. Few mainstream books, television shows, magazines, movies, and other media included sexual content. Although Kinsey's studies had been conducted and disseminated to the professional community, sexual information was not readily available to the general public.

Changes in the 1960s

These cultural conditions all began to change in the 1960s. The peace, prosperity, and contentment of the post–World War II 1950s began to give way to the rebelliousness of the baby boom generation of the 1960s. Many social, economic, technological, and political forces came together to create a synergy that changed the course of history. As Petersen (1999) notes, a number of firsts came together during 1960s. The sixties saw the birth control pill, the IUD, Freedom Riders, be-ins, sit-ins, love-ins, the Peace Corps, topless bathing suits, topless bars, water beds, lava lamps, *Hair* (the play), hippies and yippies, Playboy Clubs, Stonewall, and Woodstock all converge in a turbulent decade of social change.

Nowhere was change more evident than in issues related to sexuality. Technological advances in contraception brought widespread availability of the birth control pill. This gave women newfound freedom and control of their fertility and enabled them to reenter the workforce in ever-increasing numbers. The number of women taking birth control pills rose from 408,000 in 1961 to 6 million in 1966 (Petersen, 1999).

Masters and Johnson (1966) released their breakthrough research regarding sexual response and sexual pleasure. Men and women learned about the clitoris and multiple orgasms. Other research followed when the interest in information about sexuality became an outcry. Popular magazines of the 1950s, such as *Playboy*, were joined by *Penthouse, Screw, Cosmopolitan,* and others to meet this need (Petersen, 1999).

All of these developments helped spawn a **women's movement,** which began to question many long-standing cultural assumptions regarding the roles of men and women in society. The women's movement brought to the forefront issues such as equal rights, abortion, child care in the workplace, sexual assault, and a host of others. The ensuing debate forever changed the way men and women perceived themselves and their roles as citizens.

Styles, too, began to change. The Broadway play *Hair* focused attention on changing sex roles for men and women. It rejoiced in a newfound androgyny that liberated men from their clean-cut image and women from their bras. Men began to grow long hair and wear beads, and some women discarded their bras and exposed their midriffs. Attitudes and values about sexuality were changing faster than the society could adapt to the change.

One of the most telling legacies of the 1960s was the growing mainstream acceptance of sex as a topic of discussion. Books, films, magazines, newspapers, posters, and the evening news began to increase the level and realism of sexual content. Self-help books about sexuality proliferated. Academicians, feminists, and politicians began to seriously discuss the implications of sexuality and gender research for social policy and laws. While this was going on, average Americans were beginning to discuss their own sexuality. One of the most interesting by-products of the women's and sexual revolutions of the 1960s and early 1970s was how comfortable people became in discussing sex (Hunt, 1974; Hite, 1976).

In the 1950s, a tight sweater and coy look were very risqué.

Women's movement A force to gain full educational, social, and economic opportunities and rights for women equal to those that men are traditionally understood to have

Changes in the 1970s and 1980s: Three Illustrative Examples

The 1970s and 1980s saw a continued increase of sexual themes in the media. Not only did the amount of sexual information increase, but the content, too, became more diverse. Subjects such as homosexuality, bisexuality, and interracial sex were becoming much more noticeable in mainstream media. This new wave of sexual

Madonna is still going strong after bursting on the American pop culture scene over 20 years ago.

permissiveness was marked by changing rules about what previously had been considered private information. Three well-known media figures serve as examples here: actress/singer Madonna, designer Calvin Klein, and 1988 presidential candidate Gary Hart.

The Material Girl

Although now a mother in her 40s, Madonna ushered in a new era of mainstream hedonism and me-generation narcissism in the 1970s. Madonna's "material girl" embodied all of the elements of post-1960s sexuality: open acceptance of sexual desire, the pursuit of sex and passion, a focus on self-fulfillment, glorification of the human body as a sensual and sexual object, permission to explore bisexuality, interracial sex, and personal adornment and clothing that transcended gender conventional style. Madonna combined all of these things into one package and put that package on display in American living rooms. She represented the disparate elements of the tumultuous 1960s, the self-centered 1970s, and the androgynous 1980s in a synergistic, in-your-face assault on American sexual mores.

Although not a self-professed "women's libber" or political figure, Madonna has been one of our most visible and enduring symbols of the post-1960s–1970s American sexual revolution. While the Britney Spears and Christina Aguileras come and go, Madonna has managed to reinvent herself in each of the past three decades and remains an icon of American sexual liberation. She embodies all of the issues that many people have been struggling with most of their lives. She is part caricature, part best friend, part you or me. Almost anyone who identifies with any of the vast changes in American sexual values of the past three decades can see something of him- or herself in Madonna.

Calvin Klein's Clothing Ads

Calvin Klein has been one of the most influential businesspersons in the United States, responsible for increased acceptance of homosexuality, bisexuality, and **androgyny.** Through his clothing and, more important, his advertising, Klein ushered in an acceptance of alternative sexual lifestyles without ever conducting a study, publishing research, or delivering a speech. Klein has pushed the limits of acceptability and taste to the maximum for 25 years.

Klein's clothing style almost single-handedly transformed the boundaries of acceptable standards of dress for men. Klein ushered in denim chic. His casual look helped men (and women) introduce the casual look into the social scene and the workplace. Today, we often see men in denim shirts or dress shirts and ties with jeans or a casual sport coat in the fanciest of locations—the ballet, opera, theater, and most restaurants and clubs. Klein-influenced attire is accepted in all but the most formal of workplaces. This represents a milestone in gender role expectations for men. More and more, men are realizing that being a man doesn't have to include strict adherence to a dress code of the past.

Klein's advertising, however, had even more of an impact on the fabric of sexuality than his clothing did. From the start, Klein's ads pushed the advertising industry to the limits. He exposed flesh—exposed naked backs, buttocks, and breasts. He posed his models suggestively and flaunted the merchandising of

Androgyny Exhibiting both male and female traits

sex in society 17.1

Reactions to the Material Girl

Students' reactions to Madonna tend to be polarized. Love her or hate her, she is a current icon of a changing society.

"Madonna—wow, is she hot." (male, age 22)

"Madonna—I love her. She does what she wants, says what she wants. She's a real bitch, but cool." (female, age 21)

"She's hot, but I wouldn't screw her. She probably has AIDS." (male, age 22)

"I love her. She's definitely a '90s woman." (female, age 19)

"What a slut." (female, age 19)

"I wish I could be more like her. She's so confident and assertive. She knows what she wants and goes after it." (female, age 18)

"I think she's gross. She'd sleep with anybody." (female, age 29)

"I like her attitudes about sex. She's exploring all of the possibilities and apologizing for nothing. She's got guts." (female, age 35)

"She's my ultimate fantasy lady, but I don't think I'd want to marry her." (male, age 23)

products through sex. Even when he wasn't exposing flesh, he was emphasizing the allure of young, nubile bodies; the curve of a hip in skin-tight jeans, the slope of a neck from a denim shirt wide open at the collar, the span of a set of shoulders, or the bulge of a bicep. All of these images are Klein trademarks.

Another of Klein's impacts was with his models. He imprinted first homosexuality, then bisexuality, and most recently androgyny onto the American advertising and marketing scene. Klein's male models of the 1970s were hunks—well-built, with bulging arms and chiseled abdomens. His men of the 1970s turned on male and female viewers alike. His eroticism was always double-edged: It mimicked the sex role behavior of gay men and was a turn-on to heterosexual women. Gay men admired Klein's hunks with their tight buns, broad shoulders, and clean-shaven, healthy look. Straight women admired them for the same look.

Klein's more recent group shots left lingering questions about who was cavorting with whom in the ads. Were the men cavorting with the women, the other men, or both? Were the women wistfully admiring the men or the other women, or both? It was clear who the men were and who the women were. The object of their affection, however, was in doubt.

One of Klein's more recent advertising themes is of a sort of emaciated androgyny. The men and the women are cast in muted tones—blacks, blues, grays. Most of the models look thin and in need of some personal grooming. This has been referred to as a "heroin chic" look.

Calvin Klein's trademark advertisements reflect the merchandizing of products through sex.

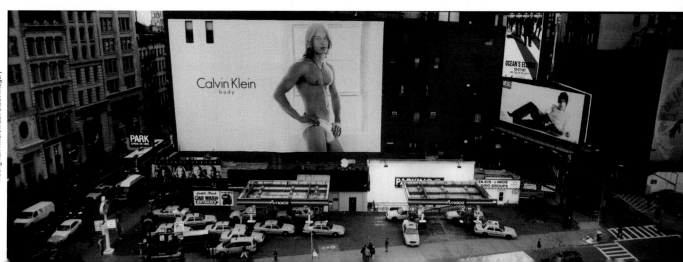

A 1995 Klein campaign raised the ire of media watchdog groups that claimed he crossed the line from bad taste into harmful promotion of a life-threatening lifestyle and look. This advertising campaign used adolescent boys in various seductive poses amid backdrops reminiscent of someone's den. An anonymous voice in the background asked the boys, "Do you like to pose?" The campaign, critics claim, bordered on "kiddie porn" and smacked of pedophilia (Martin, 1995). Whatever one feels about Klein and his various campaigns over the past two decades, his images and ideas undoubtedly helped shape American perceptions about what is sexy and sensual.

Physical Wellness

Critics of media portrayals of what is sensual, beautiful, and sexual claim these set unrealistic standards of perfection and a physical ideal that is unattainable for most people. Proponents of sexy media themes and personalities view these positively. The widespread interest in lifting weights, exercising, and eating healthfully comes in part from images of physical beauty personified by models and popular media personalities (such as Madonna), who promote these behaviors as contributing to their sexiness. You can scarcely pass a women's or men's magazine that doesn't portray the virtues of working out to sculpt a "sexy" body. In a sense, then, the fitness craze, which generally enhances physical wellness, is fueled by the same sexual climate that has also produced many negative sexual images.

Monkey Business

A presidential aspirant finishes our trilogy of symbols of an evolving American sexuality of the past 30 years. Gary Hart was a Democratic Party candidate for president of the United States in 1988. One of the front-runners in the campaign, he had a good chance to earn the Democrats' endorsement for president. All of that changed on the fateful morning of May 3, 1987, when the headline of the *Miami Herald* read, "Miami Woman Linked to Hart" (Bradlee, 1997).

Gary Hart—candidate for president, respectable congressman, businessman, husband, father, with all-American good looks and a charismatic personality— was caught by photographers with Donna Rice, his associate, sitting on his lap on the deck of the yacht *Monkey Business.* Reporters revealed that Rice had stayed overnight in Hart's Capitol Hill house.

This may not seem like a big deal today. As a culture, we seem to have been desensitized to such carryings-on. In 1988, however, it represented a tremendous change in the evolution of American sexual values and the way in which the media covered events and the lives of public figures. Prior to Hart's affair, the personal sex lives of political and other (such as sports) figures were off-limits. The media stayed away from reporting on sexual behavior, especially if this activity was out of public view. It was not allowed on air, in print, or as a subject of an interview.

Stories that we read about today, such as the pro football player with the Dallas Cowboys drug/prostitution case and President Clinton's alleged affairs, never would have been aired in the past. We would not know about them. The unwritten rules of the game were that certain aspects of celebrities' lives were off-limits to the media and not available to the public.

That all changed with the Gary Hart case. Leaking of the story and the subsequent in-depth coverage, complete with front-page photos, broke new ground. The rules had changed. One newspaper's decision about allowing the story to be printed changed the way the U.S. media would report the news from then on. It also set the stage for how information of that nature would be handled in the future.

It also opened the floodgates for a new way of sexual information to be disseminated to the American public. Sexual behavior, drug use behavior, and the like, began to be carried over the airwaves into every small town, big city, and suburban living room. This was the beginning of the in-your-face talk shows, newsmagazine programs, and shock jocks that now are prominent on the American media landscape.

Madonna, Klein, and Hart broke new cultural ground by pushing sexual standards to the limit. They set the stage for allowable behavior and media coverage. What makes their emergence as sexual standard-bearers different from those that came before them is timing. The sweeping changes they created in entertainment, advertising, and media reporting came at a time when the United States was ushering in the first wave of massive technological changes.

Changes in the 1990s and 2000s

Two Illustrative Examples

Two events more than any that occurred during this period of American sexual history have defined sex for sale at the end of the 20th century and the beginning of the 21st century. Both involve money—specifically, the huge amounts of money to be made from subscription Internet services. The first was the use of one such service, *The Drudge Report*, to release speculation of the Bill Clinton–Monica Lewinsky affair. The second is the proliferation of Internet subscriber pornography sites. To understand both, we first need to understand the impact of technological innovations over the past 20 years.

The Impact of Technological Innovations

Stern and Handel (2002) propose that the one constant in the relationship between sexuality and the changing technological landscape is sexuality. Americans have been interested in exploring their sexuality since they landed on the shores of the new world.

Sexuality has historically been expressed through all forms of communication technology, from print (magazines, newspapers, books, and the like), to telegraph, telephone, radio, television, movies, non-Internet computer, and most recently the Internet (Stern & Handel, 2002). Americans' interest in sexuality hasn't changed; it has merely evolved and become more visible as new technologies have emerged and evolved. As Petersen (1999, p. 486) points out, "From Edison's kinetoscope, which had given us the nickel image of *The Kiss,* to today's seemingly unlimited Internet potential, Americans have increasingly made sex visible. The electric lights that had taken sex out of the shadows now provided not a sewer but a pulsing, sensuous, sane environment, a carnal consensus for the millennium."

The 1990s and early 2000s brought a new wave of information technology that included affordable cable television, videocassette and digital videodisc (DVD) players, personal computers (PCs), home videocassette recorders, and high-speed Internet access.

These new technologies were different from all those that had preceded them. The three qualities that set them apart from all the others were power, personal use, and low cost. Cable television brought the world into our living rooms. With more than 100 channels today, we are literally flooded with visual information and data from around the world. For the first time in history, with the Gulf War in 1990, we were spectators in one of our wars as we watched it unfold on television on real time as it actually happened. There were no time delays, no papers to read, nothing to mull over. We simply sat back and watched our country wage war, without editing or tape delay as in Vietnam and previous conflicts.

In 1999, a national survey found that over a third of all 2- to 7-year-olds and over two-thirds of all 8- to 18-year-olds had a television in their own bedrooms. Many of those televisions were hooked up to cable TV services and videocassette recorders (Roberts, 2000). The number of people in the United States who subscribe to cable television has risen steadily over the past few years. In 2000, 70 percent of all homes in the United States had direct to home pay cable television service (U.S. Department of Labor, 2003). Sales of cable television services in the United States rose by 16 percent in 2001. Worldwide, close to 50 million homes had direct to home cable television service. Sales are projected to reach 80 million (U.S. Department of Labor, 2003). Home VCR costs have decreased markedly in the past decade. In 1996, more than 84 percent of all homes in the United States owned at least one VCR, and 39 percent owned two or more.

In addition to the power of the media, these technologies ushered in a new era of personal accessibility and efficiency in delivering sexual content. Cable television and personal computers have become as common as the telephone. Cable television made available pay-per-view movies, X-rated programming, and a host of other innovations that have the potential to bring sexual content along with other topics into our homes 24 hours a day.

Combined with the power of the home computer is the Internet. The personal computer took the nation by storm in the early 1990s, and introduction of the Internet offered Americans the opportunity to connect instantly with millions of users worldwide. The personal computer industry has grown more than 400 percent since 1990. In 1996, 40 percent of U.S. homes had at least one personal computer (Lagnado, 1996). In 1999, more than half of all U.S. households had at least one personal computer, and more than 56 percent of all households were online (Brown, 2002). The Internet makes it possible to move information and communicate far more effectively and with more people in more ways than ever before in the history of civilization.

The sweeping acceptance of these technologies and their sheer power in moving volumes of information and images into U.S. homes opened the floodgate to another wave of sexual communication. Stern and Handel (2002) consider this new state of technological evolution provided by high-speed Internet connectivity as very efficacious in delivering sexuality-related information, entertainment, and services.

One positive aspect of this second wave is its ability to provide accurate, non-biased information on sexuality (Edwards, 1996). As Fisher and Barak (2002) point out, Internet-based sexuality education programs can offer significant resources and expert instruction, and they can reach massive audiences in a very cost-effective manner. The Internet also opens up many exciting venues for conducting sex research. Mustanski (2002) explains that the anonymity and accessibility of the Internet, along with access to very large sample sizes, make sexual survey research very attractive.

On the down side, the Internet is so large and powerful that it is almost impossible to police. It brings graphic, sadomasochistic, live video clips into the living room. It connects 45-year-old pedophiles with potential victims through **chat rooms.**

Chat rooms Live e-mail discussion lines in which a person can communicate with others by typing messages

Couple this technology with a much more permissive culture, and you have an entirely different sexual landscape today than at any time in U.S. history. It is a no-holds-barred culture in which almost anything goes—and much of it goes into our living rooms, bedrooms, and offices via these new technologies. Although all of these things existed before 1990, now the low cost has allowed Americans to be exposed to almost any sexual idea, theme, or image in the privacy of the home. Nearly anything goes—especially if it sells. Our two examples give contrasting views of this new climate.

The Drudge Report

Matt Drudge, 30-year-old computer geek, burst onto the American scene on January 18, 1998, when he published a story in his online gossip column, *The Drudge Report*, about the then-alleged affair between President Bill Clinton and Monica Lewinsky. What makes this case unique isn't the details of the affair. As we know, presidents have been having affairs and using their power, influence, and office to attract women for decades. What is unique about this particular affair is that it was released to the world through an entirely new medium: a subscriber-based online news outlet, *The Drudge Report*.

In 1995, Drudge, a man with a dream of becoming the first nationally recognized online gossip columnist, started his business from scratch. Working from his apartment, his newsletter (www.drudgereport.com) grew to include an estimated 85,000 paid subscribers. Drudge was signed by America On-Line (AOL), at the time one of the nation's largest Internet service providers, to publish the newsletter for it. Drudge gained notoriety for many cases, particularly one where he made allegations that a well-known White House aide, Sidney Blumenthal, was a wife beater.

Critics of Drudge cite his admitted "80 percent" accuracy rate as substandard for mainstream news reporting. Most mainstream media outlets will not publish a story with a 20 percent margin for error. Furthermore, they claim that anyone with a penchant for gossip, a computer, and a Web site can post such "news" on the Internet. The Internet, with the potential to reach billions of subscribers worldwide in an instant, is a relatively unsupervised medium. Anyone can create a Web site and post news without peer review or supervision. Proponents of online news outlets claim that mainstream media outlets are too conservative, sit on stories too long, and protect political and other figures.

In the Clinton–Lewinsky case, Drudge's claim that the media was sitting on the story (he found out about the affair through unnamed reports of supposed tapes Linda Tripp had made of telephone conversations with Monica Lewinsky) proved true. It was only after the public furor created by Drudge's report that the mainstream news media released the story. Drudge's popularity worldwide soared following the release of the story. Subscriptions to his newsletter soared, and his newfound notoriety included his reporting being picked by Agence France Presse (the world's oldest news wire service) as one of the century's top 10 media events.

Emotional Wellness

Not only is sexual information available in unprecedented amounts, but sexual counseling, therapy, and self-help also are within the average person's reach. As sex comes into the open, so does sexual healing. Online chat rooms, self-help groups, and other computerized services offer increasing opportunities for dealing with sexual concerns and problems.

Web sites are available catering to all people and interests. Gay people who need help to come out of the closet can find help and link up with others around the country or around the corner. Transgendered people no longer have to feel alone. They have their own Web sites and referral networks a mere mouse-click away. Although electronic resources will never take the place of a live helping relationship, the technological innovations and resources available to average individuals can greatly improve their emotional wellness by providing easy access to information and services that were not available a decade ago.

Subscriber Internet Services

One of the most fascinating outgrowths of the new technologies regarding sexuality is the burgeoning development of subscriber Internet services. Subscriber Internet services are similar to cable television premium channels and pay-per-view services. With cable television, subscribers can pay for a menu of related channels (a group of movie channels, for instance) or an individual channel (Home Box Office [HBO] is a good example). In addition, subscribers can pay for a single event (pay-per-view) available to all subscribers to the service or just to subscribers of a specific channel (who can buy a boxing match, auto race, specific movie, and so forth).

Adult-oriented Internet sites are following the same model. Most of these sites allow "visitors" to enter their sites and sample their wares. In most cases, the sites provide enough tantalizing X-rated samples of pages included in the overall site to give the visitor a sense of what lies within the entire site. If the person likes the site, he or she can "subscribe" for a monthly fee. Fees range from a few dollars a month to over $50 for some of the more exotic sites.

For the price of a subscription, most sites provide members with the following features: X-rated still photos, short video clips, full-length video films, chat rooms (to chat with the site sponsor and/or other members), dating services, merchandise (sex aids, books, magazines, videos, and more), and links, to name the most common. In most cases, the site sponsor usually is featured in the photos, videos, and chat. Sites are sponsored by porn stars, swinging couples, exotic dancers and strippers, and a host of "amateurs" (self-proclaimed "boy and girl next door" types). All sites are blocked to nonmembers and those under the age of consent (varies from 18 to 21 years old).

Membership sales to subscriber adult Internet sites have become the next frontier in sex for sale in the United States and the world. Danni Ashe, a former stripper and a pioneer in this medium, hosts one of the most widely subscribed sites on the Web. Ashe started Danni's Hard Drive in 1995 from her bedroom as a hobby. It has grown into a medium-sized corporation with 42 employees, a 15,000-square-foot office/studio, and over 4.5 million users per month. In 2001, Danni's Hard Drive was expected to make between $7 and $8 million in profit (Lewis, 2001).

Danni's Hard Drive is by no means a fluke. Rather, it is a harbinger for how sex will be sold in the future. Subscriber Internet sex sites are among the most profitable forms of business being conducted either on or off the Web. What makes them unique is that they do not rely on advertising. Instead of being driven by selling advertisements and the needs and wants of advertisers, subscriber sites turn enough profits to be self-sustaining. Indeed, most premier subscriber sex sites have profit margins of more than 20 percent (which is unheard of in most sales-related businesses). Start-up costs are generally low, and most subscriber sex sites turn profitable after just 6 months. In comparison, Amazon.com, probably the most well-known retail site on the Web, was still nowhere near profitable 4 *years* after it started (Lewis, 2001).

More than 200,000 sexually explicit Internet sites were available in 2001, and experts estimated that 40 percent of adult Internet users spent at least 90 minutes online viewing porn per week. According to Greg Clayman, the president of Video-secrets.com, a company that provides streaming video to Danni's Hard Drive and other large-scale Internet subscriber sites, it seems that people use the Internet to do three primary things: check e-mail, check investments, and check pornography (Lewis, 2001). Of the $2 billion paid for online content in the United States last year, $1.4 billion was for pornography.

Internet subscriber sex sites have survived the crash of the dot.com economy, a severely depressed stock market, a weak economy, and war in the Middle East to thrive when other e-businesses are shutting down. Many business analysts find such success a mystery, but when you view it as part of the evolving sex-for-sale phenomenon that has been with us since the dawn of recorded history, it makes perfect sense. Consumers of these products can shop at home. They can preview what they might be interested in buying and purchase it online, without leaving their house. They can view, interact with, and download sexually explicit material in the privacy of their own homes where the average buyer feels most comfortable.

Although both Internet subscriber sex sites and *The Drudge Report* illustrate the most recent evolution of sex for sale adapting to technological innovation, we fully expect that by the time we go to press, yet another technological breakthrough will have emerged, with those who sell sex following closely on its heels.

Social Wellness

Many argue that the current sexual climate in the United States impacts negatively on our social wellness as individuals and as a culture. Everything from child rearing to productivity in the workplace, they say, becomes harder as parents, employers, and government have to compete against the lure and distraction of sexual availability. It is more difficult, they argue, to uphold standards of decency and social relationships in the face of a no-holds-barred societal attitude toward sex.

Others disagree. They argue that greater sexual freedom and availability of sexual information and services empowers people and fosters understanding of their sexuality. Social wellness, they say, is thereby enhanced because sexuality, a natural part of life, is allowed its full expression. This allows people to understand their sexuality better and develop higher levels of social wellness.

Pornography, Erotica, and Obscenity

One of the major concerns about the increasing availability of sexual information and images in the media and over the Internet is the easy access to pornography, erotica, and obscene materials. In past decades, restricting access to this material was much easier. Keeping it away from minors, as well as adults who did not desire that type of exposure, was simple. Today it is much more difficult. The debate concerning what is pornographic, erotic, or obscene has reopened and intensified. Although *pornography, erotica,* and *obscenity* have been used interchangeably, these terms mean entirely different things.

Pornography

Derived from the Latin roots *porne* (prostitute) and *graphos* (depicting), **pornography** literally means a depiction, in writing or pictures, of prostitutes or prostitution. It refers more commonly to any depiction of lewd material or erotic behavior designed to cause sexual arousal. In U.S. culture, the connotation of pornography and pornographic materials is usually negative, even though most people admit they get sexually excited while viewing it.

Pornography A depiction of lewd material or erotic behavior designed to cause sexual arousal

Erotica

Derived from the Greek word *erotikos* (love poem), **erotic** means devoted to or tending to arouse sexual love or desire. Erotic materials depict beauty, love, sensuousness, voluptuousness, and the like. In U.S. culture (and most others around the world), the depiction of erotica and erotic materials tends to be positive. This judgment is subjective, however. Some people do not distinguish pornography from erotica and lump them together.

Erotic Devoted to arousing sexual love or desire

In real life, separating some pornographic materials from erotica is difficult. Often, the context of the material helps to define it. For instance, one could view two films, an X-rated porn film and a sex ed video. Each film portrays a heterosexual couple having sex. Both films have graphic displays of nudity, masturbation, oral sex, and intercourse in various positions. What is the difference? Are the films pornographic or erotic?

The porno film makes little mention of love or expressions of caring. The relationship between the partners may be unknown or casual. The sexual acts may be forced or seemingly initiated by one partner for his or her own gratification. The genitalia are overemphasized, with close-ups of the coupled genitalia. Most porn films end with a mandatory, degrading ejaculation in the face of the female.

The sex ed video emphasizes communication. The couple talks to each other. They ask what each desires, whether something feels good, and the like. They take their time. Their intent is mutual pleasuring. They equally participate and initiate. The narration describes what is happening. The partners proceed through the various acts and show their appreciation, caring, and kindness. These videos do not include genital close-ups and orgasm. They do not show "in-your-face" ejaculation.

One could almost use a continuum to evaluate sexually explicit materials. Pornographic materials would represent one extreme, and instructional sex ed materials would be at the other end, with erotica in the middle. To complicate matters, one must also consider whether the material is obscene.

Obscenity

Obscenity Material that is abhorrent to moral virtue and accepted norms of social behavior

Obscenity is derived from the Latin word *obscenus*, which means dirty, filthy, and disgusting. Obscene materials repel the senses and are abhorrent to morality, virtue, and accepted norms of societal behavior. In 1966, the U.S. Supreme Court defined obscene materials as meeting three criteria:

- The dominant theme had to appeal to a purely erotic interest in sex.
- The material had to be offensive to contemporary community standards.
- The material had to be without serious literary, artistic, political, or scientific value.

This definition posed serious difficulties in interpretation, and numerous challenges have been brought to bear. In 1973, the Supreme Court reversed its ruling using the three original criteria. In *Miller v. California*, the Court decided that only one criterion was necessary to define obscenity: local community standards. Each community had to decide for itself whether specific materials were offensive by its standards. The producers, actors, distributors, and sellers of materials that a community defines as obscene are all subject to prosecution even if the materials were produced in another community. This criterion is still in effect today. It is troubling because it gives a vocal minority in a community the ability to declare anything from skimpy bathing suits to Michelangelo's *Venus de Milo* obscene.

In general, materials described as erotic are not perceived as obscene and usually are not the target of prosecution. Obscene materials, in contrast, are considered to be subcategories of pornography. The overwhelming majority of Americans believe that adults should have access to sexually explicit material, both erotic and pornographic, depicting sexual activity between consenting adults (Diamond & Dannemiller, 1989).

Support for obscene materials is much less. These materials usually depict themes other than sexual activity between consenting adults. Materials that involve children, rape, sadomasochism, and similar themes are more often those that fail to meet community standards.

Ain't Nobody's Business If We Do

Peter McWilliams's book *Ain't Nobody's Business If We Do* is based on a single idea: You should be allowed to do whatever you want with your own person and property, as long as you don't physically harm the person or property of a nonconsenting other.

Simple. Seemingly guaranteed to us by that remarkable document known as the United States Constitution and its even more remarkable Bill of Rights. And yet, it's not the way things are.

Roughly half of the arrests and court cases in the United States each year involve consensual crimes—actions that are against the law but directly harm no one's person or property except, possibly, the "criminal's."

More than 750,000 people are in jail right now because of something they did, something that did not physically harm the person or property of another. In addition, more than 3 million people are on parole or probation for consensual crimes. Furthermore, more than 4 million people are arrested each year for doing something that hurts no one but, potentially, themselves.

The injustice doesn't end there, of course. Throwing people in jail is the extreme. If you can throw people in jail for something, you can fire them for the same reason. You can evict them from their apartments. You can deny them credit. You can expel them from schools. You can strip away their civil rights, confiscate their property, and destroy their lives—just because they're different.

At what point does behavior become so unacceptable that we should tell our government to lock people up? The answer, as explored in this book: We lock people up only when they physically harm the person or property of a nonconsenting other.

Go to McWilliams's Web site for the book: http://crime.about.com/gi/dynamic/offsite.htm?site=http%3A%2F%2Fwww.mcwilliams.com%2Fbooks%2Faint%2F101.htm. Or visit his home page, www.mcwilliams.com, to read more about his ideas regarding our sexual (and other) personal freedoms and how they are threatened.

How do you feel about laws that target consensual behavior that harms no one? What are you willing to do to protect these freedoms?

Prostitution

Prostitution has been around since the dawn of civilization. The earliest written accounts are in the Bible. Jesus himself took time to protect a prostitute from a stone-throwing crowd who would persecute her. Prostitution is illegal in the United States except in Nevada, where it is regulated and limited to certain counties. In Nevada and other places where prostitution is legal, prostitutes are called *sex workers,* and they are employed in the sex worker industry. Prostitution is legal in many European, Asian, African, and South American countries, where it is considered a victimless crime.

Small numbers of prostitutes in the United States have organized in an attempt to try to legalize it in all 50 states. Legalization, they believe, will help protect prostitutes, ensure better working conditions, extend benefits such as disability and Social Security, and help them reduce their risk for contracting a variety of sexually transmitted diseases, including HIV (Shrage, 1996; Prostitutes' Education Network, 2003). It also will free police to spend more time on other forms of crime, relieve the courts of a tremendous burden, and allow women to use their bodies the way they want to.

Although people tend to assume that all prostitutes are women, men and women alike engage in exchanging sex for money, food, shelter, drugs, or other resources. They can be subcategorized. Prostitutes who literally solicit clients off the streets are called *hookers* (females) and *hustlers* (males), although the labels

Prostitution The exchange of sexual services for money

case study 17.2

Edgar: Paying for Sex

Edgar, 43, married, identifies as Hispanic.

Married for 20 years, Edgar has two children, ages 13 and 16. He is a middle manager in an insurance company. He describes his relationship with his wife as intimate and committed but feels the passion in their relationship died several years ago. Although they have sex about once a week or every other week, it isn't very exciting and he wants more. He frequents massage parlors about twice a month, paying for a massage that includes masturbation and usually fellatio.

I guess you could say that sex for me has never been all that exciting. Except for the prostitutes I used to pay for when I was in Vietnam, I was sexually inexperienced. I didn't have sex until I enlisted in the army at 18 and went to Vietnam. When I returned, I got a job in an insurance company and went to college at night.

I met my wife at the insurance company during the first month I worked there, and we got married about a year after that. The first year or so, things were OK. My wife wasn't very interested in sex, and we probably had intercourse about once a week that first year. She's pretty conservative and isn't into oral sex or anything kinky. I really didn't know what to expect of married life. My dad never really talked about sex with me, and I was too embarrassed to talk to my friends about it in much detail. My first son was born after a year, and things slowed down a little more with my wife.

I was in New York for a training program for my current job. I guess it was about 10 years ago. I remember walking around Times Square and going into the bookstores and bars. I passed a massage parlor, and the guy out front was passing out coupons for a special deal. I said, "What the heck," and went in. I had been curious about these massage parlors and was feeling horny. No one there knew me, so I took a chance. I picked out my masseuse and went into our little room.

After undressing, she started to rub my back, and before long her touches became a lot more intimate. She asked if I wanted her to jerk me off, and I said yes. I had to pay her a little more but it was worth it. The next night I went into a different place and found out I could get a blow job for about $20. The masseuse there was unattractive, but, boy, could she give head. It reminded me of my experiences in Vietnam.

When I returned home to Virginia from my training program, I began to seek out massage parlors in Richmond and other places within a reasonable drive from my home. I've been doing this at least once a month more than 10 years. My wife doesn't know, and the cost isn't too much. I'm basically happily married and love my kids. I wish I had more sex with my wife and she was into oral sex, but I don't think she'll change. She won't even talk about seeing a sex therapist, so I keep doing what I'm doing. I don't have a problem with it, and it probably keeps my marriage going.

could apply to either gender. These prostitutes also are known as *streetwalkers.* They generally are at the lower end of the social order of prostitutes. Street hustlers and hookers are frequently addicted to drugs, are runaways, or have other economic or personal problems that force them into the often violent world of streetwalking.

Street prostitutes solicit customers who walk or drive by them. Streetwalkers usually negotiate with their clients and then have sex with them either in their car or at a local hotel or motel where short-stay rooms are available at reasonable rates. Some hustlers and hookers solicit clients in truck stop parking areas and have sex with their clients in their rigs.

In urban areas, many street hookers and hustlers are runaways—adolescents who have run away from home or have been forced out by their parents or caregivers. Many have run away from abusive home environments and are willing to

sex in society 17.3

The HIV Highway

They call it the HIV highway. In reality, it is a transcontinental highway linking the several sub-Saharan African countries. It is more like a dirt road than a highway. It is a symbol of the old Africa, where time has stood still and traditions live on. The HIV highway got its name because of health officials' belief that it has been a main conduit of infection with the deadly virus. The highway has countless roadside stops where prostitutes ply their trade.

This is the same trade they have pursued throughout the history of the road. The main difference is that now most of them are infected with HIV. These factors make sex along the trans-Africa highway a deadly behavior:

- Condom use by the truck drivers and the prostitutes is practically nonexistent.
- Anal intercourse is common.

- The coexistence of genital ulcer disease (STDs that cause genital ulcers such as chancroid and syphilis) is common in the women and their customers.
- A final tragic note is the reluctance of these men to use condoms with their wives once they have been notified of their HIV seropositivity. Many of them perceive condom use as both unmanly and a sure sign of promiscuity.

The governments of sub-Saharan nations have instituted a massive STD/HIV prevention program to try to combat the problem. They have literally set up prevention service on the road. They have worked with the prostitutes to try to have them organize and institute greater compliance with use of condoms. They have used educational strategies ranging from one-to-one counseling to massive governmental media campaigns.

---

risk the dangers of the streets over the sure harm of the environments from which they escaped. Many of the gay youth hooking and hustling on the streets ran away from persecution for their sexual orientation.

Streetwalking has many unwritten rules, which concern respecting other prostitutes' work areas (also known as "turf"), outwitting undercover police officers, avoiding sadists and murderers, and trying to avoid STDs/HIV. Because of these "rules," streetwalkers often work for pimps (a type of business agent) who help control some of these problems in exchange for a share of the profits.

Street pimps vary in their approach to working with hookers and hustlers. Some provide valuable protection and care for their workers to some extent. Others are thinly disguised sadists and criminals who dominate their hookers and hustlers through drugs, violence, and fear. In the netherworld of streetwalking, violence and death are never far away.

Brothel A house of prostitution

Brothels

Prior to 1920, large **brothels** could be found in every major American city. Many were elegant facilities where customers (overwhelmingly male) could have a drink, eat dinner, play cards, socialize with peers and the prostitutes, and have sex. Typically, brothels were set up like hotels, with socializing downstairs and sex negotiated in upstairs rooms. Repeat business was the norm, and clients were generally recruited by word of mouth (Petersen, 1999). As a result of legislation and the sweeping moral reform of the early 1920s, most brothels were closed, driving prostitution into the streets or the massage parlors. Brothels still exist in Nevada and, on a much smaller scale, most major metropolitan areas.

Ben Edwards/GettyImages

Prostitution is one of the world's oldest professions.

Massage Parlors

Prostitutes who work in massage parlors are referred to as *hookers* and *hustlers* but also may be known as *masseuses*. Most massage parlors are fronts for houses of prostitution, where, in addition to a massage, clients are able to receive masturbation, oral sex, and sometimes sexual intercourse.

Most clients of massage parlors walk in off the street and pay cash for a massage and either masturbation or oral sex. Their visit usually lasts 30 minutes and costs anywhere from $20 to $50. Massage parlors usually have procedures that help screen for potential undercover police activities. For example, they require that customers sign a form indicating that they are not police officers. Clients pay for the massage in advance, with no mention of sexual "extras" until the later stages of the massage. The overwhelming majority of prostitutes working in massage parlors is female.

Escort Services

In theory, escort services involve the legal practice of "escorting" a client to dinner, a show, a political affair, and the like, for a fee. In reality, most escort services derive their primary business through "out-call" male and female prostitution. Escort services advertise in telephone books, newspapers, and magazines. Many clients are referred by other satisfied customers. Customers call and are matched with the type of "escort" they desire. Escorts come to the client's residence or hotel and negotiate sexual activity (O'Kane, 1994).

Prostitutes who work for escort services are referred to as *call girls* or *call boys*, as well as escorts. Escort services may be run by a pimp or madam who works the phones and arranges the meetings. Some escort services are run by groups of prostitutes who schedule appointments based on availability and referral. Many call girls and call boys work independently after they establish their own client base.

In general, call girls and call boys are at the top of the status hierarchy of prostitutes. They typically charge from $50 to $200 an hour or between $500 and $1,000 a night. Call girls and call boys work through telephone calls, personal meetings, and referrals. Because they are not on the street, they are not subject to the control and fees associated with pimps. If call persons are not in business for themselves, they have a madam or pimp scheduling for them.

Periodically, high-priced call girls are arrested, and their high-profile clients make the headlines. Sydney Biddle-Barrows, the "Mayflower Madam," and Heidi Fleiss are two examples. In each case, the "madam" was a well-educated, respectable woman of noble upbringing (well-heeled families from New York and Los Angeles, respectively). Both told of enterprising entrepreneurs who earned a living catering to the sexual needs of the rich and famous. The clientele included famous actors (and actresses), politicians, judges, businesspersons, and assorted celebrities.

Exotic Dancers, Strippers, and Live Sex Performers

Bars and clubs dedicated to providing adult entertainment from dancers have proliferated in the 1990s. These may be bars (which have licenses to sell and offer alcoholic beverages and are open to the general public) or "gentlemen's clubs" (which do not have licenses to sell liquor and are open to members only). The activities of establishments licensed to sell liquor are regulated by agencies such as the Bureau of Alcohol, Tobacco and Firearms (AFT). These establishments usually

case study 17.3

Kim: Working Her Way Through College as an Exotic Dancer

Kim, 23, single, lesbian, identifies as Korean American.

Last year my lover Danielle convinced me to apply for a job as an exotic dancer at a local men's club. She had been doing it for a few months, and the money was great. She said that with my exotic Asian looks I'd make a fortune in tips if I was willing to act a little. I didn't want to do it, but Danielle said she'd be there a lot to make sure nobody hassled me when I danced. Besides, she said, if I got the job, they occasionally had two girls dance at the same time, and we could try this if I wanted to.

I got the job, and the money really was good, and the bouncers kind of adopted me because they knew I was Danielle's lover.

I was a nervous wreck the first night I had to dance. The first set was a near-disaster. I didn't want to make eye contact with the customers because I thought they'd know I wasn't straight, and I was worried that they'd really be obnoxious. I didn't dance too well, either. I think I earned about $7 in tips, mostly out of sympathy.

The next night was better. I had a couple of drinks before going on, and Danielle was there, so I danced for her. She told me to relax and fantasize that she was the only person in the bar. It started to be a real a turn-on, and I relaxed and really got into the music. The guys in the bar went crazy and were all holding dollar bills to stick into my G-string. That was a real turn-off, but the manager and the bouncers made sure that things didn't get out of hand. They told me to smile, and if I let the guys touch my breasts and butt, I'd get more tips. I took their advice and brought home close to $300 that first night. I average about $150 in tips on a typical night.

I don't really like it when the customers proposition me, but it comes with the territory. I'd say about 30 percent of the guys hit on me, but I've learned how to cope with it by smiling, telling them I like guys but love women, and move on. Most of them can deal with that, and it probably feeds their fantasies when they go home and jerk off or have sex with their wives.

Danielle and I have talked about opening a bar of our own when we graduate this year. We want to do something upscale that caters to women's fantasies and dance in the club together as well as manage the place. There is a ton of money to be made in this line of work.

Critical Thinking

Dancers and club operators would describe what they do as providing erotic entertainment and not engaging in sexual activities with customers. How would you characterize Kim's behavior at work?

Use your Virtual Workbook to explore your answer to this question at **http://health.wadsworth.com/blonna1.**

---

are under a stricter code than clubs, which usually are regulated by local ordinances. Because of this, clubs usually tend to offer more risqué forms of entertainment ranging from totally nude dancing to lap and couch dancing.

About 2,500 gentlemen's clubs have been established around the United States. The industry has gotten so large that it has its own trade publication, *Stripper* magazine. The revenues generated from these clubs are staggering: from $500,000 a year for the average club to more than $5 million for a well-run club.

Once called *go-go dancers,* the entertainment provided by strippers and exotic dancers has changed in the 1990s. Go-go dancers and strippers of the past usually performed on a stage, or literally in a cage, separated from their customers. Appreciative customers sometimes threw money onto the stage or offered to buy the dancer a drink and offer a tip.

In the 1990s, dancers have come off the stage and cages and onto the bars, tabletops, couches, and laps of customers in these clubs. Nowadays exotic dancers typically dance along the bar, discarding items of clothing as they stop to tease customers, who are allowed to slip their tips (usually folded dollar bills) into the dancer's top or G-string (a skimpy thong covering her pubic area). Dancers (at least those desiring larger tips) usually allow customers to feel their breasts, buttocks, and vulva fleetingly while passing along their tips.

Most dancers earn between $10 and $20 an hour and rely heavily on tips to make up the bulk of their earnings. Many of the larger gentlemen's clubs employ big-name, hard-core film actresses as feature performers. The nation's top five or six porn actresses can earn $15,000 to $20,000 per week (four shows a night) to dance at the larger clubs. The next half-dozen famous actresses earn about $8,000 to $15,000 to dance in these clubs. Club owners use film credits and magazine spreads to market their performers (Schlosser, 1997).

Many states have laws regulating a dancer's attire and may require her to wear pantyhose and keep her top on or at least hold it up against her breasts. Customers are not allowed to fondle the dancers, with the exception of inserting dollar bills into their G-strings or tops. Any sexual exchange between dancer and customer is not allowed, as this behavior constitutes prostitution, and bars usually hire bouncers to ensure that neither customers nor dancers violate this rule.

Exotic dancers in clubs often leave the bar to dance one-on-one with customers. Lap dancers usually straddle a customer and dance suggestively against his crotch. Couch dancers usually take a customer to a private couch, where they kneel on top of him or over him and dance suggestively in a more private ambiance. The objective of lap dancing and couch dancing in many instances is to offer the customer the opportunity literally to be masturbated to the point of orgasm by the dancer's motions without her ever using her hand. Such dancing usually requires an extra fee ($20 and up) and is timed (if the customer hasn't "come" or wants more stimulation, he has to buy more time).

Live sex shows usually take place in a theater environment but often occur in a bar or club. One or more couples literally have sex on stage, on the floor, or on the bar while the customers watch, often masturbating as they become aroused.

Although dancing and live sex shows are not the same as prostitution, the performers often are prostitutes and are willing to arrange sex for pay sessions with customers at a later time. Live sex shows now are available on the Internet. A customer can sign on in Iowa and be a member of the audience in a live sex show in Amsterdam.

Environmental/Occupational Wellness

Some communities have organized to restrict sex industry outlets to nonresidential sectors rather than eliminate X-rated bookstores, bars, and other establishments. Other communities have banned them outright. The issue of community boundaries regarding the sex industry directly affects sex workers themselves. Sex workers are employed in a variety of work sites. Some, such as X-rated movie houses, bookstores, massage parlors, and escort services, are legal and protected under law. Others, such as prostitution and nude dancing, are illegal in most states. Sex workers, particularly those working illegally, are at increased risk for a variety of problems ranging from disease to unfair labor practices. Many sex workers are calling for unionization as a way to increase work-site-based protections. In the majority of non-sex-based business, participating in sexually oriented activities (Internet use, telephone sex, and the like), even on lunch or break time, is grounds for dismissal. Many corporations and other workplaces routinely screen workers' computer and telephone records to monitor such activities.

Tech Sex

Whereas prostitution entails sexual contact with a live person, tech sex—sexual activity that connects with some form of technology—is masturbatory sex. It is designed to excite and arouse, leading to release of tension through masturbation. The same technological innovations that make sexual information available have opened new outlets for purveyors of impersonal sex for sale. These include sex talk lines, interactive cable TV sex, interactive computer sex, and computer sex chat rooms. These differ from ordinary pornography and erotica because the customer connects to a live human being via the phone, television, or computer. It is the ultimate sex of the 1990s–2000s technological revolution.

Telephone Sex

Every night, between the hours of 9:00 P.M. and 1:00 A.M., approximately 250,000 people in the United States dial a commercial phone sex number. The average call lasts 6 to 8 minutes and costs anywhere from $0.89 to $4 a minute. In 1996, Americans spent between $750 million and $1 billion on telephone sex (Schlosser, 1997).

A customer buys telephone sex by dialing a 900 number. A new scam uses a free 800 number to mask a 900 pay-per-call service. When the 800 number is called, the caller is identified through caller ID, and the 900 pay-per-call provider bills the incoming number for the call ("Call for a Crackdown," 1994).

In 1991, the Federal Communications Commission (FCC) restricted the type of calls that could be made using 900 numbers. It banned all domestic calls it considered "obscene communications for commercial purposes." Because the ban does not extend to overseas calls, however, this loophole has created a burgeoning foreign market for telephone sex. Phone sex calls are routed to out-of-the-way places such as Aruba, the Mariana Islands, Guyana, and the Dominican Republic, where operators are standing by to take your call and cater to your every whim (Schlosser, 1997).

In 1993, telephone companies earned nearly $900 million from international services. An estimated 90 percent of those revenues came from phone-sex lines. These foreign revenues are shared among the domestic American company, its foreign phone company, and telephone sex providers. Some small countries have started their own telephone companies to get a bigger chunk of the market (*Economist*, 1994; "Adult Video," 1995).

Once customers' connections are established, they are billed per minute to their telephone bill. A person can engage in heterosexual talk, homosexual talk, bisexual talk, or group talk. It is anonymous, graphic, expensive—and an illusion. Phone sex practitioners are trained to keep customers talking, to cater to their every fantasy. Because it is impersonal and anonymous, they are tempted to say things that normally are taboo.

The typical telephone sex customer is a "lonely heart" seeking conversation. Often, the sexual content of the call is of secondary importance. Anyone, however, is capable of becoming hooked on phone sex. Most telephone "actresses"—as they are referred to—are housewives, accountants, secretaries, bank tellers, senior citizens, and various other women seeking to earn a little extra income (Schlosser, 1997).

Although it is a seemingly innocent form of sexual contact, telephone sex has become a major problem. It is a difficult form of sexual exchange to control. Minors have easy access to these services, and the costs can add up. The media are full of stories of parents opening up their phone bills and being surprised by Junior's 900-number bill for hundreds of dollars.

Also, pedophiles and other sex offenders often use Internet access to identify and lure their victims. They can gain access to potential victims by establishing relationships with phone sex providers to illegally trace their victim's telephone numbers through caller ID.

Is Sex Selling to You?

Most states have laws that forbid selling sex. But there are definitely no laws forbidding using sex to sell. You are constantly bombarded by ads using sex to grab your attention. This activity will help you increase your awareness of just how often sex is used to sell a product to you and help you decide whether you want to support the products using this tactic.

For the next month, every time you thumb through a magazine, look at the newspaper, or view any other print material that has advertisements, look for the ads that use sex to sell. The sex part may be in the form of a couple embracing, a sexy guy wearing no shirt, and so forth. Evaluate what they are trying to sell and whether the product is really related to the picture. Put a Post-it or some type of marker on the page with your evaluation and stack all evaluated material in one place. At the end of the month, look at all of the pages you have marked. Were the majority of ads just using sex to sell the product? Do you agree with this technique? If not, are these products you will avoid buying because of their blatant use of sex in a commercial way? Are these ads influencing the way you view sexuality?

Commercial Television

Two trends within commercial television programming are of note concerning the dissemination of sexually explicit material and messages: the relaxation of restrictions on presenting sexual themes (particularly regarding the spoken word) and the creation of music video.

Commercial television closely regulates overt visual sexual programming. Total frontal nudity and sexual behavior without clothes are prohibited. Partial nudity is regulated but has a much wider berth than it did 20 years ago. Shows such as *Baywatch* and the morning workout shows feature scantily clad lifeguards and athletes with bulging swimsuits and plunging tank tops. In soap operas, lovemaking is depicted but involves the participants in bed under the covers, or

healthy sex hints 17.1

Television Rating Guide

In response to the 1996 Telecommunications Law, a voluntary committee made up of executives from the television and movie industries was established. In December 1997, the task force, led by Jack Valenti, the chief of the Motion Picture Association of America (MPAA), presented a set of guidelines to rate television programs.

Valenti's group presented ratings that are remarkably similar to those used in evaluating motion pictures. These, and the proposed TV ratings, evaluate programming by age-appropriateness. Those contesting such a rating system prefer a more content-based rating system similar to that used in Canada. The Canadian system evaluates programming based on the strength of content using a 1 to 3 scale on V (violent content), S (sexual content and nudity), and L (adult language). A program could get mixed ratings—L-1, V-3, or S-1—for instance.

These guidelines have sparked controversy among children's and parents' rights groups. The groups' major complaint centers on the ambiguity of the ratings, which are age, not content, based.

Sources: Bash (1997); Kent (1997); "U.S. TV Ratings System" (1996).

the camera cuts away as clothes begin to be shed. Although partial nudity is common, it is restricted to nongenital displays. In 1997, under pressure from the federal government, the entertainment industry proposed a set of voluntary standards to rate television programming.

The spoken word and sexual posturing while clothed are subject to much less regulation. Talk shows and soap operas are permitted to use all but the most graphic language (*fuck* is still banned, but *balls* and *screw,* among others, are permissible). Participants on panel talk shows and audience participation programs bare their soul while discussing everything from adultery to zoophilia.

The most unique addition to prime-time commercial television sex is the music video. This medium combines the power of music with implied and overt sexual themes. Undulating bodies (many partially clad) combine with seductive melodies and lyrics to offer a powerfully erotic presentation. In other cases, music combines with a kaleidoscope of disjointed violent images ranging from smashing guitars to drive-by shootings. Illicit drug use is often thrown into the mix, creating a unique mélange of sex, drugs, and music.

Cable Television and Videocassettes

A leading product that cable television subscribers request is pay-per-view and subscription sex services. The adult video market, personified by sex-on-cable providers such as Playboy, Spice, and the Adam and Eve Channel, grew from $521 million in 1994 to $664 million in 1995, with projections for continued growth ("Adult Video," 1995). In 2002, revenues from the Playboy Channel (the pay-TV Playboy service) surged by 30 percent, with sales exceeding $23 million. This surge in pay-TV services offset losses from Playboy's print and other operations (Devaney, 2002).

Recognizing the fortunes to be made in adult entertainment online, major corporations are going after these markets. For instance, General Motors earns over $150 million in revenue from adult channels on its Direct TV cable television venue. AT&T, which has withdrawn from the scandalous 900 pay telephone sex lines, is heavily invested in cable television. It handles several pay-per-view adult television channels, including the very profitable Playboy's Hot Network (Devaney, 2002).

The advent of cable television and home VCRs has almost single-handedly caused the near-extinction of the "porno movie theater." Cable television has literally brought the world of soft-core and hard-core pornography into middle America's living room. Twenty years ago, viewing pornography entailed either a trip to the local X-rated movie house or threading a super-8 film into the old family projector, setting up the screen, and hoping kids (or parents) wouldn't discover you watching the movie.

Today, virtually every cable television service provider has at least one soft-core channel that serves up late-evening viewing of "nonpenetrative" (penetration and ejaculation scenes have been edited out) versions of X-rated films. Many of the larger metropolitan-area cable television companies also offer X-rated (penetration and ejaculation are shown) channels for home viewing. These channels typically are offered for an extra charge (premium) that rarely exceeds $15 per month, thereby ensuring access to nearly all markets.

In 1996, the Federal Telecommunications Law was passed, limiting the hours for airing these channels to between 10 P.M. and 6 A.M.. All companies also are required to provide devices that deny transmission without a code that can be entered to activate the service.

The cost of the average VCR has dropped to well below $200, putting it in the range of affordability for most households. The boom in VCR sales of the 1980s and 1990s created a massive audience for marketing home movies. The fastest-

case study 17.4

Jon: Watching X-rated Videos

Jon, 18, single, gay, is white.

Jon is a college freshman in one of the author's online human sexuality classes. His written comments were composed in response to the author's queries concerning Jon's exposure to X-rated videos as an adolescent.

The first time I ever saw an X-rated video was over at my friend Tom's house. Tom had a collection of straight and gay porno and kept them hidden in the back of his closet.

Tom invited me and a couple of other friends over one night and when his parents were out, we watched one. We watched a few videos on everything including fucking, oral, anal, group, straight, gay, and interracial sex.

It was kind of weird watching it with these guys. Nobody knew I was gay, and I got real turned on by the gay scenes but was able to disguise it because of all the other stuff on the tape. I made a copy of the tape and watched it until I wore it out. I must have jerked off a couple of hundred times to that tape.

Since then I have found an X-rated video store that has gay tapes and DVDs that I rent every once in a while. I have to be very careful because nobody knows I'm gay, and I've got to hide the stuff from my roommate. I like to watch the tapes and masturbate. I don't think there is anything wrong with this. The only thing I worry about is getting caught by my roommates who are straight.

growing segment of the home videocassette market is the adult video consumer. The number of hard-core sex video rentals in the United States rose from 75 million in 1985 to 490 million in 1992. It reached an all-time high in 1996, with rentals of more than 665 million X-rated sex videos (Schlosser, 1997).

Purchases of adult videos in the United States approached that of rentals over the past decade. The X-rated video segment of the film industry is one of the most profitable and reliable forms of film production. In California alone, more than 8,000 new hard-core video titles are produced annually (Gardetta, 1988).

"Adult entertainment" has grown into a multibillion-dollar a year industry. In 2001, Americans rented more than 750 *million* adult films on video or DVD and watched millions more on cable and satellite TV and in hotel rooms (Devaney, 2002). The industry has prospered during the past 5 years, despite recessions, terrorism, and economic uncertainty. In the past few years, dozens of new studios have been popping up throughout California's San Fernando Valley, the seat of the adult film industry in the United States (Gardetta, 1998).

This dramatic rise in home video rentals and purchases has shifted the focus of consumption of these products from the seedy adult movie houses of 20 years ago to the home. It also has provided easier access for adolescent viewers.

Computer Sex

As we mentioned, more than half of U.S. households own at least one personal computer, and over 56 percent (over 30 million users) of Americans are Internet users. Most of these users are experienced PC owners who access the Internet with their home computers (Richards, 1997). Web TV (a type of Internet TV) and other non-PC Internet access devices introduced in the U.S. marketplace in 1998 are expected to add an additional 250,000 to 300,000 users. If this technology catches on, the average non-computer-literate person will have access to the World Wide Web and Internet (Richards, 1997).

case study 17.5

Ed

Ed, 41, married, is white.

Ed, a continuing education student, recalls his response to finding an X-rated video in the VCR in the family room after a sleepover his 14-year-old son had the night before.

I was cleaning the basement family room. The VCR light was on, so I ejected the film and, much to my surprise, found an X-rated video in it. I figured my son and his friends had watched it the night before, so I talked with him about it when he came home from school. I asked him if it was his, and he said it was one of his friend's father's tapes. His buddy had brought it over for the guys to watch. I told him that I was more upset over him leaving it in the basement where his 10-year-old brother could have viewed it than the fact that he had seen it. I asked him what he thought of the movie, and he told me that it was a real turn-on.

I reemphasized to him that his mother and I still didn't want him to begin having intercourse until he was older and found a girlfriend he cared about and it would be exclusive. I also reassured him that I understood his natural curiosity about sex and sexual behavior and that masturbation was an acceptable outlet. I also wanted to be sure that he understood that X-rated films are fantasy sex and that he shouldn't confuse what he saw on some of these tapes with reality. I explained that these tapes are designed to cater to our fantasies but that real sex between two people involves talking, negotiating, and caring.

He said he understood and didn't really expect that sex would be like the film. He said that some of the stuff on the film was too kinky for him anyway. I sometimes worry that my approach is too casual, but Ed is a very responsible boy and seems to treat girls with respect. I feel that if I make too big a deal out of this, it will become a forbidden-fruit deal and he'll want to watch them even more.

Critical Thinking

Is Ed helping or hurting his son's healthy sexual development in his approach to viewing X-rated materials?

Use your Virtual Workbook to explore your answer to this question at **http://health.wadsworth.com/blonna1.**

The world of personal computers has opened up two primary access points to sexually oriented materials and adult-oriented Web site connections via the Internet and X-rated software. Until recently, the word *sex* was the most popular search term (it was supplanted by *MP3*) on the Internet (Lewis, 2001). Fisher and Barak (2002) report that the top eight Internet searches involve pornography.

Rimm's (1995) controversial study, "Marketing Pornography on the Information Superhighway," surveyed 917,410 sexually explicit pictures, descriptions, short studies, and film clips available on the Internet. Critics of this study point out that Rimm didn't actually view or count actual images on the Internet. He studied dozens of private (available to subscribers only) adult bulletin boards sites and described how sexual images were described, *not* the images themselves. From the organization of content on these private, adult bulletin boards, Rimm generalized to the Internet as a whole. This approach would be like, as Petersen (2002) puts it, studying a dozen adult bookstores in New York's Times Square and generalizing their inventory to *all* bookstores such as Barnes & Noble and Borders. In fact, for consenting (and often paying) adults, the Internet makes downloading hard-core pictures, movie clips, and stories easy.

Unfortunately, the Internet also provides access to hard-to-find materials that aren't readily available and are often illegal. This cornucopia of sexually explicit materials includes pedophilia, bondage, sadomasochism, and sex with animals (Elmer-Dewitti, 1995).

Internet-based sexually oriented materials are difficult to supervise. With more than 40 million sites (the number grows by thousands daily) and nearly universal access, the Internet provides global access to sexually oriented material. A consumer who has a connection to the Web can access sexually oriented chat rooms, still pictures (X-rated stills of anything desired, including kiddie porn), video clips (short sections of sex films), and live sex shows (the viewer becomes part of the audience from his or her living room) that can originate from anywhere around the globe. A person can connect with a live sex show from Denmark, a sadist or masochist from Asia, or a housewife selling still pictures of herself engaging in fellatio with her husband in Australia. Although this may sound too good to be true to an adult who enjoys pornography, it can cause much concern for the average parent of a teenage son or daughter. Technology is available to block minors' access to adult Internet sites. These barriers, however, work only if parents and other adults using home PCs install them and check up on them regularly. Problems remain, however, even with these technological aids in place.

Computer chat rooms share many of the characteristics of telephone sex lines. They allow intimate but nonpersonal interaction over telephone lines. Users of computer chat rooms sit at a keyboard and "chat" by typing in messages and sharing them with other users in the "room." The relative safety of sitting at a keyboard creates an environment in which "chatter" is often personal and graphic in its sexual content (Topp, 1997).

Software

The production of computer software has undergone a renaissance over the past few years. The primitive, sexually oriented software of the 1980s, which featured cartoonlike animation, has given way to the crystal-clear CD-ROM-based X-rated interactive software of the 1990s. The newest software features sound, color, life-like graphics, and the ability to move the characters into a limitless variety of sexually explicit interactions. Software technology is increasing in sophistication and quality with such speed that, by the time this page is printed, the X-rated software on the shelves of your local computer or "adult" store will be outdated.

X-rated and soft-core software is available in stores, through the mail, or can be downloaded directly onto a personal computer. It is a huge industry that is difficult to supervise. Innovative software peddlers market their wares through chat rooms on the Internet, computer and sex magazines, and shareware (public-domain software that is exchanged without cost) (Silberg, 1996).

healthy sex hints 17.2
Computer Blocking Software

Several blocking software packages are available for use with personal computers to selectively block Internet sites that transmit sexual material intended for adults. These products average about $35 retail and must be installed on the computer's hard drive. Each works in a slightly different way.

PC Magazine rated seven products and found that no single screening tool will meet the needs of every user (Kunro, 1997). The tools ranged from simple to complex to install and use. The more complex software seems to provide more comprehensive blocking capability, allowing parents to control Web sites, chat rooms, e-mail, and other applications. Some allow parents to control the amount of time children spend online and to monitor the sites visited.

All of the tested products performed well in their intended functions. *PC Magazine* found, however, that a foolproof blocking software product is impossible to develop because of the subjective nature of what parents consider objectionable and the ever-changing nature of the Internet.

Nonetheless, these products do offer a tool to help parents monitor their children's computer activity. As with all software applications, parents must continually upgrade and monitor the products to ensure that they are performing at optimal efficiency.

Sources: Munro (1997); "Is Your Kid Caught Up in the Web?" (1997); "Guarding Young Web-Surfers" (1997).

Effects of Pornography and Sexually Explicit Material

As long as pornography has been available, there have been attempts to regulate it, citing that it leads to a variety of social maladies including rape, sexual harassment, degradation and exploitation of women, and weakening of the moral fiber of America.

Two presidential commissions on pornography and obscenity have been impaneled over the past 25 years to examine the effects of viewing such material. The first commission was designated in 1970 by President Richard Nixon. The commission was charged with examining whether exposure to pornography could cause personal harm or lead to sexual violence. It found that exposure to pornography and obscene materials did not cause personal harm or contribute to sexual violence.

The second commission, impaneled by President Ronald Reagan in the early 1980s, had a similar charge. The Meese Commission found that exposure to nonviolent pornography was not harmful and did not lead to sexual aggression and violence (Attorney General's Commission on Pornography, 1986; Petersen, 1999). A secondary finding of the commission, however, touched off a great deal of controversy among human sexuality professionals. This finding was the claim that the most prevalent forms of pornography were violent in nature and that exposure to this material had a causal relationship to sexual violence.

healthy sex hints 17.3

Safe Internet Use

The Internet offers the world at your fingertips. It personifies the best and the worst of technological innovation. With a little common sense and some specific safeguards, it can be a great source of sexual information and materials. The following tips can help you surf safely.

1. Install site-blocking software. Some things on the Internet are best kept away from children.
2. Monitor your family's use of the Internet. Computers were never intended to take the place of live human interaction.
3. Establish online guidelines, and limit the amount of time children stay online.
4. Think of the computer as you would a television set. You don't want to (or want your family to) spend hours mesmerized in front of the screen. Take a walk; shoot baskets; do something interactive, such as playing Scrabble or cooking together.
5. Never give out your real name and address over the Internet, for any reason (especially on chat lines).
6. Never agree to unsupervised personal meetings with people you "meet" over the Internet. Let the person know you will meet in a neutral public place and that you will be bringing a friend.
7. If you use online sex services (view erotic materials, chat, and so forth), realize that this is fantasy sex. The reason it is a turn-on relates in part to the anonymity of the sex.
8. Like all fantasy sex, recognize that you may not want to actually experience what you discuss or view on the Internet.
9. If someone you met on the Internet has found out who you are and where you live and is trying to establish contact with you against your will, call the police immediately. Internet use is not illegal, but stalking is.
10. If you find yourself becoming addicted, disconnect, drop your online service, and get professional help.

Spiritual Wellness

Our nation's *moral fabric* is a term used by all presidents (including George W. Bush as well as Nixon and Reagan) to describe our standards as a society. It refers to our values, attitudes, and beliefs about moral issues that reflect our spiritual health as a nation. Religious leaders and others concerned with the moral fabric of America claim that the widespread availability of pornography, both online and through other sources, reflects our moral bankruptcy as a society. Our spirituality, they say, suffers when sex becomes a commodity instead of an intimate bond that connects people through love and commitment. Those who represent the opposing view cite the absence of evidence connecting greater sexual availability and permissiveness with moral decay.

These claims were instantly refuted by sex researchers and professional organizations (Board of Directors, 1987). Researchers argued that studies of the sexual content of samples of pornographic material revealed that between 4 and 16 percent contained violent themes or scenes depicting violence (Slade, 1986). Professional organizations decried the supposed causal link between viewing violent pornography and sexual violence, citing the lack of substantiating evidence within the commission's report or in the professional literature.

Intellectual Wellness

One positive outcome of greater accessibility to sexual resources coupled with the technological innovations of the past decade is the incredible explosion in information technology. Our ability to conduct research, gather information, process what we've found, and share resources has never been better. Average people working from home on a personal computer can tap into the greatest minds of our time without leaving home. This has the potential to greatly enhance our intellectual well-being. We have unprecedented access to information about any facet of sexuality, in the privacy of our own home.

Your responses to the Personal Assessment, Thought Questions, and Test Yourself! quiz questions can be logged online in your Virtual Workbook at **http://health.wadsworth.com/blonna1.**

Personal Assessment

17.1 Private Lives of Public People

1. Do the media (or anyone) have the right to divulge a private citizen's personal sexual information under any circumstances?   yes _____ no _____

2. Do the media (or any person) have the right to divulge a public figure's (person running for office, sports figure, entertainer, and so forth) personal sexual information under any circumstance?   yes _____ no _____

   If you answered yes to question 1 or 2, please describe those circumstances.

   _____

3. Does a person's personal sexuality influence his or her professional behavior?

   yes _____ no _____

4. If you answered yes to question 3, please describe how.

   _____

5. Should some sexual things be kept private regardless of the circumstances?

   yes _____ no _____

6. If you answered yes to question 5, please describe these things and why you feel this way.

   _____

17.2 Cyber-Sex Addiction Screening Test (c-SAAT)

This is an assessment developed by Shannon O'Hara, a marriage and family therapist from Los Angeles. It is designed to assess sexually compulsive Internet behavior. More than three positive answers indicate a possible need to seek help from a professional counselor specializing in this area.

1. Spending increasing amounts of time online focused on sexual or romantic intrigue or involvement

2. Involvement in multiple romantic or sexual affairs in chat rooms

3. Not considering online sexual or romantic "affairs" to be a possible violation of spousal/partnership commitments

4. Failed attempts to cut back on the frequency of online or Internet sexual and romantic involvement or interaction

5. Online use interferes with work (tired or late due to previous nights use, online while at work)

6. Online use interferes with primary relationships (minimizing or lying to partners about online activities, spending less time with family, partners)

7. Intense engagement in collecting Internet pornography

8. Engaging in fantasy online acts or experiences that would be illegal if carried out (for instance, rape, child molestation)

9. Decreased social or family interactive time due to online fantasy involvements

10. Being secretive or lying about the amount of time spent online or type of sexual/romantic fantasy activities carried out online

11. Engaging with sexual or romantic partners met online, while also involved in marital or other primary relationship

12. Increasing complaints and concern from family or friends about the amount of time spent online

13. Frequently becoming angry or extremely irritable when asked to give up online involvement to engage with partners, family, or friends

14. Primary focus of sexual or romantic life becomes increasingly related to computer activity (including pornographic CD-ROM use)

Source: Courtesy of Dr. Robert Weiss, LCSW.

Thought Questions

1. How are pornography, obscenity, and erotica different?

2. What is the significance of the Gary Hart scandal in establishing a new zeitgeist concerning the media and sexuality?

3. What impact has technology had on the availability of sexuality explicit material and services?

4. What are the arguments for and against legalization of prostitution?

5. What is Peter McWilliams's position on sex laws?

6. What are some of the sexual problems associated with the Internet, and how can they be addressed?

Test Yourself!

1. Madonna's sexual significance as a media icon is that
   a. she brought the me-generation's pursuit of sex, passion, and self-fulfillment into mainstream culture.
   b. she had 10 platinum albums in the 1970s.
   c. she was the first pop singer to appear nude in *Playboy.*
   d. she was the first female pop singer to publish a book on S&M.

2. Gary Hart's contribution to using sex to sell newspapers, magazines, and television advertising is that
   a. he was the first politician to be caught in bed with his secretary.
   b. he was the first national-level politician to have his private sexual activities aired by mainstream media.
   c. he was the first presidential candidate to have sex with a campaign worker.
   d. he was the first national-level politician to father a child out of wedlock.

3. Calvin Klein was one of the first designers to use _____, the intentional blurring of gender roles in national advertising campaigns.
   a. bisexuality
   b. homosexuality
   c. androgyny
   d. omnisexuality

4. Matt Drudge ushered in a new era of media coverage of the sexual exploits of public figures with his _____ coverage of the Bill Clinton–Monica Lewinsky affair.
   a. sordid
   b. satellite
   c. documentary
   d. Internet

5. According to Petersen, Americans' pursuit of sexuality-related goods and services has always
   a. driven technological innovation.
   b. lagged behind technological innovation.
   c. been a function of good economic times.
   d. been driven by fear of law.

6. Obscene materials are generally illegal. The Supreme Court has long believed that the best judge of obscenity is
   a. the Supreme Court.
   b. local religious leaders.
   c. local community standards.
   d. the U.S. Postal Service.

7. Prostitution is legal _____ in the United States.
   a. in all states
   b. in Nevada
   c. in New York, California, and Nevada
   d. nowhere

8. Which of the following statements best characterizes the selling of sexually explicit materials and services online?
   a. It represents a small percentage of e-commerce.
   b. It represents a small and declining percentage of e-commerce.
   c. It represents a large but stable percentage of e-commerce.
   d. It represents the largest and most rapidly growing percentage of e-commerce.

9. The neighborhood pornographic movie theater
   a. has been experiencing a resurgence with a growing adult film industry.
   b. has all but disappeared due to the availability of sexually explicit materials available online and on cable television.
   c. has experienced a slow steady growth since 2000.
   d. is illegal in most states.

10. The Meese Commission, impaneled under President Reagan, found that exposure to nonviolent pornography
    a. was harmful and prevented normal sexual development.
    b. was a leading cause of the increase in date rape.
    c. was the second leading cause of rape.
    d. was not harmful and did not lead to sexual aggression and violence.

Media Menu

You can link to the following online tools by visiting
http://health.wadsworth.com/blonna1.

 InfoTrac Activity

Lewis, E. (2001, June 28). Sex education: Industry trend or event? *New Media Age*, pp. 47–56.

 Web Resources

National Task Force on Prostitution

www.bayswan.org/index.html

The Prostitutes' Education Network site, offering information about health, legislation, and other issues affecting prostitutes and sex workers. Provides many links to prostitution-related issues.

Blue Ribbon Campaign for Online Free Speech

www.eff.org/blueribbon.html

A site sponsored by the Electronic Frontier Foundation (EFF), a movement that opposes censorship on the Web. A section on the latest news from the government cites links for more information.

Sex, Censorship, and the Internet

www.eff.org/CAF/cafuiuc.html

The Electronic Frontier Foundation (EFF) is a nonprofit, nonpartisan organization working to protect fundamental civil liberties and freedom of expression on Internet. This site is geared to college-related Internet freedom issues.

Sex Laws On-Line

www.geocities.com/CapitolHill/2269

This site is a gateway to current sex laws in the United States and in other countries.

Peter McWilliams's Home Page

www.mcwilliams.com/books

If you found McWilliams's perspective interesting, you might want to review some of his other works. All are available online for free.

References

Adult video, cable market surges. (1995). *Broadcasting & Cable, 125*(13) 47.

Attorney General's Commission on Pornography. (1986). *Report on pornography and obscenity.* Washington, DC: U.S. Department of Justice.

Bash, A. (1997, August 20). Age-based TV ratings slated as first planned. *USA Today On-line* [Online].

Board of Directors of the Society for the Scientific Study of Sex. (1987). SSSS responds to the U.S. Attorney General's Commission on Pornography. *Journal of Sex Research, 23*(2), 284–285.

Bradlee, N. C. (1997). The Bradlee files. *Newsweek, 126*(13), 82–88.

Brown, J. D. (2002). Mass media influences on sexuality. *Journal of Sex Research, 38*(4), 42–45.

Call for a crackdown on the 900 billing charade [editorial]. (1994). *Business Communications Review, 24*(5), 12.

Diamond, M., & Dannemiller, J. E. (1989). Pornography and community standards in Hawaii: Comparisons with other states. *Archives of Sexual Behavior, 18,* 6.

Edwards, M. (1996). The Net and the Web: Unlimited potential to communicate sexuality issues. *SIECUS Report, 25*(1), 2–4.

Elmer-Dewitti, P. (1995, July). "On a screen near you": Cyberporn. *Time, 146*(1).

Fisher, W. A., & Barak, A. (2002). Internet pornography: A psychosocial perspective on Internet sexuality. *Journal of Sex Research, 38*(4), 312–323.

Gardetta, D. (1998, November). The LUST tycoons. *Los Angeles Magazine,* p. 141.

Guarding young Web-surfers: Don't count on special software to protect kids' privacy. (1997, September). *Consumer Reports, 62*(9), 17.

Heavy breathing: Phone sex. (1994). *Economist, 332*(7874), 71.

Hite, S. (1976). *The Hite report: A nationwide study on female sexuality.* New York: Macmillan.

Hunt, M. M. (1974). *Sexual behavior in the 1970's.* Chicago: Playboy.

Is your kid caught up in the Web? How to find the best parts and avoid the others. (1997, May). *Consumer Reports, 65*(5), 27–32.

Kent, R. E. (1907). Television ratings. *FCC-V-chip Homepage.* Available via e-mail: rekent@eecs.wsu.edu.

Lagnado, I. (1997). Is the PC party really over? *HFN: The Weekly Network for the Home Furnishing Network, 71*(3), 10.

Lewis, E. (2001, June 28). Sex education: Industry trends or event. *New Media Age,* pp. 47–56.

Martin, J. (1995, September). Calvinism. *America.*

Masters, W. H., & Johnson, V. E. (1966). *Human sexual response.* Boston: Little, Brown.

McWilliams, P. (1998). *Ain't nobody's business if you do: The absurdity of consensual crimes in a free country.* Santa Monica, CA: Prelude.

Munro, K. (1997, April 8). Filtering utilities. *PC Magazine, 16*(7), 235–238.

Mustanski, B. S. (2002). Getting wired: Exploiting the Internet for the collection of valid sexuality data. *Journal of Sex Research, 38*(4), 292–301.

O'Kane, M. (1994, March 21). All in a night's work: Male escorts. *Guardian,* pp. 2–4.

Petersen, J. R. (1999). *The century of sex: Playboy's history of the sexual revolution 1990–1999.* New York: Grove.

Prostitutes' Education Network. (2003). Home page [Online]. Available: www.bayswan.org/index.html.

Richards, K. (1997). PCs on the Web: Researcher forecasts sales drive. *HFN: The Weekly Newspaper for the Home Furnishing Network, 71*(1), 79–81.

Rimm, M. (1995, June). Marketing pornography on the information superhighway. *Georgetown Law Journal, 83,* 1849–1934.

Roberts, D. (2000). Media and youth: Access, exposure, and privatization. *Journal of Adolescent Health, 27*(2), 814.

Schlosser, E. (1997, February 10). Pornography. *U.S. News & World Report,* pp. 43–50.

Shrage, L. (1996, Spring). Prostitution and the case for decriminalization. *Dissent.*

Silberg, L. (1996). Hot for your home PC. *HFN: The Weekly Newspaper for the Home Furnishing Network, 70*(48), 47–49.

Slade, J. (1986). Violence in the hard-core pornographic film: A historical survey. *Journal of Communication, 34*(3), 148–163.

Stern, S. E., & Handel, A. D. (2002). Sexuality and mass media: The historical context of psychology's reaction to sexuality on the Internet. *Journal of Sex Research, 38*(4), 283–291.

Topp, D. (1997). Virtual immorality [Online]. Available: walraven@iadfw.net and http://web2.airmail.net/walraven/esquire.htm.

U.S. Department of Labor. (2003). Cable and other pay television services [Online]. Bureau of Labor Statistics. Available: http://stats.bls.gov/oco/cg/cgs017.htm.

U.S. TV ratings system almost finalized. (1996, November 26). *Toronto Star.*

Test Yourself! Answer Key

At the end of each chapter, you had the opportunity to test yourself on key concepts. Here are the answers to the questions, organized by chapter.

Chapter 1
1. d 2. a 3. b 4. a 5. b 6. b
7. c 8. a 9. d 10. d

Chapter 2
1. b 2. c 3. d 4. a 5. b 6. c
7. d 8. b 9. a 10. d

Chapter 3
1. a 2. c 3. d 4. b 5. a 6. b
7. c 8. a 9. a 10. b

Chapter 4
1. c 2. a 3. c 4. a 5. d 6. c
7. a 8. b 9. d 10. c

Chapter 5
1. b 2. c 3. c 4. a 5. d 6. a
7. c 8. a 9. c 10. d

Chapter 6
1. b 2. a 3. c 4. c 5. c 6. c
7. a 8. d 9. c 10. b

Chapter 7
1. b 2. b 3. c 4. c 5. a 6. d
7. c 8. a 9. d 10. c

Chapter 8
1. b 2. d 3. c 4. c 5. d 6. a
7. b 8. c 9. d 10. c

Chapter 9
1. b 2. a 3. a 4. b 5. d 6. a
7. b 8. d 9. c 10. c

Chapter 10
1. b 2. a 3. a 4. b 5. b 6. d
7. c 8. c 9. c 10. a

Chapter 11
1. b 2. b 3. a 4. c 5. a 6. b
7. a 8. c 9. a 10. b

Chapter 12
1. c 2. a 3. c 4. a 5. c 6. b
7. b 8. b 9. d 10. a

Chapter 13
1. a 2. c 3. b 4. b 5. d 6. c
7. b 8. d 9. a 10. b

Chapter 14
1. a 2. b 3. c 4. d 5. a 6. d
7. a 8. c 9. c 10. b

Chapter 15
1. b 2. c 3. a 4. b 5. c 6. d
7. a 8. c 9. b 10. b

Chapter 16
1. c 2. b 3. d 4. a 5. a 6. b
7. a 8. b 9. c 10. c

Chapter 17
1. a 2. b 3. c 4. d 5. a 6. c
7. b 8. d 9. b 10. d

Glossary

Abortion Termination of an established pregnancy through surgical or nonsurgical techniques

Abstinence Self-restraint or self-denial, as in not engaging in sexual activity

Abstinence-based curricula School programs that advocate not having sex before marriage

Acquaintance rape Forced intercourse by a person, other than a spouse, whom the victim knows

Active listening Listening with understanding and providing feedback

Actual-use effectiveness The percentage of women who get pregnant while using a contraceptive method for 1 year

Adhesions Spider-web-like bands of scar tissue that painfully bind internal organs to each other or the abdominal wall

Adolescence Time period representing the psychosocial transition from childhood to young adulthood

Afterbirth The placenta, umbilical cord, which has been cut at the baby's abdomen but attached to the placenta, and membranes expelled after the birth of a child

Aggressiveness Pursuing one's own wants and needs without regard for the rights of others

AIDS The acronym for *acquired immunodeficiency syndrome,* the end result of HIV infection

Allurin A chemical released by a mature ovum that attracts a sperm to enable conception

Amenorrhea Absence of menstruation at some time after a female has reached menses

Amniocentesis Removal of the amniotic fluid

Amniotic fluid The transparent liquid contained in the amniotic sac that protects the fetus from injury and helps maintain an even temperature

Amphetamine A central nervous system stimulant that is administered by ingestion, injection, snorting, or inhalation

Androcentrism A position of viewing the world with the male at the center

Androgens A group of naturally occurring steroid hormones produced by both men and women

Androgynous Expressing characteristics and traits considered stereotypically male and female

Anilingus Oral stimulation of the anus

Anorgasmia An inability to achieve orgasm

Anus The opening of the bowel, through which fecal matter is eliminated from the body

Areola The brownish or pink ring of tissue surrounding the nipple of the breast

Assertiveness Pursuing one's own needs and wants without infringing on others

Assisted reproductive technology (ART) Infertility interventions in which a laboratory is involved with the union of the sperm and egg

Associational brain functions Connecting together individual sensory inputs

Autoeroticism The dimension of the sex life defined by sexual desire and/or gratification experienced by a person without the direct participation of another

Autoinnoculate To self-inflict the spread of disease from one body part to another

Autonomic nervous system The part of the peripheral nervous system that is automatic and involuntary

Aversion therapy A behavior modification technique that pairs an aversive stimulus with the behavior targeted for change

Balanitis Inflammation of the glans penis

Barrier methods Nonsurgical contraceptive measures that prevent the sperm and egg from uniting

Bartholin's glands Small glands adjacent to the vaginal opening that secrete a mucus-like lubricant during arousal

Basal body temperature (BBT) The lowest body temperature of a healthy person during waking hours

Behaviorism A stimulus-response theory of personality development grounded in the belief that human personality evolves as a result of the interaction between exposure to stimuli and the responses that this exposure evokes in the person. Watson is credited with the theory, expanded later by Skinner.

Binge drinking Having four or more drinks at one sitting

Biological essentialism The position that biology is destiny and our biology explains our nature

Biological immaturity The incomplete anatomical and physiological development associated with early adolescence or preadolescence

Biological/anatomical sex Categorizing individuals based primarily on their reproductive organs, chromosome makeup, and hormone levels; traditionally, one sex is labeled male and the other female

Birth control The broadest term covering all methods designed to prevent the birth of a child

Bisexuality Forming sexual relationships with both men and women

Blastocysts Spherical clusters of cells, also known as *preembryos*, that form shortly after conception

Blood alcohol concentration (BAC) A measurement of percentage of alcohol in blood; also termed *blood alcohol level (BAL)*

Body composition The fat and nonfat components of the human body; important in assessing recommended body weight

Body language Sending intentional or unintentional messages through body postures and movements

Bonding The close physical emotional attachment between infants and their primary caregiver(s)

Breech position A birth position in which the buttocks or foot rather than the baby's head presents at the cervix

Brothel A house of prostitution

Cannula A tapered, strawlike tube used in the vacuum aspiration method of abortion

Carriers Individuals who have a given disease and are capable of passing it on but have no apparent symptoms

Celibacy Abstaining from sexual intercourse

Central nervous system The brain and spinal cord

Cervical interepithelial neoplasms (CIN) Tumors or growths within the cervical membrane tissues

Cervix The neck of the uterus, which extends into the inner end of the vagina

Cesarean delivery (c-section) The surgical form of childbirth in which an incision is made through the abdomen and uterus to deliver the baby

Chancre A painless, indurated primary lesion of early syphilis

Chancroid An STD named for the irregular and painful genital lesions it produces, caused by the bacterium *Haemophilus ducreyi*

Chat rooms Live e-mail discussion lines in which a person can communicate with others by typing messages

Childbirth Labor and delivery

Child molestation Abuse of a child by nonfamily members

Child molester One who makes indecent sexual advances to children

Child sexual abuse Any sexual contact between an adult and a child who is under 18 years of age

Chlamydia trachomatis The most prevalent sexually transmitted bacterial pathogen, causing the STD chlamydia

Circumcision Surgical removal of foreskin of penis

Clitoris A small, highly sensitive, organ located at the top of the labia minora

Cohabitation Living together without being married

Coitus Vaginal intercourse

Communication The process by which information is exchanged between individuals through a common system of symbols, signs, and behaviors

Companionate love Feelings that include deep attachment, commitment, and intimacy

Complementary relationships Relationships based on differences

Congenital syphilis The disease acquired by the fetus in the womb and present at birth

Connective tissue Tissue that supports or binds other tissue

Contraception Methods designed to prevent conception

Corpus luteum The follicle after it has released its ovum and begins to produce progesterone

Covert sensitization A type of behavior modification in which an aversive fantasy is paired with the paraphiliac fantasy in an attempt to extinguish it

Cowper's glands Bulbourethral glands, located below seminal vesicles, which produce preejaculatory fluid that lubricate vas deferens and urethra and protect sperm that are being ejaculated

Cryptorchidism Undescended testicle(s)

Culture The sum of the learned set of rules governing the behavior of people, often focused on the influences of race, class, religion, and ethnicity

Cunnilingus Oral stimulation of the clitoris or vulva

Cystitis Bladder infections

Cystoscopy Direct visual examination of interior of urethra, urinary bladder, and kidneys by inserting a cystoscope (optical viewing tube) into the urethra

Cysts An abnormal condition of fluid-filled sacs that can burst and cause pain and scarring

Declarative statement A verbal initiating technique that does not require a response to a message

Decoding The use of knowledge, memory, language, context, and personal history and experience to interpret a message

Dialogue An exchange of information in communication

Dilation and evacuation (D&E) A second-trimester abortion procedure in which the cervix is first dilated, and then the fetus removed by suction and curretage

Discharge A secretion from a bodily orifice, such as the urethra or vagina, which may or may not represent an infection

Domestic partnerships Registered relationships between gay and lesbian couples

Dyadic sex Referring to the sexual behavior of a couple, the two people in a relationship

Dysmenorrhea Painful menstruation

Dyspareunia Genital pain associated with sexual intercourse

Dysuria Burning upon urination

Ectopic pregnancy Implantation of an egg outside the womb

Effacement Thinning of the cervix during first stage of labor

Ego Rational, analytical facet of human mind, according to Freudian theory

Ejaculatory inevitability The first step in male ejaculation; beginning of smooth-muscle contractions that trigger release of ejaculate

Electromyographic Refers to measurement of muscle tension through electrical sensors at skin surface

Embryo A fertilized egg up to 8 weeks gestation

Emission The release of secretions from various organs and glands that produce male ejaculate

Emotional well-being A component of wellness that refers to being in touch with one's feelings, having the ability to express them, and being able to control them when necessary

Encoding Selecting the signs, symbols, emotions, and words to transmit a message

Endemic A 20 percent level of ongoing infection within a specific population

Endometriosis A condition in which pieces of the endometrium migrate to the fallopian tubes, ovaries, or abdominal cavity

Endometrium The inner blood lining of the uterus

Environmental well-being A component of wellness that reflects our ability to function in our immediate environment, such as home, school, and work, as well as being able to deal with the world at large

Epidemic Levels of infection in populations that exceed those normally expected for that population

Epidemiological Dealing with incidence, distribution, and control, as in STDs

Epidemiological synergy The distribution of disease caused by the effects of infection with more than one condition

Epididymis A comma-shaped structure that sits along top of each testicle and serves as storage chamber for immature sperm

Epididymitis Inflammation of the small oblong body that rests upon and beside the surface of the testes

Epidural anesthetic An injection of a drug into the spinal cord during labor to dull pain

Episiotomy A surgical procedure that facilitates childbirth by enlarging the vaginal opening through cutting the perineum

Erectile dysfunction A disturbance or disorder related to obtaining an erection

Erection Filling of the penile spongy tissue with blood during vasocongestion, resulting in a hard, erect, penis

Erogenous Capable of producing sexual excitement

Erotic Devoted to arousing sexual love or desire

Ethyl alcohol A grain alcohol that is a central nervous system depressant

Exhibitionism Deriving sexual pleasure from exposing one's genitals to unsuspecting strangers

External inhibitions Impulse control against abusing children, as influenced by surrounding people and environment

Extradyadic sex Referring to sexual behavior outside the primary relationship. This term replaces *extramarital sex*, which is confined to heterosexual marriages.

Extramarital sex Usually refers to coitus, sexual intercourse, outside marriage

Fallopian tubes Conduits connected to the uterus through which the egg passes into the uterus during ovulation. Fertilization usually takes place at the outer third of the tube.

Family planning The conscious effort of deciding to have a family, including when to have children, how many, and how far apart to space them

Family practitioners Physicians who offer comprehensive health care, including monitoring pregnancies and delivering babies

Feedback A verbal or nonverbal response sent from a person receiving a message to the person sending that message

Fellatio Oral stimulation of the penis

Female climacteric A syndrome experienced by women between about 45 and 55 years of age as a result of declining levels of estrogen production associated with menopause

Feminist theory Theories that argue that personality and identity are socially constructed. What is "correct development" for boys is different from what is deemed "correct development" for girls.

Fertilin A protein on the plasma membrane of the sperm that enables it to bind with the ovum

Fertility awareness Natural family planning

Fertilization/conception Union of the sperm and ovum

Fetal alcohol syndrome Effects on embryo and fetus of pregnant woman's alcohol consumption; symptoms include facial abnormalities, mental retardation, and nervous system damage

Fetishism Deriving sexual pleasure from inanimate objects

Fetus A fertilized egg from 8 weeks after conception to birth

Fibroadenomas Benign, solid tumors associated with fibrocystic breast disorder

Follicle An egg sac in the ovary

Frotteurism Deriving sexual pleasure from rubbing up against unsuspecting and unwilling victims

Gametes The reproductive cells—sperm and ova

Gender dysphoria The condition in which one's anatomy is inconsistent with one's gender identity

Gender identity One's personal perception and sense of being male, female, or blended

Gender polarization The belief that males and females are fundamentally different, with mutually exclusive scripts

Gender role The ways we express our gender identity—including appearance, clothing, movement, and life choices

Genital herpes An infection caused by exposure to the herpes simplex virus type 1 or type 2 through sexual contact

Genital warts An STD caused by the HPV or human papilloma virus

Gestation The period of time representing pregnancy and development of fetus from conception to birth

Glans penis The end of corpus spongiosum, which is composed of the head of the penis and the urethral opening

Gonads The primary endocrine glands in men (testes) and women (ovaries) that influence sexuality

Gonorrhea A sexually transmitted disease caused by the bacteria *Neisseria gonorrheae*

G-spot An area in the upper, rear section of the vagina named after Ernest Grafenberg, who claimed it to be an erogenous zone

Guanosine triphosphate A chemical that controls the muscular and vascular changes of erection

Gynecology The medical specialty focused on women's reproductive health

Gynecomastia Enlargement of one or both breasts in men

Hallucinogens A class of drugs that distort the perception of reality by altering the perception of all sensory inputs

Health Total mental, physical, and social well-being, not merely the absence of disease

Healthy sexuality The safe and open exploration and development of our potential as human beings

Hemispheres The two halves of the cerebrum, each controlling the functions of the opposite side of the body

Hepatitis B virus (HBV) A disease caused by contact with infected blood; often associated with unprotected sex with multiple partners

Heterosexuality Forming sexual relationships with members of the other sex

HIV The acronym for *human immunodeficiency virus*, the infection that leads to AIDS

Holistic health The process of moving toward optimal functioning across the physical, social, spiritual, emotional, and intellectual dimensions

Homologous structures Body parts that develop from the same embryonic tissue (for example, the female clitoris and the male penis)

Homosexuality Forming sexual relationships with members of the same sex

Hooking up A sexual encounter between two people who may or may not know each other well and are not seriously dating

Hormonal releasing factors Chemicals secreted by the hypothalamus that trigger the pituitary to release specific hormones

Human chorionic gonadotropin (hCG) A hormone secreted during pregnancy that shows up in the urine of pregnant women; the basis for determining pregnancy using home kits

Human papilloma virus (HPV) A condition spread through direct contact with an infected person's genital warts during sexual contact

Humanism A theory of personality development proposing that human personality development is shaped by innate desire and need for maximizing personal growth

Hydrocele Accumulation of fluid in any sac, cavity, or duct

Hymen The membrane that covers the introitus

Hypoactive sexual desire disorder A dysfunction characterized by very low or complete absence of sexual desire

Hypothalamus The part of the brain that correlates activities between the nervous centers and the pituitary gland

Hypoxyphilia Deriving sexual pleasure from activities that involve oxygen deprivation

Hysterectomy Surgical removal of uterus. In practice, a hysterectomy often is accompanied by surgical removal of fallopian tubes and sometimes also the ovaries

Hysterosalpingograms Tests that determine whether the fallopian tubes are open

Hysterotomy A surgical procedure in which the fetus and placenta are removed surgically through an abdominal incision

"I" language Taking responsibility for feelings by saying "I feel . . ." versus "You make me feel . . ."

Id Pleasure-seeking, guilt-free facet of human mind, according to Freudian theory

IDU The acronym for *injectable drug user*

Illogical thinking Thought based on inaccurate or irrational perception of information

Immunocompetence The level of efficiency of the immune system

Implantation The attachment of a fertilized egg to lining of uterus

Incest Child sexual abuse involving genetically related family members

Incidence The number of new cases of a disease during a specific time period

Incidence rates Rates of new infection used to measure the likelihood of becoming infected

Infantilism Deriving sexual pleasure from being treated like an infant

Infertility The inability to conceive after 1 year of unprotected intercourse

Inhibited male orgasm A persistent or recurrent delay in or absence of orgasm following a normal excitement phase

Intellectual well-being A component of wellness referring to the ability to process information effectively and rationally

Internal inhibitions Natural impulse control against adult–child sexual relations

Intersexual An individual possessing some degree of both male and female internal or external reproductive structures; the preferred term, replacing earlier labels of *hermaphrodite* and *pseudohermaphrodite*

Intimacy Connectedness to another person characterized by mutual caring, openness, self-disclosure, honesty, attentiveness, sharing, commitment, trust, empathy, and tenderness

Introitus The vaginal opening

In vitro fertilization (IVF) A procedure in which ova are removed from the woman's body and fertilized with sperm in a laboratory; the embryo is surgically implanted into her uterus

Labia majora The larger, outer vaginal lips

Labia minora The smaller, inner vaginal lips

Lactation The process of producing and secreting milk from the breasts

Laparoscope A medical instrument made up of a tube with a light that permits examination of reproductive structures, requiring only a small abdominal incision

Lochia The uterine discharge that is released over a period of weeks after childbirth

Lymph nodes The main drainage and filtration sites in the lymph system

Macro-environment The environment that extends beyond the micro and includes one's city, state, country, and the world at large

Male climacteric A syndrome experienced by about 5 percent of men in their 40s and 50s, characterized by diminished interest in sex, loss of appetite, fatigue, and inability to concentrate

Mammary glands Glands within the breasts that produce milk for lactation

Masturbation Individual or mutual stimulation of genitalia by hand or using other objects

Megan's Law Legislation requiring notification that a sex offender has been released and is residing in a community

Menarche The onset of the menstrual cycle in girls

Menopause The absence of a period for 12 consecutive months, without surgery or medical treatment

Metacommunication Communication about communication

Micro-environment The part of one's environment that is immediate and includes living situation, campus, neighborhood, home, and work site and family, friends, and associates who populate these places

Minilaparotomy A female sterilization procedure in which the fallopian tubes are cut to block transport of the egg

Mirroring Restating the message exactly, including body language

Monogamy Commonly used to refer to having one sexual partner, whether married to that person or not

Morbidity The relative incidence of a disease

Mortality The number of deaths during a specific time period

Motor Relating to nerve impulses going out to muscles

Myomectomy A surgical procedure that removes fibroid tumors without removing the uterus

Myometrium The muscular, middle layer of the uterus

Myotonia Involuntary skeletal muscle contractions

Nongonococcal urethritis (NGU) An infection in the urethra of males, usually caused by chlamydia bacteria

Nontraditional relationships Any relationships other than a monogamous, legal marriage between a man and a woman

Nuclear family A family made up of the mother, father, and their children

Obscenity Material that is abhorrent to moral virtue and accepted norms of social behavior

Obstetrics A medical specialization focused on pregnancy and childbirth

Occupational/vocational well-being A component of wellness that reflects our ability to use our unique skills/talents to work that is meaningful and rewarding. Our values are expressed through involvement in paid and non-paid activities that are personally rewarding for us and make a contribution to the well-being of the community at large.

Oedipal complex A psychoanalytical term (named after Oedipus in Shakespeare's play) that describes the internal struggle that 3- to 4-year-olds face as they begin to identify more with their opposite-sex parent

Open-ended questions Sentences that require information from the other person

Opportunistic infection An infection that is able to develop as a result of the body's weakened immune status

Orgasm The stage of sexual response characterized by ejaculation in males and involuntary muscular contractions followed by relaxation in both males and females

Orgasmic disorders Dysfunctions related to the orgasm phase of sexual response

Outercourse Nonpenetrative sexual activities such as massage and masturbation

Ovarian cycle A three-phased period of time covering maturation of a follicle, release of ovum, and secreting role of corpus luteum

Ovaries Two almond-shaped structures that contain and release ova and secrete the hormones estrogen and progesterone

Ovulation The release of an egg from the ovary

Paraphilia An unusual or atypical sexual behavior that becomes the focal point for an obsessive preoccupation or need

Paraphrasing Restating a message in one's own words

Passionate love Feelings characterized by intense longing for another, infatuation, ecstasy when reciprocated, and emptiness when not shared by the other

Passive listening One-way listening; provides no feedback

Pedophilia Engaging in sexual activity with or fantasizing about prepubescent children

Performance anxiety Fear, worry, or panic associated with one's perceived sexual behavior

Perimenopause A period of gradually declining estrogen levels produced by the ovaries

Perimetrium The outer lining of the uterus

Perineum In men, the erogenous area of skin extending from the base of testicles to the anal opening; in women, the area of muscle and skin between vagina and anus

Peripheral nervous system All nerves coming off of the spinal cord

Personality The collection of values, attitudes, and behavior that make us who we are

Pheromones Body chemicals that attract potential sexual partners

Phimosis A condition where a tight foreskin cannot be retracted fully

Physical well-being A component of wellness reflected in how well the body performs its intended functions

Pelvic Inflamatory Disease (PID) A generic term that can apply to any STD that produces the characteristic symptoms of infection; used to describe infection of the uterus, fallopian tubes, or ovaries resulting in fever, malaise, pain, and other symptoms

Placenta An organ that attaches to the uterine wall and serves as a conduit for oxygen and nutrients to pass to the developing fetus

Pornography A depiction of lewd material or erotic behavior designed to cause sexual arousal

Postabortion syndrome (PAS) A controversial term referring to supposed long-term negative psychological effects of abortion

Posttraumatic stress disorder (PTSD) A syndrome developing after exposure to an extremely traumatic event. Symptoms include anxiety, sleeplessness, eating disorders, depression, and hyperactive nervous system.

Pragmatics The relationship between communicators

Premarital sex Usually refers to coitus, sexual intercourse, before marriage

Premature ejaculation The persistent or recurring early onset of orgasm and ejaculation

Premenstrual syndrome (PMS) A condition preceding menstruation, characterized by a myriad of physical and psychological symptoms

Prevalence rates Rates of prevailing infection used to measure the extent of the overall threat faced by the public

Primary sex characteristics Growth of the sex organs

Prior learning Factors relating to childhood development

Prodrome Stage of a communicable disease that follows the incubation period, with nonspecific, possibly flulike symptoms

Promiscuity Frequent and indiscriminate change in sexual partners

Prostaglandins Hormones that can cause muscle contractions and have been associated with menstrual pain

Prostate gland A chestnut-sized gland connected to neck of the bladder and vas deferens, which secretes alkaline fluid and enzymes that are part of ejaculatory fluid

Prostatitis Inflammation and irritation of the prostate gland

Prostitution The exchange of sexual services for money

Protease inhibitors A group of antiviral drugs used to prevent replication of HIV-infected cells

Psychoanalytic theory Also known as Freudian theory (after its founder, Sigmund Freud), describes personality development as outgrowth of interaction of id (pleasure-seeking, guilt-free), superego (the conscience, influenced by society and parents), and ego (rational, analytical mind driven by logical thinking)

Psychosexual development The blending of sexual aspects of one's development with other psychological factors

Psychosis A severe form of mental disorder or disease affecting the total personality

Psychotropic drugs Substances that are mind altering

Puberty Biological transition from childhood to young adulthood

Pubic lice *Phthirius pubis;* small insects (metazoan) that infest the host's pubic hair

Queer theory Theories that look to explain sexual orientation and sexual identity without relying on heterosexuality as the norm

Rape Illicit sexual intercourse without consent

Rates Statistics calculated by dividing the number of cases of disease by the population at risk of infection

Refractory period The time from last orgasm to the next beginning of excitement

Reproductive readiness Pubertal development resulting in full growth of genitalia and onset of fertility

Rohypnol A depressant drug also known as the "date rape drug," because it causes loss of memory and makes women vulnerable to uninvited sexual intercourse

Role model A person whose behaviors are imitated by others

RU-486 Known as the "abortion pill"; mifepristone, a drug used to induce menstruation by blocking the absorption of progesterone and thereby preventing the uterine lining from supporting an embryo

Safe zone A fertility awareness concept that factors ovulation and length of time sperm and eggs can live as a time to avoid intercourse

Scabies A condition caused by the *Sarcoptes scabiei* parasite, which burrows under the skin and lays eggs

Scrotum A double-chambered pouch of tissue that hangs loosely from the base of the penis, containing the testicles

Secondary sex characteristics Physical traits that develop during puberty and signal sexual maturity; examples are developed breasts, armpit and pubic hair, and coarse facial hair

Self-esteem A way of looking at oneself; may be high or low

Seminal vesicles Small structures connected to vas deferens, which release fluids that nourish and buffer sperm as they are ejaculated

Sensate focus Nongenital pleasuring used to heighten sensuality without sexual activity

Sensory Relating to nerve messages coming into the brain

Sensuality Experiencing things through all five senses

Serous fluid A fluid that has the characteristics of serum

Sex surrogate A person who acts as a substitute sex partner during therapy

Sexologists Specialized researchers of sexual subjects from a variety of disciplines including psychology, biology, medicine, nursing, and health

Sexology The discipline that scientifically studies sexuality

Sexual aggression Any form of forced sexual contact, including but not limited to intercourse, without the person's consent

Sexual aversion disorder A disorder characterized by disgust and active avoidance of any genital sexual contact

Sexual coercion Any nonconsensual sexual behavior that occurs as the result of arguing, pleading, and cajoling and includes, but is not limited to, force

Sexual differentiation The processes by which the embryo/fetus develops into a male or a female; internal and external genitalia develop in distinct ways, as does the brain

Sexual dysfunction A disturbance or disorder in desire, excitement, orgasm, or resolution of the sexual response cycle

Sexual harassment Unwelcome sexual advances, requests for sexual favors, and other verbal or physical conduct of a sexual nature in the workplace or educational setting

Sexual lifestyle The interaction between types and numbers of current sex partners

Sexual masochism Deriving sexual pleasure from being humiliated or forced to suffer pain

Sexual orientation One's propensity for romantic and erotic attachments. *Heterosexuality* refers to attaching to a partner with different anatomy; *homosexuality* refers to a same-sex partner; *bisexuality* refers to attaching to both men and women

Sexual sadism Deriving sexual pleasure from inflicting pain or humiliation

Sexual victimization Depriving a person of free choice and forcing him or her to endure, observe, or comply with sexual acts

Sexuality A broad term referring to all aspects of being sexual

Sexually transmitted diseases (STDs) Diseases that are spread from person to person through sexual contact

Social well-being A component of wellness that involves connection to others through various types of relationships

Sociopath A manifestly antisocial psychopath

Somatic nervous system The part of the peripheral nervous system under voluntary control

Somatotropic drugs Substances that are body altering

Sonogram The picture of the fetus produced by an ultrasound screening

Spectatoring Becoming an outside observer of one's own sexual encounter while it is occurring

Spermatogenesis Sperm production

Spiritual well-being A component of wellness that involves feeling connected to something beyond oneself

Spirochete A mobile, flexible, corkscrew-shaped bacterium of the genus *Spirocheta*, one type of which causes syphilis

Statutory rape A person older than the legal age of consent having intercourse with a partner who is younger than the legal age of consent

Sterility The permanent inability to reproduce

Sterilization Techniques (vasectomy and tubal ligation) that prevent sperm from reaching ova

Stranger rape Forced intercourse by a person who is unknown to the target person

Suction curettage A surgical abortion procedure that removes the embryo and placenta from the uterus through suction and use of a curette

Superego The conscience, influenced by society and family, according to Freudian theory

Symmetrical relationships Relationships based on equality

Synergistic effect An enhanced, unpredictable drug effect caused by combining two or more substances

Syphilis An STD caused by the spirochete bacterium *Treponema pallidum*

Teratogenic effects Side effects of drugs and other substances that cause birth defects

Testes Two almond-shaped male gonads responsible for sperm and hormone production

Testosterone The main hormone associated with sexual desire; the most notable androgen, recognized for fueling aggressiveness in males

Thalamus The part of the brain that relays all inputs to the cerebral cortex

Theoretical effectiveness The lowest expected percentage of women who will get pregnant while using a given contraceptive method

Thriving Pattern of normal weight gain, neuromuscular development, and other developmental attributes of infants

Toxemia A highly dangerous condition during pregnancy when high blood pressure occurs

Transactional analysis (TA) Eric Berne's communication model based on three ego states—parent, adult, and child

Transcend To rise above or extend beyond ordinary limits

Transgendered The preferred term to describe individuals whose gender identity and gender role encompass both masculine and feminine qualities.

Transsexualism (a gender identity disorder) A strong and persistent cross-gender identification

Transudation The production of vaginal lubrication because of sweating of vaginal tissue engorged with blood during vasocongestion

Transvestic fetishism Deriving sexual pleasure from wearing women's clothing

Tubal ligation A female sterilization procedure in which a surgical instrument is used to cut and tie back the fallopian tubes to block passage of the ova and thereby prevent fertilization

T-zone Transformation zone of the cervix, where columnar epithelial tissue of the uterus meets with squamous tissue of the vagina

Urethra The tube through which urine (and semen for males) passes from the bladder to outside the body

Urethral opening The opening to the urethra, lying behind the clitoris and in front of the vaginal opening

Urethritis Inflammation and irritation of urethra

Uterine fibroid tumors Noncancerous solid growths on the endometrium or in the walls of the uterus

Uterus Also called the womb, a fist-sized muscular structure that houses the developing fetus during gestation

Vacuum aspiration An induced abortion procedure in which uterine contents are removed by suction; used for early abortions

Vagina A tubular organ connecting to the uterus, which serves both reproductive and erotic functions

Vaginismus Painful, involuntary contractions of the outer third of the vagina during attempted penetration

Vaginitis Inflammation and irritation of the vagina

Varicocele An enlarged vein in the scrotum impairing blood flow

Vas deferens A tube extending from testicles to prostate gland, where it converts into urethra; responsible for transporting sperm and other ejaculatory fluid

Vasectomy A male contraceptive method resulting in sterilization by cutting and tying off the vas deferens

Vasectomy The surgical sterilization of the male that involves cutting and tying off the vas deferens

Vasocongestion The movement of blood flow into the genitals resulting in a variety of responses including erection in men and lubrication in women

Vesicles Fluid-filled blisters

Vestibule The area within the labia minora that includes the hymen, introitus, and urethral opening

Viability A gestational weight of the fetus of at least 500 grams and/or age of 24 weeks of age

Viagra The drug sildenafil, prescribed for the treatment of erectile disorder

Voyeurism Deriving sexual pleasure from observing unsuspecting individuals undressing or engaging in sexual activities

Vulva The external female genitalia

Wellness The state of optimal health and well-being

Widowhood The period of time between loss of spouse and remarriage

Women's movement A force to gain full educational, social, and economic opportunities and rights for women equal to those that men are traditionally understood to have

Yes/no questions A verbal initiating technique involving a question that requires only a yes or no response

Credits

This page constitutes an extension of the copyright page. We have made every effort to trace the ownership of all copyrighted material and to secure permission from copyright holders. In the event of any question arising as to the use of any material, we will be pleased to make the necessary corrections in future printings. Thanks are due to the following authors, publishers, and agents for permission to use the material indicated.

Chapter 1

5: Courtesy of Richard Blonna/Jean Levitan **9:** © AP Wide World Photos/Mark J. Terrill **18:** © Fitness & Wellness, Inc. **18:** © Fitness & Wellness, Inc. **18:** © Fitness & Wellness, Inc. **18:** © Adrian Lyon/GettyImages

Chapter 2

36 (all): © Susan Lerner 1999/Joel Gordon Photography **41:** © Digital Vision/Fotosearch **41:** © ImageState/Fotosearch **41:** © Joel Gordon Photography **41:** © Joel Gordon Photography **43:** © Digital Vision/GettyImages **58:** © Robin Nelson/PhotoEdit, Inc.

Chapter 3

76: Courtesy of Richard Blonna/Jean Levitan **77:** © Tim Pannell/CORBIS

Chapter 4

97: © Arthur Tilley/GettyImages **104:** © Christoph Wilhelm/GettyImages **104:** © Scholastic Studio 10/IndexStock **105:** © Peter Cade/GettyImages **113:** Courtesy of Janet Pollak **121 (both):** Courtesy of Donald R. Laub, M.D.

Chapter 5

134: Courtesy of Richard Blonna/Jean Levitan **135:** © Michael Newman/PhotoEdit, Inc. **137:** © Myrleen Ferguson Cate/PhotoEdit, Inc. **138:** © Lawrence Manning/CORBIS **146:** © Suza Scalora/GettyImages **146:** © Tony Freeman/PhotoEdit, Inc. **161:** © Color Day Production/GettyImages

Chapter 6

169: © Bill Aron/PhotoEdit, Inc. **170:** © Jacobs Stock Photography/GettyImages

184: © Spencer Grant/PhotoEdit, Inc. **186:** © ROB & SAS/CORBIS

Chapter 7

209: © Paul Franciscus **211:** © Paul Vozdic/GettyImages **216:** © Fitness & Wellness, Inc.

Chapter 8

242: © Thinkstock/GettyImages **246:** © Anthony Saint James/GettyImages

Chapter 9

277: © Edward Holub/CORBIS **277:** © Foreverart.com **281:** © Bruce Strong

Chapter 10

294: © Brooke Slezak/GettyImages **300:** © Ghislain & Marie David de Lossy/GettyImages **307:** © Ian Logan/GettyImages

Chapter 11

329: © Ryan McVay/GettyImages **330:** © Benelux Press/GettyImages

Chapter 12

354: © Fitness & Wellness, Inc. **361:** © Image Source/CORBIS **366:** © Visual Image Source Limited/Index Stock Imagery **383:** © Pixland/Index Stock Imagery **384:** Courtesy of Milex Products, Inc., Chicago, Illinois

Chapter 13

397: © Digital Vision/GettyImages **401:** Courtesy of Richard Blonna/Jean Levitan

404: Photographs from Lennart Nilsson, *A Child is Born,* © 1966, 1977 Dell Publishing Company, Inc. **405:** Photographs from Lennart Nilsson, *A Child is Born,* © 1966, 1977 Dell Publishing Company, Inc.; Art by Raychel Ciemma **412:** © Keith Brofsky/GettyImages

Chapter 14

436: © Charles Thatcher/GettyImages **439:** © Joel Gordon Photography **440:** © Joel Gordon Photography **441:** © Michael Newman/PhotoEdit, Inc. **443:** © Joel Gordon Photography **446:** © Peter Ardito/Index Stock Imagery **448:** © Reuters/CORBIS **450:** © Michael Newman/PhotoEdit, Inc.

Chapter 15

485: © Centers for Disease Control and Prevention **486:** © Centers for Disease Control and Prevention **487:** © Centers for Disease Control and Prevention **488:** © Centers for Disease Control and Prevention **495:** © Centers for Disease Control and Prevention **498:** © Centers for Disease Control and Prevention **501:** © Centers for Disease Control and Prevention

Chapter 16

523: © Jonathan Nourok/PhotoEdit, Inc. **532:** © Brad Markel/Liaison/GettyImages **534:** © Bruce Ayres/GettyImages

Chapter 17

555: © Photodisc Collection/GettyImages **556:** © Dave Hogan/GettyImages **557:** © Heungman Kwan/Index Stock Imagery **567:** © Ben Edwards/GettyImages

Index